# Head Injury: An Evidence-Based Approach

# Head Injury: An Evidence-Based Approach

Edited by Dexter Mueller

hayle
medical

New York

Hayle Medical,
750 Third Avenue, 9th Floor,
New York, NY 10017, USA


Visit us on the World Wide Web at:
www.haylemedical.com

ISBN: 978-1-63241-848-7

**Cataloging-in-Publication Data**

Head injury : an evidence-based approach / edited by Dexter Mueller.
    p. cm.
Includes bibliographical references and index.
ISBN 978-1-63241-848-7
1. Head--Wounds and injuries. 2. Evidence-based medicine.
3. Clinical medicine--Decision making. I. Mueller, Dexter.
RD521 .H43 2020
617.510 44--dc21

# Table of Contents

# Preface

Head injury is any injury that results in trauma to the skull or brain, due to falls, accidents or physical assault. Head injury can be conspicuous or inconspicuous. In an open head injury, the skull may be broken or cracked open, leading to bleeding. Besides the more apparent nature of the injury, it may present itself with symptoms such as sleepiness, abnormal behavior, severe headaches, vomiting, mismatched pupil sizes and localized paralysis in certain parts of the body. Many of these problems may not be immediately apparent and may develop later in life. Sometimes, a head injury can result in the destruction or degeneration of brain cells leading to brain damage. Several imaging techniques can aid in detecting and assessing the extent of brain damage, such as MRI, CT scan, PET, magnetic resonance spectroscopy, single-photon emission tomography, etc. Most head injuries though benign need close monitoring for complications such as intracranial bleeding. Neurosurgical evaluation is useful when the brain sustains severe damage. Treatment strives to control elevated intracranial pressure by using paralytics, sedation and cerebrospinal fluid diversion. The second line of strategy may involve barbiturate coma, decompressive craniectomy, hypertonic saline and hypothermia. This book contains some path-breaking studies in head injuries. It provides an evidence-based approach to the management of head injury. It will serve as a valuable source of reference for graduate and post graduate students.

This book is a result of research of several months to collate the most relevant data in the field.

When I was approached with the idea of this book and the proposal to edit it, I was overwhelmed. It gave me an opportunity to reach out to all those who share a common interest with me in this field. I had 3 main parameters for editing this text:

1. Accuracy – The data and information provided in this book should be up-to-date and valuable to the readers.

2. Structure – The data must be presented in a structured format for easy understanding and better grasping of the readers.

3. Universal Approach – This book not only targets students but also experts and innovators in the field, thus my aim was to present topics which are of use to all.

Thus, it took me a couple of months to finish the editing of this book.

I would like to make a special mention of my publisher who considered me worthy of this opportunity and also supported me throughout the editing process. I would also like to thank the editing team at the back-end who extended their help whenever required.

**Editor**

# Complications of Treating Terrible Triad Injury of the Elbow

**Hong-wei Chen**[1]*[9], **Guo-dong Liu**[2]*[9], **Li-jun Wu**[3]

1 Department of Orthopedics, Wenzhou Medical College-Affiliated Yiwu Central Hospital, Yiwu, Zhejiang, China, 2 Department 8, Research Institute of Surgery, Daping Hospital, Third Military Medical University, Chongqing, P.R. China, 3 Department of Orthopedics, Wenzhou Medical College-Affiliated Second Hospital, Wenzhou, Zhejiang, China; Institute of Digital Medicine, Wenzhou Medical College, Wenzhou, Zhejiang, China

## Abstract

*Objective:* Terrible triad injury of the elbow (TTIE), comprising elbow dislocation with radial head and coronoid process fracture, is notoriously challenging to treat and has typically been associated with complications and poor outcomes. The objective of this systematic review was to summarize the most recent available evidence regarding functional outcomes and complications following surgical management of TTIE.

*Methods:* Medline, EMBASE, Cochrane Library, and Google Scholar were searched to identify relevant studies, which were included if they were retrospective or prospective in design, involved participants who had TTIE, and were published in English. Outcomes of interest were functional outcomes and complications.

*Results:* Sixteen studies, involving 312 patients, were included in the systematic review. Mean follow up after surgery was typically 25 to 30 months. Mean Mayo elbow performance scores ranged from 78 to 95. Mean Broberg-Morrey scores ranged from 76 to 90. Mean DASH scores ranged from 9 to 31. The proportion of patients who required reoperation due to complications ranged from 0 to 54.5% (overall = 70/312 [22.4%]). Most of these complications were related to hardware fixation problems, joint stiffness, joint instability, and ulnar neuropathy. The most common complications that did not require reoperation were heterotopic ossification (39/312 [12.5%] patients) and arthrosis (35/312 [11.2%] patients).

*Conclusions:* The results of this systematic review indicate that functional outcomes after surgery for TTIE are generally satisfactory and that complications are common. Further research is warranted to determine which surgical techniques optimize functional outcomes and reduce the risk of complications.

**Editor:** Sanjoy Bhattacharya, Bascom Palmer Eye Institute, University of Miami School of Medicine, United States of America

**Funding:** This study was supported by National Natural Science Foundation of China (81271663) and General Program of Science and Technology Department of Zhejiang Province (2013C33216). The funders had no role in study design, data collection and analysis, decision to publish, or preparation of the manuscript.

**Competing Interests:** The authors have declared that no competing interests exist.

\* E-mail: chw6988@aliyun.com (HC); aryastark@126.com (GL)

9 These authors contributed equally to this work.

## Introduction

The combination of elbow dislocation with both radial head and coronoid process fracture is notoriously challenging to treat and, as such, has been termed "terrible triad" injury of the elbow (TTIE) [1]. This type of elbow injury is typically due to low or high energy falls onto an outstretched hand, which results in valgus and axial compression of the supinated forearm [2]. This leads to failure of the lateral collateral ligament complex (the medial collateral ligament may also fail), dislocation of the elbow, and consequent fracture of the radial head and coronoid process [2,3]. As a result of these injuries, the elbow is left in an unstable state that invariably requires surgical intervention. Unfortunately, due to the complexity of injury, outcomes have traditionally been poor, with long-term complications including stiffness, pain, arthritis, and joint instability [4].

The aim of surgery in managing TTIE is the restoration of stability of the humeroulnar and humeroradial joints, thus facilitating early postoperative elbow motion to reduce the

likelihood of long-term joint stiffness or disability [3,5]. Clearly, to optimize the chances of success, such surgery must adequately account for all three injury components of the terrible triad [3]. Over the years various reports have described surgical management of these fractures, with there being differences in the surgical approach used, the means of fixation, and the type of implant used in cases requiring replacement arthroplasty of the radial head [2,3]. To date, however, there is no consensus as to the optimal means of surgical management. In 2011, Rodriguez-Martin and colleagues [6] published the results of a systematic review summarizing injuring patterns, treatment, and outcomes (including complications) in patients with TTIE. On the basis of findings from five studies included in the review (all published before 2009), the authors made a number of recommendations regarding the management of TTIE. Since publication of Rodriguez-Martin's [6] article, the findings from a considerable number of additional studies on this topic have been published. Such studies clearly reflect the most current treatment practices. As a consequence, we decided to perform a systematic review of the literature to gain a more comprehensive understanding of complications and functional outcomes in patients with TTIE following surgical repair.

## Materials and Methods

### Search Strategy

Medline, EMBASE, Cochrane Library, and Google Scholar were searched on 31 July 2013 using combinations of the following search terms: elbow triad terrible, coronoid fracture, radial fracture, elbow fracture, and elbow dislocation.

### Study Selection

Studies were considered for inclusion in the review if they involved participants who met the criteria for TTIE (i.e., elbow dislocation, radial head fracture, and coronoid process fracture), and were published in English. Studies were excluded from the review if they included patients with injuries other than TTIE or if they were published in the form of letters, comments, editorials, or case reports. References lists of pertinent articles were hand searched to identify other potentially relevant studies.

### Data Extraction

Data were extracted by two independent reviewers who consulted with a third reviewer to resolve any disagreements. The following data/information were extracted from each eligible study: author details, number, sex, and age of patients, length of follow up, Mason classification for radial head fractures [7], Regan-Morrey classification for coronoid fractures [8], functional outcomes (Mayo elbow performance scores [1], Broberg-Morrey scores [9], and Disabilities of the Arm, Shoulder and Hand (DASH) scores [10]), and any complications.

### Outcome Measures

The outcomes measures of interest were functional outcomes and complications.

## Results

### Study Selection

A total of 125 studies were identified in the initial search (Figure 1). Of these, 23 underwent full text review, 7 were excluded for various reasons (outlined in Figure 1), and 16 [11–26] were included in the systematic review.

### Study Characteristics

The main characteristics of the studies included in the systematic review are summarized in Table 1. All studies, except for that reported by Zeiders and Patel [15], were retrospective in design. The number of patients in the studies ranged from 6 to 40 (total = 312). Most (13 of 16) studies reporting information on patient sex included a majority (>50%) of male patients. Most studies reported that the mean age of patients was 40 to 49 years. The mean length of follow up ranged from 13.6 to 64 months, although 25 to 30 months follow up was most common.

### Functional Outcomes

8 of 16 studies included assessment of Mayo elbow performance scores, which ranged (mean) from 78 to 95 (Table 2). Two studies [21,23] reported that mean scores excellent, whereas mean scores in the remainder of the studies were good. Overall, for the studies reporting individual patient results (N = 155 patients), 61 (39%) patients had excellent scores, 66 (43%) had good scores, 23 (15%) had fair scores, and 5 (3%) had poor scores. 7 of 16 studies

included assessment of Broberg-Morrey Scores, which ranged (mean) from 76 to 90. Two studies [22,25] reported that mean scores excellent, whereas mean scores in the remainder of the studies were good. Overall, for the studies reporting individual patient results (N = 98 patients), 27 (28%) patients had excellent scores, 39 (40%) had good scores, 24 (24%) had fair scores, and 8 (8%) had poor scores. 8 of 16 studies reported DASH scores, which ranged (mean) from 9 to 31.

### Complications

The complications reported in the studies included in the systematic review are summarized in Table 3. The proportion of patients who required reoperation ranged from 0 to 54.5%, with most studies reporting that approximately 30% of patients experienced the need for reoperation. No patients required reoperation in 3 studies [15,16,23]. Overall, 70 of 312 (22.4%) patients experienced complications requiring reoperation. Complications requiring reoperation were typically because of problems related to hardware/fixation, joint stiffness, joint instability, or ulnar neuropathy. There were few instances of wound infection. The following is a brief summary of the results from studies in which >1 patient experienced the same complication. Leigh et al. [24] reported that 2 of 23 (8.7%) patients experienced symptomatic nonunion of the radial head and neck or were unable to regain a functional range of motion despite >6 months of rehabilitation. Garrigues et al. [22] reported that 3 of 40 (7.5%) patients experienced limited flexion, residual instability, or had an oversized radial prosthesis. Seijas et al. [18] reported that 3 of 18 (16.7%) experienced dislocation and that 2 of 18 (11.1%) patients experienced Essex-Lopresti lesions. Winter et al. [17] reported that 2 of 13 (15.4%) patients experienced a lack of appropriate physiotherapy necessitating lateral arthrolysis. Lindehovius et al. [25] reported that 2 of 18 (11.1%) patients experienced joint stiffness or ulnar neuropathy. Forthman et al. [26] reported that 4 of 22 (18.2%) patients experienced ulnar neuropathy and that 3 of 22 (13.6%) patients experienced joint stiffness. Egol et al. [14] reported that 2 of 37 (5.4%) patients experienced joint stiffness. Pugh et al. [12] reported that 4 of 36 (11.1%) patients experienced limited range of motion and that 2 of 36 (5.6%) patients experienced radioulnar synostosis. Ring et al. [11] reported that 5 of 11 (45.4%) patients experienced redislocation.

The most common complications that did not require reoperation were heterotopic ossification (reported by 39 of 312 [12.5%] patients in 10 of 16 studies) and arthrosis (reported by 35 of 312 [11.2%] patients in 4 of 16 studies). In the study reported by Toros et al. [23], 6 of 16 (37.5%) patients experienced grade I arthrosis. In the study reported by Garrigues et al. [22], 5 of 40 (12.5%) patients experienced heterotropic ossification. In the study reported by Seijas et al. [18], 4 of 18 (22.2%) patients experienced heterotropic ossification. In the study reported by Lindenhovius et al. [25], 9 of 18 (50.0%) patients experienced grade I arthrosis and 3 (16.7%) experienced grade II arthrosis. In the study reported by Forthman et al. [26], 6 of 22 (27.3%) patients experienced grade I arthrosis and 1 (4.5%) experienced grade II arthrosis. In the study reported by Egol et al. [14], 18 of 37 (48.6%) patients experienced heterotopic ossification. In the study reported by Ring et al. [11], 10 of 11 (90.9%) patients experienced ulnohumeral arthrosis.

## Discussion

In this systematic review, we examined functional outcomes and complications after surgical repair of TTIE. A total of 16 studies, almost exclusively retrospective in design, involving more than 300 patients were found to be eligible for inclusion in our review.

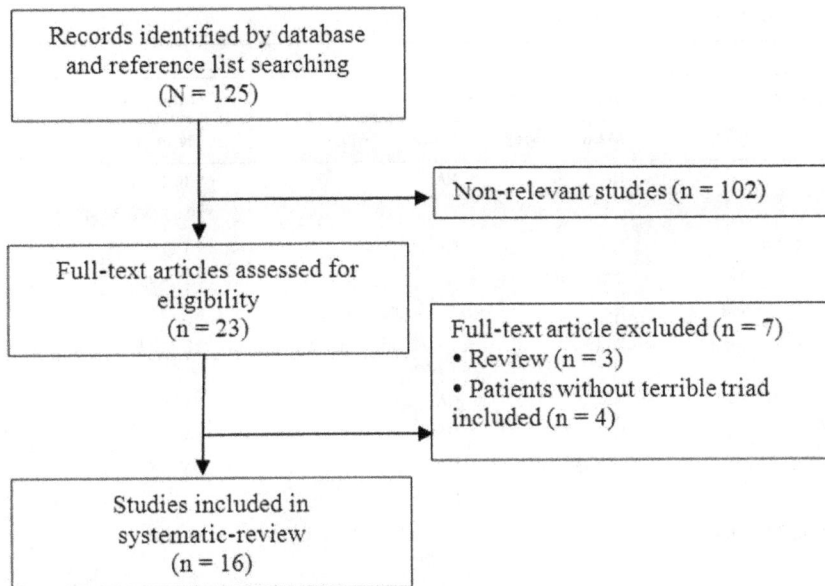

**Figure 1. Flow diagram of study selection.**

Overall, functional outcomes were satisfactory, whereas complications (including both those requiring reoperation and those not requiring reoperation) were relatively common.

We found that functional outcomes, as determined by assessing Mayo elbow performance, Broberg-Murray, and/or DASH scores were consistently satisfactory. Indeed, with regards to Mayo elbow performance and Broberg-Murray scores, approximately 70% or more of patients had good to excellent scores. Further, less than 10% of patients had poor scores. The findings of our systematic review are consistent with those of an earlier systematic review of studies published before 2009, in which the majority of Mayo elbow performance and Broberg-Murray scores were excellent or good [6]. Hence, application of current surgical strategies/ technology would appear to have maintained, rather than

**Table 1.** Characteristics of studies included in the systematic review.

| 1st Author (year) | Patients, number | Sex, % male | Mean Age (range), years | Mean Follow-up (range), months | Radial Head Fracture Classification[a] | Coronoid Fracture Classification[b] |
|---|---|---|---|---|---|---|
| Leigh (2012) | 23 | 52.2 | 43.5 (19–67) | 40.6 (16–73) | I–III | I–III |
| Toros (2012) | 16 | 68.8 | 34 (24–50) | 34.5 (14–110) | II–III | I–II |
| Garrigues (2011) | 40 | 55 | 48 (22–76) | 24 (18–53) | NA | I–III |
| Jeong (2010) | 13 | 53.8 | 43.8 (15–76) | 25 (18–41) | I–III | I–III[c] |
| Wang (2010) | 8 | 75 | 39 (20–52) | NA | II–III | I–II |
| Chemama (2010) | 13 | 84.6 | NA | 63 (15–128) | I–III | I–II |
| Seijas (2009) | 18 | 44.4 | 45 (17–77) | 13.6 (4–38) | II–III | I–II |
| Winter (2009) | 13 | 69.2 | 40 (18–77) | 25 (15–48) | Non-reparable fracture | No fracture or I |
| Pai (2009) | 6 | 100 | 26–54 | 26.4 (12–36) | NA | I |
| Lindenhovius (2008) | 18 | 66.7 | 47 (22–76) | 29 (10–53) | II–III | II |
| Zeiders (2008) | 32 | NA | NA | 36 (12–60) | NA | NA |
| Egol (2007) | 37 | 40.5 | Male: 49 (28–68) | 27 (12–105) | I–III | I–III |
| | | | Female: 57 (32–79) | | | |
| Forthman (2007) | 22 | 63.6 | 48 (24–75) | 29 (12–53) | II–III | II |
| van Riet (2005) | 6 | 66.7 | 42 (27–58) | 64 (18–112) | NA | II–III |
| Pugh (2004) | 36 | 61.1 | 41.4 (13–76) | 34 (20–65) | I–IV | I–III |
| Ring (2002) | 11 | 54.5 | 49 (17–67) | NA | II–III | II |

NA, not available.
[a]Based on Mason Classification.
[b]Based on Regan-Morrey Classification.
[c]Based on O'Driscoll Classification.

**Table 2.** Summary of functional outcomes for studies included in the systematic review.

| 1st author (year) | Mayo Elbow Performance Scores | | Broberg-Morrey Scores | | DASH Scores |
| | Mean (range) | Detail | Mean (range) | Detail | Mean (range) |
|---|---|---|---|---|---|
| Leigh (2012) | NA | NA | NA | NA | 9.16 (0–18.3)[a] |
| | | | | | 10.83 (6.7–37.9)[b] |
| Toros (2012) | 92.8 (85–100) | 9 excellent; 7 good | NA | NA | 9.1 (0–32) |
| Garrigues (2011) | NA | NA | 90 (64–100) | NA | 16 (0–43) |
| Jeong (2010) | 95 (85–100) | 10 excellent; 3 good | NA | 10 excellent; 3 good | NA |
| Wang (2010) | 78 (55–95) | 2 excellent; 3 good; 2 fair; 1 poor | 76 (51–95) | 1 excellent; 3 good; 3 fair; 1 poor | 31 (0–72) |
| Chemama (2010) | 87 (75–100) | 4 excellent; 10 good | NA | NA | NA |
| Seijas (2009) | NA | NA | NA | NA | NA |
| Winter (2009) | NA | NA | 86.5 (55–100) | NA | NA |
| Pai (2009) | NA | NA | NA | NA | NA |
| Lindenhovius (2008) | 88 (65–100) | 6 excellent; 8 good; 2 fair; 0 poor | 90 (64–100) | 5 excellent; 10 good; 3 fair; 0 poor | 15 (0–43) |
| Zeiders (2008) | NA | NA | NA | NA | 23 (19–28) |
| Egol (2007) | 81 (45–100) | 7 excellent; 12 good; 9 fair; 1 poor | 77 (33–100) | 3 excellent; 10 good; 12 fair; 4 poor | 28 (0–72) |
| Forthman (2007) | 89 (65–100) | 7 excellent; 9 good; 1 fair; 0 poor | 88 (53–100) | 6 excellent, 11 good, 3 fair, 2 poor | 13.3 (0–43) |
| van Riet (2005) | NA | 1 excellent; 1 good; 2 fair; 2 poor | NA | NA | NA |
| Pugh (2004) | 88 (45–100) | 15 excellent; 13 good; 7 fair; 1 poor | NA | NA | NA |
| Ring (2002) | NA | NA | 76 (34–98) | 2 excellent; 2 good; 3 fair; 1 poorNA | |

DASH, Disabilities of the Arm, Shoulder and Hand; NA, not available.
[a]DASH score for radial head repair group.
[b]DASH score for radial head replacement group.

increased, the proportion of patients experiencing positive outcomes after management of TTIE. Further refinement of surgical/management strategies in the future will hopefully decrease the proportion of patients who experience fair or poor outcomes.

Although a relatively high proportion of patients had satisfactory functional outcomes, many patients experienced complications, including ulnar neuropathy, elbow joint stiffness, heterotopic ossification, and arthrosis. Indeed, overall, slightly less than one-third of patients required reoperation due to complication(s), typically due to instability or stiffness-related problems. There was no clear chronological trend in the occurrence of complications i.e., the rate of complications did not obviously decrease with time/presumable advances in management strategies/technology. This is despite the publication of an algorithm for the surgical management of TTIE and excellent review on the topic by Mathew et al. in 2009 [2]. Interestingly, 3 studies did not report that any patients required reoperation for the management of complications [15,16,23]. Two of these studies [16,23], however, included a small number (≤16) of patients. The other study, reported by Zeiders and Patel [15] involved 32 patients who were operated on following preoperative planning using three-dimensional computerized tomographic reconstruction and use of a treatment algorithm. Several patients in this study experienced heterotopic ossification; however, there was no mention of any complications requiring reoperation. This is unusual for a study involving a relatively (for this injury) large number of patients. In general, the continuing high rate of complications experienced by patients after surgical management of TTIE is concerning and

signifies that further refinement of surgical approaches and preoperative and postoperative management are needed.

Our systematic review has several limitations that should be considered when interpreting the findings. Firstly, all except for 1 study [15] were retrospective in design. As such, the overall strength of evidence from these studies is not of the highest quality. Evidence from additional prospective studies would be welcome. Secondly, although our review included a relatively large number of studies (N = 16), the overall number of patients was not particularly high at just over 300. Although results from larger scale studies would provide more definitive evidence, such studies are unlikely to occur because terrible triad injuries of the elbow are not sufficiently common. Finally, the studies included in our review lacked homogeneity in a number of areas. Surgical approaches and management varied between studies, as did type of radial head and coronoid fractures, and the length of follow up. These differences may have affected both functional outcomes and complications to some extent. We must emphasize, however, that despite the lack of homogeneity, the overall results were quite compelling in that functional outcomes were consistently satisfactory for most patients and that complications were common.

In summary, the results of this systematic review indicate that most patients experience satisfactory functional outcomes following surgery for TTIE. Unfortunately, a relatively high proportion of patients continue to experience complications after surgery that often requires reoperation. Further refinements in surgical techniques and pre and postoperative management are needed to reduce complications.

**Table 3.** Summary of complications reported in studies included in the systematic review.

| 1st author (year) | Reoperations, number (%) | Number of Patients, Indication for Reoperation (Method of Reoperation) | Number of Patients, Complications Not Requiring Reoperation (Complication Management) |
|---|---|---|---|
| Leigh (2012) | 6 (26.1) | 2, symptomatic nonunion of repaired radial head and neck fracture (radial head replacement) | None |
| | | 1, migration of Kirschner wire for radial head fixation (Kirschner wire removal) | |
| | | 1, persistent joint subluxation due to no initial repair of LCL complex (LCL complex repair + downsize radial head implant) | |
| | | 1, deep infection (surgical washout + antibiotics) | |
| | | 2, unable to regain functional range of motion despite >6 months rehab (removal of metalware + circumferential capsular release) | |
| Toros (2012) | 0 (0) | None | 6, grade I arthrosis[a] |
| | | | 4, ulnar neuropathy |
| | | | NA, heterotopic ossification |
| Garrigues (2011) | 11 (27.5) | 3, residual instability for 18 months (1 total elbow arthroplasty, 2 NA) | 5, heterotopic ossification |
| | | 3, oversized radial prosthesis (NA) | 4, nonunion |
| | | 5, capsulectomy (3 ulnar nerve transposition due to limited flexion prior to capsulectomy, 2 NA) | 3, failed fixation |
| | | | 3, malunion |
| Jeong (2010) | 1 (7.7) | 1, ulnar neuropathy (ulnar nerve release) | 2, heterotopic ossification |
| Wang (2010) | 2 (25.0) | 1, broken Kirschner wire for fixation of humeroradial joint (Kirschner wire removal) | 3, residual subluxation |
| | | 1, pain and extension deficit due to plate (olecranon fixation plate removed) | 2, heterotopic ossification |
| Chemama (2010) | 2 (15.4) | 1, persistent instability due to disinserted MCL (ligament repair + external fixation) | 1, osteoarthritis |
| | | 1, severe pain on the lateral column (Swanson metal radial head prosthesis removal; ulnocarpal impingement subsequently noted) | |
| Seijas (2009) | 6 (33.3) | 2, Essex-Lopresti lesion (Darrach's osteotomy) | 4, heterotopic ossification |
| | | 1, arthritic degeneration <1 year (total elbow arthroplasty) | 4, mechanical blocking of pronation and supination |
| | | 3, unnoticed dislocation (1 external fixator, 2 Kirschner wires) | 2, transient ulnar nerve injury |
| Winter (2009) | 6 (46.2) | 1, subluxation to due to overstuffing of the implant (NA) | 1, medial dislocation due to fall after surgery (simple closed reduction) |
| | | 1, radial head prosthesis disassembly due to overstuffing of the implant (NA) | 1, heterotopic ossification |
| | | 1, deep infection (hardware removal) | |
| | | 2, lack of appropriate physiotherapy (lateral arthrolysis) | |
| | | 1, capitellar erosion (NA) | |
| Pai (2009) | 0 (0) | None | 1, radial neuropraxia |
| | | | 1, mild stiffness |
| | | | 1, mild osteoarthritis of radiocapitellar joint |
| Lindenhovius (2008) | 5 (27.8) | 2, stiffness (1 elbow release + ulnar nerve transposition, 1 elbow release + ulnar nerve release + excision of anterior and posterior heterotopic bone) | 9, grade I arthrosis[a] |
| | | 2, ulnar neuropathy (ulnar nerve transposition) | 3, grade II arthrosis[a] |
| | | 1, wound infection (surgical debridement + irrigation) | |
| | | 1, sustained distal humerus fracture (open reduction + internal fixation) | |
| Zeiders (2008) | 0 (0) | None | 3, heterotopic ossification |
| Forthman (2007) | 9 (40.9) | 4, ulnar neuropathy (ulnar nerve transposition) | 6, grade I arthrosis[a] |
| | | 3, stiffness (contracture release) | 1, grade II arthrosis[a] |
| | | 1, instability due to noncompliance + inappropriate arm use (total elbow arthroplasty) | |
| | | 1, dislocation due to accident (interposition arthroplasty) | |

**Table 3.** Cont.

| 1st author (year) | Reoperations, number (%) | Number of Patients, Indication for Reoperation (Method of Reoperation) | Number of Patients, Complications Not Requiring Reoperation (Complication Management) |
|---|---|---|---|
| Egol (2007) | 5 (17.2) | 1, ulnohumeral articulation resubluxation (external fixator replacement + radial head excision and replacement + elbow release) | 18, heterotopic ossification |
| | | (radial head replacement) | 3, ulnar nerve neuritis |
| | | 1, painful prosthesis loosening (radial head prosthesis removal) | 1, complex regional pain syndrome (stellate ganglion block) |
| | | 2, stiffness (elbow release) | |
| | | 1, NA (elbow release + radial head replacement) | |
| van Riet (2005) | 3 (50.0) | 1, severe pain and limited range of motion (total elbow arthroplasty) | 1, heterotopic ossification |
| | | 1, instability (additional LCL reconstruction via semitendinosus) | 1, resorption of coronoid graft + severe osteoarthritis |
| | | 1, irritated pin sites in external fixator (hardware removal + elbow release) | |
| Pugh (2004) | 8 (22.2) | 4, limited range of motion (hardware removal + elbow release) | 3, heterotopic ossification |
| | | 2, radioulnar synostosis (synostosis resection + contracture release + metal radial head removal) | |
| | | 1, posterolateral rotator instability (articulated external fixator) | |
| | | 1, wound infection (surgical debridement + antibiotics) | |
| Ring (2002) | 6 (54.5) | 1, radioulnar synostosis (synostosis resection + elbow capsular release) | 1, neuropathic arthropathy |
| | | 5, redislocation (4 fixation of ulnohumeral joint with pins, 1 total elbow arthroplasty) | 10, ulnohumeral arthrosis[a] |

LCL: lateral collateral ligament; MCL, medial collateral ligament; NA: not available.
[a]Based on Broberg and Morrey criteria.

## Author Contributions

Conceived and designed the experiments: HC. Performed the experiments: HC GL LW. Analyzed the data: HC GL LW. Wrote the paper: HC.

## References

1. Morrey BF, Sanchez-Sotelo J (2009) The elbow and its disorders. Philadelphia, PA: Saunders/Elsevier. xx, 1211 p. p.
2. Mathew PK, Athwal GS, King GJ (2009) Terrible triad injury of the elbow: current concepts. J Am Acad Orthop Surg 17: 137–151.
3. Dodds SD, Fishler T (2013) Terrible triad of the elbow. Orthop Clin North Am 44: 47–58.
4. Rockwood CA, Green DP (1996) Rockwood and Green's fractures in adults. Philadelphia: Lippincott-Raven.
5. Pipicelli JG, Chinchalkar SJ, Grewal R, Athwal GS (2011) Rehabilitation considerations in the management of terrible triad injury to the elbow. Tech Hand Up Extrem Surg 15: 198–208.
6. Rodriguez-Martin J, Pretell-Mazzini J, Andres-Esteban EM, Larrainzar-Garijo R (2011) Outcomes after terrible triads of the elbow treated with the current surgical protocols. A review. Int Orthop 35: 851–860.
7. Mason ML (1954) Some observations on fractures of the head of the radius with a review of one hundred cases. Br J Surg 42: 123–132.
8. Regan W, Morrey B (1989) Fractures of the coronoid process of the ulna. J Bone Joint Surg Am 71: 1348–1354.
9. Broberg MA, Morrey BF (1986) Results of delayed excision of the radial head after fracture. J Bone Joint Surg Am 68: 669–674.
10. Hudak PL, Amadio PC, Bombardier C (1996) Development of an upper extremity outcome measure: the DASH (disabilities of the arm, shoulder and hand) [corrected]. The Upper Extremity Collaborative Group (UECG). Am J Ind Med 29: 602–608.
11. Ring D, Jupiter JB, Zilberfarb J (2002) Posterior dislocation of the elbow with fractures of the radial head and coronoid. J Bone Joint Surg Am 84-A: 547–551.
12. Pugh DM, Wild LM, Schemitsch EH, King GJ, McKee MD (2004) Standard surgical protocol to treat elbow dislocations with radial head and coronoid fractures. J Bone Joint Surg Am 86-A: 1122–1130.
13. van Riet RP, Morrey BF, O'Driscoll SW (2005) Use of osteochondral bone graft in coronoid fractures. J Shoulder Elbow Surg 14: 519–523.
14. Egol KA, Immerman I, Paksima N, Tejwani N, Koval KJ (2007) Fracture-dislocation of the elbow functional outcome following treatment with a standardized protocol. Bull NYU Hosp Jt Dis 65: 263–270.
15. Zeiders GJ, Patel MK (2008) Management of unstable elbows following complex fracture-dislocations—the "terrible triad" injury. J Bone Joint Surg Am 90 Suppl 4: 75–84.
16. Pai V, Pai V (2009) Use of suture anchors for coronoid fractures in the terrible triad of the elbow. J Orthop Surg (Hong Kong) 17: 31–35.
17. Winter M, Chuinard C, Cikes A, Pelegri C, Bronsard N, et al. (2009) Surgical management of elbow dislocation associated with non-reparable fractures of the radial head. Chir Main 28: 158–167.
18. Seijas R, Ares-Rodriguez O, Orellana A, Albareda D, Collado D, et al. (2009) Terrible triad of the elbow. J Orthop Surg (Hong Kong) 17: 335–339.
19. Chemama B, Bonnevialle N, Peter O, Mansat P, Bonnevialle P (2010) Terrible triad injury of the elbow: how to improve outcomes? Orthop Traumatol Surg Res 96: 147–154.
20. Wang YX, Huang LX, Ma SH (2010) Surgical treatment of "terrible triad of the elbow": technique and outcome. Orthop Surg 2: 141–148.
21. Jeong WK, Oh JK, Hwang JH, Hwang SM, Lee WS (2010) Results of terrible triads in the elbow: the advantage of primary restoration of medial structure. J Orthop Sci 15: 612–619.
22. Garrigues GE, Wray WH, 3rd, Lindenhovius AL, Ring DC, Ruch DS (2011) Fixation of the coronoid process in elbow fracture-dislocations. J Bone Joint Surg Am 93: 1873–1881.
23. Toros T, Ozaksar K, Sugun TS, Kayalar M, Bal E, et al. (2012) The effect of medial side repair in terrible triad injury of the elbow. Acta Orthop Traumatol Turc 46: 96–101.
24. Leigh WB, Ball CM (2012) Radial head reconstruction versus replacement in the treatment of terrible triad injuries of the elbow. J Shoulder Elbow Surg 21: 1336–1341.

# 2

# Subject-Specific Increases in Serum S-100B Distinguish Sports-Related Concussion from Sports-Related Exertion

Karin Kiechle[1], Jeffrey J. Bazarian[2]*, Kian Merchant-Borna[2], Veit Stoecklein[3], Eric Rozen[4], Brian Blyth[2], Jason H. Huang[5], Samantha Dayawansa[5], Karl Kanz[1], Peter Biberthaler[6]

1 Department of Trauma Surgery, Klinikum der Universität München, Ludwig-Maximilians Universität, München, Germany, 2 Department of Emergency Medicine, University of Rochester Medical Center, Rochester, New York, United States of America, 3 Department of Neurosurgery, Klinikum der Universität München, Ludwig-Maximilians Universität, München, Germany, 4 Department of Athletics and Recreation, University of Rochester, Rochester, New York, United States of America, 5 Department of Neurosurgery, University of Rochester Medical Center, Rochester, New York, United States of America, 6 Department of Trauma Surgery, Technical University of Munich, München, Germany

## Abstract

**Background:** The on-field diagnosis of sports-related concussion (SRC) is complicated by the lack of an accurate and objective marker of brain injury.

**Purpose:** To compare subject-specific changes in the astroglial protein, S100B, before and after SRC among collegiate and semi-professional contact sport athletes, and compare these changes to differences in S100B before and after non-contact exertion.

**Study Design:** Longitudinal cohort study.

**Methods:** From 2009–2011, we performed a prospective study of athletes from Munich, Germany, and Rochester, New York, USA. Serum S100B was measured in all SRC athletes at pre-season baseline, within 3 hours of injury, and at days 2, 3 and 7 post-SRC. Among a subset of athletes, S100B was measured after non-contact exertion but before injury. All samples were collected identically and analyzed using an automated electrochemiluminescent assay to quantify serum S100B levels.

**Results:** Forty-six athletes (30 Munich, 16 Rochester) underwent baseline testing. Thirty underwent additional post-exertion S100B testing. Twenty-two athletes (16 Rochester, 6 Munich) sustained a SRC, and 17 had S100B testing within 3 hours post-injury. The mean 3-hour post-SRC S100B was significantly higher than pre-season baseline (0.099±0.008 µg/L vs. 0.058±0.006 µg/L, p = 0.0002). Mean post-exertion S100B was not significantly different than the preseason baseline. S100B levels at post-injury days 2, 3 and 7 were significantly lower than the 3-hour level, and not different than baseline. Both the absolute change and proportional increase in S100B 3-hour post-injury were accurate discriminators of SRC from non-contact exertion without SRC (AUC 0.772 and 0.904, respectively). A 3-hour post-concussion S100B >0.122 µg/L and a proportional S100B increase of >45.9% over baseline were both 96.7% specific for SRC.

**Conclusions:** Relative and absolute increases in serum S100B can accurately distinguish SRC from sports-related exertion, and may be a useful adjunct to the diagnosis of SRC.

**Editor:** Charles C. Caldwell, University of Cincinnati, United States of America

**Funding:** This study was supported by National Institutes of Health grant K24HD064754. The funders had no role in study design, data collection and analysis, decision to publish, or preparation of the manuscript.

**Competing Interests:** The authors have the following competing interests: Bazarian and Blyth: Patent pending, "Method of Diagnosing Mild Traumatic Brain Injury", US serial number 61/467,224. This patent involves the use the peripheral protein Apolipoprotein A1 to aid in the diagnosis of concussion. Bazarian: Consulting Banyan Biomarkers, Roche Diagnostics.

* E-mail: jeff_bazarian@urmc.rochester.edu

## Introduction

Sports-related concussions (SRC) are common in both the United States and Germany. In the US, the Centers for Disease Control and Prevention estimates that there are 1.6–3.8 million SRC per year [1], with the highest concussion rates found among contact sports such as ice hockey, football, soccer, and basketball [2]. While there are no similar cumulative figures for Germany, a recent epidemiological survey found the overall incidence of traumatic brain injuries (TBI) to be 330/100,000 inhabitants and

that 6.3% of these were due to sports [3,4]. With the current German population at just over 81.5 million, that translates into over 268,000 sports TBIs per year.

After a concussion, most athletes recover within 7–10 days [5], but up to 10% have post-concussion symptoms such as headache and dizziness lasting longer than 7 days [6,7]. In addition, multiple concussions are thought to be linked to the early onset of neurodegeneration, known as chronic traumatic encephalopathy [8]. Existing concussion management guidelines are designed to mitigate these risks and involve primarily rest [5]. However, the effect of these guidelines on reducing long-term disability depends entirely on recognizing that a concussion has occurred in the first place. While sideline tools such as SAC [9], SCAT 2 [5], and SCAT 3 [10] are designed to assist coaches and certified athletic trainers in identifying the mental status changes (loss of consciousness, amnesia, confusion) that are the hallmark of this injury, unrecognized or unreported concussions are still quite common, occurring in over half of injured high school football players queried via a confidential survey [11]. An objective parameter that can be easily and rapidly measured on-site could optimize the identification and clinical management of concussed athletes.

Serum S100B has emerged as a potential candidate in this regard. S100B is a 21 kDa dimeric protein expressed primarily by brain astrocytes and belongs to a multigenic family of calcium-binding proteins [12–14]. Its primary clinical role in concussion management has been to help identify the approximately 5% of concussion patients that have intracranial hemorrhage on head CT scan. Although S100B's specificity for abnormal head CT is low (40%), its high sensitivity (99%) [15–17] has led to its adoption as a clinical tool to screen for head injured patient requiring a head CT scan (pre-head CT screen) in several countries in Europe and Asia.

Enthusiasm for the use of S100B to aid in the diagnosis of concussion, however, has been tempered by significant overlap between levels in healthy individuals and in athletes who have had a concussion. Using cutoffs derived from comparing these two groups, only very high S100B levels—rarely seen after concussion–are considered abnormal, making this test appear clinically useless in a sports setting. However, small but significant post-concussion increases can be revealed by comparing S100B values not among groups, but in *individual athletes* before injury to that after injury. This kind of study is expensive and labor-intensive to perform because one cannot predict which athletes will get injured during a season; serum must be obtained from several hundred athletes in order to accrue pre and post-concussion samples in 20–30 athletes.

A second problem for using S100B clinically is the observation that serum levels rise not only after concussion but also after a game in which no concussion was observed [18–21]. Explanations for this observation range from exertion-related release of small amounts of S100B from melanocytes, chondrocytes and adipocytes [12], to occult or unreported brain injury, or a combination of the two. In order to separate the effect of these two processes on S100B, one needs to compare S100B increases in concussed athletes to that in a group of athletes undergoing exertion but not body contact in whom the risk of even occult brain injury is very low.

In an effort to unlock the diagnostic potential of S100B, we sought to compare subject-specific changes in S100B before and after concussion among collegiate and semi-professional athletes. Our secondary aim was to compare these changes to differences in S100B before and after non-contact exertion. By using an intra-subject, before-and-after study design, we minimized the effect that individual-level variation in baseline S100B levels has on obscuring group-level post-concussion increases. In addition, by examining S100B changes in a reference group not undergoing sports-related contact, we sought to minimize the probability that S100B elevations in the comparison group are due to occult brain injury.

## Methods

We performed a longitudinal cohort study of contact sport athletes in Munich and Rochester between 2009 and 2011.

### Ethics Statement

The study was approved by the ethics committees of the Ludwig Maximilians University in Munich, Germany and at the Rochester Institute of Technology and University of Rochester in Rochester, NY, USA. Voluntary participation was solicited through communication with athletic directors, coaches, and athletes. All participating athletes completed written informed consent forms before inclusion in the study, which described the purpose, objective, and details of the testing and research participation.

### Inclusion and Exclusion Criteria

Athletes were eligible for inclusion if they were ≥18 years of age and active participants in contact sport teams affiliated with the Ludwig Maximilians University in Munich, Germany, or with the University of Rochester or Rochester Institute of Technology in Rochester, New York.

The University of Rochester participates in several National Collegiate Athletic Association (NCAA) Division III sports including the following contact sports: football, soccer, and basketball. In addition, the University of Rochester provides orthopedic and trauma care to hockey players at Rochester Institute of Technology (men participate in NCAA Division I and women, at the time of the study, in Division III). Athletes from these teams were eligible to participate. Although German universities don't participate in US-style collegiate athletic organizations, the Ludwig Maximilians University provides orthopedic and trauma care to the Straubing Tigers Ice Hockey Club which is a semi-professional ice hockey team that currently plays in the Deutsche Eishockey Liga (*German National Ice Hockey League*). Athletes from this team were eligible to participate in the current study.

Athletes who sustained a moderate or severe TBI (determined by a hospital GCS of 3–12) were excluded from the study. Athletes who sustained a concussion within two weeks of baseline (ie: during the off-season or during a non-sport activity) were also excluded. History of prior head injury was determined by self-report using a previously validated survey tool[22].

### Serum Sampling

Among Rochester athletes, baseline samples were collected on all participating athletes but analyzed for S100B only in those who subsequently developed concussion. Samples were collected within 3 hours of SRC and at days 2, 3 and 7 post-concussion. Among Munich athletes, baseline samples were collected and analyzed for S100B in all participants, then again after a period of exertion (but before injury), and finally on the subset who suffered a concussion, also within 3 hours of injury (**Table 1**). Exertion consisted of non-contact ice-hockey skating drills. Post exertion testing was limited to Munich athletes principally for reasons of convenience. The Straubing Tigers had the largest number of participating athletes of any single participating team, as well and a regular practice schedule made in advance. These factors facilitated post-exertion serum sample with a minimum of study personnel. Because members of Straubing Tigers were frequently on the road, post-concussion serum was not obtained from Munich athletes beyond the 3-hour time point.The study group thus consisted of athletes with S100B samples obtained before and after concussion, and the comparison group consisted of athletes with S100B samples obtained before and after non-contact exertion.

**Table 1.** Study overview.

| Munich Athletes (n) | | Rochester Athletes (n) |
|---|---|---|
| 30 | Pre-season (resting) S100B | 16 |
| 30 | Post-exertion S100B | 0 |
| 6 | Concussion | 16 |
| 6 | 3-hours Post-Concussion S100B | 11 |
| 0 | 2 days Post-Concussion S100B | 16 |
| 0 | 3 days Post-Concussion S100B | 15 |
| 0 | 7 days Post-Concussion S100B | 16 |

Athletes were considered concussed if they had an injury witnessed by an on-field coach or certified athletic trainer meeting the definition of concussion defined by the Sport Concussion Assessment Tool 2 (SCAT2) [5]. This definition consists of an injury resulting in any one or more of the following: symptoms (such as headache), physical signs (such as unsteadiness), impaired brain function (such as confusion), or abnormal behavior.

Methods for obtaining and handling serum were identical at both sites. Four milliliters of venous blood was drawn into sterile Vacuatiner serum separator tubes and immediately placed on 0°C ice. Within 60 minutes, the blood was centrifuged (3000 rpm, 10 minutes), and the serum separated and stored at −80°C until sample analysis.

## Serum S100B Measurement

Serum S100B concentrations were determined by electrochemoluminometric immunoassay (ELECSYS® S100, ROCHE Diagnostics, Mannheim, Germany) with a detection limit of 0.005–39 µg/L, according to the manufacturer's instructions.. Briefly, two monoclonal antibodies directed against the beta-chain of the S100 dimer were incubated with 20 µl of sample for 9 minutes. Streptavidin-coated microparticles were added, and the mixture was incubated for an additional 9 minutes in order to form a solidified immunocomplex. The reaction mixture was transferred to a measurement cell where the beads were magnetically captured on an elctrode surface, and unbound components were removed by washing. A defined voltage was applied to the electrode to initiate the electrochemiluminescent reaction and the resultant light emission was measured using a photomultiplier. Serum S100B concentrations were reported as µg/L of serum and reported as mean values ± SD. Reference range of S100B is 0.02 to 0.15 µg/L [23].

## Analysis

Serum S100B concentrations before and after SRC, as well as before and after non-contact exertion, were compared using paired t-tests. Changes in S100B concentrations among all concussed athletes were compared using paired and unpaired t-tests. Receiver operating characteristic (ROC) analyses were performed to evaluate S100B's classification accuracy for SRC [24]. In these analyses, S100B levels within 3 hours of concussion were compared to S100B levels after non-contact exertion. We examined the ROC of the post-SRC or post-exertion S100B value as well as the proportional change in post-concussion/exertion S100B relative to preseason (baseline). The proportional change was defined as [(post-exertion or 3-hour post-SRC S100B − baseline S100B)/baseline S100B]. Analyses were performed using

SAS®Software Version 9.3 (SAS Institute Inc., Cary, NC, USA) and GraphPad Prism Version 5.02 for Windows (GraphPad Software, La Jolla California USA). A p-value of ≤0.05 was considered statistically significant.

This study was designed to to detect clinically-relevant increases in S100B. Because the sample size was fixed by the number of concussed subjects (46), we report here the power this sample size had to detect clinically relevant S100B increases. Cliniclaly-relevant increases were defined based on prior studies reporting baseline S100B levels in athletes ranging from 0.11–0.22 ug/L (SD range 0.04–0.04 ug/L) that increased by 36–64% after exertion[20,25]. Thus, assuming a Type I error of 0.05, mean baseline S100B level of 0.11 ug/L, and SD in mean baseline S100B of 0.05 ug/L, 46 sujbects provides 96% power to detect an increase of 25% or greater in mean baseline S100B levels.

## Results

Thirty Munich athletes agreed to participate, providing baseline and post-exertion serum samples. All of these samples were analyzed for S100B. Six of these athletes suffered a SRC during the study period (**Table 1**). A total of 306 Rochester athletes agreed to participate, providing baseline (but not post-exertion) serum samples. Sixteen of these athletes suffered a SRC during the study period. Only the serum samples from the 16 concussed Rochester athletes were analyzed for S100B at baseline and after SRC. The initial, within-3-hour serum sample was not obtained in five of these 16 athletes because the SRC occurred during a game outside the Rochester area; however, subsequent samples were obtained at the later time points.

Forty-six athletes (30 from Munich and 16 from Rochester) had baseline samples, as well as post-exertion and/or post-SRC samples, analyzed for S100B. The mean age of all athletes was 25.4 years and 89% were male (**Table 2**). The mean age of Munich athletes was significantly greater than the mean age of Rochester athletes (28.4±0.82 years vs. 19.8±0.34 years, p< 0.001). The mean baseline S100B concentration among Munich athletes was not significantly different than the mean baseline concentration among Rochester athletes (0.070±0.03 µg/L vs. 0.068±0.04 µg/L, p = 0.85).

Among the 30 Munich athletes who underwent post-exertion S100B testing, there was no difference in mean post-exertion S100B level compared to baseline (0.071±0.03 µg/L vs. 0.070±0.03 µg/L, p = 0.87) (**Figure 1**). Proportional post-exertion changes in S100B ranged from −35 to +50%. The mean proportional post-exertion S100B change was +2.7%.

During the study period, 22 athletes (17 male and 5 female; 16 from Rochester and 6 from Munich) suffered a SRC, of which serum samples were collected within 3-hours of injury from 17 individuals (11 from Rochester and 6 from Munich). None of these concussions were accompanied by other extracranial fractures or lacerations. Among these 17 athletes, the mean S100B level within 3 hours of injury was significantly higher than baseline (0.099±0.008 µg/L vs. 0.058±0.006 µg/L, paired t-test p< 0.0001; **Figure 1**). Proportional post-SRC changes in S100B ranged from −14 to +180%. The mean post-SRC S100B change was +81.2%. Longitudinal S100B levels measured post-injury days 2, 3 and 7 were not significantly different than baseline, although they were all significantly lower than the 3-hour post injury level (**Figure 2**).

The ROC using the absolute value 3-hour post-injury/ exertional S100B value revealed an AUC of 0.772 (95% CI: 0.64, 0.91). However the AUC using the proportional increase in post-injury/exertional S100B level over baseline was higher

**Table 2.** Subject characteristics.

| Characteristic | Munich Athletes (n = 30) | Rochester Athletes (n = 16) | Combined Cohort (n = 46) |
|---|---|---|---|
| Age, Mean Years (SD) | 28.4 (4.5) | 19.8 (1.4) | 25.4 (5.5) |
| Male, N (%) | 30 (100) | 11(68.8) | 41 (89.1) |
| Race | | | |
|   Caucasian, N (%) | 30 (100) | 14 (87.5) | 44 (95.7) |
|   African American/European, N (%) | 0 | 2 (12.5) | 2 (4.3) |
| Sport | | | |
|   Ice Hockey, N (%) | 30 (100) | 4 (25) | 34 (73.9) |
|   Soccer, N (%) | 0 | 3 (18.8) | 3 (6.5) |
|   Football, N (%) | 0 | 8 (50) | 8 (17.4) |
|   Basketball, N (%) | 0 | 1 (6.2) | 1 (2.2) |
| Baseline S100B, mean µg/L (SD)* | 0.070 (.03) | 0.068 (.04) | 0.070 (.03) |

*T-test to assess difference between Munich and Rochester cohorts at baseline, p = 0.85.

(0.904, 95% CI: 0.80, 1.0; **Figure 3**). Cutoff values that maximize sensitivity and specificity for SRC diagnosis are shown in **Table 3**. A 3-hour post-concussion S100B level of >0.122 µg/L and a proportional S100B increase of >45.9% over baseline were both 96.7% specific for concussion.

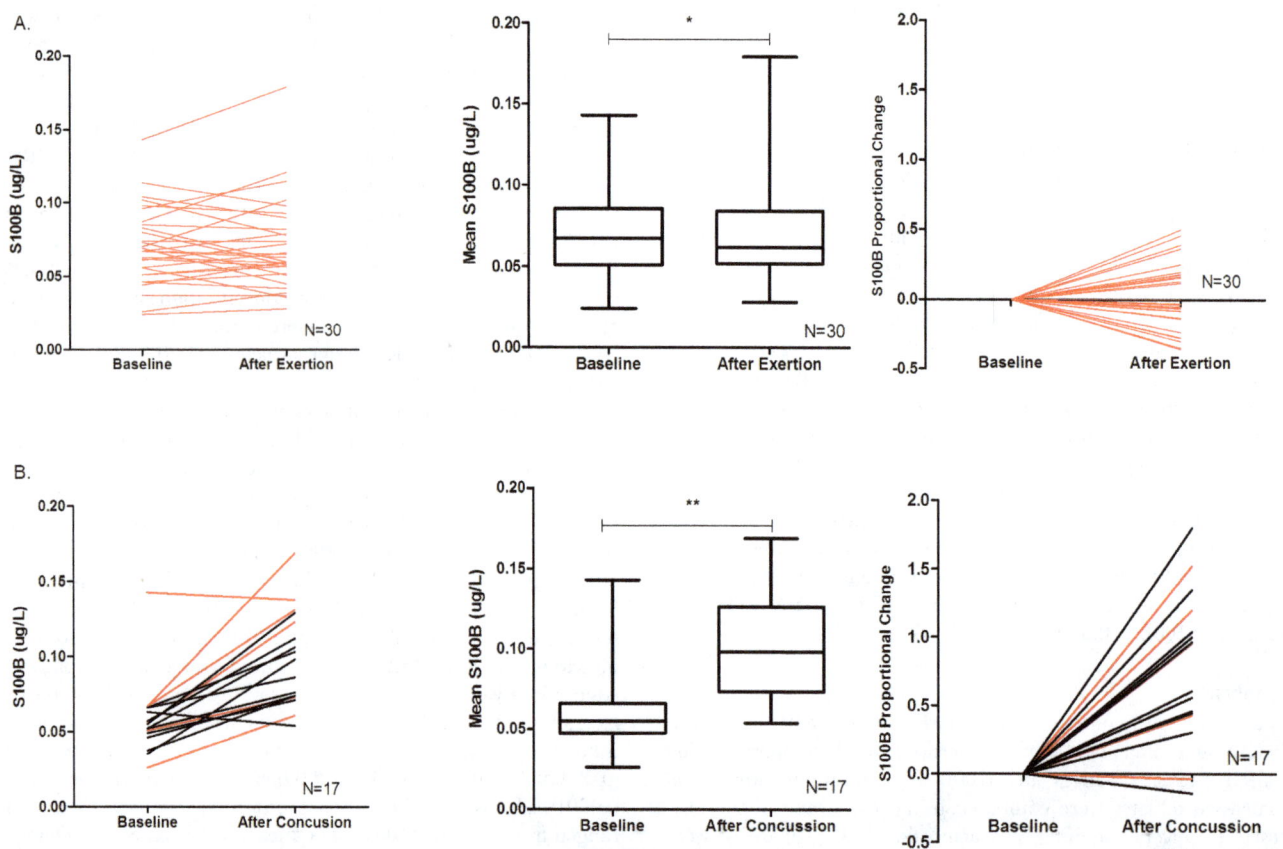

Figure 1. S100B Changes after non-contact exertion and sports-related concussion. **A**: Absolute (Left) and proportional (right) changes in S100B levels after non-contact exertion among individal athletes. The proportional change is defined as (post-exertion or 3-hour post-SRC S100B – baseline S100B)/baseline S100B (range: −35% to +50%; mean proportional change =+2.7%). The mean post-exertional S100B concentration (0.071±0.03 µg/L) was not significantly different from mean baseline (0.070±0.03 µg/L, *p = 0.87, Middle). **B**: Absolute (Left) and proportional (right) changes in S100B levels within 3 hours of SRC among individual athletes. The mean post-SRC S100B concentration within 3 hours of concussion (0.099±0.008 µg/L) was significantly higher than that at baseline (0.058±0.006 µg/L, **p = 0.0002, Middle). Proportional change (right) ranged from −14% to +180%; mean proportional change +81.2%). Munich athletes are designated in red, Rochester athletes in black.

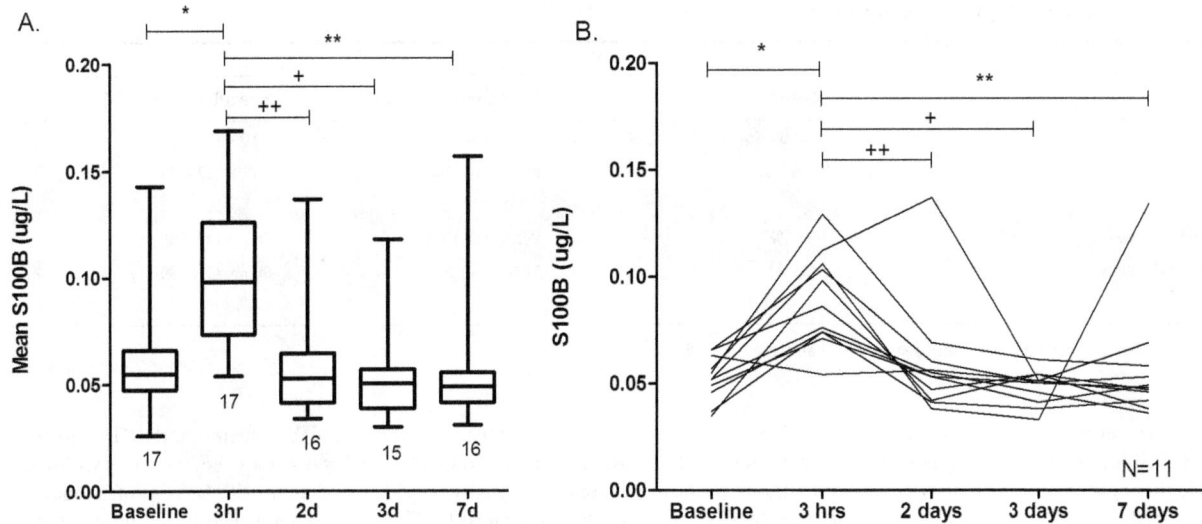

**Figure 2. Longitudinal changes in S100B before and after sports-related concussion. A**: Mean changes in S100B levels among all concussed athletes at baseline and at four time points after injury. The number of athletes included in determining the mean at each time point is indicated below each box plot. The mean S100B concentration within 3 hours of SRC ($0.099 \pm 0.032$ µg/L) was significantly higher than that at baseline ($0.058 \pm 0.025$ µg/L, *$p < 0.0001$) using a paired t-test. The 3 hour S100B level was also higher than that at 2 days ($0.059 \pm 0.03$ µg/L, ++$p = 0.0004$), 3 days ($0.052 \pm 0.02$ µg/L, +$p < 0.0001$), and 7 days ($0.059 \pm 0.03$ µg/L, **$p = 0.001$) post-SRC using unpaired t-tests. **B**: Longitudinal changes in S100B levels among concussed athletes who had baseline and all four post-SRC S100B measurements. All 11 of these athletes were from the Unviersity of Rochester. The mean S100B level within 3 hours of SRC ($0.099 \pm 0.032$ µg/L) was significantly higher than that at baseline ($0.058 \pm 0.025$ µg/L, *$p < 0.0001$), and higher than that at 2 days ($0.059 \pm 0.027$ µg/L, ++$p = 0.0047$), 3 days ($0.048 \pm 0.008$ µg/L, +$p = 0.0002$), and 7 days ($0.056 \pm 0.027$ µg/L, **$p = 0.0058$) post-SRC using paired t-tests.

## Discussion

The current approach to diagnosing SRC is complicated by the subjective nature of the current sideline assessment tools as well as by symptom minimization among athletes motivated to remain in the game [11]. The lack of an objective and accurate diagnostic aid hinders efforts to minimize both the short and long-term consequences of SRC.

In the current study, we have demonstrated that elevated S100B measured within 3 hours of injury is an accurate discriminator of

SRC from sport-related exertion. Classification accuracy is greatly enhanced if the post-injury value is compared to a pre-season baseline. This will come as little surprise to those accustomed to comparing an injured athlete's post-concussion cognitive test scores to their pre-season scores. Unlike tests of cognition, however, measurements of serum S100B are less likely to be affected by stress, sleep deprivation, and pain. Moreover, baseline levels can't be manipulated by athletes trying to minimize the effects of potential future concussions. On the other hand, unlike cognitive performance, which can remain abnormal for weeks

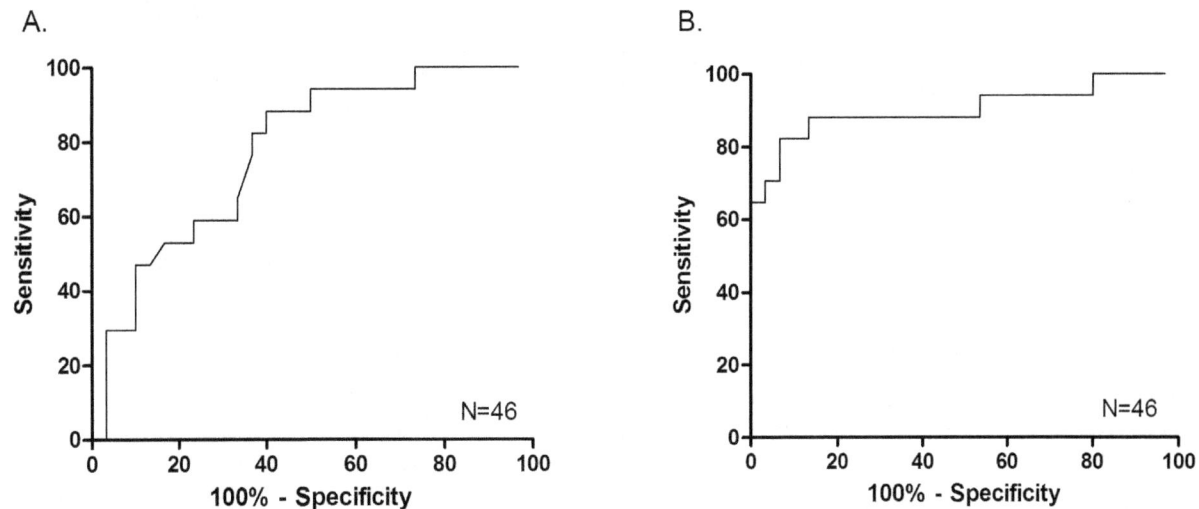

**Figure 3. Diagnostic accuracy of S100B for sports-related concussion. A**: The ROC using the 3-hour post-SRC value or the post-exertion S100B value revealed an AUC of 0.772 (95% CI: 0.64, 0.91). B: The AUC using the proportional increase in post-SRC/exertional S100B level over baseline was 0.904 (95% CI: 0.80, 1.0).

**Table 3.** Concussion classification using S100B.

| | Cutoff | Sensitivity (95% CI) | Specificity (95% CI) |
|---|---|---|---|
| 3-hour S100B | 0.0605 µg/L[†] | 94.1% (71,100) | 50.0% (31, 69) |
| | 0.122 µg/L[‡] | 29.4% (10, 56) | 96.7% (83,100) |
| Proportional Change | −3.5%[†] | 94.1% (71,100) | 46.7% (28, 66) |
| in 3-hour S100B relative | 45.9%[‡] | 70.6% (44, 90) | 96.7% (83, 100) |
| to baseline | | | |

Cutoff values shown are those that maximize sensitivity (†) and specificity (‡).

after concussion, serum S100B levels are cleared rapidly [26]; in our study S100B levels were back to baseline by day 2 after SRC. Thus, while the initial 3 hour level may be a useful adjunct to the diagnosis of SRC, subsequent S100B levels can't be used as a diagnostic aid, and will not be helpful in determining when an athlete is recovered and ready to return to contact sports.

Based on our preliminary findings, an S100B level of > 0.122 µg/L or a proportional S100B increase of >45.9% over baseline measured within 3 hours of injury is quite specific for SRC, while a level <0.0605 µg/L or a proportional decrease of > 3.5% essentially rules it out. Six concussed athletes had serum drawn within 15 minutes of injury (5 of 6 were elevated) suggesting that sampling could be done on the sideline, relatively soon after injury. The prompt measurement of S100B is ideal, given the relatively short biological half-life of S100B. Pending confirmation in larger studies, these results suggest that S100B could be used to aid in the sideline diagnosis of SRC.

However, several practical issues remain. Although used clinically in Germany, S100B testing has not been approved by the FDA for use in the US. In addition, there is currently no portable, point of care assay for S100B measurement, making sideline testing problematic. The Roche Elecsys® analyzer used in the current study is the size of a large desktop printer and requires a centrifuged venous blood sample. Point of care test devices that require a finger stick sample of blood are, however, currently under development [27]. The rollout of these devices would allow athletic trainers to collect baseline as well as post injury S100B levels in a training room or athletic field. Baseline finger stick S100B testing could become integrated into the required pre-participation physical exam that is part of collegiate and secondary sports participation in both the US and Germany. This idea may not be so implausible given the 2010 NCAA regulations in the US requiring pre-participation blood testing for the sickle cell trait[28]. The effort required to overcome these obstacles would be more than offset by the potential benefits of accurately diagnosing and managing an injury to the brain affecting millions of athletes around the world.

While our study has many strengths, including a before-and-after design and a comparison group with a very low risk of occult brain injury, there are several limitations. The primary results involved combining data from two seemingly distinct cohorts; one from Munich and one from Rochester. Although athletes in both cohorts consisted of young adults playing their sport at a highly competitive level, the cohorts differed with respect to age, gender, and sport. They also differed with respect to concussion

prevalance; 20% for the Munich athletes and <1% for the Rochester athletes. This difference may be due in part to the increased concussion risk associated with semi-professional ice hockey but more likely reflects differences in play time. Munich athletes played 8 months a year while the collegiate athletes in Rochester played for only 2–3 months. Because each player served as their own control, these differences were unlikley to bias the main results. Moreover, the mean baseline S100B levels are nearly identical in the two cohorts, as were the patterns of post-injury S100B change (**Table 2 and Figure 1**). These observations underscore the legitimacy of analyzing the groups together. Finally, all of the SRCs in our study were isolated injuries to the head, without the potentially confounding effects of extracranial injuries on S100B elevations. Although others have demonstrated that the contribution of extracranial S100B to overall serum levels is negligible [29], our results should be applied with caution to SRCs accompanied by significant extracrainal injuries such as fractures.

In summary, current sideline diagnosis of SRC relies on athlete self-report or trainer/coach recognition using SAC, SCAT 2, or SCAT 3. Despite this, unrecognized or unreported concussions are still quite common. Our results suggest that serum S100B measured within 3 hours of a sports-related injury can accurately distinguish SRC from sports-related exertion. The accuracy of this prediction is enhanced if the post-injury level is compared to a pre-season baseline level, much in the same way that cognitive test scores are currently interpreted. Serum S100B >0.122 µg/L or a proportional S100B increase of >45.9% over baseline are highly specific (96.7%) for SRC. These results suggest that serum S100B may be a useful adjunct to the diagnosis of SRC.

## Acknowledgments

The authors gratefully acknowledge the assistance Kirsten Ross, Christine Nabinger and Stephanie Amalfe who coordinated enrollment and study-related activities; and Akshata Nayak, Ming Ji, and Emily Tuttle who assisted with serum sample measurement.

## Author Contributions

Conceived and designed the experiments: K Kiechle JJB PB. Performed the experiments: K Kiechle JJB PB. Analyzed the data: K Kiechle JJB PB BB JHH SD KMB. Contributed reagents/materials/analysis tools: JJB PB BB K Kanz. Wrote the paper: K Kiechle JJB PB BB JHH SD VS K Kanz ER KMB. Statistical analysis: K Kiechle JJB KMB. Supervision: JJB PB ER.

# References

1. Prevention CCfDC (2007) Nonfatal traumatic brain injuries from sports and recreation activities–United States, 2001-2005. MMWR - Morbidity & Mortality Weekly Report 56: 733–737.

2. Marar MN, Fields SK, Comstock DR (2012) Epidemiology of Concussions Among United States High School Athletes in 20 Sports. The American Journal of Sports Medicine 40: 747–755.

3. Rickels E vWK, Wenzlaff P (2011) Treatment of traumatic brain injury in Germany. Unfallchirurg 114: 417–423.

4. Rickels E, von Wild K, Wenzlaff P (2010) Head injury in Germany: A population-based prospective study on epidemiology, causes, treatment and outcome of all degrees of head-injury severity in two distinct areas. Brain Injury 24: 1491–1504.

5. McCrory P, Meeuwisse W, Johnston K, Dvorak J, Aubry M, et al. (2009) Consensus statement on concussion in sport: the 3rd International Conference on Concussion in Sport held in Zurich, November 2008. Journal of Athletic Training 44: 434–448.

6. Echemendia RJ, Putukian M, Mackin RS, Julian L, Shoss N (2001) Neuropsychological test performance prior to and following sports-related mild traumatic brain injury. Clinical Journal of Sport Medicine 11: 23–31.

7. McCrea M, Randolph C, Barr WB, Hammeke TA, Marshall SW, et al. (2013) Incidence, Clinical Course, and Predictors of Prolonged Recovery Time Following Sport-Related Concussion in High School and College Athletes. Journal of the International Neuropsychological Society 19: 22–33.

8. McKee AC, Cantu RC, Nowinski CJ, Hedley-Whyte ET, Gavett BE, et al. (2009) Chronic traumatic encephalopathy in athletes: progressive tauopathy after repetitive head injury. Journal of Neuropathology & Experimental Neurology 68: 709–735.

9. McCrea M, Kelly JP, Randolph C, Kluge J, Bartolic E, et al. (1998) Standardized assessment of concussion (SAC): on-site mental status evaluation of the athlete. The Journal of head trauma rehabilitation 13(2): 27–35.

10. McCrory P, Meeuwisse WH, Aubry M, Cantu RC, Dvorak J, et al. (2013) Consensus statement on concussion in sport: the 4th International Conference on Concussion in Sport, Zurich, November 2012. Journal of Athletic Training 48: 554–575.

11. McCrea M, Hammeke T, Olsen G, Leo P, Guskiewicz K (2004) Unreported Concussion in High School Football Players Implications for Prevention. Clin J Sport Med 14: 13–17.

12. Zimmer DB, Cornwall EH, Landar A, Song W (1995) The S100 protein family: history, function, and expression. Brain Research Bulletin 37: 417–429.

13. Donato R (2003) Intracellular and extracellular roles of S100 proteins. Microscopy Research & Technique 60: 540–551.

14. Marenholz I, Heizmann CW, Fritz G (2004) S100 proteins in mouse and man: from evolution to function and pathology (including an update of the nomenclature). Biochemical & Biophysical Research Communications 322: 1111–1122.

15. Unden J, Romner B (2010) Can low serum levels of S100B predict normal CT findings after minor head injury in adults?: an evidence-based review and meta-analysis. Journal of Head Trauma Rehabilitation 25: 228–240.

16. Biberthaler P, Linsenmeier U, Pfeifer KJ, Kroetz M, Mussack T, et al. (2006) Serum S-100B concentration provides additional information fot the indication of computed tomography in patients after minor head injury: a prospective multicenter study. Shock 25: 446–453.

17. Bazarian JJ, Blyth BJ, He H, Mookerjee S, Jones C, et al. (2013) Classification Accuracy of Serum Apo A-I and S100B for the Diagnosis of Mild Traumatic Brain Injury and Prediction of Abnormal Initial Head Computed Tomography Scan. Journal of Neurotrauma 30: 1747–1754.

18. Otto M, Holthusen S, Bahn E, Sohnchen N, Wiltfang J, et al. (2000) Boxing and running lead to a rise in serum levels of S-100B protein. International Journal of Sports Medicine 21: 551–555.

19. Hasselblatt M, Mooren FC, Von Ahsen N, Keyvani K, Fromme A, et al. (2004) Serum S100beta increases in marathon runners reflect extracranial release rather than glial damage. Neurology 62: 1634–1636.

20. Stalnacke BM, Tegner Y, Sojka P (2003) Playing Ice Hockey and Basketball Increases Serum Levels of S-100B in Elite Players; A Pilot Study. Clinical Journal of Sport Medicine 13: 292–302.

21. Stalnacke BM, Tegner Y, Sojka P (2004) Playing soccer increases serum concentration of the biochemical markers of brain damage S-100B and neuron-specific enolase in elite players: a pilot study. Brain Injury 18: 899–909.

22. Corrigan JD, Bogner J (2007) Initial reliability and validity of the Ohio State University TBI Identification Method. Journal of Head Trauma Rehabilitation 22: 318–329.

23. Ben Abdesselam O, Vally J, Adem C, Foglietti M-J, Beaudeux J-L (2003) Reference values for serum S-100B protein depend on the race of individuals. Clinical Chemistry 49: 836–837.

24. Tang W, Hua H, Tu XM (2012) Applied Categorical and Count Data Analysis. Boca Raton, FL: CRC Press, Taylor & Francis Group.

25. Stalnacke BM, Ohlsson A, Tegner Y, Sojka P (2006) Serum concentrations of two biochemical markers of brain tissue damage S-100B and neurone specific enolase are increased in elite female soccer players after a competitive game. British Journal of Sports Medicine 40: 313–316.

26. Towend W (2006) Rapid Elimination of protein S-100B from Serum after Minor Head Trauma. Journal of Neuotrauma 23: 149–155.

27. FierceBiomarkers (2012) A*STAR's Institute of Microelectronics and SFC Fluidics Collaborate To Develop Point-of-Need Traumatic Brain Injury Diagnostic Device. FierceBiotech Research Channel.

28. Bonham VL, Dover GJ, Brody LC (2010) Screening student athletes for sickle cell trait–a social and clinical experiment. New England Journal of Medicine 363: 997–999.

29. Pham N, Fazio V, Cucullo L, Teng Q, Biberthaler P, et al. (2010) Extracranial sources of S100B do not affect serum levels.[Erratum appears in PLoS One. 2010;5(10). doi: 10.1371/annotation/bdcb41f2-a320-4401-a6ab-86e71738597e]. PLoS ONE [Electronic Resource] 5.

# 3

# Trauma-Associated Tinnitus: Audiological, Demographic and Clinical Characteristics

Peter M. Kreuzer[1]*, Michael Landgrebe[1,2], Martin Schecklmann[1], Susanne Staudinger[1], Berthold Langguth[1], The TRI Database Study Group[¶]

1 Department of Psychiatry and Psychotherapy, University of Regensburg, Regensburg, Germany, 2 Department of Psychiatry, Psychosomatic Medicine and Psychotherapy, Sozialstiftung Bamberg, Bamberg, Germany

## Abstract

*Background:* Tinnitus can result from different etiologies. Frequently, patients report the development of tinnitus after traumatic injuries. However, to which extent this specific etiologic factor plays a role for the phenomenology of tinnitus is still incompletely understood. Additionally, it remains a matter of debate whether the etiology of tinnitus constitutes a relevant criterion for defining tinnitus subtypes.

*Objective:* By investigating a worldwide sample of tinnitus patients derived from the Tinnitus Research Initiative (TRI) Database, we aimed to identify differences in demographic, clinical and audiological characteristics between tinnitus patients with and without preceding trauma.

*Materials:* A total of 1,604 patients were investigated. Assessment included demographic data, tinnitus related clinical data, audiological data, the Tinnitus Handicap Inventory, the Tinnitus Questionnaire, the Beck Depression Inventory, various numeric tinnitus rating scales, and the World Health Organisation Quality of Life Scale (WHOQoL).

*Results:* Our data clearly indicate differences between tinnitus patients with and without trauma at tinnitus onset. Patients suffering from trauma-associated tinnitus suffer from a higher mental burden than tinnitus patients presenting with phantom perceptions based on other or unknown etiologic factors. This is especially the case for patients with whiplash and head trauma. Patients with posttraumatic noise-related tinnitus experience more frequently hyperacousis, were younger, had longer tinnitus duration, and were more frequently of male gender.

*Conclusions:* Trauma before tinnitus onset seems to represent a relevant criterion for subtypization of tinnitus. Patients with posttraumatic tinnitus may require specific diagnostic and therapeutic management. A more systematic and – at best - standardized assessment for hearing related sequelae of trauma is needed for a better understanding of the underlying pathophysiology and for developing more tailored treatment approaches as well.

**Editor:** Xi (Erick) Lin, Emory Univ. School of Medicine, United States of America

**Funding:** The study was supported by the Tinnitus Research Initiative/TRI (www.tinnitusresearch.org). All authors confirm no conflicts of interest in regard to the manuscript. The funders had no role in study design, data collection and analysis, decision to publish, or preparation of the manuscript.

**Competing Interests:** The authors have declared that no competing interests exist.

* E-mail: peter.kreuzer@medbo.de

¶ Membership of The TRI Database Study Group is provided in the Acknowledgments

## Introduction

Each year, approximately 1–2 million people experience a traumatic brain injury (= TBI) in the United States [1,2]. Apart from that, TBI is found among the most common war related injuries due to blast and concussion [3]. Recent studies revealed that 15.8% of service members in the Iraq war experienced traumatic brain injury [4,5], in combat team samples an even higher prevalence ranging up to 22.8% was reported [6].

Trauma to the head – especially to the ear – is often associated with tinnitus [7], defined as an intermittent or constant sound sensation which cannot be attributed to an external sound source. In military personnel with TBI up to 38% reported comorbid tinnitus complaints [8]. A random sample of the Iraq war records revealed that 71% of soldiers experienced loud noises and that

15.6% had tinnitus [9,10]. According to the American Tinnitus Association 3 to 4 million veterans suffer from tinnitus and compensation payments for combat related hearing loss [10] and tinnitus account for approximately US$ 1.2 billion per year [11]. But also in civil populations acoustic trauma is among the most frequently reported triggers for the development of chronic tinnitus [12,13].

Notably, many different types of trauma can precede tinnitus onset. Noise trauma typically causes damage to the inner ear, and as a consequence leads to tinnitus [14]. Brain injuries can cause a variety of auditory symptoms such as hearing loss, tinnitus, and central deficits indicating the vulnerability of the auditory pathways to traumatic injury [15]. Moreover, also neck [16] injuries and emotional trauma [17,18] are well known triggers of tinnitus [19,20]. Therefore, we investigated the categories "noise trauma", "whiplash", and "head trauma", and its combinations with regard to a large sample of tinnitus patients presenting in specialized tinnitus centers worldwide. The term "post-traumatic" or "trauma-associated" as mentioned in the present manuscript does not refer to the psychological aspects of trauma in the sense of "posttraumatic stress (disorder)". It is rather applied to subsume the trauma categories "noise trauma", "whiplash", and "head trauma" (without further specification of its extent).

Tinnitus can vary in its phenomenological characteristics and in the amount of the related distress. It can cause severe distress on individuals and it has been shown to be correlated with sleeping disorders [21], depression [18,22] and anxiety [23,24,25,26,27,28,29,30]. It may affect the individual's concentration and ability for attentional focusing and working memory [31,32]. Development of tinnitus may even end up in suicidal attempts [33,34,35,36]. Perceptual characteristics such as tinnitus loudness [37] or tinnitus frequency [38] only explain to a small extent the amount of tinnitus suffering. Other relevant factors include age at onset [39], personality factors [40] and coping behavior [41]. It has also been proposed that etiologic factors such as head and neck injuries related to tinnitus onset may exert an influence on the amount of tinnitus complaints [16].

In order to find out whether trauma and especially the different types of trauma at tinnitus onset are of relevance for perceptual, demographic and clinical characteristics of tinnitus a large worldwide sample of patients presenting at specialized tinnitus clinics has been investigated. The main objectives were to 1) to determine the percentage of cases of chronic tinnitus related to different types of trauma; 2) to describe the characteristics of these population and 3) to compare these characteristics with tinnitus patients whose tinnitus onset was not associated with trauma.

## Materials and Methods

The data presented in this study derive from the Tinnitus Research Initiative Database [42]. Data management was conducted according to the Data Handling Plan (TRI-DHP V07, May 9th, 2011). Data analysis was conducted according to the Standard Operating Procedure (TRI-SA V01, May 9th, 2011), thereby following a study-specific Statistical Analysis Plan (SAP-008, 20/12/2011) that was written according to the SAP template (TRI-SAP V01, May 9th, 2011). All documents can be accessed under http://database.tinnitusresearch.org/. Analysis details can be found at the end of this section.

The default dataset import (November 1st, 2011) from the Tinnitus Research Initiative (TRI) Database consisted of 2,184 patients (see figure 1). Patients presented between 2005 and 2011 at different tinnitus centres worldwide (mainly from Brasil and Europe; center specific analysis could not be done due to irregular frequencies for the single trauma types with respect to centres; more detailed information about contributing tinnitus centres can be found at http://database.tinnitusresearch.org/en/map/map_en.php). Patients gave written informed consent to record their data in the database and to perform analyses with the data. The project has been approved by the local ethics committee of the Medical Faculty of the University of Regensburg. The database project is coordinated by the department of psychiatry and psychotherapy of the University of Regensburg, Germany, and the database server is located at the ManaTheam GmbH in Regensburg.

The variable "onset related event" was deduced from the question of the Tinnitus Sample Case History Questionnaire (TSCHQ; 45) "Was the initial onset of your tinnitus related to:" with the pre-formulated answers "loud blast of sound", "whiplash", "change in hearing", "stress", "head trauma", and "other". Patients who did not answer the TSCHQ were excluded from analysis resulting in a sample of 1,604 patients (see figure 1). Patients were grouped according to their self-reported onset related events (see figure 1).

We built the five categories "no trauma", "noise trauma", "whiplash", and "head trauma", and "other tinnitus related onset". If one patient reported multiple events including one single trauma this patient was subsumed to the group of this trauma. Patients with multiple traumata were excluded from primary analysis (n = 23; 1.4%) (see figure 1).

Assessment was performed before the first consultation in the tinnitus clinics and included the Tinnitus Sample Case History Questionnaire (TSCHQ), the Tinnitus Handicap Inventory (THI) [43], the Tinnitus Questionnaire (TQ) [44], the Beck Depression Inventory (BDI) [45], and four domains of the World Health Organisation Quality of Life Scale (WHOQoL). The different domains of the WHOQOL measure 1st "physical health", in particular activities of daily living, dependence on medicinal substances and medical aids, energy and fatigue, mobility, pain and discomfort, sleep and rest, work capacity; 2nd "psychological health", in particular bodily image and appearance, negative/positive feelings, self-esteem, spirituality/religion/personal beliefs, thinking, learning, memory and concentration; 3rd "social relationships", in particular personal relationships, social support, sexual activity; and 4th "environmental factors", in particular financial resources, freedom, physical safety and security, health and social care, home environment, opportunities for acquiring new information and skills, opportunities for recreation, physical environment, and transport [46].

Subjectively perceived loudness, discomfort, annoyance, ignorability, and unpleasantness were assessed by numeric rating scales (range: 0–10).

In addition to these variables, we were interested in the demographic characteristics age, gender and age at tinnitus onset. Furthermore, we investigated the tinnitus duration until presentation at our clinic, the way of onset (gradual/abrupt), number of preceding treatments until presentation, tinnitus characteristics such as pulsatile or non-pulsatile sound perception, tonal or noise-like tinnitus, the possibility of masking the tinnitus by music or sounds and the ability of modulating the tinnitus by somatic manoeuvres. Comorbid symptoms of tinnitus such as headaches, vertigo/dizziness, temporomandibular disorders, neck pain or other pain symptoms were asked for. Hyperacousis was checked by the following TSCHQ-items (number 28 and 29): a) "Do you have a problem tolerating sounds because they often seem much too loud? That is, do you often find too loud or hurtful sounds which other people around you find quite comfortable?" with the predetermined response possibilities "never/rarely/sometimes/usually/always" and b) "Do sounds cause you pain or physical discomfort? "yes/no/I don't know".

In addition, current psychiatric treatment was assessed. The mean hearing level (dB hearing level (pure tone audiogram) over eight frequencies (0.125/0.250/0.500/1/2/4/6/8 kHz) of both ears was documented and averaged."

If no data were available at the screening visit (first consultation), we used data from the baseline visit of a clinical intervention. If both screening and baseline data were available we used the mean of both time points. For statistical analyses we used analyses of variance (ANOVAs) for continuous variables (e.g., age) and chi-square-tests for categorical variables (e.g., gender) with the variable onset (no trauma/noise/whiplash/head/other) as group variable (table 1). Significance threshold was set to a Bonferroni corrected

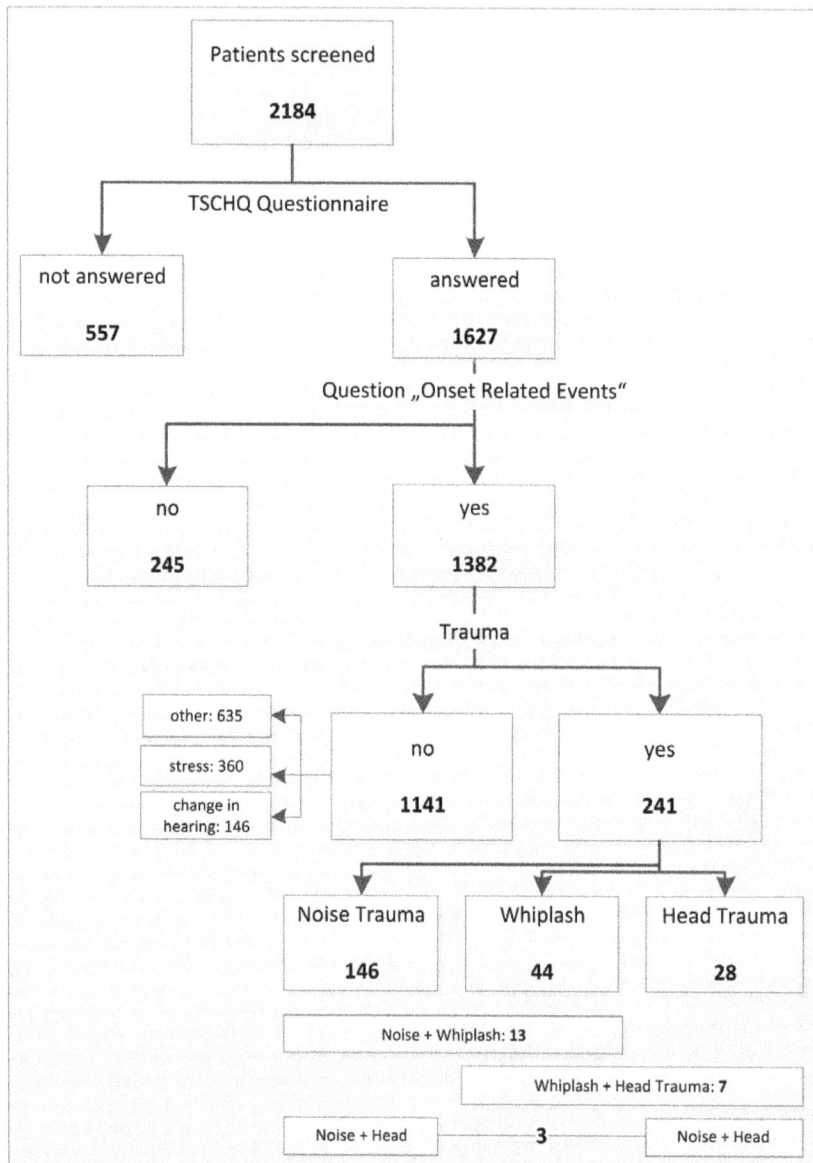

**Figure 1. Patients' flowchart, data provided in absolute numbers.**

level of 0.0016 (0.0016 = 0.05/31 included variables). In case of significant results in the ANOVA, post-hoc tests were performed by using t-tests for continuous variables and using z-standardized residuals of the frequencies of the single cells of the chi-square-tests for categorical variables. These post-hoc tests are displayed graphically (figure 2 to 5). For post-hoc tests significance threshold was set to an uncorrected level of 0.05.

## Results

A total of 1,604 patients answered the TSCHQ-Question concerning onset-related events thus providing a self-report of possible triggering factors of the phantom perception. 241 individuals reported a trauma-associated tinnitus onset. 146 reported a history of noise trauma, 44 a history of whiplash, and 28 a history of head trauma as an *isolated* trigger for their tinnitus. Detailed information is given in figure 1.

We found significant group effects for the variables age at presentation, age at onset, gender, tinnitus duration, vertigo/dizziness, neck pain, other pain symptoms, current psychiatric treatment, TQ, THI, BDI, WHOQOL domain 1 and 4, and both hyperacousis-questions regarding "sound toleration" and "sounds causing pain and physical discomfort".

Groups did not differ for the variables "number of preceding treatments", "pulsatile vs. non-pulsatile tinnitus character", "tonal/noise-like/cricket-like tinnitus", "maskability", "somatic modulation", "headache", "temporomandibular joint disorders (TMJD)", "hearing level", WHOQOL domains 2 and 3, and the five numeric tinnitus rating scales regarding the aspects "loudness", "discomfort", "annoyance", "ignorability", and "unpleasantness".

As patients with multiple trauma history (n = 23; see figure 1) have been excluded from analysis as described in the methods section of this manuscript, we additionally calculated thirty (as shown in table 1) group contrasts of single trauma cases vs.

**Table 1.** Sample characteristics and clinical assessment scales (given as mean±standard deviation); significant results after Bonferroni correction for multiple testing are highlighted in bold letters.

| | no trauma | noise | whiplash | head | other | F/$\chi^2$ | df | p |
|---|---|---|---|---|---|---|---|---|
| sample characteristics | | | | | | | | |
| **age at presentation** | **54.3±13.8** | **49.3±15.1** | **54.4±8.1** | **47.6±14.6** | **52.9±12.8** | **4.589** | **4** | **.001** |
| **age at tinnitus onset** | **45.3±15.2** | **36.2±15.3** | **47.4±8.5** | **41.2±16.5** | **44.3±13.6** | **11.820** | **4** | **<.000** |
| **gender (female/male)** | **94/151** | **32/114** | **12/32** | **10/18** | **447/693** | **18.606** | **4** | **.001** |
| tinnitus and audiologic characteristics | | | | | | | | |
| **duration in months** | **103.7±108.7** | **144.5±135.5** | **75.1±82.7** | **75.6±69.0** | **95.6±104.0** | **7.096** | **4** | **<.000** |
| preceding treatments | 2.61±1.040 | 2.77±1.159 | 3.05±1.011 | 2.54±1.170 | 2.78±1.052 | 2.806 | 4 | .042 |
| pulsatile (no/yes with heartbeat/yes other than heartbeat) | 196/22/19 | 115/11/18 | 32/4/6 | 22/3/1 | 899/123/106 | 5.861 | 8 | .663 |
| tone/noise/crickets/other | 120/46/54/19 | 85/30/18/11 | 19/8/6/10 | 14/8/3/3 | 616/204/210/97 | 21.432 | 12 | .044 |
| maskable (no/yes) | 55/161 | 22/104 | 5/30 | 7/13 | 244/734 | 6.750 | 4 | .150 |
| somatic modulation (no/yes) | 169/71 | 97/48 | 19/23 | 15/12 | 751/377 | 11.626 | 4 | .020 |
| headache (no/yes) | 155/81 | 82/60 | 21/22 | 8/17 | 686/426 | 14.544 | 4 | .006 |
| **vertigo/dizziness (no/yes)** | **179/57** | **86/53** | **19/23** | **11/15** | **732/369** | **25.953** | **4** | **<.000** |
| temporomandibular disorder (no/yes) | 196/42 | 108/34 | 26/17 | 15/8 | 874/237 | 13.173 | 4 | .010 |
| **neck pain (no/yes)** | **123/119** | **61/82** | **5/38** | **10/17** | **482/630** | **23.573** | **4** | **<.000** |
| **other pain (no/yes)** | **169/70** | **87/57** | **19/22** | **12/16** | **632/465** | **20.258** | **4** | **<.000** |
| **current psychiatric treatment (no/yes)** | **226/17** | **125/20** | **35/8** | **17/10** | **945/180** | **24.156** | **4** | **<.000** |
| **sound tolerance (low/high)** | **178/63** | **73/73** | **28/15** | **16/11** | **732/398** | **23.025** | **4** | **<.000** |
| **painful sounds (no/yes)** | **133/85** | **49/87** | **11/23** | **9/18** | **441/569** | **31.384** | **4** | **<.000** |
| hearing level (median HL) | 23.2±20.31 | 21.4±13.38 | 18.8±11.83 | 18.7±9.92 | 20.7±13.51 | 1.395 | 4 | .233 |
| tinnitus questionnaires | | | | | | | | |
| **TQ** | **36.2±18.53** | **42.5±18.14** | **49.2±14.74** | **51.8±20.81** | **40.6±17.37** | **7.090** | **4** | **<.000** |
| **THI** | **42.8±24.82** | **51.5±23.44** | **55.3±23.70** | **60.7±24.44** | **48.0±22.55** | **6.770** | **4** | **<.000** |
| **BDI** | **9.8±8.72** | **11.6±8.07** | **15.4±10.20** | **15.6±9.19** | **11.1±8.56** | **5.733** | **4** | **<.000** |
| **WHOQOL domain 1** | **14.7±3.27** | **13.9±3.22** | **12.7±3.51** | **12.5±3.63** | **14.4±2.98** | **4.735** | **4** | **.001** |
| WHOQOL domain 2 | 14.2±2.98 | 13.9±2.52 | 12.6±2.66 | 12.6±2.78 | 14.0±2.74 | 3.154 | 4 | .014 |
| WHOQOL domain 3 | 15.0±3.22 | 13.9±3.03 | 13.3±3.27 | 13.5±2.38 | 14.5±3.17 | 3.094 | 4 | .015 |
| **WHOQOL domain 4** | **15.7±2.80** | **15.0±2.56** | **14.7±2.90** | **13.5±3.06** | **15.8±2.37** | **6.487** | **4** | **<.000** |
| numeric rating scales | | | | | | | | |
| loudness | 6.2±2.34 | 6.4±2.34 | 6.9±2.16 | 6.9±2.29 | 6.4±2.13 | 1.472 | 4 | .208 |
| discomfort | 6.9±2.55 | 7.0±2.29 | 7.7±1.94 | 7.4±2.15 | 7.0±2.26 | 1.359 | 4 | .246 |
| annoyance | 6.4±2.62 | 6.5±2.36 | 7.4±2.05 | 7.3±2.23 | 6.6±2.34 | 2.009 | 4 | .091 |
| ignorability | 6.6±2.90 | 6.6±2.71 | 7.7±2.03 | 7.2±2.87 | 6.7±2.57 | 1.774 | 4 | .131 |
| unpleasantness | 6.5±2.61 | 6.6±2.45 | 7.5±1.81 | 7.2±2.29 | 6.6±2.37 | 2.046 | 4 | .086 |

multiple trauma cases (n = 218; subsuming all patients with noise or head trauma or whiplash) resulting in no significant results (lowest p-values = .017 and.028 (uncorrected for multiple comparisons) for the items "preceding treatment approaches" and tinnitus questionnaire total score, respectively.

Comprehensive information about clinical characteristics, questionnaire ratings and audiological data is given in table 1.

## Discussion

### Occurrence of Tinnitus Onset Related Traumata

With a percentage of 4.9% (= (44+28+7)/1604; see figure 1) patients suffering from a tinnitus induced by whiplash or head trauma (or a combination) represent only a small subsample in our database derived from several tinnitus centers worldwide participating in the Tinnitus Research Initiative (TRI). In an earlier study, Folmer and Griest reported a prevalence of a history of head and neck trauma in more than 10 percent of the patients presenting in the specialized tinnitus clinic in Portland, Oregon [16]. Vice versa, in the literature there is evidence that tinnitus is found to be highly prevalent in patients with a history of trauma. Flint et al. investigated the incidence of persisting auditory and vestibular sequelae in a group of 30 young adults (aged 21–45 years) recovering from traumatic brain injury, that had taken place previously (range 19 months to 27 years). A variety of sequelae to TBI were reported including tinnitus (53%), vestibular dysfunction (83%), abnormal facial sensory symptoms (27%) and intolerance to loud/sudden noises (87%) [19]. Ten (33%) participants demon-

## Age at Onset

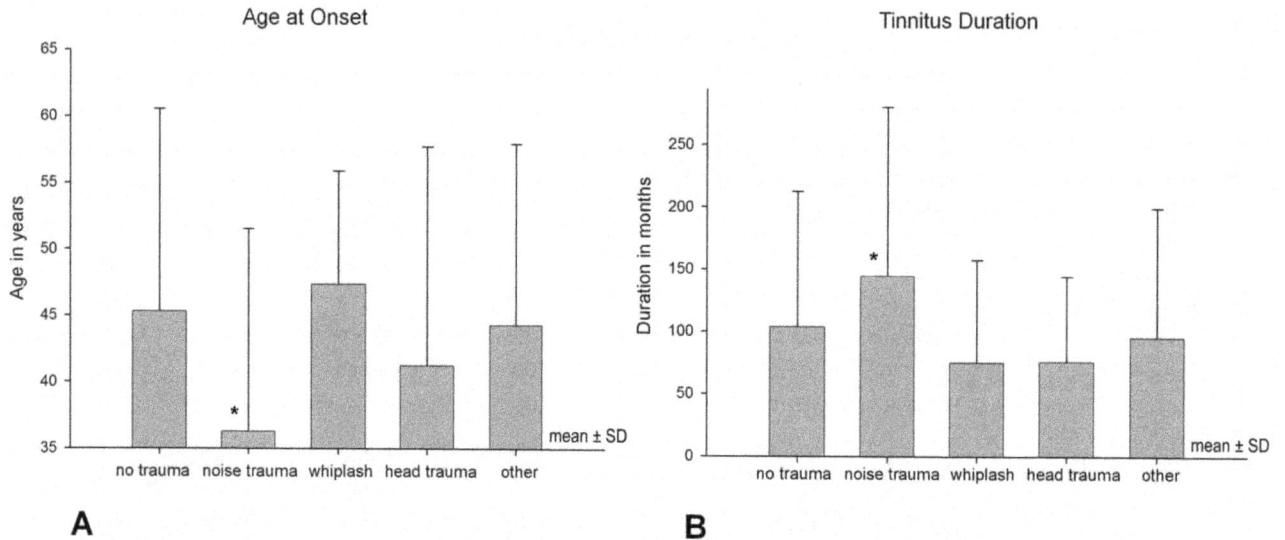

## Tinnitus Duration

**A**                                                                    **B**

**Figure 2. Age at Tinnitus Onset and Tinnitus Duration (mean ± SD). A** * Statistically significant between-groups contrasts (p<0.001) to groups "no trauma", "whiplash", and "other". **B** * Statistically significant between-groups contrasts (p<0.005) to groups "no trauma", "whiplash", "head trauma" and "other".

strated significant sensorineural hearing impairment in addition to speech recognition performance significantly worse than would have been predicted from their hearing impairment [19].

But also in total, given the high prevalence of head, neck and noise trauma and the frequent occurrence of tinnitus after these traumas the rate of reported trauma at tinnitus onset in our sample is very low. Different explanations may account for this finding: a) trauma at tinnitus onset may be underreported by patients especially when there was a delay between trauma and tinnitus onset; b) patients with posttraumatic tinnitus may be preferentially encountered in specific settings such as military medicine or occupational medicine; c) posttraumatic tinnitus might be

underestimated by treating physicians with respect to other trauma-related symptoms and therefore these patients might not be referred to tinnitus clinics and be underrepresented in this study population; d) Patients with trauma-associated tinnitus experience tinnitus frequently but rarely present themselves to specialized tinnitus centres because they do not suffer a lot from it compared to other trauma-related impairments; The last explanation is rather unlikely as in our study sample patients with trauma-associated tinnitus showed greater symptom-related burden (see figure 4).

We are aware that our study can only provide a vague estimation of the prevalence of trauma preceding tinnitus onset. First, our analyses rely entirely on patients' self reports; secondly even if our sample is large and derives from many centers world-wide it is biased since it reflects the patient population in specialized tinnitus clinics. Therefore, further prospective and population based studies are needed for a more precise estimation of the prevalence of trauma before tinnitus onset.

### Summary of the TRI Database Findings

Posttraumatic tinnitus was associated with higher distress levels reflected by higher scores in TQ, THI, BDI, and WHOQoL subscores 1 and 4 as compared to tinnitus patients without trauma at tinnitus onset. These findings reached statistical significance for whiplash and head trauma (TQ, THI, BDI, WHOQOL Dom1 and Dom4) (see figures 4 and 5). This is in line with the findings of the study of Folmer and Griest, who reported both higher Tinnitus Severity Index Scores. However, these authors found also more pronounced tinnitus loudness (measured by 1-to-10 scales and tinnitus matching) in patients suffering from trauma-associated tinnitus [16]. Whereas, our data did not show any effects in tinnitus ratings as elicited by numeric rating scales. In addition, these patients reported greater difficulties with concentration, memory, and clear thinking [16]. Possibly, trauma-associated tinnitus might constitute a subtype connected with higher symptom-related distress levels. Another explanation would be that the higher impairment of posttraumatic tinnitus is not directly associated with a specific trauma associated pathophysiology but rather reflects dysfunctional coping strategies. A "fateful" tinnitus

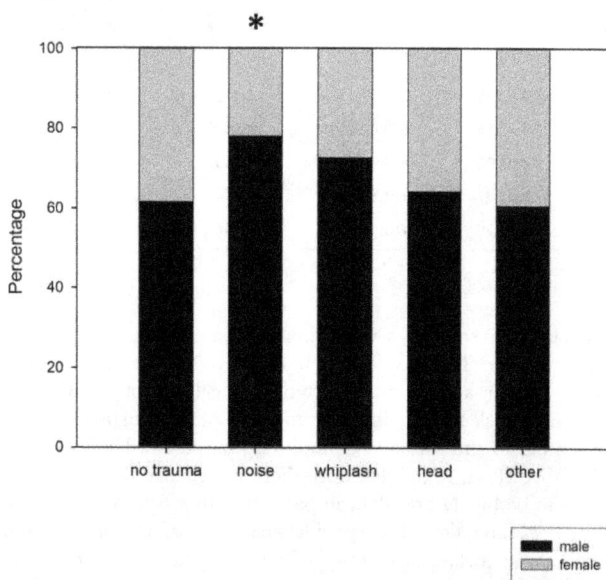

**Figure 3. Gender distribution shown in percentage of male/ female patients.** * Proportion of male patients higher than statistically expected.

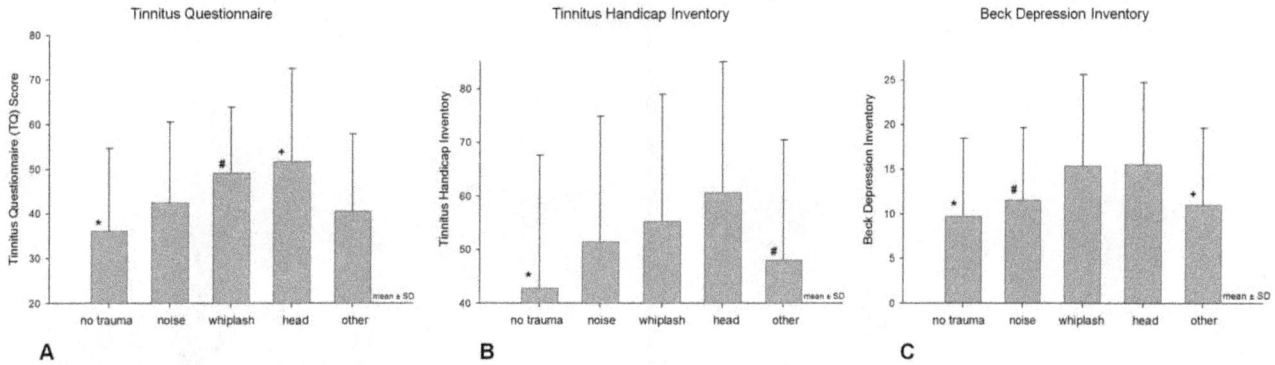

**Figure 4. Clinical Questionnaire Assessment Scales at Presentation (mean ± SD). A** * Statistically significant between-groups contrasts to all other groups (p<0.005). # Statistically significant between-groups contrasts to groups "no trauma", "noise", and "other" (p<0.05). + Statistically significant between-groups contrasts to groups "no trauma" and "other" (p<0.05). **B** * Statistically significant between-groups contrasts to all other groups (p<0.005). # Statistically significant between-groups contrasts to groups "no trauma", "whiplash", and "head" (p<0.05). **C** * Statistically significant between-groups contrasts to all other groups (p<0.05). # Statistically significant between-groups contrasts to groups "no trauma", "whiplash", and "head" (p<0.05). + Statistically significant between-groups contrasts to groups "no trauma", "whiplash", and "head" (p<0.05).

onset without any triggering factors might be tolerable, habituable and integrable more easily than a trauma-associated onset which is often accompanied by strong emotions such as surprise, helplessness, pain, and fear, especially when the trauma has not been caused by the patient but by a second party. In many of these cases, patients suffer not only from a bodily damage but tend to regard themselves as "victims" and spend much time with ruminating thoughts about the traumatic event and its preventability such as "If I hadn't gone there and wouldn't have done that... I would not have met this...". Similarly, the expectation for compensation payments may influence habituation. These dysfunctional coping strategies may particularly explain the elevated depression scores in the BDI after head and whiplash trauma. The participation rate in psychiatric treatment reflects this situation, indicating that trauma patients in our sample underwent current psychiatric treatment more frequently than patients without trauma-related onset (see table 1). However, this finding might be biased by psychiatric trauma consequences unrelated to tinnitus. Also, the WHOQOL Quality of Life Questionnaires showed similar patterns like the THI, TQ, and BDI. Apparently, trauma patients as a whole suffered from a more pronounced impairment of their quality of life than tinnitus patients of other etiologies. This pattern was similar for all of the four WHOQOL domains (see Figure 5).

Patients without tinnitus related onset events (including trauma and non-trauma events) reported less frequently that sounds can cause them pain or physical discomfort (see figure 6). Furthermore, the tolerance to loud or hurtful sounds is reduced especially in the subgroup of noise trauma patients (see figure 6). As patient groups did not differ in their hearing levels, recruitment phenomena are considered unlikely to account for these symptoms. In particular, there was no significant between-groups contrast of hearing loss levels at 4 kHz (F = 0.906; df = 4; p = 0.460) and no at the remaining frequencies either (F = 1.414; df = 4; p = 0.227) suggesting that no typical c5-dip [47] was present in noise trauma patients. Rather, the impairment assessed by both questionnaire items suggests a more frequent occurrence of hyperacousis in patients with noise related posttraumatic tinnitus, thus indicating differences in central auditory processing [48]. In this regard our findings of an increased rate of hyperacousis in posttraumatic tinnitus correspond well with earlier studies demonstrating high rates of intolerance to loud sounds after TBI [19]. These findings indicate that in TBI in addition to potential cochlear damage the

direct impact on the central auditory pathways is relevant for the etiology of posttraumatic tinnitus. As also mentioned above, no difference in cumulative hearing loss between patients with trauma and non-trauma-groups was observed in our study (see table 1). On a descriptive level, patients without a history of trauma showed higher levels of cumulative hearing loss than patients affected by noise trauma but this difference did not reach significance. This is surprising because it has been reported that acoustic trauma and blast injuries result typically in high-frequency hearing loss [15,47]. However, Nicolas-Puel et al. reported similar findings in a sample of 555 patients attending the specialized Tinnitus Clinic in Montpellier, France. Patients with a reported history of noise trauma (17% of the total sample) showed symmetrical hearing loss without differences in lateralization of the tinnitus percept. As in our study, this subset of patients was mainly male and on average 10 years younger than other tinnitus patients. Possibly, young men tend to live an active life and execute risky behavior more frequently thus undergoing an increased risk for accidents. In this French study hearing loss of patients with noise trauma was significantly less pronounced than that measured in the other patients [49]. The observed less pronounced hearing loss in tinnitus patients with noise trauma may be a hint for the relevance of the temporal dynamics of hearing loss for tinnitus generation. As compared with slowly progressing hearing loss in presbyacousis, noise trauma causes a sudden hearing impairment which might trigger specific neuroplastic mechanisms in the brain which in turn induce tinnitus. The induced tinnitus may then persist, even if hearing function recovers in many patients.

Further studies in humans and experimental studies in animals demonstrate that the extent of permanent threshold shift after trauma is variable and may depend on the type of trauma. Nölle et al. reported in a sample of 31 patients (24–56 years) after a history of blunt head trauma that initial sensorineural hearing loss (as a result of the inner ear fluid concussion) was transiently perceived only. Auditory brainstem responses (ABR) were normal in all patients, but 76% experienced lowered loudness discomfort levels. The authors stated that blunt trauma of the head can lead to auditory dysfunction, probably as a result of diffuse axonal injury of the central auditory pathway [50]. In contrast, Nageris et al. reported in a sample of 73 patients exposed to physical trauma in case of explosion, that 78% experienced high-frequency accentuated sensorineural hearing loss with only 7% improving over time [51]. Apparently, the correlation of head and acoustic

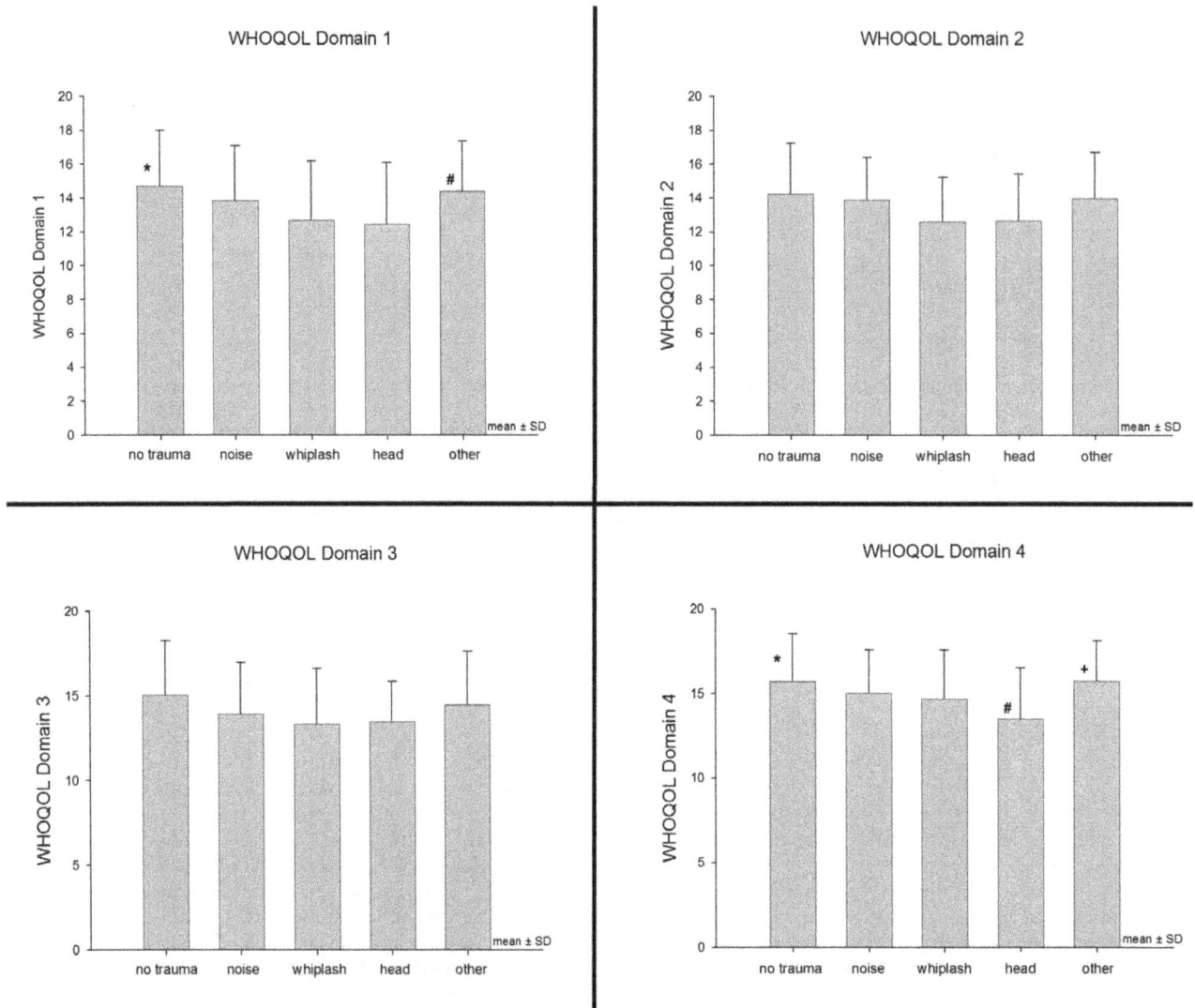

**Figure 5. WHOQOL Questionnaire. Domain 1** * Statistically significant between-groups contrasts(p<0.05) to groups "noise", "whiplash", and "head". # Statistically significant between-groups contrasts (p<0.05) to groups "whiplash" and "head". **Domain 4** * Statistically significant between-groups contrasts (p<0.05) to groups "noise" and "head". # Statistically significant between-groups contrasts (p<0.05) to groups "noise", "whiplash", and "head". + Statistically significant between-groups contrast (p<0.05) to group "noise".

trauma with hearing loss strongly depends on the specific form of trauma and its *extent*, so a more detailed, structured and - at best - standardized assessment of trauma-related information is considered vital for the drawing of outlines both in post-trauma research and the definition of therapeutic needs and the prediction of clinical outcomes.

In view of the findings described above patients with noise trauma are more frequently of male gender. Those with a history of noise trauma are younger and describe an earlier onset and longer tinnitus duration at first consultation in a contributing tinnitus center of the TRI consortium. This is well in line with the findings of Nicolas-Puel *et al.*, from a sample presenting at the tinnitus clinic in Montpellier. The patients presenting with noise-induced tinnitus were reported to be mainly male and on average were 10 years younger than other tinnitus patients. In contrast to our results, these patients were reported to differ also in their perceptional characteristics mainly suffering from bilateral high-pitched "whistling" tinnitus in correlation with their high-

frequency hearing loss [52]. Especially in young people relevant noise exposure from recreational activities is expected. Between 50 and 70% of young people who expose themselves to loud recreational noise have temporarily experienced tinnitus [53]. Up to 75% of Disc jockeys develop tinnitus, They develop hearing loss both at high frequencies and at low frequencies and have tinnitus of the same sound spectra [54].

A further clinical observation was the fact that patients suffering from trauma-associated tinnitus reported pain symptoms more frequently than other non-trauma-patients. Whiplash patients indicated coincidence of neck pain at a significantly higher rate than all other groups (see figure 6). Vertigo and dizziness were more prevalent in patients suffering from tinnitus associated with whiplash and head trauma as already reported in the literature [55]. These findings support the notion of a generally strong correlation of tinnitus and pain syndromes [56] which might be even more pronounced in patients with trauma-associated tinnitus and merits careful prospective observational studies in the future.

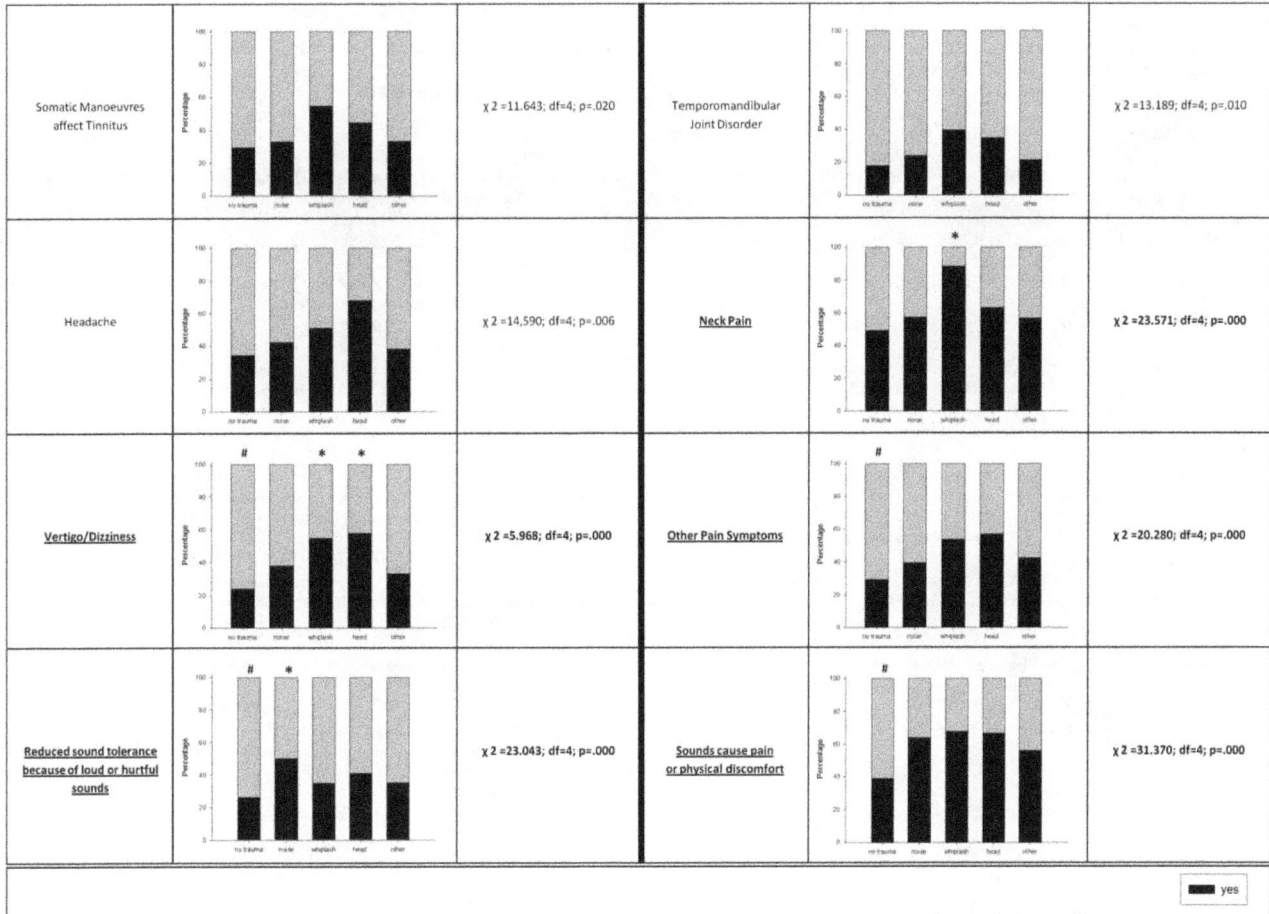

**Figure 6. Percentage of accompanying factors of tinnitus with respect to different trauma-associated and non-trauma-associated tinnitus patients' groups.** Significant results (after Bonferroni correction for multiple testing) are highlighted in bold and underlined letters; * higher proportion of patients with yes-answer than expected; # lower proportion of patients with yes-answer than expected.

## Conclusion and Outlook

Our data clearly indicate differences between tinnitus patients with and without trauma at tinnitus onset. Patients suffering from trauma-associated tinnitus suffer from a higher mental burden than tinnitus patients presenting with phantom perceptions based on other or unknown etiologic factors. This is especially the case for patients with whiplash and head trauma. Patients with posttraumatic noise-related tinnitus experience more frequently hyperacousis, were younger, had longer tinnitus duration, and more frequently male.

Thus, trauma before tinnitus onset seems to represent a relevant criterion for subtypization of tinnitus. Patients with posttraumatic tinnitus may require specific diagnostic and therapeutic management. A more systematic and – at best - standardized assessment for hearing related sequelae of trauma is needed for a better understanding of the underlying pathophysiology and for developing more tailored treatment approaches as well.

## Acknowledgments

We want to thank Sandra Pfluegl, Helene Niebling, Jarmila Gerxhaliu-Holan and Constantin Martin for their help and effort in collecting and handling data. The members of The TRI Database Study Group are: Veronika Vielsmeier, Tobias Kleinjung, Astrid Lehner, Timm B. Poeppl, Ricardo Figueiredo, Andréia Azevedo, Ana Carolina Binetti, Ana Belén Elgoyhen, Marcelo Rates, Claudia Coelho, Sven Vanneste, Dirk de Ridder, Paul van de Heyning, Florian Zeman, Markus Mohr, Michael Koller.

## Author Contributions

Conceived and designed the experiments: PMK ML BL. Performed the experiments: PMK ML BL. Analyzed the data: MS SS. Wrote the paper: PMK ML MS BL. The data analysed in this study derive from the Tinnitus Research Iniative (TRI) Database. All members of the TRI Database Study Group contributed data.

## References

1. Thurman D, Guerrero J (1999) Trends in hospitalization associated with traumatic brain injury. JAMA 282: 954–957.
2. Thurman DJ, Alverson C, Dunn KA, Guerrero J, Sniezek JE (1999) Traumatic brain injury in the United States: A public health perspective. J Head Trauma Rehabil 14: 602–615.
3. Warden D (2006) Military TBI during the Iraq and Afghanistan wars. J Head Trauma Rehabil 21: 398–402.
4. MacGregor AJ, Dougherty AL, Galarneau MR (2011) Injury-specific correlates of combat-related traumatic brain injury in Operation Iraqi Freedom. J Head Trauma Rehabil 26: 312–318.
5. MacGregor AJ, Shaffer RA, Dougherty AL, Galarneau MR, Raman R, et al. (2010) Prevalence and psychological correlates of traumatic brain injury in operation iraqi freedom. J Head Trauma Rehabil 25: 1–8.

6. Terrio H, Brenner LA, Ivins BJ, Cho JM, Helmick K, et al. (2009) Traumatic brain injury screening: preliminary findings in a US Army Brigade Combat Team. J Head Trauma Rehabil 24: 14–23.

7. Sindhusake D, Golding M, Wigney D, Newall P, Jakobsen K, et al. (2004) Factors predicting severity of tinnitus: a population-based assessment. J Am Acad Audiol 15: 269–280.

8. Lew HL, Jerger JF, Guillory SB, Henry JA (2007) Auditory dysfunction in traumatic brain injury. J Rehabil Res Dev 44: 921–928.

9. Geckle L, Lee R (2004) Soldier perceptions of deployment environmental exposures. Albuquerque: NM: Force Health Protection Conference.

10. Mao JC, Pace E, Pierozynski P, Kou Z, Shen Y, et al. (2011) Blast-Induced Tinnitus and Hearing Loss in Rats: Behavioral and Imaging Assays. J Neurotrauma.

11. Yankaskas K (2012) Prelude: Noise-induced tinnitus and hearing loss in the military. Hear Res.

12. Axelsson A, Sandh A (1985) Tinnitus in noise-induced hearing loss. Br J Audiol 19: 271–276.

13. Leske MC (1981) Prevalence estimates of communicative disorders in the U.S. Language, hearing and vestibular disorders. ASHA 23: 229–237.

14. Bauer CA, Brozoski TJ (2001) Assessing tinnitus and prospective tinnitus therapeutics using a psychophysical animal model. J Assoc Res Otolaryngol 2: 54–64.

15. Fausti SA, Wilmington DJ, Gallun FJ, Myers PJ, Henry JA (2009) Auditory and vestibular dysfunction associated with blast-related traumatic brain injury. J Rehabil Res Dev 46: 797–810.

16. Folmer RL, Griest SE (2003) Chronic tinnitus resulting from head or neck injuries. Laryngoscope 113: 821–827.

17. Hinton DE, Chhean D, Pich V, Hofmann SG, Barlow DH (2006) Tinnitus among Cambodian refugees: relationship to PTSD severity. J Trauma Stress 19: 541–546.

18. Langguth B, Landgrebe M, Kleinjung T, Sand GP, Hajak G (2011) Tinnitus and depression. World J Biol Psychiatry 12: 489–500.

19. Jury MA, Flynn MC (2001) Auditory and vestibular sequelae to traumatic brain injury: a pilot study. N Z Med J 114: 286–288.

20. Moller A, Langguth B, de Ridder D, Kleinjung T (2011) Textbook of Tinnitus.: Springer.

21. Cronlein T, Langguth B, Geisler P, Hajak G (2007) Tinnitus and insomnia. Prog Brain Res 166: 227–233.

22. Dobie RA (2003) Depression and tinnitus. Otolaryngol Clin North Am 36: 383–388.

23. Belli S, Belli H, Bahcebasi T, Ozcetin A, Alpay E, et al. (2008) Assessment of psychopathological aspects and psychiatric comorbidities in patients affected by tinnitus. Eur Arch Otorhinolaryngol 265: 279–285.

24. Folmer RL, Griest SE, Meikle MB, Martin WH (1999) Tinnitus severity, loudness, and depression. Otolaryngol Head Neck Surg 121: 48–51.

25. Malouff JM, Schutte NS, Zucker LA (2011) Tinnitus-related distress: A review of recent findings. Curr Psychiatry Rep 13: 31–36.

26. Marciano E, Carrabba L, Giannini P, Sementina C, Verde P, et al. (2003) Psychiatric comorbidity in a population of outpatients affected by tinnitus. Int J Audiol 42: 4–9.

27. Andersson G, Freijd A, Baguley DM, Idrizbegovic E (2009) Tinnitus distress, anxiety, depression, and hearing problems among cochlear implant patients with tinnitus. J Am Acad Audiol 20: 315–319.

28. Crocetti A, Forti S, Ambrosetti U, Bo LD (2009) Questionnaires to evaluate anxiety and depressive levels in tinnitus patients. Otolaryngol Head Neck Surg 140: 403–405.

29. Halford JB, Anderson SD (1991) Anxiety and depression in tinnitus sufferers. J Psychosom Res 35: 383–390.

30. Hesser H, Andersson G (2009) The role of anxiety sensitivity and behavioral avoidance in tinnitus disability. Int J Audiol 48: 295–299.

31. Rossiter S, Stevens C, Walker G (2006) Tinnitus and its effect on working memory and attention. J Speech Lang Hear Res 49: 150–160.

32. Stevens C, Walker G, Boyer M, Gallagher M (2007) Severe tinnitus and its effect on selective and divided attention. Int J Audiol 46: 208–216.

33. Jacobson GP, McCaslin DL (2001) A search for evidence of a direct relationship between tinnitus and suicide. J Am Acad Audiol 12: 493–496.

34. Lewis JE (2002) Tinnitus and suicide. J Am Acad Audiol 13: 339; author reply 339–341.

35. Lewis JE, Stephens SD, McKenna L (1994) Tinnitus and suicide. Clin Otolaryngol Allied Sci 19: 50–54.

36. Turner O, Windfuhr K, Kapur N (2007) Suicide in deaf populations: a literature review. Ann Gen Psychiatry 6: 26.

37. Hiller W, Goebel G (2006) Factors influencing tinnitus loudness and annoyance. Arch Otolaryngol Head Neck Surg 132: 1323–1330.

38. Adamchic I, Hauptmann C, Tass PA (2012) Changes of oscillatory activity in pitch processing network and related tinnitus relief induced by acoustic CR neuromodulation. Front Syst Neurosci 6: 18.

39. Schlee W, Kleinjung T, Hiller W, Goebel G, Kolassa IT, et al. (2011) Does tinnitus distress depend on age of onset? PLoS One 6: e27379.

40. Langguth B, Kleinjung T, Fischer B, Hajak G, Eichhammer P, et al. (2007) Tinnitus severity, depression, and the big five personality traits. Prog Brain Res 166: 221–225.

41. Budd RJ, Pugh R (1996) Tinnitus coping style and its relationship to tinnitus severity and emotional distress. J Psychosom Res 41: 327–335.

42. Landgrebe M, Zeman F, Koller M, Eberl Y, Mohr M, et al. (2010) The Tinnitus Research Initiative (TRI) database: a new approach for delineation of tinnitus subtypes and generation of predictors for treatment outcome. BMC Med Inform Decis Mak 10: 42.

43. Newman CW, Jacobson GP, Spitzer JB (1996) Development of the Tinnitus Handicap Inventory. Arch Otolaryngol Head Neck Surg 122: 143–148.

44. Hallam RS, Jakes SC, Hinchcliffe R (1988) Cognitive variables in tinnitus annoyance. Br J Clin Psychol 27 (Pt 3): 213–222.

45. Steer RA, Beck AT, Riskind JH, Brown G (1986) Differentiation of depressive disorders from generalized anxiety by the Beck Depression Inventory. J Clin Psychol 42: 475–478.

46. WHOQOL-BREF: Introduction, Administration, Scoring. (1996) World's Health Organization. Geneva, Switzerland.

47. Shida S, Yoshida M (1990) [Clinical observation on the dip location of industrial deafness and physiological consideration on the dip origin]. Nihon Jibiinkoka Gakkai Kaiho 93: 1823–1831.

48. Gu JW, Halpin CF, Nam EC, Levine RA, Melcher JR (2010) Tinnitus, diminished sound-level tolerance, and elevated auditory activity in humans with clinically normal hearing sensitivity. J Neurophysiol 104: 3361–3370.

49. Nicolas-Puel C, Akbaraly T, Lloyd R, Berr C, Uziel A, et al. (2006) Characteristics of tinnitus in a population of 555 patients: specificities of tinnitus induced by noise trauma. Int Tinnitus J 12: 64–70.

50. Nolle C, Todt I, Seidl RO, Ernst A (2004) Pathophysiological changes of the central auditory pathway after blunt trauma of the head. J Neurotrauma 21: 251–258.

51. Nageris BI, Attias J, Shemesh R (2008) Otologic and audiologic lesions due to blast injury. J Basic Clin Physiol Pharmacol 19: 185–191.

52. Nicolas-Puel C, Akbaraly T, Lloyd R, Berr C, Uziel A, et al. (2006) Characteristics of tinnitus in a population of 555 patients: specificities of tinnitus induced by noise trauma. Int Tinnitus J 12: 64–70.

53. Quintanilla-Dieck Mde L, Artunduaga MA, Eavey RD (2009) Intentional exposure to loud music: the second MTV.com survey reveals an opportunity to educate. J Pediatr 155: 550–555.

54. Potier M, Hoquet C, Lloyd R, Nicolas-Puel C, Uziel A, et al. (2009) The risks of amplified music for disc-jockeys working in nightclubs. Ear Hear 30: 291–293.

55. Boniver R (2002) Temporomandibular joint dysfunction in whiplash injuries: association with tinnitus and vertigo. Int Tinnitus J 8: 129–131.

56. De Ridder D, Elgoyhen AB, Romo R, Langguth B (2011) Phantom percepts: Tinnitus and pain as persisting aversive memory networks. Proc Natl Acad Sci U S A 108: 8075–8080.

# 4

# Amelioration of Acute Sequelae of Blast Induced Mild Traumatic Brain Injury by N-Acetyl Cysteine

**Michael E. Hoffer**[1]*[◊], **Carey Balaban**[2◊], **Martin D. Slade**[3], **Jack W. Tsao**[4], **Barry Hoffer**[5]

**1** Spatial Orientation Center, Department of Otolaryngology, Naval Medical Center San Diego, San Diego, California, United States of America, **2** Departments of Otolaryngology, Neurobiology, Communication Sciences and Disorders, and Bioengineering, University of Pittsburgh, Pittsburgh, Pennsylvania, United States of America, **3** Department of Internal Medicine, Yale University, New Haven, Connecticut, United States of America, **4** Wounded, Ill and Injured Directorate (M9), US Navy Bureau of Medicine and Surgery, Washington, D.C., United States of America, **5** Department of Neurosurgery, Case Western University, Cleveland, Ohio, United States of America

## Abstract

*Background:* Mild traumatic brain injury (mTBI) secondary to blast exposure is the most common battlefield injury in Southwest Asia. There has been little prospective work in the combat setting to test the efficacy of new countermeasures. The goal of this study was to compare the efficacy of N-acetyl cysteine (NAC) versus placebo on the symptoms associated with blast exposure mTBI in a combat setting.

*Methods:* This study was a randomized double blind, placebo-controlled study that was conducted on active duty service members at a forward deployed field hospital in Iraq. All symptomatic U.S. service members who were exposed to significant ordnance blast and who met the criteria for mTBI were offered participation in the study and 81 individuals agreed to participate. Individuals underwent a baseline evaluation and then were randomly assigned to receive either N-acetyl cysteine (NAC) or placebo for seven days. Each subject was re-evaluated at 3 and 7 days. Outcome measures were the presence of the following sequelae of mTBI: dizziness, hearing loss, headache, memory loss, sleep disturbances, and neurocognitive dysfunction. The resolution of these symptoms seven days after the blast exposure was the main outcome measure in this study. Logistic regression on the outcome of 'no day 7 symptoms' indicated that NAC treatment was significantly better than placebo (OR = 3.6, p = 0.006). Secondary analysis revealed subjects receiving NAC within 24 hours of blast had an 86% chance of symptom resolution with no reported side effects versus 42% for those seen early who received placebo.

*Conclusion:* This study, conducted in an active theatre of war, demonstrates that NAC, a safe pharmaceutical countermeasure, has beneficial effects on the severity and resolution of sequelae of blast induced mTBI. This is the first demonstration of an effective short term countermeasure for mTBI. Further work on long term outcomes and the potential use of NAC in civilian mTBI is warranted.

**Editor:** Michael Fehlings, University of Toronto, Canada

**Funding:** Supported by the Department of Defense. The funders had no role in study design, data collection and analysis, decision to publish, or preparation of the manuscript.

**Competing Interests:** The authors have declared that no competing interests exist.

* E-mail: Michael.hoffer@med.navy.mil

◊ These authors contributed equally to this work.

## Introduction

Mild traumatic brain injury (mTBI) is the most common injury seen in the current conflicts in Iraq and Afghanistan and an increasingly common injury in modern society. An estimated 19.5–22.8% of all returning deployed troops suffer from mTBI [1]. The most common cause of mTBI is blast exposure from improvised explosive devices (IEDs) or other explosive ordinances. Over the last three decades the mechanisms, characteristics, diagnostic schemes, and treatment strategies for blunt head trauma have been studied extensively. Unfortunately, many of the lessons learned from blunt head trauma cannot be applied automatically to blast injured subjects [2].

Disentangling the neurological features of mTBI from PTSD is important for improving diagnosis and treatment of low-level blast injuries [3]. Many previous studies were conducted well after the actual blast injury and focused on the role of mTBI as a precursor of PTSD [1,4]. Diagnosis of mTBI requires a documented traumatic event, with a transient loss or alteration of consciousness, accompanied by at least one of a list of neurologic, neurotologic, or cognitive symptoms [5]. One highly prevalent symptom is dizziness, a subjective marker of balance dysfunction.

N-acetylcysteine (NAC) is a logical choice for a field-based clinical trial. NAC is the active agent in Mucomyst, an FDA approved medication with a forty-year safety history. NAC is an effective neuroprotective agent in animal ischemia-reperfusion cerebral stroke models [6,7,8], a rodent closed head trauma model [9], a sensory nerve axotomy model [10] and inner ear neuronal death after noise exposure [11,12]. Although these neuroprotective effects of NAC appear to be mediated by both antioxidant and anti-inflammatory effects [7,8,13,14,15], NAC also acts indirectly at metabotropic glutamate receptors to counteract cocaine-induced disruption of nucleus accumbens [16]. Further, oral NAC and placebo preparations have been utilized on over 1000 Marines and Sailors in on-going approved clinical investigations to test protection from noise-induced hearing loss. Finally, NAC has limited capability to cross the normal blood-brain barrier [13], which suggests that it can preferentially enter tissue at sites of post-traumatic barrier disruption.

This protocol administered a loading dose of NAC to exposed U.S. Service members within 0–72 hours after blast exposure and followed a set of subjective and objective outcome measures of mTBI. The addition of NAC to standard treatment produced a much higher rate of symptom resolution than placebo at seven treatment days.

## Materials and Methods

### Overview

The study is the first double blind, placebo controlled study examining mTBI to take place during active combat. It was subject to design constraints because the participants were active duty personnel who never departed from an active combat zone. Diagnosis and treatment of mTBI were delivered by medical personnel in a medical facility within that active combat zone. Operational manpower needs and military policy precluded follow-up beyond the initial seven day treatment period. Enrollment in the study ended with the conclusion of combat operations in Western Iraq. A flow diagram for the study is shown in Figure 1.

### Ethics

The protocol was approved by the Joint Theatre Trauma and Research Office in Baghdad, Iraq and the theatre Institutional Review Board (IRB) at Brooke Army Medical Center.

### Detailed Methods

The protocol for this trial and supporting CONSORT checklist are available as supporting information; see Checklist S1 and Protocol S1. The study was conducted at Al Taqaddum Level II Medical Facility (TQ) in Iraq. US Military Service members exposed to a significant blast in the Al Anbar province of Iraq were evaluated at TQ as rapidly as feasible (given operational and weather concerns). The October 2007 Joint Service Surgeon General and DoD Health Affairs criteria were utilized to diagnose mTBI [5]. Briefly, this definition specifies that there is an exposure, a brief alteration of consciousness, and then manifestation of any one of a number of mTBI symptoms. Exposure was defined as feeling a blast wave or being in a vehicle that was damaged by a blast wave. Alteration of consciousness required a report by another individual on the scene. Balance dysfunction, confusion, headache, sensorineural hearing loss, impaired memory and sleep disturbances were considered as mTBI symptoms. Individuals with moderate to severe TBI, significant orthopedic injuries, or those requiring computerized tomography scans, evacuation from theatre, or emergent surgeries were excluded from this study.

All subjects underwent a comprehensive history and physical exam by the Principal Investigator (PI). A finding of balance dysfunction required subjective dizziness, an abnormal head thrust test (abnormal eye motion after quick turning of the subjects head by the investigator [17]), an abnormal Romberg/tandem Romberg test (excessive swaying or falling while attempting to stand still with eyes closed and arms extended [18]), and an abnormal dynamic gait index (DGI) score (a dedicated set of walking tasks scored by the PI [19]) of <22. Criteria for resolution of balance dysfunction were no subjective dizziness, normal head thrust and Romberg tests, and a normal DGI. Audiometric testing identified hearing loss and its resolution. Confusion, headache, sleep disturbances, and impaired memory were based upon self-reports; resolution of these symptoms required a report that "I feel as good as before the blast." Sleep disorders were difficult to assess because many subjects were sleep deprived upon arrival; they were diagnosed when clinical judgment indicated that initial exhaustion was eliminated.

All subjects diagnosed with mTBI were given standard treatment for signs and symptoms as needed, which was identical to treatment administered for mTBI in US military and civilian hospitals. Treatment included an individualized exercise program, symptomatic headache medications (non-narcotic medicine such as topiramate, sumatriptin, and ibuprofen to treat associated symptoms), low level of activity with proper rest, and controlled mental stimulation. All subjects were also informed about the study and offered an opportunity to participate. All individuals were advised that participation was voluntary and would have no impact on their ability to receive care or on their ability to receive standard of care for their injury. All individuals who desired to consider participating were given an informed consent form to read and allowed ample opportunity to ask questions. Those agreeing to participate completed the IRB approved informed consent document. All participants received a pre-randomized bottle containing 500 mg tablets of either NAC or placebo, prepared by the pharmacy of a major United States Military Medical Center. Assignment was based solely on order of accession into the study. Simple randomization was utilized to create an assignment list (randomization schedule) for subjects to be assigned to either the Placebo or NAC group as no interim analyses were to be conducted and this method assures that each treatment assignment is completely unpredictable [20]. The randomization schedule was created prior to subject accrual and resulted in a 49·4% to 50·6% split in subjects between the two groups. Participants, providers, and evaluators were all blinded to which treatment group each subject was assigned.

The 4 gram loading dose was witnessed and then bottles were name labeled and given to the subject's corpsman, medic or a nurse (for subjects remaining at TQ). Beginning 18–24 hours after the loading dose, subjects were given 4 grams daily (in two divided doses of 2 gm morning and night) for 4 days. The dose was then reduced to 3 gm daily [in two divided doses of 1.5 gm morning and night]. Every dose was witnessed by a corpsman, medic, nurse, or doctor.

The Controlled Oral Word Association Test (COWA) [21], animal naming (AN), and timed Trail Making Tests (TMT) A and B [22,23,24,25] were administered as neuropsychological tests of executive function. Normative TMT data were estimated from published age-normed data [26], assuming an equal mixture of 18–24 and 25–34 year old groups. The initial clinical assessment, history, physical, DGI, hearing, and neuropsychology tests were repeated at three and seven days after enrollment.

The study was designed originally to examine the effects of NAC versus placebo in subjects also receiving standard treatment

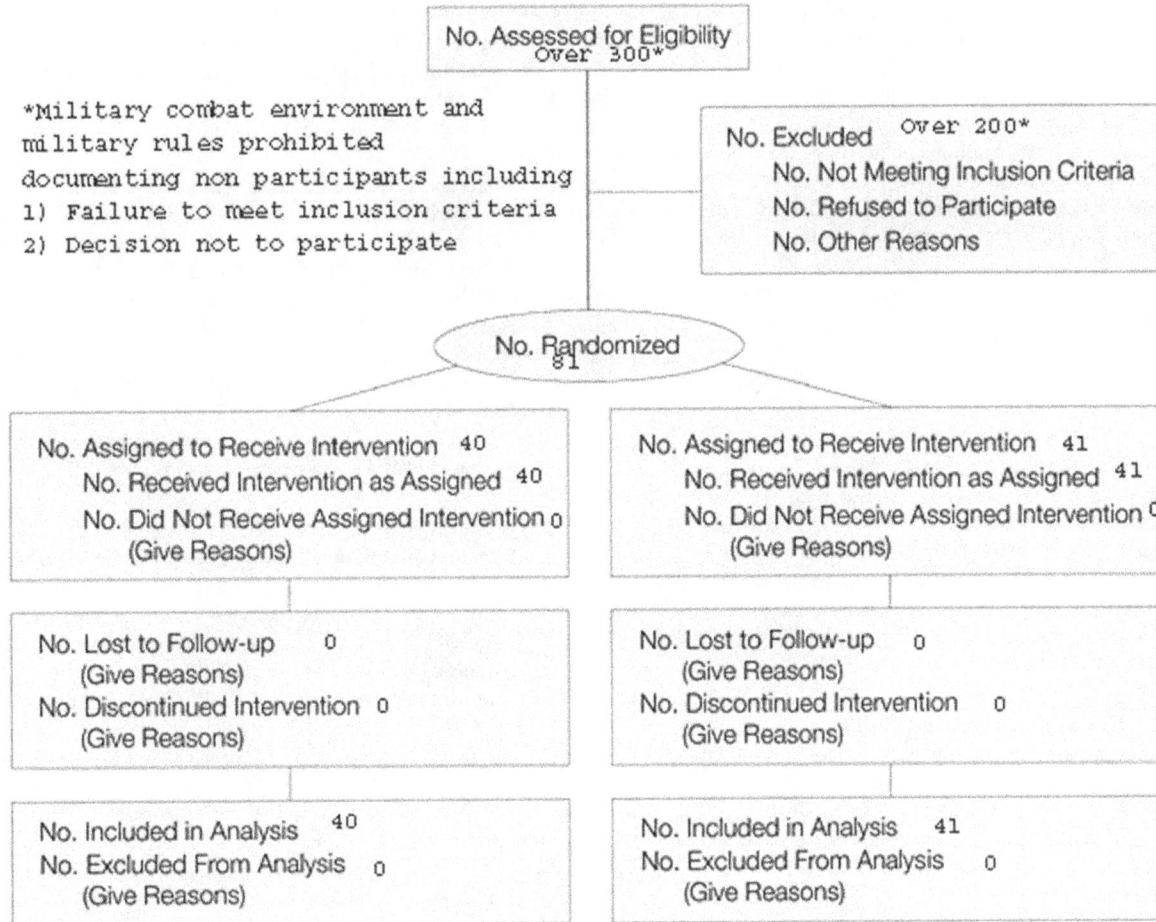

**Figure 1. Consort Flow Diagram.**

(measured exercise program and non-narcotic headache medicines). Because availability of transportation in the combat zone affected a patient's arrival time at TQ, we also examined secondarily the impact of early (within 24 hours) versus delayed (26–72 hours after injury) diagnosis and treatment on outcomes. Time of arrival at TQ was based purely on distance of the injury from TQ and the safety and availability of transportation back to TQ. While it is impossible to control for all confounders between the early and late group, it should be noted that individuals in both groups came from the same sets of combat units, were doing the same duty, and were living under the same conditions. The primary endpoint was the percentage of subjects free of all symptoms of mild TBI on D7 where D7 was defined 7 days since the loading dose of medication was given. It was assumed that 80% of subjects in the placebo arm of the study would still have at least one symptom on day 7. The study was sized to determine if NAC was able to reduce that 80% to 50%, hence only 50% of subjects would still have a symptom of mild TBI on day 7, with a 95% level of confidence, 80% power, and a 1:1 ratio of control to experimental subjects. Based upon these criterion, 38 subjects were required in each arm of the study [27]. Secondary endpoints were balance dysfunction resolution, absence of headache, confusion, memory problems, abnormal sleep, trail making A, trail making B, controlled oral word association (COWA), and animal naming (AN) all on day 7, as well as the percentage of subjects free of all symptoms of mild TBI three days post initial treatment.

Student t-tests were utilized to determine differences between groups for age, distance from blast and number of blast exposures at time of assignment for treatment. Pooled variance determined significance unless group variances were significantly different, in which case Satterthwaite's method was used. MLR and Least Significant Differences (LSD) tests were used for multiple comparisons. Fisher's exact test was used to test group differences for categorical variables of sex and job title.

For the primary analysis, unadjusted logistic regression was used to model the effect of NAC on resolution of symptoms D7. For secondary analyses, multivariate logistic regression modeled the effects of NAC, early treatment, number of previous blast occurrences, age, distance from blast, as well as all two-way interactions, on resolution of symptoms on D7. Parsimonious models [28] were constructed utilizing a backward elimination strategy with a significance level to stay of $\alpha = 0.05$. In a similar manner, multivariate linear regression modeled predictors of the number of D7 symptoms. Parallel analyses of day 3 data revealed no significant effects.

## Results

### General subject characteristics

Eighty-one subjects participated in the study (eighty males and one female). The age range was 18–43 years of age with a median age of 22 years. The subject demographic data (Table 1) did not differ between the NAC and the placebo groups, between subjects treated early (≤24 hours) or late (26–72 hours) after injury, or between any of the four treatment groups defined by combinations of these factors. The groups did not differ with respect to other medicines being utilized. Neither alcohol nor drug abuse were factors because the study was conducted in a controlled combat setting. Theatre guidelines prohibited a detailed documentation or tracking of those who declined participation but over 1/3 of those seen declined to participate in the trial. No participant suffered unintended effects, side effects, or harm. In particular, no GI upset was reported.

All subjects in the study had objective clinical evidence of balance dysfunction. Table 2 summarizes the distribution of additional mTBI symptoms. Only one subject had an isolated finding of balance dysfunction. Hearing loss, headache and confusion were the next most prevalent features.

## Symptom emergence during the study

The prevalence of mTBI symptoms varied with the latency between blast exposure and examination. Hearing loss emerged on subsequent study days in 3 subjects, headache developed in 8 subjects, memory problems in 2 subjects and abnormal sleep in 10 subjects. Symptoms persisting at D7 are shown in Table 3.

## Treatment effects

The NAC group was significantly more likely to have symptom resolution D7 (OR = 3.60, p = 0.0062, $R^2 = 0.37$). In secondary analyses, both NAC treatment and early treatment initiation contributed independently to symptom resolution (Figure 2, left panels). There were independent main effects of both NAC treatment ($F_{1,\,78} = 10·28$, p<0.01) and treatment initiation time ($F_{1,\,78} = 10·91$, p<0.01) on the number of D7 symptoms ($R^2 = 0.21$). The early treatment group given NAC had the fewest D7 symptoms (p<0·01, $R^2 = 0.24$ re: each other group by LSD tests). The early treatment group without NAC showed fewer symptoms than the late treatment group without NAC (p<0.05). The late treatment group given NAC showed an intermediate number of symptoms that did not differ significantly from either early or late treatment groups without NAC There were no significant treatment group differences in the total number of symptoms upon entry ($R^2 = 0.03$) or on treatment day 3 ($R^2 = 0.04$).

Logistic regression on the outcome of 'no D7 symptoms' confirmed that NAC treatment was significantly better than placebo (p<0.005) and early intervention was significantly better than later intervention (p<0.005, max-rescaled $R^2 = 0.37$)). The odds of complete symptom resolution for Group B (early treatment

with NAC) were greater than the other groups (Tables 4 and 5, p<0.001). Parsimonious logistic regression models for balance dysfunction resolution and the absence of headache on day seven also showed significant effects for NAC and early treatment initiation (p<0.05), with no significant effects of covariates or interactions.

Confusion resolved markedly after early treatment; 59/60 subjects treated early had no confusion D7, compared with only 14/21 subjects treated later (exact test, p<0.001). The parsimonious logistic regression model showed that D7 confusion was predicted by both the time of treatment (p<0.05) and the distance from the blast (p<0.05). No significant effects emerged in the parsimonious logistic regression models for hearing loss, memory problems and abnormal sleep. Despite the low prevalence of abnormal sleep in this series, it was significantly less likely (exact test, p = 0.029) in the NAC treated subject population on day seven (1/41) than in the placebo treated subjects (7/40).

## Neuropsychological treatment effects

Results on entry were significantly poorer than published normative Trail making Test A and B (TMTA and TMTB) data for subjects who were in the age ranges of 18–34 years [26] (Table 6, z-tests, p<0.001). Controlled oral word association (COWA) and animal naming (AN) were within normal limits.

NAC administration restored normal TMT performance within 7 days after blast-induced mild traumatic brain injury (mTBI) (Table 7). The D7 MLR showed TMTA (F(1,74) = 6.64, p<0.05) and TMTB (F(1,74) = 4.866, p<0.05) scores were improved significantly by NAC treatment and scores for the NAC treated groups were equivalent to age-based norms. The D7 TMT scores for groups that did not receive NAC remained impaired. The D7 COWA and AN results showed no group differences (Tables 8 and 9).

The D7 TMT performance paralleled the resolution of mTBI symptoms. Times were significantly shorter in symptom-free subjects (Bonferroni-adjusted t-tests, p<0.05). Subjects who were symptom free on D7 had normal TMTA and TMTB times, while the symptomatic subjects had prolonged times.

**TM perforation and outcomes.** TM perforation is a common combat-related blast injury [29,30,31,32] that may indicate the magnitude of shock wave exposure [30,33,34] and be a proxy for blast over-pressure intensity [28,29]. The number of symptoms and TMT test results at time of entry (day 0) were unaffected by TM status. TM perforation and NAC treatment status were both significant predictors of the number of day 3 symptoms (ANOVA, F(1,78) = 33.51, p<0.001 and F(1,78) = 4.64,

**Table 1.** Study Group Characteristics.

| Continuous Covariates | Treatment Before 24 Hours | | | | Treatment After (26–72 Hours) | | | |
|---|---|---|---|---|---|---|---|---|
| | Group A: -NAC Control(n = 31) | | Group B: +NAC (n = 29) | | Group C: -NAC Control (n = 9) | | Group D: +NAC (n = 12) | |
| | Mean | Std Dev | Mean | Std Dev | Mean | Std Dev | Mean | Std Dev |
| Age | 23.58 | 4.16 | 24.92 | 6.52 | 25.42 | 6.19 | 27.68 | 6.96 |
| Distance from blast (feet)[†] | 17.42 | 7.40 | 16.79 | 5.18 | 14.67 | 2.69 | 15.83 | 4.69 |
| Number of Blast Exposures (inclusive) | 2.23 | 3.60 | 1.45 | 1.21 | 1.89 | 1.69 | 6.58 | 8.31[‡] |

[†]include vehicle dimensions (74/81 participants) and IED distance.
[‡]Greater variance reflects the random inclusion of the two oldest individuals in the study population.

**Table 2.** Distribution of mTBI Symptoms Co-morbid with Balance Dysfunction: Entry to Study.

| Number of Symptoms | Hearing loss | Headache | Confusion | Memory Problem | Sleep Abnormal | Number of Subjects |
|---|---|---|---|---|---|---|
| 1 | − | − | − | − | − | 1 |
| 2 | + | − | − | − | − | 6 |
| | − | + | − | − | − | 6 |
| | − | + | − | − | − | 6 |
| 3 | − | + | − | + | − | 7 |
| | − | + | + | − | − | 6 |
| | + | − | − | − | + | 1 |
| | + | + | − | − | − | 8 |
| | + | − | − | + | − | 2 |
| | + | − | + | − | − | 13 |
| 4 | + | − | + | + | − | 1 |
| | + | + | + | − | − | 17 |
| | + | + | − | + | − | 7 |
| | + | + | − | − | + | 1 |
| 5 | + | + | + | − | + | 1 |
| Subjects Symptomatic | 57 | 53 | 42 | 17 | 3 | 81 |

$p = 0.034$, respectively). For the early treatment initiation group, the reduction of D7 symptoms by NAC treatment was independent of TM status (ANOVA, $F (1, 56) = 12.19$, $p = 0.001$). NAC treatment also produced significantly better resolution (no D7 symptoms) than placebo (logistic regression, $p < 0.005$).

## Discussion

This is the first prospective, double-blinded, placebo-controlled randomized study to focus on the acute treatment of combat blast-related mTBI in a forward war zone. Supplementation of standard therapy with oral NAC had a significant impact on neuropsychological test results, number of mTBI symptoms, and complete symptom resolution by day seven of treatment when compared to placebo. Moreover, the pill form of NAC, the active ingredient in the FDA approved medication "Mucomyst", produced no side effects in blast mTBI subjects. Although the study was powered only to examine the effects of NAC, there was a statistically significant secondary finding that standard treatment initiation

**Table 3.** Unresolved mTBI Symptom Patterns on Treatment Day 7.

| Number of Symptoms | Balance dysfunction | Hearing loss | Headache | Confusion | Memory Problem | Sleep Abnormal | Number of Subjects |
|---|---|---|---|---|---|---|---|
| 1 | − | + | − | − | − | − | 3 |
| | − | − | + | − | − | − | 4 |
| | − | − | − | + | − | − | 3 |
| | + | − | − | − | − | − | 4 |
| 2 | − | − | + | − | − | + | 1 |
| | − | + | + | − | − | − | 2 |
| | − | − | + | + | − | − | 1 |
| | + | − | − | − | − | + | 3 |
| | + | + | − | − | − | − | 3 |
| | + | − | + | − | − | − | 6 |
| 3 | − | + | + | + | − | − | 1 |
| | + | + | + | − | − | − | 3 |
| | + | − | + | − | − | + | 2 |
| | + | − | + | + | − | − | 2 |
| 4 | + | − | + | + | − | + | 1 |
| 5 | + | + | + | − | + | + | 1 |
| Subjects Symptomatic | 25 | 13 | 24 | 8 | 1 | 8 | 40 |

## Symptom Resolution on Day 7 in the Treatment Groups

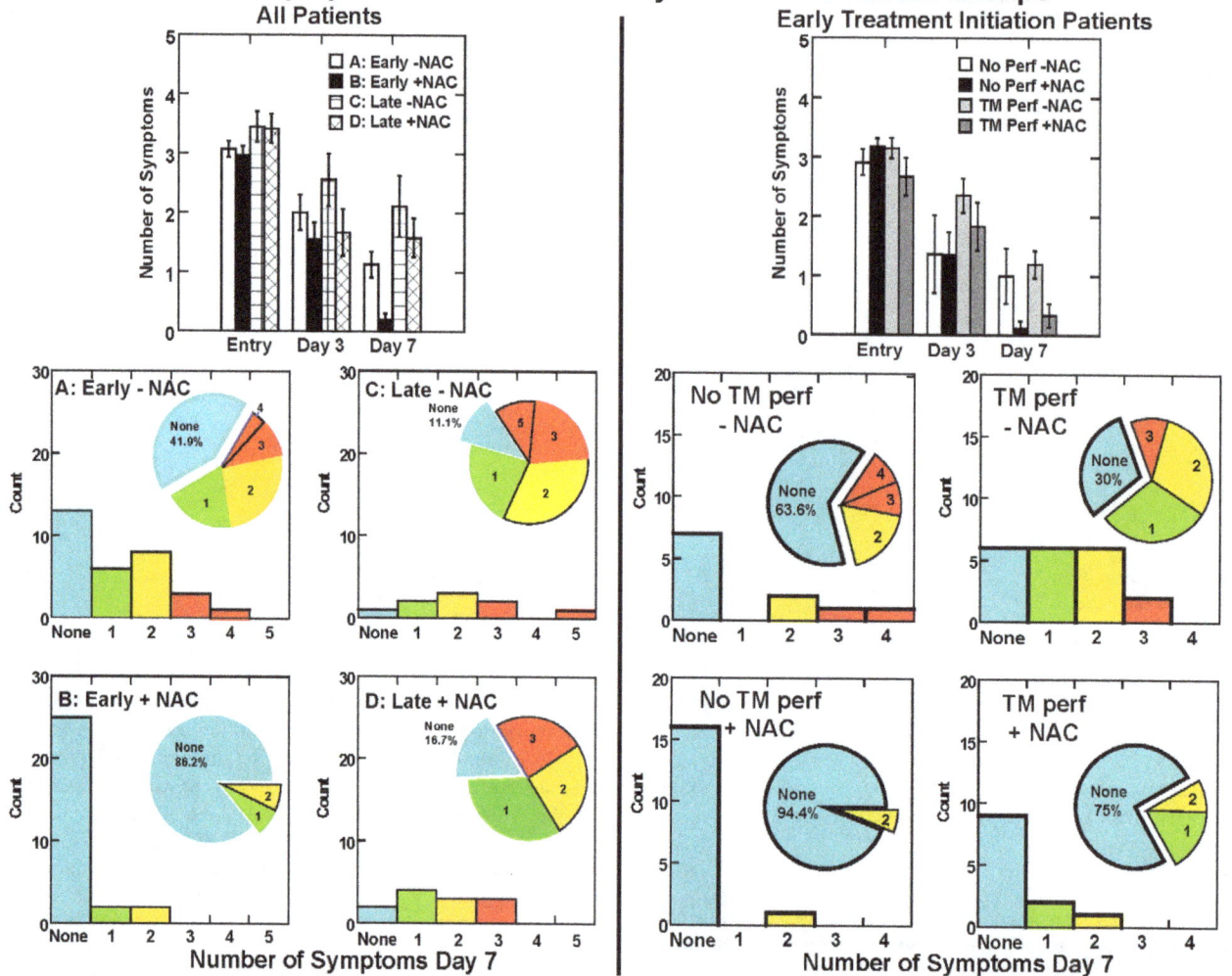

**Figure 2. The number of symptoms for four groups of patients.** The upper left panel shows results for all patients in the study. The upper right graph illustrates the impact of tympanic membrane perforations in the patients seen within 24 hours of blast exposure The distribution of the data on day 7 are shown for each group in the lower graphs, with a pie chart to indicate the percentage with no residual symptoms.

within 24 hours had an independent benefit on neurological but not on neuropsychological outcome measures (TMT). A possible explanation for this difference is that the outcome measures assess the status of different neuronal circuitry components. The additive effects of NAC and early treatment produced 86% mTBI

symptom resolution within seven days. Factors such as number of previous blast exposures, age and distance from the blast did not influence treatment outcomes significantly.

Headache and balance dysfunction are major clinical issues that arise acutely after blast exposure, impede return to duty, and can

**Table 4.** Treatment Effects: Day 7 Symptoms.

| Timing of Treatment | Treatment | n | No Symptoms- Day 7 | | | No Symptoms (Excluding Residual hearing loss-Day 7 | | |
|---|---|---|---|---|---|---|---|---|
| | | | Odds Ratio* | Max Rescaled R2 | Pr>ChiSq | Odds Ratio* | Max Rescaled R2 | Pr>ChiSq |
| After 24 hours | Placebo | 9 | 1 (reference) | 0.38 | 0.0002 | 1 (reference) | 0.34 | 0.0005 |
| After 24 hours | NAC | 12 | 1.60 (0.12, 20.99) | | | 2.67 (0.23, 31.07) | | |
| Before 24 hours | Placebo | 31 | 5.05 (0.56, 45.64) | | | 5.78 (0.64, 52.03) | | |
| Before 24 hours | NAC | 29 | 38.40 (3.88, 379.68) | | | 38.40 (3.88, 379.68) | | |

*95% Confidence Interval.

**Table 5.** Treatment Effects: Day 7 Symptoms.

| Timing of Treatment | Treatment | n | No Balance Dysfunction - Day 7 | | | No Headache -Day 7 | | |
|---|---|---|---|---|---|---|---|---|
| | | | Odds Ratio* | Max Rescaled R2 | Pr>ChiSq | Odds Ratio* | Max Rescaled R2 | Pr>ChiSq |
| After 24 hours | Placebo | 9 | 1 (reference) | 0.21 | 0.0185 | 1 (reference) | 0.25 | 0.0117 |
| After 24 hours | NAC | 12 | 4.00 (0.64, 25.02) | | | 2.80 (0.46, 16.93) | | |
| Before 24 hours | Placebo | 31 | 3.17 (0.66, 15.12) | | | 3.64 (0.76, 17.46) | | |
| Before 24 hours | NAC | 29 | 17.33 (2.78, 108.06) | | | 27.00 (3.67, 198.69) | | |

*95% Confidence Interval.

persist chronically [1,4,35]. Because they seriously impair performance in a combat environment, the initiation of standard treatment with oral NAC within 24 hours of mTBI is likely to have a definitive impact on battlefield end-strength and the readiness of troops in theater.

Performance on TMT neuropsychological tests was impacted significantly by blast mTBI and ameliorated by NAC administration. The initial test times were prolonged significantly at enrollment. NAC administration within 72 hours of injury produced normal D7 TMT times, but performance remained abnormal for subject groups that received only standard therapy. Because all subjects were tested on the same schedule and the reliability of repeated TRAIL making tests [25] is well documented, test-retest effects are not a confounding factor. Hence, TMTs are useful for documenting and monitoring cognitive status changes in acute blast mTBI.

The efficacy of NAC in early treatment of blast mTBI is consistent with its efficacy as a neuroprotective agent in ischemia-reperfusion cerebral stroke [6,7,8], closed head trauma [9], sensory nerve axotomy [10] and in the prevention of mitochondrial damage and loss of dendritic spines in hippocampal neurons [36] in animal models of closed head trauma and ischemia-reperfusion brain injury. A single, low level shock wave exposure to rodents can produce persistent biochemical changes in the hippocampus and cerebral cortex, accompanied by apoptotic cell death [37,38,39]. Even relatively low exposures produce very small parenchymal and subarachoid hemorrhages in 30–40% of exposed animals [40]. These findings suggest that vascular primary injury contributes to symptoms of mTBI, with slower development of neuronal damage [41]. Post-treatment with NAC has afforded protection against neuronal death in animal models. These neuroprotective effects reflect known antioxidant and anti-inflammatory effects [7,8,13,14,15,36]. The cellular bases for memory and regulation of motivation properties within the

nucleus accumbens may be improved by NAC activating neuronal cysteine-glutamate exchange and indirect effects on mGluR2/3 and mGluR5 [16] transmission. Finally, enhanced local bioavailability of NAC may be a natural consequence of vascular disruption in mTBI. Because NAC has limited capability to cross the normal blood-brain barrier [13], increased local brain permeability during vascular remodeling [42] may facilitate selective delivery to affected sites. A delayed opening of the blood-brain barrier from neuroinflammatory responses [42,43], could create longer-term therapeutic opportunities.

Early symptomatic treatment initiation produced improvement that was statistically independent of effects of NAC treatment. The early and late subjects came from the same set of combat units with a shared history of living environment, combat exposure and similar clinical presentations. Although we believe that the time of enrollment was determined only by distance from TQ and availability of transport, it is impossible to know if there were unknown confounders between the two groups. However, we believe that the improvement seen in early subjects can be attributed to the concurrent standard symptomatic medical treatment and balance rehabilitation exercises begun earlier in the early treatment group. Exercise, in particular, can have neuroprotective pharmacomimetic effects on structures such as the hippocampus, possibly mediated by trophic factors [44].

Clinical trials in an active combat theater are subject to outside factors for "early termination" that do not arise in standard clinical environments. For this study, the opportunity for subject enrollment ended when combat operations terminated in this part of Iraq, prior to reaching the pre-determined number of enrollees for the trial. Because the available data were powered sufficiently to test the effects of NAC, we proceeded with analysis after all patients completed the protocol. The enthusiasm about the large treatment effect must be tempered by a recent review of the Cochran database [45], showing that studies with relatively small

**Table 6.** Neuropsychological Tests: TMT at Study Entry.

| Timing of Treatment | Treatment | n | Trail Making A (seconds) – At entry to study | | | Trail Making B (seconds) – At entry to Study | | |
|---|---|---|---|---|---|---|---|---|
| | | | Mean (Standard Deviation) | $R^2$ | Pr>F | Mean (Standard Deviation) | $R^2$ | Pr>F |
| After 24 hours | Placebo | 9 | 38.4 (19.9)** | 0.04 | 0.4243 | 62.2 (24.4)** | 0.01 | 0.8941 |
| After 24 hours | NAC | 12 | 37.4 (20.7)** | | | 70.3 (45.9)** | | |
| Before 24 hours | Placebo | 30 | 31.4 (11.3)** | | | 66.5 (20.8)** | | |
| Before 24 hours | NAC | 27 | 32.4 (9.2)** | | | 69.0 (21.7)** | | |

**Table 7.** Neuropsychological tests: TMT at Day 7.

| Timing of Treatment | Treatment | n | Trail Making A (seconds) – Day 7 | | | Trail Making B (seconds) – Day 7 | | |
|---|---|---|---|---|---|---|---|---|
| | | | Mean (Standard Deviation) | $R^2$ | Pr>F | Mean (Standard Deviation) | $R^2$ | Pr>F |
| After 24 hours | Placebo | 9 | 34.2 (18.3)** | 0.09 | 0.0633 | 63.6 (16.3)** | 0.07 | 0.1504 |
| After 24 hours | NAC | 12 | 23.4 (4.9) | | | 50.2 (15.9) | | |
| Before 24 hours | Placebo | 30 | 27.0 (12.0)* | | | 56.2 (20.1)* | | |
| Before 24 hours | NAC | 27 | 23.5 (7.7) | | | 49.1 (17.1) | | |

*$p<0.05$ or **$p<0.01$ by z-test versus TMTA (23.7±7.8 seconds (S.D.)) or TMTB.

patient numbers and large odds ratios often show smaller odds ratios when the study is repeated. In this regard, we do note that the lower bounds of the 95% confidence intervals for early NAC treatment are reasonably large. It also should be noted that although we were able to draw some statistical conclusions the study was not powered to look at early vs. late treatment which argues for caution in interpreting that data.

One must be cautious to assert the therapeutic implications of NAC treatment for TBI within the limited scope of this study. While the results are very promising, the study was limited to evaluating a relatively small but representative sample of combat troops with acute mild head trauma and other minor injuries over one week of treatment. Some additional caveats are also inherent in the far-front battlefield environment. For example, study participants came from the same set of combat units with similar environmental exposure histories, living conditions (including the same forward operating bases), training, missions, and combat environments; combat personnel are predominantly males in their twenties. Therefore, it is prudent to consider several caveats for our findings. The study results do not imply any benefit for moderate or severe head trauma with significant surgical injuries. Because only one female was enrolled, the study may not generalize to all females. Although the study endpoint was only D7 there is some evidence to suggest that these effects may be long lasting. Tweedie, et al [46] have shown that mTBI triggers biochemical cascades within the first 24 hours which produce long term sequelae. Their work suggests that it is important to interrupt these cascades as early as possible. D7 resolution may indicate the lack of significant apoptotic and inflammatory changes in both grey and white matter. Nevertheless, the effects of treatment on longer term outcomes will need to be the subject of further study in a larger number of subjects.

The study can then, at least, be interpreted in a narrow fashion as showing a benefit of using NAC and early intervention for blast mTBI in an acute combat setting after mild blast exposure. The study brings up the intriguing possibility that NAC may be useful in other mTBI settings, but before this conclusion be reached much more study in the area and using this agent is required.

## Summary and Conclusions

We report the first double blinded placebo- controlled randomized study of a pharmaceutical countermeasure for the symptoms of blast-induced mTBI. All 81 subjects were seen within 72 hours of blast exposure by the same clinician-investigator at a forward location in an active combat zone. All medications and treatments were witnessed by a nurse, corpsman, or medic. The outcomes demonstrate that supplementation with oral NAC had a significant impact on neuropsychological test results, number of mTBI symptoms, and complete symptom resolution by day seven of treatment when compared to placebo. A secondary finding was that standard treatment initiation within 24 hours had an independent benefit on the neurological but not on neuropsychological outcome measures. Early treatment with NAC and standard therapy administered by a provider with expertise in mTBI care resulted in a seven day symptom resolution rate of 86% as compared to 11% in those receiving the same standard care by the same provider but who received placebo and began therapy between 24–72 hours after blast exposure. Additionally it should be noted that during this trial the pill form of NAC, the active ingredient in the FDA approved medication Mucomyst, produced no side effects in blast mTBI subjects. Mucomyst has an excellent safety profile in over forty years of use in hospitals worldwide. As such use of this medicine appears to be the first described pharmaceutical countermeasure for mTBI. These results while promising are still preliminary. This outcome needs to be supported by other studies of NAC for this pathophysiology examining neurosensory symptoms over a variety of time points both acute and chronic. Additionally, these findings argue for

**Table 8.** Neuropsychological Tests: COWA and Animal Naming at Study Entry.

| Timing of Treatment | Treatment | n | COWA – At entry to study | | | Animal Naming – At entry to Study | | |
|---|---|---|---|---|---|---|---|---|
| | | | Mean (Standard Deviation) | $R^2$ | Pr>F | Mean (Standard Deviation) | $R^2$ | Pr>F |
| After 24 hours | Placebo | 9 | 30.6 (8.0) | 0.07 | 0.1245 | 17.4 (3.4) | 0.02 | 0.7787 |
| After 24 hours | NAC | 12 | 35.3 (8.3) | | | 19.7 (6.5) | | |
| Before 24 hours | Placebo | 30 | 39.3 (11.2) | | | 19.4 (6.1) | | |
| Before 24 hours | NAC | 27 | 35.3 (10.1) | | | 19.9 (6.9) | | |

**Table 9.** Neuropsychological Tests: COWA and Animal Naming at Day 7.

| Timing of Treatment | Treatment | n | COWA – Day 7 Mean (Standard Deviation) | $R^2$ | Pr>F | Animal Naming – Day 7 Mean (Standard Deviation) | $R^2$ | Pr>F |
|---|---|---|---|---|---|---|---|---|
| After 24 hours | Placebo | 9 | 35.6 (11.7) | 0.03 | 0.5222 | 19.4 (7.7) | 0.03 | 0.5994 |
| After 24 hours | NAC | 12 | 40.8 (9.4) | | | 22.3 (6.3) | | |
| Before 24 hours | Placebo | 30 | 38.6 (15.6) | | | 21.2 (6.0) | | |
| Before 24 hours | NAC | 27 | 42.3 (11.1) | | | 22.5 (6.1) | | |

investigations of this therapy for other causes of traumatic brain injury.

## Acknowledgments

The authors would like to thank J.D. Malone, CAPT MC USN (ret) for advice on this manuscript and Alicia B. Janos, BA and Jeannine B. Mielke, PhD for assistance with choice of the cognitive tests used. The authors would like to thank and acknowledge the pioneering work on NAC after noise-induced trauma in our lab by Ronald Jackson, PhD and Rick Kopke, COL MC USA (ret).

Disclaimer: The views expressed in this article are those of the author(s) and do not necessarily reflect the official policy or position of the Department of the Navy, Department of Defense, or the U.S. Government.

## Author Contributions

Conceived and designed the experiments: MEH CB. Performed the experiments: MEH. Analyzed the data: CB MS JT BH. Contributed reagents/materials/analysis tools: CB JT. Wrote the paper: MEH CB MS JT BH.

## References

1. Terrio H, Brenner LA, Ivins BJ, Cho JM, Helmick K, et al. (2009) Traumatic brain injury screening: preliminary findings in a US Army Brigade Combat Team. J Head Trauma Rehabil 24: 14–23.
2. Elder GA, Cristian A (2009) Blast-related mild traumatic brain injury: mechanisms of injury and impact on clinical care. Mt Sinai J Med 76: 111–118.
3. Bryant RA (2008) Disentangling mild traumatic brain injury and stress reactions. New England Journal of Medicine 358: 525–526.
4. Hoge CW, McGurk D, Thomas JL, Cox AL, Engel CC, et al. (2008) Mild traumatic brain injury in U.S. Soldiers returning from Iraq. N Engl J Med 358: 453–463.
5. French LM, Mouratidis M, Dicianno B, Impink B (2009) Traumatic brain injury. In: Pasquina PF, Cooper RA, editors. Care of the Combat Amputee. Washington, D.C.: Borden Institute. pp. 399–414.
6. Cuzzocrea S, Mazzon E, Costantino G, Serraino I, Dugo L, et al. (2000) Beneficial effects of n-acetylcysteine on ischaemic brain injury. British Journal of Pharmacology 130: 1219–1226.
7. Khan M, Sekhon B, Jatana M, Giri S, Gilg AG, et al. (2004) Administration of N-acetylcysteine after focal cerebral ischemia protects brain and reduces inflammation in a rat model of experimental stroke. Journal of Neuroscience Research 76: 519–527.
8. Sekhon B, Sekhon C, Khan M, Patel SJ, Singh I, et al. (2003) N-Acetyl cysteine protects against injury in a rat model of focal cerebral ischemia. Brain Research 971: 1–8.
9. Hicdonmez T, Kanter M, Tiryaki M, Parsak T, Cobanoglu S (2006) Neuroprotective effects of N-acetylcysteine on experimental closed head trauma in rats. Neurochemistry Research 31: 473–481.
10. Hart AM, Terenghi G, Kellerth J-O, Wiberg M (2004) Sensory neuroprotection, mitochondrial preservation, and therapeutic potential of N-acetyl-cysteine after nerve injury. Neuroscience 125: 91–101.
11. Bielefeld EC, Kopke RD, Jackson RL, Coleman JK, Liu J, et al. (2007) Noise protection with N-acetyl-l-cysteine (NAC) using a variety of noise exposures, NAC doses, and routes of administration. Acta Otolaryngol 127: 914–919.
12. Kopke RD, Jackson RL, Coleman JK, Liu J, Bielefeld EC, et al. (2007) NAC for noise: from the bench top to the clinic. Hearing Research 226: 114–125.
13. Gilgun-Sherki Y, Rosenbaum Z, Melamed E, Offen D (2002) Antioxidant therapy in acute central nervous system injury: current state. Pharmacological Reviews 54: 271–284.
14. Pahan K, Sheikh FG, Namboodiri AMS, Singh I (1998) N-acetyl cysteine inhibits induction of NO production by endotoxin or cytokine stimulated rat peritoneal macrophages, $C_6$ glial cells and astrocytes. Free Radical Biology & Medicine 24: 39–48.
15. Santangelo F (2003) Intracellular thiol concentration modulating inflammatory response: influence on the regulation of cell functions through cysteine prodrug approach. Current Medicinal Chemistry 10: 2599–2610.
16. Moussawi K, Pacchioni A, Moran M, Olive MF, Gass JT, et al. (2009) N-Acetylcysteine reverses cocaine-induced metaplasticity. Nature Neuroscience 12: 182–189.
17. Schubert MC, Tusa RJ, Grine LE, Herdman SJ (2004) Optimizing the sensitivity of the head thrust test for identifying vestibular hypofunction. Phys Ther 84: 151–158.
18. Agrawal Y, Carey JP, Hoffman HJ, Sklare DA, Schubert MC (2011) The modified Romberg Balance Test: normative data in U.S. adults. Otol Neurotol 32: 309–311.
19. Marchetti GF, Whitney SL, Blatt PJ, Morris LO, Vance JM (2008) Temporal and spatial characteristics of gait during performance of the Dynamic Gait Index in people with and people without balance or vestibular disorders. Phys Ther 88: 640–651.
20. Pocock SJ (1983) Clinical Trials: A Practical Approach. London: Wiley-Blackwell. 266 p.
21. Ruff RM, Light RH, Parker SB, Levin HS (1996) Benton Controlled Oral Word Association Test: reliability and updated norms. Clinical Neuropsychol 11: 329–338.
22. Reitan RM (1992) Trail Making Test Manual for Administration and Scoring. Tucson, AZ: Ralph M. Reitan.
23. Spreen O, Strauss E (1998) Language tests. In: Spreen O, Strauss E, editors. Compendium of Neuropsychological Tests Second ed. New York: Oxford University Press. pp. 447–459.
24. Tombaugh TN, Rees L, McIntyre N (1998) Visual, visuomotor, and auditory tests. In: Spreen O, Strauss E, editors. A Compendium of Neuropsychological Tests. Second ed. New York: Oxford University Press. pp. 481–551.
25. Wagner S, Helmreich I, Dahmen N, Lieb K, Tadic A (2011) Reliability of three alternate forms of the Trail Making Tests A and B. Archives of Clinical Neuropsychology 26: 314–321.
26. Tombaugh TN (2004) Trail Making Test A and B: Normative data stratified by age and education. Archives of Clinical Neuropsychology 19: 203–214.
27. Dupont WD, Plummer WD (1990) Power and sample size calculations: a review and computer program. Controlled Clinical Trials 11: 116–128.
28. Gabaix X, Laibson D (2008) The Seven Properties of Good Models. In: Caplin A, Schotter A, editors. The Foundations of Positive and Normative Economics. New York: Oxford University Press. pp. 292–299.
29. Cave KM, Cornish EM, Chandler DW (2007) Blast injury of the ear: clinical update from the global war on terror. Military Medicine 172: 726–730.
30. Garth RJN (1994) Blast injury of the auditory system: a review of mechanisms and pathology. J Laryngol Otol 108: 925–929.
31. Lew HL, Jerger JF, Guillory SB, Henry JA (2007) Auditory dysfunction in traumatic brain injury. J Rehab Research, Development 44: 921–928.
32. Ritenour AE, Wickley A, Ritenour JS, Kriete BR, Blackbourne LH, et al. (2008) Tympanic membrane perforation and hearing loss from blast overpressure in

Operation Enduring Freedom and Operation Iraqi Freedom wounded. J Trauma 64: S174–S178.

33. James DJ, Pickett VC, Burden KJ, Cheesman A (1982) The response of the human ear to blast. Part 1: The effect on the ear drum of a short duration, fast rising pressure wave. Army Weapons Research Establishment/Chemical Defense Establishment Report No. 04/82.

34. Jensen JH, Bonding P (1993) Experimental pressure induced rupture of the tympanic membrane in man. Acta Otolaryngol 113: 62–67.

35. Hoffer ME, Balaban CD, Gottschall KR, Balough BJ, Maddox MR, et al. (2010) Blast exposure: vestibular consequences and associated characteristics. Otology & Neurotology 31: 232–236.

36. Tsai S-Y, Hayashi T, Harvey BK, Wang Y, Wu WW, et al. (2009) Sigma-1 receptors regulate hippocampal dendritic spine formation via a free radical-sensitive mechanism involving Rac1·GTP pathway PNAS doi:10.1073/pnas.0909089106.

37. Saljo A, Bao F, Hamberger A, Haglid KG, Hansson HA (2001) Exposure to short-lasting impulse noise causes microglial and astroglial cell activation in the adult rat brain. Pathophysiology 8: 105–111.

38. Saljo A, Huang YL, Hansson HA (2003) Impulse noise transiently increased the permeability of nerve and glial cell membranes, an effect accentuated by a recent brain injury. J Neurotrauma 20: 787–794.

39. Saljo A, Jingshan S, Hamberger A, Hansson HA, Haglid KG (2002) Exposure to short-lasting impulse noise causes neuronal c-Jun expression and induction of apoptosis in the adult rat brain. J Neurotrauma 19: 985–991.

40. Saljo A, Arrhen F, Bolouri H, Mayorga M, Hamberger A (2008) Neuropathology and pressure in the pig brain resulting from low-impulse noise exposure. J Neurotrauma 25: 1397–1406.

41. Balaban CD (2012) Blast-Induced Mild Traumatic Brain Injury: A Translational Scientific Approach. In: Giordano J, Waters P, editors. Brain Injury and Stroke: Pathology and Implications for Care. Arlington, VA: Potomac Institute Press. In press.

42. Rubovitch V, Ten-Bosch M, Zohar O, Harrison CR, Tempel-Brami C, et al. (2011) A mouse model of blast-induced mild traumatic brain injury. Exp Neurol 232: 280–289.

43. De Vries H, Kuiper J, De Boer AG, Van Berkel TJC, Breimer DD (1996) The blood-brain barrier in neuroinflammatory diseases. Pharmacological Reviews 49: 143–154.

44. Stranahan AM, Zhou Y, Martin B, Maudsley S (2009) Pharmacomimetics of exercise: novel approaches for hippocampally-targeted neuroprotective efforts. Current Medicinal Chemistry 16: 4668–4678.

45. Pereira TV, Horwitz RI, Ioannidis JPA (2012) Empirical evaluation of very large treatment effects of medical interventions. JAMA 308: 1676–1684.

46. Tweedie D, Milman A, Holloway HW, Li Y, Harvey BK, et al. (2007) Apoptotic and behavioral sequelae of mild brain trauma in mice. J Neurosci Res 85: 805–815.

# 5

# Mechanisms of Team-Sport-Related Brain Injuries in Children 5 to 19 Years Old: Opportunities for Prevention

Michael D. Cusimano[1,2]*, Newton Cho[1], Khizer Amin[1], Mariam Shirazi[1], Steven R. McFaull[3], Minh T. Do[3], Matthew C. Wong[1], Kelly Russell[1]

1 Injury Prevention Research Office, St. Michael's Hospital, University of Toronto, Toronto, Canada, 2 Division of Neurosurgery, St. Michael's Hospital, University of Toronto, Toronto, Canada, 3 Health Surveillance and Epidemiology Division, Public Health Agency of Canada, Ottawa, Canada

## Abstract

*Background:* There is a gap in knowledge about the mechanisms of sports-related brain injuries. The objective of this study was to determine the mechanisms of brain injuries among children and youth participating in team sports.

*Methods:* We conducted a retrospective case series of brain injuries suffered by children participating in team sports. The Canadian Hospitals Injury Reporting and Prevention Program (CHIRPP) database was searched for brain injury cases among 5–19 year-olds playing ice hockey, soccer, American football (football), basketball, baseball, or rugby between 1990 and 2009. Mechanisms of injury were classified as "struck by player," "struck by object," "struck by sport implement," "struck surface," and "other." A descriptive analysis was performed.

*Results:* There were 12,799 brain injuries related to six team sports (16.2% of all brain injuries registered in CHIRPP). Males represented 81% of injuries and the mean age was 13.2 years. Ice hockey accounted for the greatest number of brain injuries (44.3%), followed by soccer (19.0%) and football (12.9%). In ice hockey, rugby, and basketball, striking another player was the most common injury mechanism. Football, basketball, and soccer also demonstrated high proportions of injuries due to contact with an object (e.g., post) among younger players. In baseball, a common mechanism in the 5–9 year-old group was being hit with a bat as a result of standing too close to the batter (26.1% males, 28.3% females).

*Interpretation:* Many sports-related brain injury mechanisms are preventable. The results suggest that further efforts aimed at universal rule changes, safer playing environments, and the education of coaches, players, and parents should be targeted in maximizing prevention of sport-related brain injury using a multifaceted approach.

**Editor:** John E. Mendelson, California Pacific Medicial Center Research Institute, United States of America

**Funding:** This research was supported by Canadian Institute of Health Research Strategic Team Grant in Applied Injury Research #TIR-103946. The funders had no role in study design, data collection and analysis, decision to publish, or preparation of the manuscript. http://www.cihr-irsc.gc.ca/e/193.html

**Competing Interests:** The authors have declared that no competing interests exist.

* E-mail: cusimanom@smh.ca

## Introduction

Participation in sport is a valuable contributor to physical and mental well-being [1]; however, involvement in many sports is also associated with an increased risk of brain injury [2]. This is particularly concerning for children and youth, who are at risk of long-term cognitive deficits following sports-related traumatic brain injury [3]. There is a relatively high rate of youth sport participation and sport-related brain injuries [4], and currently there is no definitive treatment to ensure complete recovery.

Existing literature concerning paediatric team sports head injury prevention is incomplete, as most is targeted towards a few sports, including ice hockey [4–8]. Furthermore, literature that includes other sports has not identified key mechanisms of injury [9], or if mechanisms were addressed, it has been limited to a single Canadian province [10], sport [11], or league/institution [12]. A better understanding of brain injury mechanisms across sports is needed. This study provides a comprehensive comparative analysis of injury mechanisms across different sports amongst a large population of children aged 5–19 years. The objective of this study was to provide descriptions of team sport brain injury mechanisms in Canadian children and youth.

## Methods

Ethical approval was granted by the Research Ethics Board at St. Michael's Hospital, Toronto, Canada. This study utilized de-identified, administrative data and the ethics committee approved the waiver of consent.

In 1990, the Canadian Hospitals Injury Reporting and Prevention Program (CHIRPP) was developed as an emergency department (ED)-based injury surveillance system [13].CHIRPP currently operates in the EDs of 11 paediatric and 4 general Canadian hospitals. CHIRPP provides information such as what the patient was doing at the time of injury, injury cause, when and where the injury occurred, and the age and sex of the patient. ED staff report open-ended details regarding the nature of injury and fixed-choice details on the injured body part and treatment. The validity of CHIRPP has been previously established [14,15].

The CHIRPP database (1990–2009) was searched for individuals 5–19 years old who presented with a brain injury ("minor closed head injury", "concussion", "intracranial injury") while participating in ice hockey (hockey), soccer, American football (football), basketball, baseball, or rugby. Ringette and lacrosse were excluded because of the paucity of players and brain injuries. The extracted variables included age, sex, year, team sport, treatment (admitted/non-admitted), context (informal versus organized), a narrative description of the injury mechanism, and postal code. Sport context was categorized by organized and informal sport. Informal sport was defined as sport that was not regulated by third-party individuals including referees, coaches, or teachers. In contrast, organized sport was defined as sport in a setting in which formal regulation by a referee, coach, or teacher was present. Postal codes were used to determine community type (rural versus urban) [16]. Specific mechanisms of injury codes were developed by two research assistants (e.g.; "checked into boards from behind" or "hit by pitch while batting"). The specific mechanism of injury was then coded for the first 200 cases for each sport independently by the two research assistants using the developed coding list based on the narrative descriptions provided for each case. After establishing inter-coder agreement, the two research assistants applied the resulting codes to the remaining cases. Once coding was complete, proportions of injuries attributable to the specific mechanistic codes were determined. These specific mechanistic codes were also categorized into one of five categories: 'struck by player', 'struck by object' (in the environment i.e., net, post), 'struck by sport implement' (i.e., ball, stick), 'struck (playing) surface', and 'other'.

A descriptive analysis was conducted where normally distributed continuous variables were presented as means and standard deviations and dichotomous and polychotomous variables presented as proportions with associated 95% confidence intervals [17]. A chi-square test was performed to determine if there was an association between community type and sport context. Results were stratified by sport, sex, age group (5–9, 10–14, and 15–19 years), and helmet use. Helmet use data was analyzed for ice hockey, football, and baseball. Inter-coder reliability was evaluated by calculating chance-corrected Cohen's Kappa values [18].

## Results

A total of 12,799 team sport brain injuries were identified (16.2% of all CHIRPP reported brain injuries). Hockey accounted for the majority of brain injuries (Figure 1). Overall, 81.4% of the injured players were male and the mean age was 13.2 years (SD 2.8). Each sport had specific months where injuries peaked (Figure 2). Half of all brain injuries occurred during the fall/winter season (October–February: 51.3%), while fewer occurred during the summer (June–August: 13.6%). The highest proportion of brain injuries occurred on weekends (Saturday: 18.2%; Sunday: 17.8%). Approximately half of all brain injuries presented between 16:00–22:59 (52.1%). Informal team sports had a peak in the number of brain injuries during the early afternoon and evening; conversely, organized sports had the most number of brain injuries in the early evening (Figure 3). Almost all brain injuries occurred in urban areas (92.2%). Similar proportions of injuries were seen in organized and informal settings within each community type (rural informal: 23.8%; rural organized: 76.2%; urban informal: 25.9%; urban organized: 74.1%; $\chi^2 = 2.02$, p = 0.16). The proportion of injuries caused by striking another player increased as players aged (Figure 4).

## Ice Hockey

Ice hockey accounted for 5675 (44.3%) of all brain injuries (Table 1) with most occurring among 10–14 year-olds. Being struck by another player was the predominant mechanism (Table 1); specifically, checking into the boards among 10–14 year-olds (males: 36.3%, 95% CI: 34.7–38.0; females: 24.1%, 95% CI: 20.1, 29.6) and 15–19 year-olds (males: 33.2, 95% CI: 30.9, 35.8; females: 26.8%, 95% CI: 21.5, 34.5). Checking from behind resulted in approximately 10% of injuries among 10–14 year-olds (males: 10.6%, 95% CI: 9.7, 11.8; females: 8.3%, 95% CI: 6.2, 12.6) and 15–19 year-olds (males: 9.6, 95% CI: 8.3, 11.4%; females: 9.8%, 95% CI: 7.0, 14.5). The 5–9 year-old group was characterized by falls (males: 34.7%, 95% CI: 31.0, 39.0; females: 48.8%. 95% CI: 37.0, 65.0). Helmet usage was lowest among younger hockey players (70.4%; 95% CI: 66.7, 74.0) and increased to 78.6% (95% CI: 77.2, 79.9) among 10–19 year-olds. Being struck by a player was the most common mechanism of injury in both helmeted and non-helmeted players (Table 2).

## Soccer

Soccer resulted in 2435 (19.0%) brain injuries (Table 1), with most occurring among 10–14 year-olds. Being struck by another player was one of the main mechanisms (Table 1), especially in the form of collisions (including head-to-head collisions) among 10–14 year-olds (males: 21.9%, 95% CI: 19.4, 25.1; females: 23.1%, 95% CI: 19.8, 27.4) and 15–19 year-olds (males: 37.6%, 95% CI: 32.7, 43.6; females: 31.3%, 95% CI: 26.8, 37.0). Injury due to the ball was common among 5–9 year-olds (males: 20.6%, 95% CI: 17.5, 24.9; females: 29.9%, 95% CI: 22.8, 41.7) and 10–14 year-olds (males: 21.3%, 95% CI: 18.8, 24.5; females: 30.5%, 95% CI: 26.8, 35.1). Players 5–9 years old had a greater proportion of injuries due to striking an object in the environment, such as the net or post (Table 1). Females 15–19 years old had a greater number of injuries than males of the same age group. A greater proportion of females were injured by the ball than males (females: 26.6%, 95% CI: 24.0, 29.8; males: 17.2%, 95% CI: 15.5, 19.3). Brain injuries from kicks to the head increased with age (5–9 year-olds: 2.2%, 95% CI: 1.5, 4.3; 15–19 year-olds: 9.7%, 95% CI: 7.9, 12.6).

## Football

Football was the third leading cause of brain injuries (N = 1,651, 12.9%; Table 1) with most occurring among 10–14 year-olds. Striking another player was the main mechanism of injury (Table 1). Specifically, tackling was the predominant mechanism and increased with age. The second most common mechanism was non-tackling collision/contact with other players and also increased with age, particularly head-to-head/body collisions among 15–19 year-olds (males: 25.3%, 95% CI: 22.1, 29.4; females: 12.5%, 95% CI: 8.4, 33.5). Injuries due to striking an object in the environment were most frequent among 5–9 year-olds (Table 1). Helmet use increased from 12.5% (95% CI: 8.8, 21.6) among 5–9 year-olds to 57.5% (95% CI: 53.6, 61.6) among 15–19 year-olds. Regardless of helmet status, being struck by a player was the most common mechanism (Table 2).

## Basketball

Basketball resulted in 1,482 (11.6%) brain injuries (Table 1) with the greatest number occurring among 10–14 year-olds. The proportions of injuries due to collision/contact with other players increased with age, especially elbowing (5–9 year-olds: 0%; 15–19 year-olds: 11.2%, 95% CI: 8.9, 15.1). Striking an object in the environment occurred most often among 5–9 year-olds (Table 1).

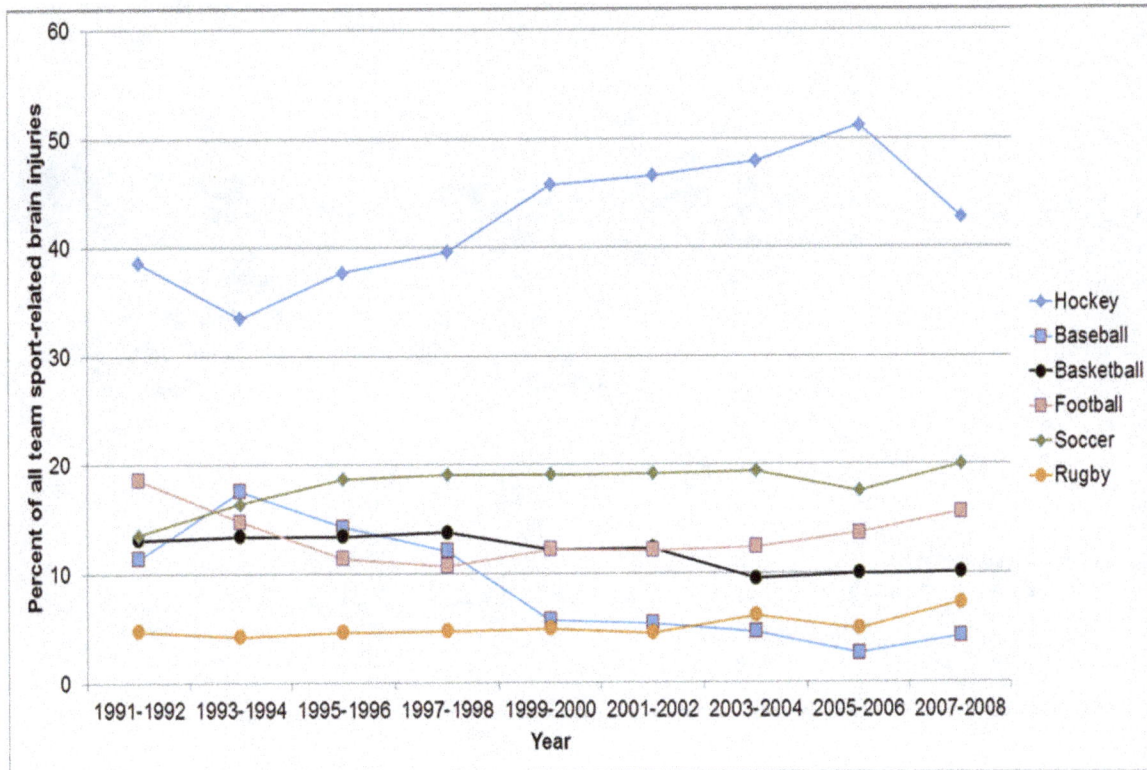

**Figure 1. Relative frequencies of brain injuries in each sport by year of incident.**

## Baseball

Baseball resulted in 835 (6.5%) brain injuries (Table 1) with most occurring among 10–14 year-olds. The most common mechanism in 10–19 year-olds was being hit by the baseball (males: 58.0%, 95% CI: 53.4, 63.0; females: 70.1%, 95% CI: 62.9, 77.0). Being hit by the bat was common among 5–9 year-olds (males: 53.8%, 95% CI: 47.9, 60.5; females: 60.9%, 95% CI: 48.4, 74.8) and often due to being too close to the batter (males: 26.1%,

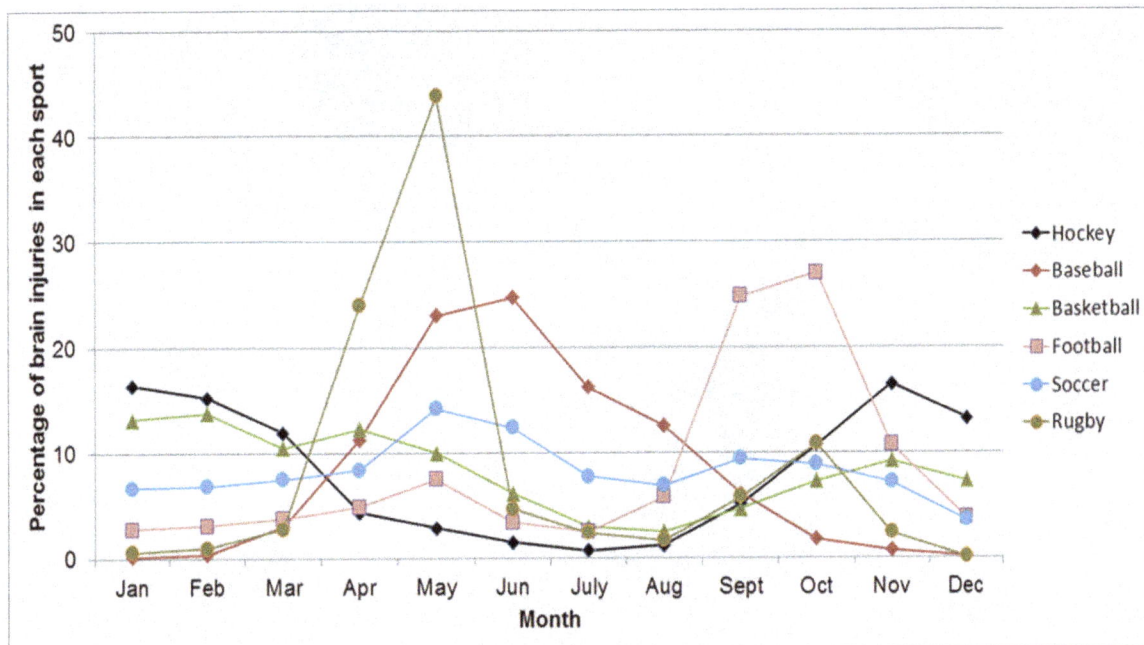

**Figure 2. Relative frequencies of brain injuries in each sport by month of incident.**

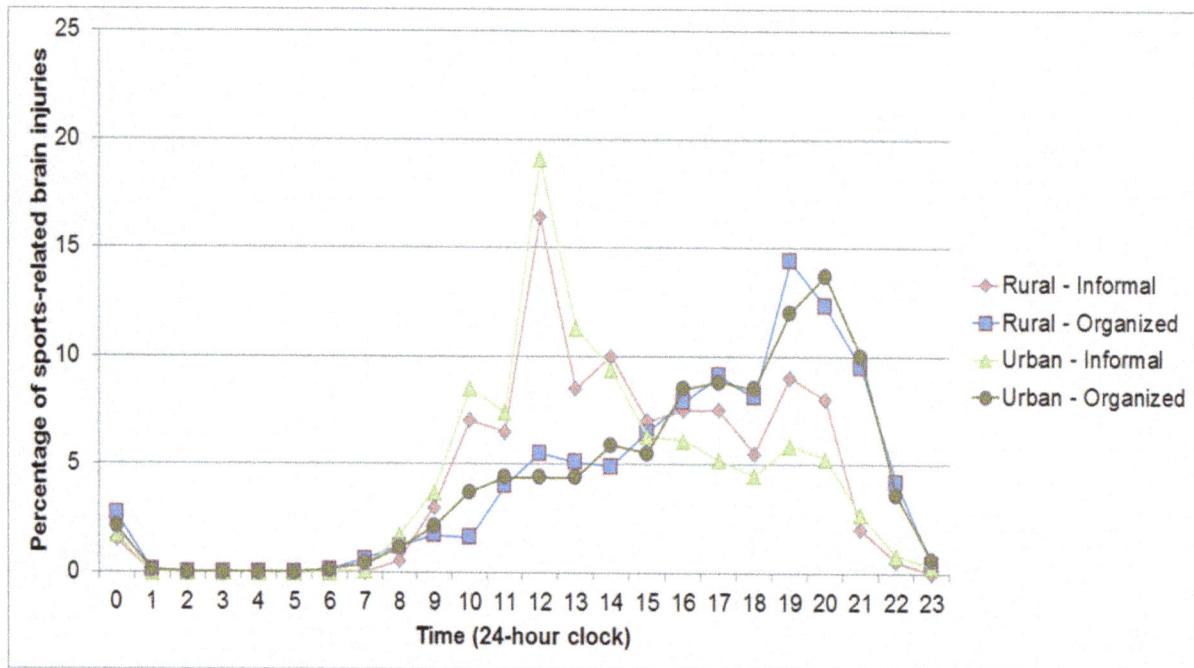

**Figure 3. Relative frequencies of brain injuries in each community-context situation by hour of incident.**

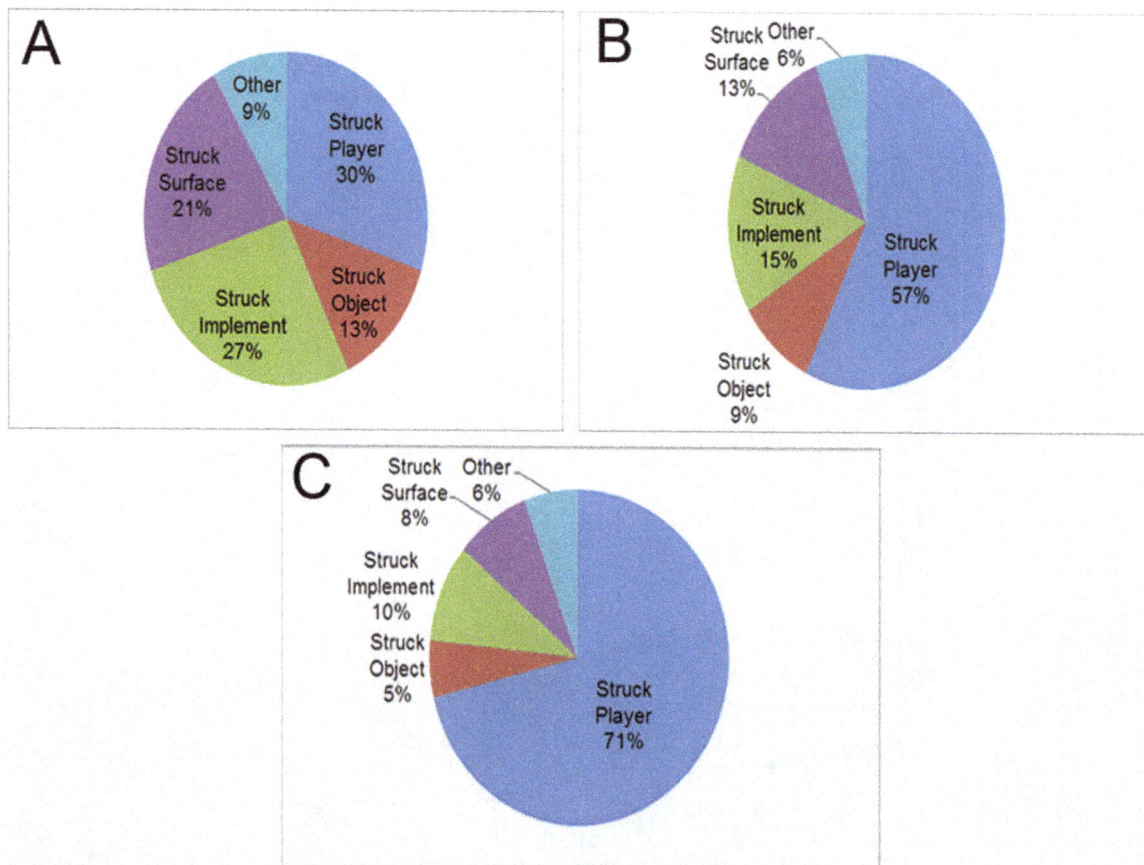

**Figure 4. Relative frequencies of brain injury mechanism by age group.**

**Table 1.** Proportions and 95% CI of brain injury mechanisms among team sports organized by age between 1990–2009 in the Canadian Hospitals Injury Reporting and Prevention Program.

| | N | 5–9 years old N (%; 95% CI) | 10–14 years old N (%; 95% CI) | 15–19 years old N (%; 95% CI) |
|---|---|---|---|---|
| **Ice Hockey** | 5 675 | 591 | 3543 | 1541 |
| Struck by player | | 225 (38.1; 34.5, 42.3) | 2293 (64.7; 63.2, 66.3) | 1074 (69.7; 67.4, 72.0) |
| Struck by object | | 101 (17.1; 14.5, 20.6) | 389 (11.0; 10.0, 12.1) | 133 (8.6; 7.4, 10.3) |
| Struck by sport implement | | 37 (6.3; 4.9, 8.9) | 236 (6.7; 5.9, 7.6) | 112 (7.3; 6.2, 8.8) |
| Struck surface | | 129 (21.8; 18.9, 25.6) | 297 (8.4; 7.6, 9.4) | 101 (6.6; 5.5, 8.0) |
| Other | | 99 (16.8; 14.2, 20.3) | 328 (9.3; 8.4, 10.3) | 121 (7.9; 6.7, 9.4) |
| **Soccer** | 2 435 | 543 | 1274 | 618 |
| Struck by player | | 183 (33.7; 30.1, 38.0) | 609 (47.8; 45.2, 50.6) | 419 (67.8; 64.1, 71.5) |
| Struck by object | | 68 (12.5; 10.3, 15.9) | 94 (7.4; 6.2, 9.1) | 17 (2.8; 2.0, 4.7) |
| Struck by sport implement | | 120 (22.1; 19.1, 26.1) | 315 (24.7; 22.6, 27.3) | 118 (19.1; 16.4, 22.7) |
| Struck surface | | 148 (27.3; 23.9, 31.4) | 224 (17.6; 15.7, 19.9) | 54 (8.7; 7.0, 11.6) |
| Other | | 24 (4.4; 3.3, 6.9) | 32 (2.5; 1.9, 3.7) | 10 (1.6; 1.1, 3.4) |
| **Football** | 1 651 | 112 | 965 | 574 |
| Struck by player | | 50 (44.6; 36.8, 54.8) | 721 (74.7; 71.9, 77.4) | 483 (84.2; 81.0, 87.0) |
| Struck by object | | 25 (22.3; 16.8, 32.3) | 73 (7.6; 6.2, 9.6) | 18 (3.1; 2.3, 5.3) |
| Struck by sport implement | | 4 (3.6; 2.4, 11.0) | 24 (2.5; 1.8, 3.9) | 15 (2.6; 1.9, 4.7) |
| Struck surface | | 29 (25.9; 19.9, 36.0) | 124 (12.9; 11.1, 15.3) | 38 (6.6; 5.1, 9.3) |
| Other | | 4 (3.6; 2.4, 11.0) | 23 (2.4; 1.8, 3.8) | 20 (3.5; 2.5, 5.7) |
| **Basketball** | 1 482 | 151 | 920 | 411 |
| Struck by player | | 39 (25.8; 20.4, 34.3) | 378 (41.1; 38.1, 44.4) | 245 (59.6; 55.0, 64.4) |
| Struck by object | | 19 (12.6; 9.2, 20.7) | 90 (9.8; 8.2, 12.1) | 28 (6.8; 5.1, 10.2) |
| Struck by sport implement | | 34 (22.5; 17.5, 30.9) | 171 (18.6; 16.4, 21.4) | 34 (8.3; 6.4, 11.8) |
| Struck surface | | 51 (33.8; 27.6, 42.9) | 260 (28.3; 25.6, 31.4) | 98 (23.8; 20.3, 28.6) |
| Other | | 8 (5.3; 3.6, 11.6) | 21 (2.3; 1.7, 3.7) | 6 (1.5; 1.0, 3.8) |
| **Baseball** | 835 | 280 | 443 | 112 |
| Struck by player | | 13 (4.6; 3.3, 8.6) | 46 (10.4; 8.2, 14.0) | 20 (17.9; 13.1, 27.5) |
| Struck by object | | 3 (1.01; 0.1, 4.9) | 7 (1.6; 1.1, 3.8) | 4 (3.6; 2.4, 11.0) |
| Struck by sport implement | | 256 (91.4; 87.7, 94.2) | 366 (86.6; 78.9, 85.9) | 77 (68.8; 60.3, 77.0) |
| Struck surface | | 1 (0.4; 0.4, 3.1) | 7 (1.6; 1.1, 3.8) | 2 (1.8; 1.4, 8.7) |
| Other | | 7 (2.5; 1.7, 6.0) | 17 (3.8; 2.8, 6.6) | 9 (8.0; 5.5, 16.5) |
| **Rugby** | 721 | 5 | 175 | 541 |
| Struck by player | | 2 (40.0; 25.1, 84.2) | 147 (84.0; 78.1, 88.8) | 464 (85.8; 82.6, 88.5) |
| Struck by object | | 0 | 0 | 5 (0.9; 0.6, 2.6) |
| Struck by sport implement | | 0 | 2 (1.1; 0.9, 5.7) | 3 (0.6; 0.4, 2.1) |
| Struck surface | | 2 (40.0; 25.1, 84.2) | 12 (6.9; 4.8, 12.8) | 14 (2.6; 1.8, 4.7) |
| Other | | 1 (20.0; 15.8, 75.0) | 14 (8.0; 5.6, 14.2) | 55 (10.2; 8.2, 13.4) |

95% CI: 21.5, 32.7; females: 28.3%, 95% CI: 20.0, 45.3). The proportion of brain injuries caused by player collisions increased with age, but only 0.6% of brain injuries were a result of sliding collisions. Overall, 6.7% of players wore a helmet, and helmet use increased to 15.2% of 15–19 year-olds. Being struck by an implement was the most common mechanism among helmeted and non-helmeted players (Table 2).

## Rugby

There were 721 (5.6%) brain injuries in rugby (Table 1) with most occurring among 15–19 year-olds. Striking another player was the main mechanism of injury (Table 1). More specifically, the main mechanisms in this age group were being tackled or tackling another player (males: 48.5%, 95% CI: 43.7, 53.9; females: 51.7%, 95% CI: 45.0, 59.4), head-to-head collisions (males: 10.2%, 95% CI, 7.9, 14.3; females: 7.3%, 95% CI, 5.1, 13.3), and head-to-knee collisions (males: 9.1%, 95% CI, 7.0, 13.0; females: 5.1%, 95% CI, 3.5, 10.6).

## Reliability

Cohen's Kappa values calculated for each sport were greater than 0.87 (range: 0.87 to 0.95) and interpreted as almost perfect agreement [19].

**Table 2.** Proportions and 95% CI of brain injury mechanisms among team sports organized by protective equipment use between 1990–2009 in the Canadian Hospitals Injury Reporting and Prevention Program.

| | N | Helmet N (%; 95% CI) | No protective equipment N (%; 95% CI) | Other protective equipment N (%; 95% CI) | Unspecified N (%; 95% CI) |
|---|---|---|---|---|---|
| **Ice Hockey** | 5675 | 4412 (77.7) | 99 (1.7) | 508 (9.0) | 656 (11.6) |
| Struck by player | | 2965 (67.2; 65.8, 68.6) | 18 (18.2; 13.2, 28.6) | 276 (54.3; 50.2, 58.8) | 333 (50.8; 47.1, 54.7) |
| Struck by object | | 463 (10.5; 9.7, 11.5) | 10 (10.1; 6.9, 19.6) | 87 (17.1; 14.4, 21.0) | 63 (9.6; 7.8, 12.4) |
| Struck by sport implement | | 255 (5.8; 5.2, 6.6) | 27 (27.3; 20.8, 38.2) | 44 (8.7; 6.8, 11.8) | 59 (9.0; 7.3, 11.7) |
| Struck surface | | 349 (7.9; 7.2, 8.8) | 24 (24.2; 18.2, 35.1) | 56 (11.0; 8.9, 14.4) | 98 (14.9; 12.7, 18.1) |
| Other | | 380 (8.6; 7.9, 9.5) | 20 (20.2; 14.9, 30.8) | 45 (8.9; 7.0, 12.0) | 103 (15.7; 13.4, 19.0) |
| **Football** | 1651 | 713 (43.2) | 212 (12.8) | 67 (4.1) | 659 (39.9) |
| Struck by player | | 660 (92.6; 90.4, 94.3) | 129 (60.8; 54.5, 67.5) | 62 (92.5; 84.1, 96.9) | 403 (61.2; 57.5, 64.9) |
| Struck by object | | 3 (0.4; 0.3, 1.6) | 32 (15.1; 11.6, 21.4) | 0 (0) | 81 (12.3; 10.3, 15.3) |
| Struck by sport implement | | 8 (1.1; 0.8, 2.6) | 11 (5.2; 3.6, 10.1) | 2 (3.0; 2.3, 14.0) | 22 (3.3; 2.5, 5.4) |
| Struck surface | | 16 (2.2; 1.6, 3.9) | 36 (17.0; 13.2, 23.4) | 2 (3.0; 2.3, 14.0) | 137 (20.8; 18.1, 24.3) |
| Other | | 26 (3.6; 2.7, 5.6) | 4 (1.9; 1.3, 6.0) | 1 (1.5; 1.5, 12.0) | 16 (2.4; 1.7, 4.3) |
| **Baseball** | 835 | 56 (6.7) | 106 (12.7) | 54 (6.5) | 619 (74.1) |
| Struck by player | | 11 (19.6; 13.6, 34.7) | 8 (7.5; 5.1, 16.2) | 12 (22.2; 15.5, 37.7) | 48 (7.8; 6.2, 10.5) |
| Struck by object | | 1 (1.8; 1.8, 14.1) | 1 (0.9; 1.0, 7.9) | 1 (1.9; 1.8, 14.6) | 11 (1.8; 1.2, 3.6) |
| Struck by sport implement | | 41 (73.2; 61.6, 83.7) | 90 (84.9; 77.3, 90.7) | 39 (72.2; 60.4, 83.0) | 529 (85.5; 82.5, 88.1) |
| Struck surface | | 1 (1.8; 1.8, 14.1) | 2 (1.9; 1.5, 9.1) | 1 (1.9; 1.8, 14.6) | 6 (1.0; 0.7, 2.5) |
| Other | | 2 (3.6; 2.7, 16.4) | 5 (4.7; 3.2, 12.8) | 1 (1.9; 1.8, 14.6) | 25 (4.0; 3.0, 6.3) |

## Discussion

The majority of team sport brain injuries occurred among males, between October and February, and among hockey players (likely due to the high participation in Canada). A large number of individuals who suffered injuries in informal sports injuries presented to the ED in the early afternoon. This may be due to injuries sustained on the school yard during recess and after school. In hockey, checking into the boards and falls were the most common mechanisms for players older than and younger than 10 years old, respectively. Soccer-related injuries among older players were characterized by player collisions and kicks to the head, while younger children tended to be struck by an object in the environment (e.g., goal post). In football, tackling was the predominant mechanism and similar findings have been observed elsewhere [12]. In basketball, proportions of injuries due to player collisions/contact including elbowing increased with age. In football and basketball, younger players tended to strike fixed structures. In baseball, the main mechanism was being struck by the baseball or bat. Injuries suffered by 5–9 year-olds were characterized mainly by being hit by the bat, often because of standing too close to the batter. Rugby was mainly characterized by player collisions.

Our research provides a baseline level of understanding for mechanisms of injury and highlights important areas of concern for the prevention of team sport-related brain injuries. Body checking has previously been identified as a risk factor for ice hockey injury [4,20,21]. We found that it was specifically checking into the boards that caused the greatest proportion of brain injuries, and that 10% of brain injuries were caused by checking into the boards from behind. This is despite rules prohibiting this action for the past twenty years. Our results support increased efforts to completely remove checking from behind. Leagues that disallow body-checking have demonstrated a significant reduction in injuries, and our findings further support the idea that making these manoeuvres illegal has the potential to reduce injuries [20]. In soccer, enforcement of stricter penalties for high kicks may reduce the frequent number of injuries due to kicks to the head. Similar efforts to reduce player-to-player intentional contact in football, rugby, basketball and soccer may also provide benefit.

Education is an important component of a multifaceted approach to injury prevention in sports. Such education should not only manifest itself as general information about brain injury, but also include very sport-specific messaging that addresses the common mechanisms of brain injury in specific sports. This education should be mandatory to participate in the organized sport and be aimed at players, coaches, trainers, officials, and parents at all levels. Furthermore, education can also aim to support rule changes in sports that may help to reduce injuries such as reducing body checking [4]. Skill improvement such as teaching younger hockey players proper skating technique could diminish fall-related brain injuries. In soccer, education about high kicks, scissor kicks, and heading the ball in close proximity to other players should be key targets for education. In baseball, education around creating safe distances from a batter, and mandatory helmets, especially for younger players is important. A systematic review in rugby shows that such educational efforts should be universally mandated and be combined with other efforts such as rule changes to be most effective [22].

Equipment and environmental changes are important avenues for prevention of youth brain injuries. Proper and mandatory universal helmet use and properly supervised no-stand zones for young and recreational baseball players hold significant promise for injury reduction. Making all goal posts and fixed structures in the vicinity of playing surfaces padded and mobile so as to lessen impact forces could reduce brain injury in soccer, basketball, and possibly hockey as well. In rugby, mouth guards and headgear are of limited benefit in reducing neurological injuries [22]; more research is needed to determine whether head protectors would reduce brain injuries in soccer and basketball. We found that helmeted and non-helmeted players were injured by similar mechanisms in ice hockey, football, and baseball, suggesting that other modalities of prevention need to be instituted in addition to personal protective equipment.

## Implications

Our results provide a basis for the modification of existing programs to incorporate multifaceted approaches addressing universal rule changes, safer playing environments, personal protective equipment use, education and economic programs. Some states have introduced laws to mandate such changes [23], but this strategy's effectiveness has not been evaluated. Economic incentives, such as improved insurance rates for sports with improved safety, should also be explored. As brain injury occurrence comes to greater public awareness, lawsuits that demand accountability from organizations and leagues will create pressure for change. Monitoring systems for the frequency/pattern of injuries should be implemented at a national or provincial level. Independent bodies that can monitor brain injury rates and efforts to reduce them should be established at the national or provincial level of all organized sports. Such bodies should be accountable to a higher level of national audit and have the authority and resources to implement changes to make that particular sport as safe as possible for as many participants as possible. Further research is needed to understand the mechanisms of traumatic brain injury in sports.

## Limitations

This study had several limitations. Firstly, the total number of youth playing each sport was unavailable thus sport, sex, age, or mechanism-specific injury rates were not calculated. As of 2010, Statistics Canada reported that there were 5 616 700 children in Canada aged 14 and under [25]. The Canadian Fitness and Lifestyle Research Institute found that in the year between March 2010 and April 2011, 38% of Canadian children aged 5–17 played soccer within the last year, followed by hockey/ringette (23%), swimming (17%), basketball (15%), and baseball (10%) [24]. This means that roughly 2 000 000 played soccer, 1 300 000 played hockey/ringette, 840 000 played basketball, and 560 000 played

baseball in 2010. This indicates that many children are at risk for suffering sport-related traumatic brain injury and that appropriate understanding of how they are getting injured is important to prevent these injuries. In this regard, more consistently available information on sports participation is essential to aid future research. This information can help with calculating injury rates but also aid in injury surveillance and the evaluation of injury prevention strategies.

The CHIRPP database is limited to brain injuries presenting to EDs so any injuries that did not present to the ED would have been missed. Fatal injuries were also not included in CHIRPP, but pediatric sport-related fatalities are rare [26], and a recent paper has further demonstrated the representativeness of CHIRPP for injury profiling [27]. Additionally, the mechanism of injury was provided in a text field and had to be coded by two individuals. Some narratives where unclear; however, the individuals consulted each other on unclear cases. A descriptive analysis was performed without multivariate modelling; however, the results were stratified by age groups and sex. Although there may be residual confounding by age group since the effect of exact age was not examined, previous papers have stratified by age as we did in the current paper [10,11].

Additionally, there may certainly be differences depending on the position being played; however, positional information was not consistently available in CHIRPP. As a result, we were unable to resolve these differences in this study. Future studies should focus on differences in the frequencies, proportions, and severity of injuries sustained in varying positions within specific sports.

## Conclusion

This study is the first to comprehensively analyze mechanisms of injury of pediatric team sports brain injuries. Intervention should be aimed at educating players, the public, and sport organizations about the most common mechanisms of injuries. Differences in mechanisms across sports and ages should help tailor future prevention efforts. Ultimately, a multifaceted approach in all sports holds promise for prevention of brain injury.

## Author Contributions

Acquisition and preparation of data: SRM MTD. Critical revision of manuscript: MDC NC KA MS SRM MTD MCW KR. Conceived and designed the experiments: MDC NC MCW. Analyzed the data: MDC NC KA MS MCW KR. Wrote the paper: MDC NC KA MS KR.

## References

1. Warburton DE, Nicol CW, Bredin SS (2006) Health benefits of physical activity: the evidence. CMAJ 174: 801–809.
2. Langlois JA, Rutland-Brown W, Wald MM (2006) The epidemiology and impact of traumatic brain injury: a brief overview. J Head Trauma Rehabil 21: 375–378.
3. Benz B, Ritz A, Kiesow S (1999) Influence of age-related factors on long-term outcome after traumatic brain injury (TBI) in children: a review of recent literature and some preliminary findings. Restor Neurol Neurosci 14: 135–141.
4. Macpherson A, Rothman L, Howard A (2006) Body-checking rules and childhood injuries in ice hockey. Pediatrics 117: e143-e147.
5. Emery CA, Meeuwisse WH (2006) Injury rates, risk factors, and mechanisms of injury in minor hockey. Am J Sports Med 34: 1960–1969.
6. Juhn MS, Brolinson PG, Duffey T, Stockard A, Vangelos ZA, et al. (2002) Position statement: Violence and injury in ice hockey. Clin J Sport Med 12: 46–51.
7. Goodman D, Gaetz M, Meichenbaum D (2001) Concussions in hockey: there is cause for concern. Med Sci Sports Exerc 33: 2004–2009.
8. Emery CA, Hagel B, Decloe M, Carly M (2009) Risk factors for injury and severe injury in youth ice hockey: as systematic review of the literature. Inj Prev 16: 113–118.
9. Delaney JS (2004) Head injuries presenting to emergency departments in the United states from 1990 to 1999 for ice hockey, soccer, and football. Clin J Sport Med 14: 80–87.

10. Kelly KD, Lissel HL, Rowe BH, Vincenten JA, Voaklander DC (2001) Sport and recreation-related head injuries treated in the emergency department. Clin J Sport Med 11: 77–81.
11. Giannotti M, Al-Sahab B, McFaull S, Tamim H (2010) Epidemiology of acute head injuries in Canadian children and youth soccer players. Injury 41: 907–912.
12. Delaney JS, Puni V, Rouah F (2006) Mechanisms of injury for concussions in university football, ice hockey, and soccer: a pilot study. Clin J Sport Med 16: 162–165.
13. Public, Health, Agency, of, Canada Canadian Hospitals Injury Reporting and Prevention Program (CHIRPP).
14. Pickett W, Brison RJ, Mackenzie SG, Garner M, King MA, et al. (2000) Youth injury data in the Canadian Hospitals Injury Reporting and Prevention Program: do they represent the Canadian experience? Inj Prev 6: 9–15.
15. Macarthur C, Dougherty G, Pless IB (1997) Reliability and validity of proxy respondent information about childhood injury: an assessment of a Canadian surveillance system. Am J Epidemiol 145: 834–841.
16. Hassan A, Pearce NJ, Mathers J, Veugelers PJ, Hirsch GM, et al. (2009) The effect of place of residence on access to invasive cardiac services following acute myocardial infarction. Can J Cardiol 25: 207–212.
17. Agresti A, Coull BA (1998) Approximate is better than 'exact' for interval estimation of binomial proportions. Am Stat 52: 119–126.
18. Cohen J (1960) A coefficient of agreement for nominal scales. Educ Psychol Meas 20: 37–46.

19. Landis JR, Koch GG (1977) The measurement of observer agreement for categorical data. Biometrics 33: 159–174.

20. Emery CA, Kang J, Shrier I, Goulet C, Hagel BE, et al. (2010) Risk of injury associated with body checking among youth ice hockey players. JAMA 303: 2265–2272.

21. Cusimano MD, Taback NA, McFaull SR, Hodgins R, Bekele TM, et al. (2011) Effect of bodychecking on rate of injuries among minor hockey players. Open Med 5: e57–65.

22. Cusimano M, Nassiri F, Chang Y (2010) The effectiveness of interventions to reduce neurological injuries in rugby union. Neurosurgery 67: 1404–1418.

23. Injury TB Zackery Lystedt Law - House Bill 1824.

24. Canadian Fitness & Lifestyle Research Institute (2011) Getting Kids Active! 2010 Physical Activity Monitor: Facts and Figures.

25. Statistics Canada, Section 2: Age and sex (2010). Available: http://www.statcan.gc.ca/pub/91-215-x/2010000/part-partie2-eng.htm.Accessed 12 January 2013.

26. Turk EE, Riedel A, Püeschel K (2008) Natural and traumatic sports-related fatalities: a 10-year retrospective study. Br J Sports Med 42: 604–208.

27. Kang J, Hagel B, Emery CA, Senger T, Meeuwisse W (2012). Assessing the representativeness of Canadian Hospitals Injury Reporting and Prevention Programme (CHIRPP) sport and receational injury data in Calgary, Canada. Int J Inj Contr Saf Promot 1–8.

# 6

# Contrast-Enhanced FLAIR (Fluid-Attenuated Inversion Recovery) for Evaluating Mild Traumatic Brain Injury

Soo Chin Kim[1,2], Sun-Won Park[1,2]*, Inseon Ryoo[2,3], Seung Chai Jung[2,4], Tae Jin Yun[2,5], Seung Hong Choi[2,5], Ji-hoon Kim[2,5], Chul-Ho Sohn[2,5]

1 Department of Radiology, Seoul Metropolitan Government - Seoul National University Boramae medical center, Seoul, Korea, 2 Department of Radiology, Seoul National University College of Medicine, Seoul, Korea, 3 Department of Radiology, Korea University Guro Hospital, Seoul, Korea, 4 Department of Radiology, Asan Medical Center, Seoul, Korea, 5 Department of Radiology, Seoul National University Hospital, Seoul, Korea

## Abstract

*Purpose:* To evaluate whether adding a contrast-enhanced fluid-attenuated inversion recovery (FLAIR) sequence to routine magnetic resonance imaging (MRI) can detect additional abnormalities in the brains of symptomatic patients with mild traumatic brain injury.

*Materials and Methods:* Fifty-four patients with persistent symptoms following mild closed head injury were included in our retrospective study (M:F = 32:22, mean age: 59.8±16.4, age range: 26–84 years). All MRI examinations were obtained within 14 days after head trauma (mean: 3.2±4.1 days, range: 0.2–14 days). Two neuroradiologists recorded (1) the presence of traumatic brain lesions on MR images with and without contrast-enhanced FLAIR images and (2) the pattern and location of meningeal enhancement depicted on contrast-enhanced FLAIR images. The number of additional traumatic brain lesions diagnosed with contrast-enhanced FLAIR was recorded. Correlations between meningeal enhancement and clinical findings were also evaluated.

*Results:* Traumatic brain lesions were detected on routine image sequences in 25 patients. Three additional cases of brain abnormality were detected with the contrast-enhanced FLAIR images. Meningeal enhancement was identified on contrast-enhanced FLAIR images in 9 cases while the other routine image sequences showed no findings of traumatic brain injury. Overall, the additional contrast-enhanced FLAIR images revealed more extensive abnormalities than routine imaging in 37 cases (p<0.001). In multivariate logistic regression analysis, subdural hematoma and posttraumatic loss of consciousness showed a significant association with meningeal enhancement on contrast-enhanced FLAIR images, with odds ratios 13.068 (95% confidence interval 2.037 to 83.852), and 15.487 (95% confidence interval 2.545 to 94.228), respectively.

*Conclusion:* Meningeal enhancement on contrast-enhanced FLAIR images can help detect traumatic brain lesions as well as additional abnormalities not identified on routine unenhanced MRI. Therefore contrast-enhanced FLAIR MR imaging is recommended when a contrast MR study is indicated in a patient with a symptomatic prior closed mild head injury.

**Editor:** Anna-Leena Sirén, University of Wuerzburg, Germany

**Funding:** The authors have no support or funding to report.

**Competing Interests:** The authors have declared that no competing interests exist.

* Email: swpark8802@gmail.com

## Introduction

Traumatic brain injury (TBI) often leads to neurocognitive deficits and neurobehavioral abnormalities. Even with mild traumatic brain injury, many patients have long-term neuro-logic or neuropsychologic abnormalities [1], [2]. As a result, imaging evaluation for detection of traumatic lesions has drawn much attention. Many prior studies have reported that magnetic resonance imaging (MRI) can reveal traumatic lesions responsible for clinical symptoms and signs in patients with negative computed tomography (CT) examinations [3]. Currently, susceptibility-weighted imaging (SWI) is more sensitive than conventional MR imaging for the detection of microhemorrhages [4], [5]. Diffusion tensor imaging (DTI) has emerged as a valuable additional technique to evaluate traumatic brain abnormalities [6–10]. However, these specialized advanced sequences require long imaging time leading to an increased incidence of movement artifacts [11], [12], and requirement of special imaging hardware.

The fluid-attenuated inversion recovery (FLAIR) is a special inversion recovery sequence using a long repetition time (TR) and echo time (TE) and an inversion time that effectively suppresses signals from free water in cerebrospinal fluid (CSF), thus allowing to highlight hyperintense lesions adjacent to CSF containing spaces. Although FLAIR images are heavily T2-weighted images, these MR images also have mild T1-weighting, which is responsible for contrast enhancement. Because of the combination of T2 prolongation, the usual mechanism for hyperintense lesion on FLAIR images, and T1 shortening from contrast material with CSF signal suppression, contrast-enhanced FLAIR MR imaging is highly sensitive to the detection of subtle cortical abnormalities such as meningeal infection, inflammation and metastases [13–

**Table 1.** The summary of demographic and clinical characteristics of patients.

| Variable | Value |
| --- | --- |
| **Patients (n)** | 54 |
| **Age (years)** | |
| Mean | 59.8 (±16.4) |
| Median (range) | 63 |
| **Sex (women/men)** | 22/32 |
| **Underlying disease (n)** | |
| No | 34 |
| Yes | 20 |
| Diabetes mellitus | 8 |
| Hypertension | 7 |
| Alzheimer's disease | 3 |
| Past history of stroke | 2 |
| **Time interval (days)** | |
| 0–3 | 37 |
| 4–7 | 10 |
| 8–14 | 7 |
| **Reason** | |
| Fall | 33 |
| Traffic accident | 17 |
| Violence | 4 |
| **GCS** | |
| 13 | 3 |
| 14 | 3 |
| 15 | 48 |
| **Post-traumatic amnesia (n)** | 12 |
| **Post-traumatic LOC (n)** | 24 |

Note — GCS indicates Glasgow Coma Score; LOC, loss of consciousness.

15]. Goo et al. reported the case demonstrating abnormal meningeal enhancement in patient with a subdural hematoma on contrast-enhanced FLAIR MR image [16]. However, to our knowledge, the clinical importance of this sequence in patients with head trauma has not been evaluated thus far.

Therefore, the purpose of the present study was to evaluate whether contrast-enhanced FLAIR MR imaging can help detect abnormalities in the brains of symptomatic subjects after mild traumatic brain injury and to determine the usefulness of additional contrast-enhanced FLAIR MR imaging.

## Materials and Methods

This retrospective study was approved by the institutional review board of Seoul Metropolitan Government - Seoul National University Boramae medical center, and patients' informed consent was waived.

### Patient Population

By using a computerized search of our hospital's medical records from October 2010 to February 2012, we identified 91 consecutive patients who visited our emergency department and had undergone brain MR examination because of persistent symptoms following mild closed head injury. Inclusion criteria for the mild traumatic brain injury were based on the American

Congress of Rehabilitation Medicine [Glasgow Coma Score of 13–15, post-traumatic loss of consciousness (LOC) (if present) < 30 min, post-traumatic amnesia (PTA) as measured by the Galveston orientation and amnesia test (if present) <24 h]. Nineteen patients with non-contrast-enhanced MR imaging were excluded. Seven patients with no available medical record about clinical background information were also excluded. Five patients were excluded because they had history of brain surgery or prior head injury before the traumatic event. Six patients were excluded because there was an interval of >14 days between the date of their injuries and MR examinations. A total of 54 patients were included in our retrospective study (M:F = 32:22, mean age: 59.8±16.4, age range: 26–84 years). The reasons for head injury were a fall in 33 patients, traffic accident in 17 patients, violence in 4 patients. CT was performed in all patients during acute hospitalization. All CT examinations found no abnormalities. All MRI examinations were obtained within 14 days after head trauma (mean: 3.2±4.1 days, range: 0.2–14 days). The summary of demographic and clinical characteristics of patients is shown in Table 1.

### MR Imaging Technique

All studies were performed with 3 T MR imaging system (Achieva; Philips Medical Systems, Best, Netherlands) using a 16-channel head coil. Following the acquisition of sagittal scout T1-

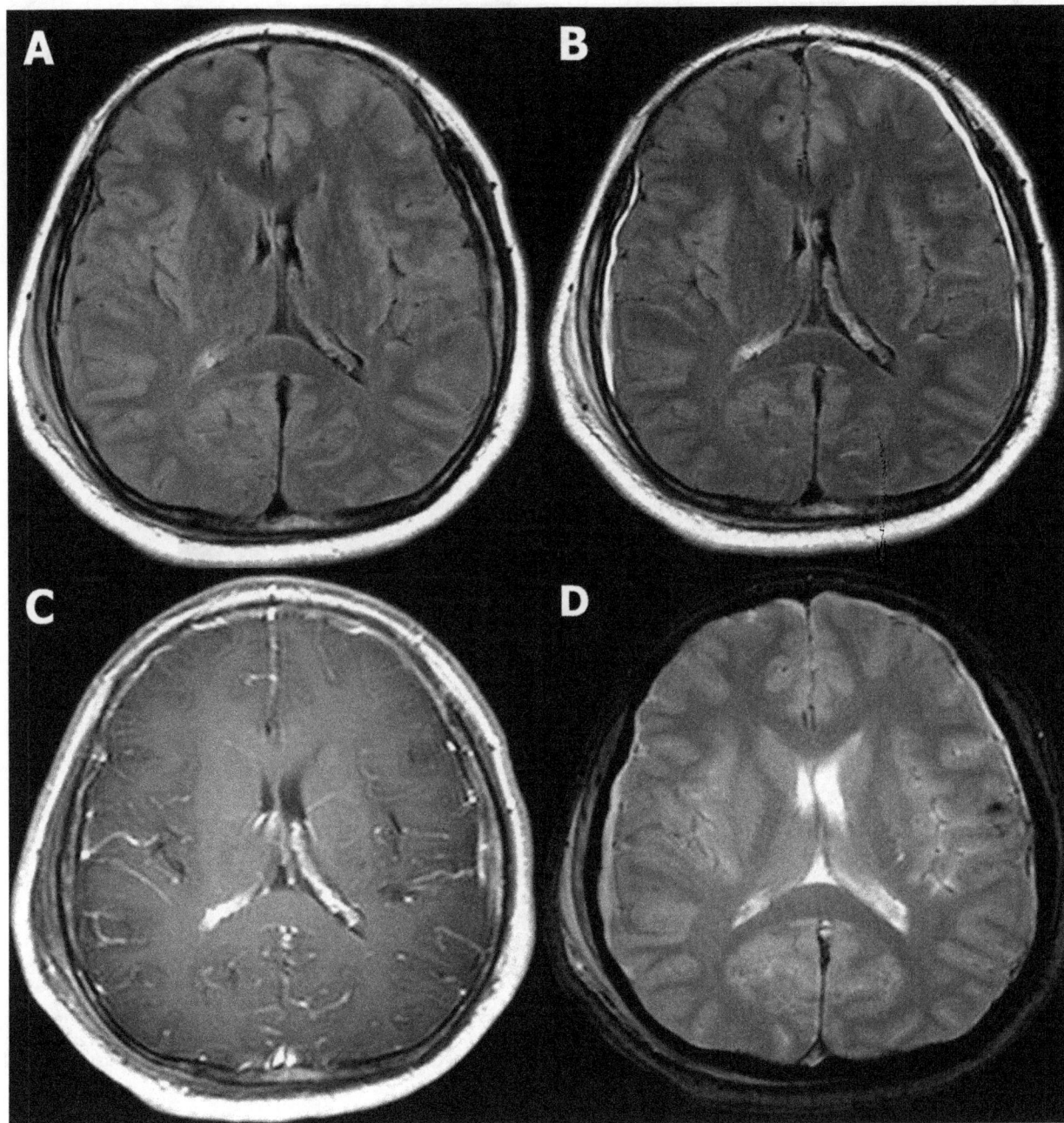

**Figure 1. A 67-year- old male patient with a history of fall down 4 hours ago.** Initial GCS score was 13. The duration of posttraumatic amnesia was 1 hour. (A) Unenhanced FLAIR MR image shows small amount of subdural hemorrhage with iso-signal intensity in Rt. parietal convexity. (B) contrast-enhanced FLAIR MR image clearly demonstrates meningeal enhancement along not only right convexity but also Lt. side. (C) contrast-enhanced T1 weighted image shows no definite enhancement. (D) GRE image depicts hemosiderin deposition only in Lt. cerebral cortex.

weighted images, spine-echo T2-weighted (TR/TEeff 3000/100 ms), spine-echo T1-weighted (TR/TE 260/10 ms; FA 70°), GRE T2*-weighted (TR/TE 724/16 ms; flip angle 18), and T2-FLAIR (TR/TEeff/TI 11000/120/2800 ms) were obtained. After the intravenous administration of 0.1 mmol/kg body weight gadobutrol (Gadovist, Bayer Schering Pharma, Berlin, Germany) over 1 minute, spine-echo T1-weighted and T2-FLAIR images were obtained. The acquisition time for contrast-enhanced FLAIR MR images was 2 minutes 40 seconds to 3 minutes 10 seconds (identical to non-contrast-enhanced FLAIR MR). All images were acquired with a section thickness of 5 mm, an intersection gap of

2 mm, a field of view of 18×18–22×22 cm, and a matrix of 256×192.

## Image analysis

Two experienced neuroradiologists (K.S.C. and R.Y.S. with 6 years of experience) reviewed the anonymized brain images by the consensus method. At the first session, they evaluated 50% of the cases using 2D T1, T2, FLAIR, GRE, and contrast-enhanced T1-weighted images as a routine image sequence and the other 50% using the combination of routine images and contrast-enhanced FLAIR images. After a 4-week interval, the cases were switched

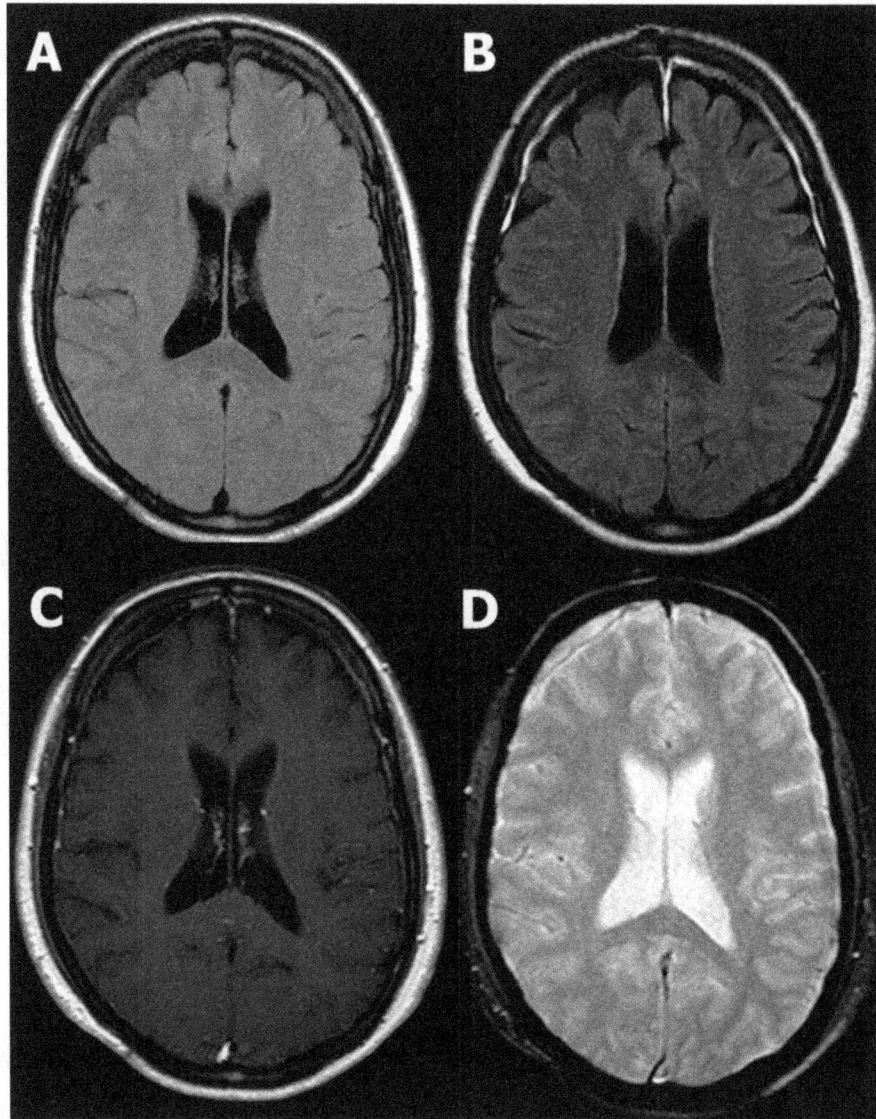

**Figure 2. A 60-year- old female patient with a history of assault 10 hours ago.** Initial GCS score was 15. The duration of posttraumatic amnesia was 3 hours. (B) Contrast-enhanced FLAIR MR image helped to detect small amount of subdural hemorrhage in both frontal convexity which was initially missed, after reviewing meningeal enhancement. No demonstrable abnormality was found on unenhanced FLAIR (A), contrast-enhanced T1 weighted (C) and GRE (D) MR images.

and read again. Each case was assessed for the presence or absence of traumatic brain lesions. Then each lesion was further described as follows: epidural hematoma (EH), subdural hematoma (SDH), subarachnoid hemorrhage (SAH)/intraventricular hemorrhage (IVH), brain contusion/intraparenchymal hemorrhage, and diffuse axonal injury (DAI). In addition, reviewers recorded the presence or absence and location of meningeal enhancement on the contrast-enhanced FLAIR images, dividing them into 3 categories: diffuse meningeal enhancement along both cerebral convexities; localized enhancement over part of 1 cerebral convexity; and enhancement along the falx only. In the localized meningeal convexity enhancement group, the location of meningeal enhancement was matched against the site of injury from medical records and/or scalp hematoma or laceration site demonstrated on imaging.

## Statistical Analysis

All statistical analyses were performed using the SPSS statistical software program (version 20.0, Chicago, III, USA). Comparison of the number of patients with traumatic brain lesions demonstrated on routine images and on the combination of routine images and contrast-enhanced FLAIR image was analyzed using the McNemar test. The unpaired student's $t$-test was used to determine whether the age and time interval of the group that showed meningeal enhancement on contrast-enhanced FLAIR images differed significantly from those of the group showing negative findings. Associations between the clinical values and meningeal enhancement on contrast-enhanced FLAIR were also evaluated by using logistic regression analysis. The data for each parameter were assessed for normality with the Kolmogorov-Smirnov test. In all tests, $P$ values less than 0.05 were considered statistically significant.

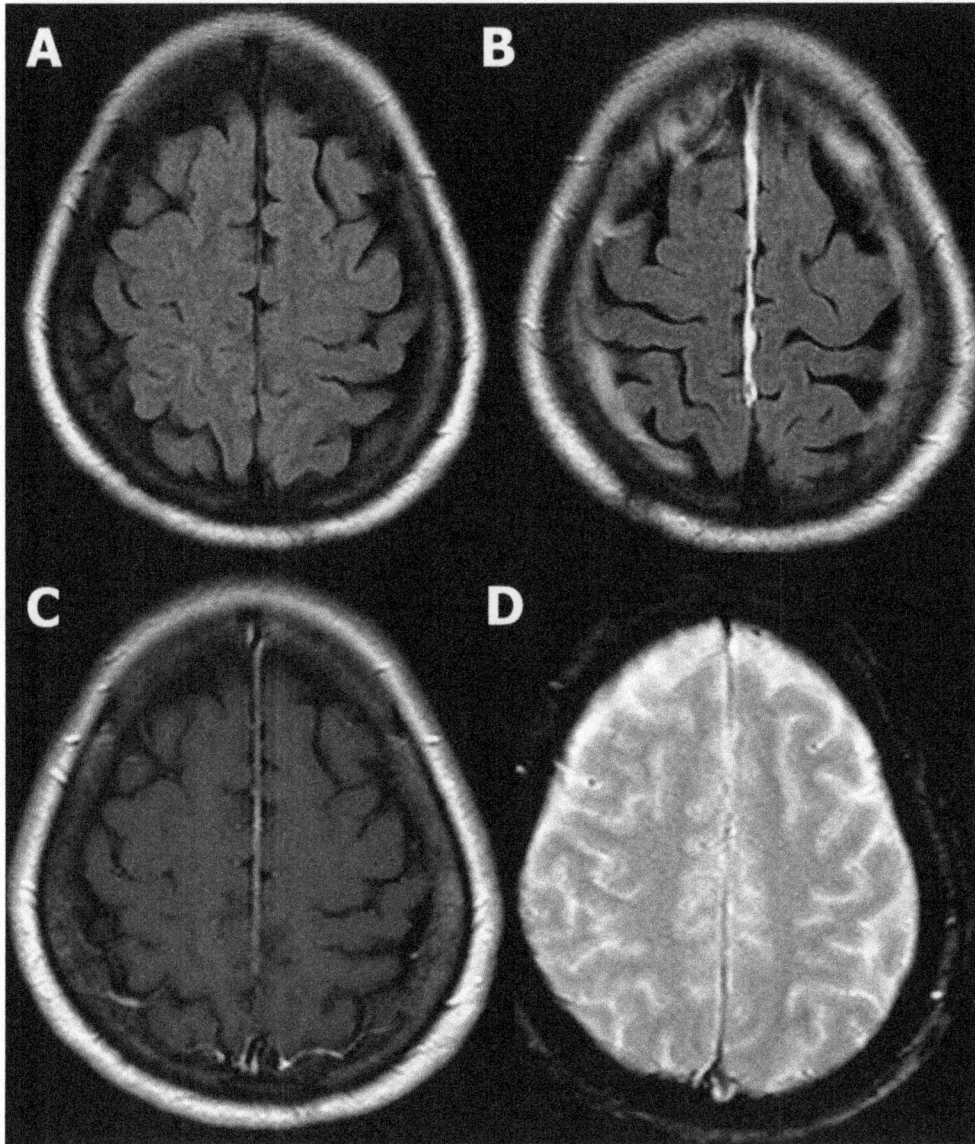

**Figure 3. A 63-year- old female patient with a history of fall down 2 days ago.** Initial GCS score was 15. She had transient episode of loss of consciousness less than 30 min. The duration of posttraumatic amnesia was 2 hours. (B) Only contrast-enhanced FLAIR MR image reveals abnormal finding – meningeal enhancement along falx. No demonstrable abnormality was found on unenhanced FLAIR (A), contrast-enhanced T1 weighted (C) and GRE (D) MR images.

## Results

Twenty-five patients with traumatic brain lesions were identified among 54 total patients after reviewing routine MRI imaging sequences. Out of the 25 patients, 22 patients showed SDH, 13 patients had SAH/IVH, 9 patients demonstrated brain contusion/intraparenchymal hemorrhage, and 3 patients had DAI. Meanwhile, 28 patients with traumatic brain lesions were detected on routine image sequence plus contrast-enhanced FLAIR (Figure 1, 2). Two patients with minimal amounts of SDH and 1 patient with SAH were additionally detected on routine image sequences in retrospect after the findings were depicted on contrast-enhanced FLAIR images (p = 0.25). In 9 patients, only contrast-enhanced FLAIR images demonstrated abnormal meningeal enhancement confined to the falx while the other routine image sequences showed no findings of traumatic brain injury (Figure 3). Overall,

the combination sequence detected 37 patients with abnormalities, significantly more than on routine images alone (p<0.001) (Table 2, Figure 4).

A total of 32 patients demonstrated meningeal enhancement on contrast-enhanced FLAIR images. With regard to the location of meningeal enhancement, 12 patients showed diffuse meningeal enhancement, 8 patients had localized convexity meningeal enhancement, and 12 patients showed meningeal enhancement only along the falx (Table 3). Out of the 8 patients who showed localized convexity meningeal enhancement, the enhancing meningeal site was opposite the injured area in 6 patients (contrecoup). In 1 patient, the site of meningeal enhancement was not obviously related to the area of injury. The exact site of injury could not be located in other patients.

Table 4 shows the results from logistic regression analyses. At univariate analysis, the following clinical entities showed a

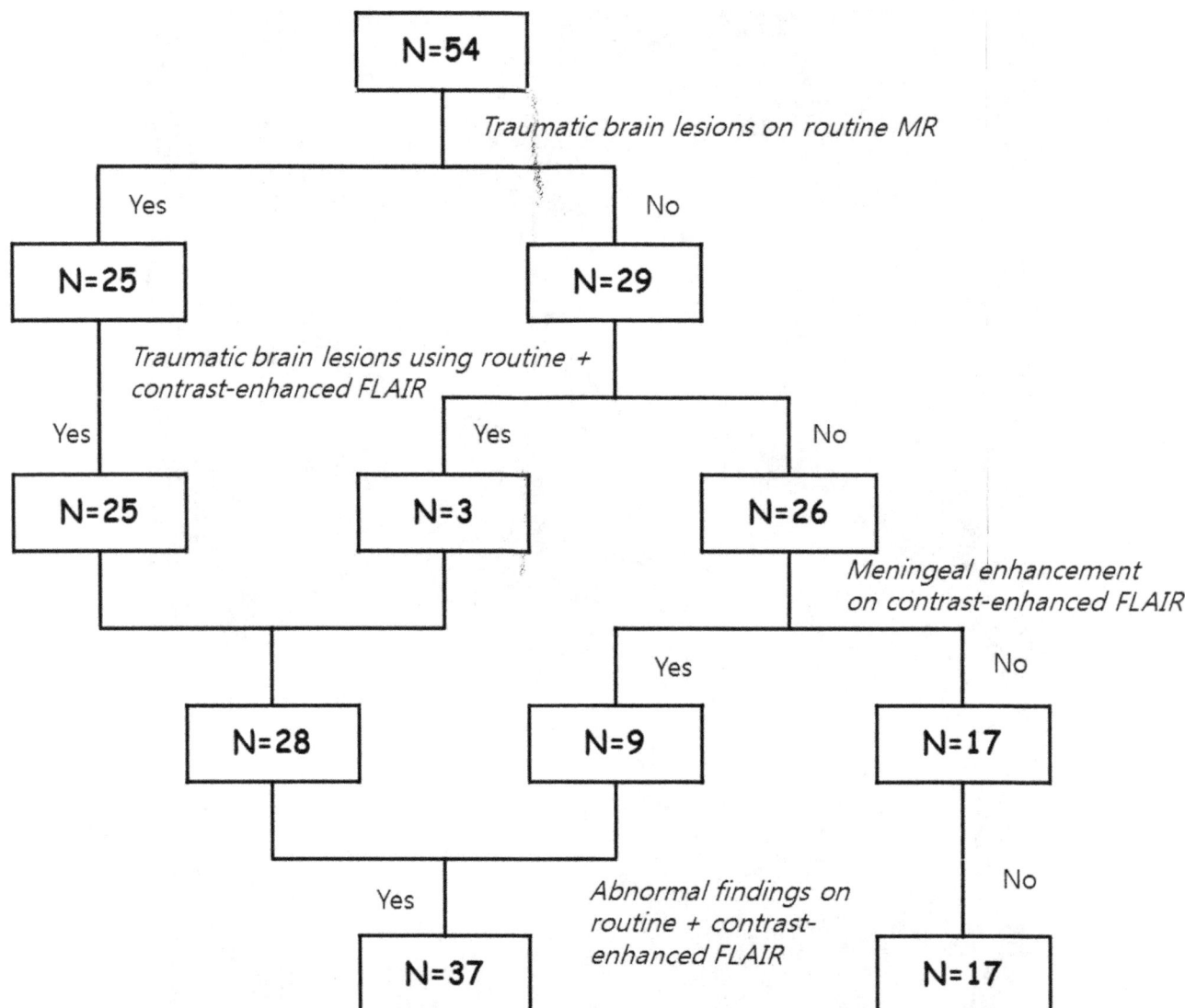

**Figure 4. Diagram of the study results.**

significant association with meningeal enhancement on contrast-enhanced FLAIR images: SAH/IVH, SDH, posttraumatic LOC, and PTA. In multivariate logistic regression analysis, SDH, and posttraumatic LOC still remained significant, with odds ratios 13.068 (95% confidence interval 2.037 to 83.852), and 15.487 (95% confidence interval 2.545 to 94.228), respectively. In subgroup analysis which was used to evaluate the association between the subgroup showing enhancement confined to the falx and the group without any meningeal enhancement, univariate analyses revealed that SDH, posttraumatic LOC and PTA were related to the meningeal enhancement (Table 5). Multivariate analysis showed that SDH and LOC were significantly correlated with the enhancement, with odds ratios 6.878 (95% confidence interval 1.084 to 43.633), and 10.545 (95% confidence interval 1.973 to 56.375), respectively (Table 5).

## Discussion

Our study verified the benefit of contrast-enhanced FLAIR images in detecting traumatic brain injury. In 32 patients, contrast-enhanced FLAIR images clearly demonstrated thick

linear enhancement of the dura. Normal dura mater shows only thin, linear, and discontinuous enhancement on contrast enhanced T1-weighted MR images due to lack of sufficient water to generate the T1 shortening required for vivid enhancement. When water accumulates within the dura mater, contrast enhancement can occur [17]. It is well known that various benign or malignant conditions, including intracranial hypotension, granulomatous disease, and metastatic disease can be associated with dural enhancement on contrast-enhanced T1-weighted MR images [17], [18]. In addition, many prior studies have demonstrated that patients who have undergone intracranial surgery show postoperative dural enhancement [19] [19–23]. This is held to be due to a local inflammatory response initiated by the bleeding from surgical violation of the dura [21], [1].

Little is known about the relationship between meningeal changes and brain trauma. Sze reported enhancement of the meninges as a result of bleeding into the subarachnoid space after subarachnoid hemorrhage from a presumed aneurysm. The researcher suggested that any process that causes bleeding into the CSF can result in abnormal meningeal enhancement [18].

**Table 2.** Comparison of the number of patients with traumatic brain lesions demonstrated on routine images and on the combination of routine images and contrast-enhanced fluid-attenuated inversion recovery (FLAIR) image.

| | T2+T1+GRE+FLAIR+ Contrast-enhanced T1WI | Plus contrast-enhanced FLAIR |
|---|---|---|
| **1) Patient with TBI (n/54)*** | **25** | **28** |
| EH | 0 | 0 |
| SAH/IVH | 13 | 14 |
| SDH | 22 | 24 |
| Brain contusion/intraparenchymal hemorrhage | 9 | 9 |
| DAI | 3 | 3 |
| **p = 0.250** | | |
| **1) + Patient with only meningeal enhancement on contrast-enhanced FLAIR (n/54)*** | **25+0** | **28+9** |
| **p<0.001** | | |

*Number of patients with traumatic brain lesions among a total of 54 patients.
Note − TBI indicates traumatic brain injury; EH, epidural hemorrhage; SAH, subarachnoid hemorrhage; IVH, intraventricular hemorrhage; SDH, subdural hemorrhage; DAI, diffuse axonal injury.

Similarly, according to pathological-anatomical studies, SDHs are actually intradural hematomas, where the dura comprises the outer layer and the inner layer is formed by the arachnoid, covered by a thin layer of dura border cells [24–27]. Early dural enhancement without associated thickening of the meninges is probably caused by vascular congestion and/or increased vascular permeability in the outer dural layer [19], [21].

In our study, 23 out of 28 patients who had any traumatic brain lesions showed meningeal enhancement, while only 5 patients with traumatic brain lesions showed no enhancement. Our results showed association between the presence of SAH or SDH and meningeal enhancement, consistent with the findings of prior studies [6], [19], [21].

According to Mathews et al., contrast-enhanced fast FLAIR images can depict lower concentrations of gadolinium compared with T1-weighted images. The finding that slow-flowing blood is not usually hyperintense on contrast-enhanced fast FLAIR images allows clearer distinction between enhancing meninges or superficial parenchyma and enhancing cortical veins [14]. In our study, the low concentrations of contrast material associated with minor meningeal or venous injury, or with small hemorrhages from trauma, caused prominent meningeal enhancement on contrast-enhanced FLAIR images, as opposed to the equivocal enhancement seen on contrast-enhanced T1-weighted images, which may be confused with cortical veins. The brighter enhancement aided in the detection of additional traumatic brain lesions. In 2 SDHs and 1 SAH, which were initially missed with routine image sequences, prominent meningeal enhancement on contrast-enhanced FLAIR images pointed to small amounts of hemorrhage around the enhancing or opposite convexity on routine image sequences. We expect that the additional finding that the focal convexity meningeal enhancement was usually in a contrecoup location opposite the trauma site may help radiologists to find more lesions.

Interestingly, we found 9 patients without traumatic brain lesions on routine image sequences and only meningeal enhancement along the falx on contrast-enhanced FLAIR images. Traumatic interhemispheric subdural hematoma (ISH) is a known

**Table 3.** The location of meningeal enhancement on contrast-enhanced fluid-attenuated inversion recovery (FLAIR) image and the number of patients with traumatic brain lesions.

| Factor | Positive meningeal enhancement | | | | Negative*(n = 22/54) |
|---|---|---|---|---|---|
| | Diffuse (n = 12/54) | Localized (n = 8/54) | Falx cerebri (n = 12/54) | Total (n = 32/54) | |
| **TBI (n/28)†** | 12 | 8 | 3 | 23 | 5 |
| SAH/IVH | 7 | 5 | 0 | 12 | 2 |
| SDH | 10 | 7 | 2 | 19 | 5 |
| Brain contusion/intraparenchymal hemorrhage | 6 | 1 | 0 | 7 | 2 |
| DAI | 0 | 1 | 1 | 2 | 1 |
| **TI (days)‡** | 4.3±4.3 | 0.9±1.4 | 2.9±5.3 | 2.9±4.4 | 3.5±3.9 |

*Number of patients who showed no meningeal enhancement on contrast-enhanced FLAIR images among a total of 54 patients.
†Number of patients out of 28 patients who were identified as having a TBI using the combination of routine images and contrast-enhanced FLAIR image.
‡The data are the means ± standard deviations.
Note − TBI indicates traumatic brain injury; SAH, subarachnoid hemorrhage; IVH, intraventricular hemorrhage; SDH, subdural hemorrhage; DAI, diffuse axonal injury; TI, time interval.

**Table 4.** Association between meningeal enhancement on contrast-enhanced fluid-attenuated inversion recovery (FLAIR) images and clinical values.

| Variable | Univariate Analysis | | Multivariate Analysis | |
|---|---|---|---|---|
| | **Odds Ratio** | **PValue** | **Odds Ratio** | **PValue** |
| SAH/IVH | **6.000 (1.187, 30.324)** | **0.030** | 2.356 (0.278, 19.981) | 0.432 |
| SDH | **4.969 (1.465, 16.856)** | **0.010** | **13.068 (2.037, 83.852)** | **0.007** |
| Brain contusion/intraparenchymal hemorrhage | 2.800 (0.523, 14.992) | 0.229 | ... | ... |
| DAI | 1.4 (0.119, 16.459) | 0.789 | ... | ... |
| Posttraumatic LOC | **11.217 (2.753, 45.697)** | **0.001** | **15.487 (2.545, 94.228)** | **0.003** |
| PTA | **9.545 (1.122, 81.198)** | **0.039** | 12.640 (0.925,172.788) | 0.057 |
| Age* | ... | 0.558 | ... | ... |
| TI* | ... | 0.651 | ... | ... |
| GCS | | 0.716 | ... | ... |
| GCS (15) | 1 | | ... | ... |
| GCS (14) | 0.000 | 0.999 | ... | ... |
| GCS (13) | 0.357 (0.030, 4.214) | 0.414 | ... | ... |

*Determined with the unpaired student's t-test.
Note — SAH indicates subarachnoid hemorrhage; IVH, intraventricular hemorrhage; SDH, subdural hemorrhage; DAI, diffuse axonal injury; LOC, loss of consciousness; PTA, post-traumatic amnesia; TI, time interval; GCS, Glasgow Coma Score.

but uncommon complication of head trauma. It is most likely due to laceration of either the parafalcine or parasagittal bridging veins between the medial border of the cerebral hemisphere and the sinus caused by linear brain acceleration during trauma [28], [29]. Although obvious subdural hematoma, which can be demonstrated on routine image sequences, did not arise, we presumed that minor lacerations sufficient for inducing contrast enhancement on contrast-enhanced FLAIR images occurred in the 9 patients. From our results, we found that the incidence of minor injury along the

interhemispheric fissure is not rare, as opposed to other reports on ISH.

We found that SDH and posttraumatic LOC were significantly associated with meningeal enhancement. In patients with isolated falcine enhancement, those were still statistically correlated with enhancement. Previous studies have shown poorer neuropsychologic performance after mild TBI complicated by a brain lesion compared with uncomplicated mild TBI despite similar GCS scores between these 2 TBI populations [30–32]. Therefore, we

**Table 5.** Association between meningeal enhancement confined to the falx on contrast-enhanced fluid-attenuated inversion recovery (FLAIR) images and clinical values.

| Variable | Univariate Analysis | | Multivariate Analysis | |
|---|---|---|---|---|
| | **Odds Ratio** | **PValue** | **Odds Ratio** | **PValue** |
| SAH/IVH | 0.000 | 0.998 | ... | ... |
| SDH | **5.500 (1.073, 28.198)** | **0.041** | **6.878 (1.084, 43.633)** | **0.007** |
| Brain contusion/intraparenchymal hemorrhage | 0.000 | 0.999 | ... | ... |
| DAI | 1.818 (0.151, 21.962) | 0.638 | ... | ... |
| Posttraumatic LOC | **10.320 (2.177, 48.925)** | **0.003** | **10.545 (1.973, 56.375)** | **0.003** |
| PTA | **4.286 (1.019, 18.029)** | **0.047** | 3.018 (0.530, 17.192) | 0.213 |
| Age* | ... | 0.742 | ... | ... |
| TI* | ... | 0.157 | ... | ... |
| GCS | | 0.791 | ... | ... |
| GCS (15) | 1 | | ... | ... |
| GCS (14) | 1.900 (0.156, 23.135) | 0.615 | ... | ... |
| GCS (13) | 1.900 (0.156, 23.135) | 0.615 | ... | ... |

*Determined with the unpaired student's t-test.
Note — SAH indicates subarachnoid hemorrhage; IVH, intraventricular hemorrhage; SDH, subdural hemorrhage; DAI, diffuse axonal injury; LOC, loss of consciousness; PTA, post-traumatic amnesia; TI, time interval; GCS, Glasgow Coma Score.

believe that the presence of meningeal enhancement implies clinically significant brain injury.

Our study has some limitations. First, in the present study, administration of contrast material is needed. However, many clinicians request a contrast study for various reasons, including evaluation of brain pathology other than traumatic lesion, which may cause the patient's symptoms, or for evaluation of intracranial and extracranial vessels. So, in case of contrast study was performed in patients with mild head injury, our result will be helpful. Moreover, meningeal enhancement depicted on contrast-enhanced FLAIR image can suggest trauma event when there is unclear history of head trauma. Second, the duration of meningeal enhancement was not evaluated, because in a majority of cases, follow-up MR exam was not performed. However, in 3 patients who underwent two MR examinations at 1 day and 1 week after the head injury, 2 patients showed persistent enhancement and 1 patient showed resolution of enhancement on follow-up MR exam. In a patient with 2 follow-up MR studies performed at 1 week and 2 years after the head injury, the meningeal enhancement was decreased after 1 week and resolved after 2 years. We propose that meningeal enhancement becomes less intense over time as a result of resolution of reactive changes related to the presence of blood. However, prior report of persistence of prolonged enhancement and thickening of the dura even years after surgery due to granulation tissue indicate that meningeal enhancement after trauma might be persistent after several years [23]. Third, we could not use SWI as a routine image sequence, since GRE image rather than SWI were routinely obtained in our hospital due to clinician's request during study period. SWI is more sensitive than GRE image for the detection of

microhemorrhages, but successful implementation may be difficult due to the longer acquisition time, particularly in head trauma patients who are motion-prone in clinical setting. Moreover, as SWI is more susceptible to artifacts caused by calvaria, susceptibility artifacts arising from field inhomogeneities at the interfaces between bone and tissue, the detection of small SAH and SDH may be limited. Soman et al. reported that GRE was superior to SWI with regard to T2* lesion conspicuity in one case with cortical venous thrombosis due to worsened calvarial artifacts adjacent to the T2* lesion [33].

Despite all these limitations, our study revealed that contrast-enhanced FLAIR images help detect meningeal enhancement in patients with symptomatic closed mild head injuries, and the enhancement often points to traumatic brain lesions. Further research is needed to establish the direct relation between meningeal enhancement on contrast-enhanced FLAIR images and neurocognitive consequences, but the presence of meningeal enhancement on contrast-enhanced FLAIR images may imply significant head injury. Because FLAIR images after administration of contrast material may provide additional information, contrast-enhanced FLAIR MR imaging is recommended when a contrast MR study is indicated in a patient with a symptomatic prior closed mild head injury.

## Author Contributions

Conceived and designed the experiments: SCK SWP IR SCJ. Performed the experiments: SCK SWP IR. Analyzed the data: SCK IR SHC JHK CHS. Contributed reagents/materials/analysis tools: SWP SCJ TJY SHC JHK CHS. Wrote the paper: SCK. Acquisition of data: SCK SWP IR SCJ TJY.

## References

1. Evans RW (1992) The postconcussion syndrome and the sequelae of mild head injury. Neurol Clin 10: 815–847.
2. McAllister TW (1992) Neuropsychiatric sequelae of head injuries. Psychiatr Clin North Am 15: 395–413.
3. Provenzale JM (2010) Imaging of traumatic brain injury: a review of the recent medical literature. AJR Am J Roentgenol 194: 16–19.
4. Akiyama Y, Miyata K, Harada K, Minamida Y, Nonaka T, et al. (2009) Susceptibility-weighted magnetic resonance imaging for the detection of cerebral microhemorrhage in patients with traumatic brain injury. Neurol Med Chir (Tokyo) 49: 97–99; discussion 99.
5. Scheid R, Ott DV, Roth H, Schroeter ML, von Cramon DY (2007) Comparative magnetic resonance imaging at 1.5 and 3 Tesla for the evaluation of traumatic microbleeds. J Neurotrauma 24: 1811–1816.
6. Rutgers DR, Toulgoat F, Cazejust J, Fillard P, Lasjaunias P, et al. (2008) White matter abnormalities in mild traumatic brain injury: a diffusion tensor imaging study. AJNR Am J Neuroradiol 29: 514–519.
7. Salmond CH, Menon DK, Chatfield DA, Williams GB, Pena A, et al. (2006) Diffusion tensor imaging in chronic head injury survivors: correlations with learning and memory indices. Neuroimage 29: 117–124.
8. Inglese M, Makani S, Johnson G, Cohen BA, Silver JA, et al. (2005) Diffuse axonal injury in mild traumatic brain injury: a diffusion tensor imaging study. J Neurosurg 103: 298–303.
9. Huisman TA, Schwamm LH, Schaefer PW, Koroshetz WJ, Shetty-Alva N, et al. (2004) Diffusion tensor imaging as potential biomarker of white matter injury in diffuse axonal injury. AJNR Am J Neuroradiol 25: 370–376.
10. Arfanakis K, Haughton VM, Carew JD, Rogers BP, Dempsey RJ, et al. (2002) Diffusion tensor MR imaging in diffuse axonal injury. AJNR Am J Neuroradiol 23: 794–802.
11. Gasparotti R, Pinelli L, Liserre R (2011) New MR sequences in daily practice: susceptibility weighted imaging. A pictorial essay. Insights Imaging 2: 335–347.
12. Masutani Y, Aoki S, Abe O, Hayashi N, Otomo K (2003) MR diffusion tensor imaging: recent advance and new techniques for diffusion tensor visualization. Eur J Radiol 46: 53–66.
13. Ercan N, Gultekin S, Celik H, Tali TE, Oner YA, et al. (2004) Diagnostic value of contrast-enhanced fluid-attenuated inversion recovery MR imaging of intracranial metastases. AJNR Am J Neuroradiol 25: 761–765.
14. Mathews VP, Caldemeyer KS, Lowe MJ, Greenspan SL, Weber DM, et al. (1999) Brain: gadolinium-enhanced fast fluid-attenuated inversion-recovery MR imaging. Radiology 211: 257–263.
15. Fukuoka H, Hirai T, Okuda T, Shigematsu Y, Sasao A, et al. (2010) Comparison of the added value of contrast-enhanced 3D fluid-attenuated

inversion recovery and magnetization-prepared rapid acquisition of gradient echo sequences in relation to conventional postcontrast T1-weighted images for the evaluation of leptomeningeal diseases at 3T. AJNR Am J Neuroradiol 31: 868–873.
16. Goo HW, Choi CG (2003) Post-contrast FLAIR MR imaging of the brain in children: normal and abnormal intracranial enhancement. Pediatr Radiol 33: 843–849.
17. Smirniotopoulos JG, Murphy FM, Rushing EJ, Rees JH, Schroeder JW (2007) Patterns of contrast enhancement in the brain and meninges. Radiographics 27: 525–551.
18. Sze G (1993) Diseases of the intracranial meninges: MR imaging features. AJR Am J Roentgenol 160: 727–733.
19. Dolinskas CA, Simeone FA (1998) Surgical site after resection of a meningioma. AJNR Am J Neuroradiol 19: 419–426.
20. Henegar MM, Moran CJ, Silbergeld DL (1996) Early postoperative magnetic resonance imaging following nonneoplastic cortical resection. J Neurosurg 84: 174–179.
21. Burke JW, Podrasky AE, Bradley WG, Jr. (1990) Meninges: benign postoperative enhancement on MR images. Radiology 174: 99–102.
22. Sato N, Bronen RA, Sze G, Kawamura Y, Coughlin W, et al. (1997) Postoperative changes in the brain: MR imaging findings in patients without neoplasms. Radiology 204: 839–846.
23. Elster AD, DiPersio DA (1990) Cranial postoperative site: assessment with contrast-enhanced MR imaging. Radiology 174: 93–98.
24. Haines DE (1991) On the question of a subdural space. Anat Rec 230: 3–21.
25. Haines DE, Harkey HL, al-Mefty O (1993) The "subdural" space: a new look at an outdated concept. Neurosurgery 32: 111–120.
26. Domenicucci M, Strzelecki JW, Delfini R (1998) Acute posttraumatic subdural hematomas: "intradural" computed tomographic appearance as a favorable prognostic factor. Neurosurgery 42: 51–55.
27. Atkinson JL, Lane JI, Aksamit AJ (2003) MRI depiction of chronic intradural (subdural) hematoma in evolution. J Magn Reson Imaging 17: 484–486.
28. Rapana A, Lamaida E, Pizza V, Lepore P, Caputi F, et al. (1997) Inter-hemispheric scissure, a rare location for a traumatic subdural hematoma, case report and review of the literature. Clin Neurol Neurosurg 99: 124–129.
29. Romano VA, Toffol GJ (1994) Confirmation of traumatic interhemispheric subdural hematoma by magnetic resonance imaging. J Emerg Med 12: 369–373.
30. Williams DH, Levin HS, Eisenberg HM (1990) Mild head injury classification. Neurosurgery 27: 422–428.

# 7

# Clinical Comparison of $^{99m}$Tc Exametazime and $^{123}$I Ioflupane SPECT in Patients with Chronic Mild Traumatic Brain Injury

**Andrew B. Newberg[1]\*, Mijail Serruya[2], Andrew Gepty[1], Charles Intenzo[3], Todd Lewis[4], Daniel Amen[5], David S. Russell[6,7], Nancy Wintering[1]**

1 Myrna Brind Center of Integrative Medicine, Thomas Jefferson University, Philadelphia, Pennsylvania, United States of America, 2 Department of Neurology, Thomas Jefferson University, Philadelphia, Pennsylvania, United States of America, 3 Department of Radiology, Thomas Jefferson University, Philadelphia, Pennsylvania, United States of America, 4 Magee Rehabilitation Hospital, Philadelphia, Pennsylvania, United States of America, 5 Amen Clinics, Inc., Newport Beach, California, United States of America, 6 Institute for Neurodegenerative Disorders, New Haven, Connecticut, United States of America, 7 Yale University School of Medicine, New Haven, Connecticut, United States of America

## Abstract

*Background:* This study evaluated the clinical interpretations of single photon emission computed tomography (SPECT) using a cerebral blood flow and a dopamine transporter tracer in patients with chronic mild traumatic brain injury (TBI). The goal was to determine how these two different scan might be used and compared to each other in this patient population.

*Methods and Findings:* Twenty-five patients with persistent symptoms after a mild TBI underwent SPECT with both $^{99m}$Tc exametazime to measure cerebral blood flow (CBF) and $^{123}$I ioflupane to measure dopamine transporter (DAT) binding. The scans were interpreted by two expert readers blinded to any case information and were assessed for abnormal findings in comparison to 10 controls for each type of scan. Qualitative CBF scores for each cortical and subcortical region along with DAT binding scores for the striatum were compared to each other across subjects and to controls. In addition, symptoms were compared to brain scan findings. TBI patients had an average of 6 brain regions with abnormal perfusion compared to controls who had an average of 2 abnormal regions (p<0.001). Patient with headaches had lower CBF in the right frontal lobe, and higher CBF in the left parietal lobe compared to patients without headaches. Lower CBF in the right temporal lobe correlated with poorer reported physical health. Higher DAT binding was associated with more depressive symptoms and overall poorer reported mental health. There was no clear association between CBF and DAT binding in these patients.

*Conclusions:* Overall, both scans detected abnormalities in brain function, but appear to reflect different types of physiological processes associated with chronic mild TBI symptoms. Both types of scans might have distinct uses in the evaluation of chronic TBI patients depending on the clinical scenario.

**Editor:** Emmanuel Andreas Stamatakis, University Of Cambridge, United Kingdom

**Funding:** This work was supported by a grant from GE Healthcare, Princeton, NJ. The funders had no role in study design, data collection and analysis, decision to publish, or preparation of the manuscript.

**Competing Interests:** Dr. Andrew Newberg's Institution received a grant from GE Healthcare in order to perform the study reported in the paper. However, GE Healthcare had no role in study design, data collection and analysis, decision to publish, or preparation of the manuscript. Dr. Daniel Amen is employed by the commercial company, Amen Clinics, Inc. Dr. John Russell is employed by the commercial company, Molecular Neuroimaging.

\* E-mail: Andrew.newberg@jefferson.edu

## Introduction

Traumatic Brain Injury (TBI) is a major public health concern. Although the medical community has long understood the potential detriment of head injury [1], there has been a resurgence of interest regarding the importance of TBI in individuals participating in contact sports, patients with various psychological or neurological dysfunction, and the population in general. In addition, it has been observed that TBI survivors, even those with mild injury, commonly face a range of clinical symptoms affecting functional status, cognition, and mood [2]. While not everyone with a mild brain injury has lasting symptoms, those who do often present daunting problems regarding the differential diagnosis and treatment [3,4]. Furthermore, since TBI can be heterogeneous in terms of its definition, effects, and prognosis, it is often unclear how a given TBI or multiple TBIs in the same individual will affect the brain's physiology and how such changes may affect clinical symptoms [5,6]. For those individuals managing patients with a history of TBI and persistent symptoms, knowledge of the underlying brain physiology may ultimately be highly beneficial for understanding the effects of the TBI and perhaps even target future therapy. Functional neuroimaging is increasingly considered an important clinical tool in the management of TBI patients [7–9]. This may especially be the case in patients with a history of TBI with chronic symptoms. Importantly, functional brain imaging may help remove some of the stigma associated with chronic symptoms such as headache, difficulty concentrating, or mood changes that are otherwise difficult to evaluate [10]. If a physiological basis for such symptoms can be established, patients can better understand the nature of their symptoms and hopefully be more compliant with treatment, whether it is medical, occupational, physical, or psychological. For example, post traumatic headache, which occurs in up to 70% of patients in the first year and 25% after the first year [11], is frequently debated as an entity due to a variety of factors including medicolegal influences and a pathophysiology that is not completely understood [12]. The possible pathophysiological mechanism may be related to neurogenic inflammation characterized by locally increased blood flow, plasma protein leakage from blood vessels, mast cell degranulation, and platelet aggregation [13]. This inflammation can be related to the head injury process itself or may be related to direct injury to the trigeminal afferent nerves or to the leptomeningeal or cerebrovascular structures that are innervated by trigeminal nerves [14]. The inflammatory response is likely mediated by glial cells which release a variety of cytokines that cause the release of pain modulators from trigeminal neurons ultimately resulting in headache.

Over the past two decades, a number of researchers, including our group, have focused on the utility of single photon emission computed tomography (SPECT) brain imaging to evaluate the neurophysiology of a variety of conditions and disorders. Depending on the tracer used, SPECT imaging can be useful for studying cerebral blood flow (CBF), dopamine transporter function, serotonin transporter function, as well as other processes [15–17]. Several studies have also shown that SPECT imaging of CBF can be helpful in TBI patients [18]. Specifically, CBF SPECT scans can demonstrate areas of impaired brain function which can help identify if trauma is present and which brain system or systems are most affected. Common findings on SPECT imaging in TBI patients include the following [9,15,19,20]:

- focal decreased CBF near the focal site of injury and/or opposite side (contra coup)
- asymmetrical hypoperfusion in the prefrontal, temporal, parietal or occipital lobes
- decreased CBF in the anterior temporal poles
- decreased CBF in the contralateral cerebellar perfusion.

Early studies suggested that SPECT scans may aid in understanding a TBI patient's symptomatology [21,22]. More recently, some investigators have suggested that SPECT imaging could even assist clinicians in developing treatment strategies. For example, decreased prefrontal cortex perfusion, which can be associated with executive dysfunction arguably may be helped with psychostimulants [23,24] or other interventions to enhance the function of the frontal lobes. Temporal lobe hypoperfusion has been associated with irritability and mood instability that may be improved with anticonvulsant or antidepressant medication. However, studies and case reports have reported variable success in the management of TBI patients [25,26]. Furthermore, since different pharmacological treatments have not always demonstrated a benefit in this population, future studies are required to better assess how well certain clinical and imaging findings can be used to direct therapy.

SPECT may be more useful than other structural imaging techniques such as magnetic resonance imaging (MRI) or x-ray computed tomography (CT) in TBI patients [27]. TBI patients often report symptoms such as headaches, memory loss, concentration difficulties, perceptual sensitivities, dizziness, or emotional liability, even when CT and/or MRI scans demonstrate no clear abnormalities [28,29,30]. Such patients may be labeled as somatic or malingering, especially when there are no significant neuroimaging abnormalities present. However, researchers investigating the differences between functional and structural imaging techniques have found SPECT to be more sensitive for detecting abnormalities in patients with varying degrees of TBI [31]. Thus, it is possible that patients with TBI will demonstrate functional abnormalities on SPECT imaging that may relate to their persistent clinical symptoms.

In addition to alterations in CBF, a growing amount of evidence implicates damage to neurotransmitter systems, such as the dopaminergic nervous system, in association with TBI [32]. For example, after experimental TBI, regional increases in dopamine levels at acute time points after acceleration–deceleration brain injury have been observed [33]. Interestingly, cortical tissue dopamine levels are actually depressed for up to 2 weeks post brain injury [34]. Increases in human cerebrospinal fluid (CSF) dopamine and its metabolites post-TBI appear to depend on both gender and genetic variations in the dopamine transporter (DAT). Increased dopamine metabolism may represent a compensatory response to increased tissue dopamine levels or may be due to additional direct effects of TBI on the regulation of the dopamine system. The consequences of such changes might be beneficial in that dopamine neurotransmission is restored after TBI or could potentially be deleterious due to dopamine-induced oxidative stress.

Another line of evidence regarding the dopaminergic effect of TBI is that dopamine receptor agonists often benefit patients via the promotion of central dopaminergic transmission [23,24]. This could be a sign that dopamine release is suppressed after injury, that dopamine uptake by the DAT is increased, or some combination of the two. Alternatively, dopamine activity may remain normal after injury, but this level of dopamine activity is not adequate in the face of the injury-induced disruptions. Given that a few studies have demonstrated beneficial effects with dopamine antagonists, it should also be acknowledged that TBI results in a complex series of injuries to a wide range of different brain structures. It is important to acknowledge that any systemic treatment for TBIwithout a well-defined window for therapy could be both beneficial and/or detrimental to the recovery process. For this reason, understanding the effect of TBI on dopamine transmission is crucial for developing a proper therapeutic plan and for promoting optimal recovery.

The current study was designed to evaluate for the first time CBF and dopamine transporter binding in the same patient with TBI and chronic symptoms. Two reviewers read the scans together using a visual scoring system based upon common clinical approaches to evaluating these scans so that this data could be more easily utilized in current clinical practice. Scan findings that were considered mild, moderate, or severe, could then be provided a numerical value to assist in a more quantitative analysis of the data. This approach was similar to previous comparison studies performed by our group for functional neuroimaging studies [35,36]. Thus, the overall purpose of this study was to assess the ability of $^{99m}$Tc Exametazime (Ceretec$^{TM}$; GE Healthcare) SPECT to detect changes in CBF and compare those changes to DAT binding evaluated with $^{123}$I Ioflupane (DaTscan$^{TM}$; GE Healthcare) SPECT in the same TBI patients with chronic symptoms. These scan findings were then compared to clinical symptoms and neuropsychological test measures of mood, health, and cognitive function. The goal is to help further develop the use of SPECT imaging in TBI patients presenting with chronic symptoms by determining how each of these two SPECT tracers may help clinicians better evaluate such patients.

## Materials and Methods

### Ethics Statements

This research was approved by the Thomas Jefferson University Institutional Review Board. Written informed consent, approved by the Thomas Jefferson University Institutional Review Board, was received from all patients who participated in the study. The clinical Investigation was conducted according to the principles expressed in the Declaration of Helsinki.

### Subjects Selection

Twenty-five patients (14M/11F; mean age $51 \pm 16$) with one or more prior traumatic brain injuries with chronic symptoms (see demographics in Table 1) were recruited. Subjects were recruited primarily from the Neurology Department at Thomas Jefferson University and also from the Concussion Clinic at Magee Rehabilitation Hospital both in Philadelphia. All subjects were evaluated with both $^{99m}$Tc Exametazime and $^{123}$I Ioflupane SPECT. The scans from these subjects were also compared to 10 $^{99m}$Tc Exametazime SPECT scans from control subjects with no history of head injury (5M/5F; mean age $54 \pm 6$) and 10 $^{123}$I Ioflupane SPECT scans from another group of control subjects also with no history of head injury (5M/5F; mean age $57 \pm 14$). $^{123}$I Ioflupane SPECT scans were obtained for the age and gender matched healthy control subjects from the Parkinson Progression Marker Initiative database (www.ppmi-info.org) and subjected to the identical analysis. All TBI patients had a history of at least one prior head injury over 6 months prior to the scan with continued symptoms that included memory loss or other cognitive problems (N = 20), headaches (N = 9), emotional problems such as anxiety or depression symptoms (N = 11), or other symptoms (see Table 1 for patient demographics and TBI history). Most subjects were currently employed or were students such that their TBI symptoms did not limit their capacity to function. Subjects did not have other neurological disorders or meet criteria for chronic traumatic encephalitis.

All subjects were evaluated with several neuropsychological questionnaires to assess health and emotional status including the Profile of Mood Scale (POMS) which measures six identifiable mood or affective states: Tension-Anxiety, Depression-Dejection, Anger-Hostility, Fatigue-Inertia, and Confusion-Bewilderment [37], the Spielberger State-Trait Anxiety Inventory (STAI) to measure anxiety [38], the Beck Depression Inventory (BDI) to measure depressive symptoms [39], and the Short Form-12 (SF-12) for general health [40] which is also subsequently divided into the Physical Component Score (PCS) and Mental Component Score (MCS).

### SPECT Acquisition

All scans were performed at the Thomas Jefferson University Department of Nuclear Medicine according to their standard clinical protocols. Approximately 10 minutes prior to injection, an intravenous cannula (IV) was placed in one arm. For CBF scans, each subject was injected with their eyes open and ears unoccluded in a dimly lit room with limited ambient environmental stimuli. Subjects received the recommended $^{99m}$Tc Exametazime dosage in the package insert of 370–740 MBq (10–20 mCi) intravenously. Imaging was performed on a Philips Forte dual headed SPECT scanner with ultrahigh resolution low energy collimators approximately 30 minutes after injection and acquired over 30 minutes. Images were reconstructed in the axial, sagittal, and coronal

planes using filtered back projection and Chang's attenuation correction. Within one month of the CBF SPECT scan, subjects underwent dopamine transporter SPECT imaging. For this scan, patients received 16 drops of Lugol's solution for thyroid blocking approximately 30 minutes prior to injection. Ten minutes prior to injection, an IV canula was placed in one arm. Each subject received 111 to 185 MBq (3 to 5 mCi) of $^{123}$I Ioflupane intravenously as per the package insert. They underwent scanning approximately 3 hours after injection for 45 minutes.

### Image Interpretation

All SPECT scans were interpreted by two board certified nuclear medicine physicians with extensive experience interpreting brain SPECT scans. The reviewers interpreted all the scans together by consensus in a randomized order for both the CBF and DAT SPECT scans. The reviewers were blinded to any clinical information. For the CBF scans, the assessment was performed to qualitatively rate the cerebral blood flow in the four major cortical brain regions – the frontal, temporal, parietal, and occipital lobes, as well as the anterior and posterior cingulate, caudate, basal ganglia, thalamus and cerebellum. With the left and right hemispheres included, there was a total of 18 brain regions evaluated. Each structure was rated for CBF in both the left and right hemisphere. We used a previously described approach for interpreting functional imaging scans [35,36] such that the CBF of each anatomic structure on the SPECT scan was given a score: 4 = normal activity; 3 = mildly decreased activity; 2 = moderately decreased, 1 = severely decreased; and 0 = no activity. DAT SPECT images were assessed visually using a similar semiquantitative score ranging from 4 = normal binding; 3 = mildly decreased binding; 2 = moderately decreased binding, 1 = severely decreased binding; and 0 = no binding. Four regions were evaluated, the left and right caudate, and the left and right putamen.

### Data Analysis

Initially, descriptive statistics were used regarding the number and extent of abnormal activity on the CBF and DAT binding scans from the TBI patients and controls. A linear regression model was used to compare the neuropsychological test scores to CBF scores in relevant regions for the entire cohort of TBI patients. For DAT binding scans, since there was a limited dynamic range of values given only 4 relevant brain regions, a t-test was used to compare those patients with highest and lowest quartiles of the neuropsychological test scores to the overall striatal DAT binding. Significant findings were cross validated with non-parametric tests (Wilcoxon Two Sample Test for comparison of groups and Spearman rank analysis for correlations) to account for possible skewness of the data. Finally, the activity for the CBF scans and DAT binding were compared to each other particularly in the basal ganglia, but also between the frontal regions on CBF scans and the basal ganglia on the DAT scans. Where indicated, correction for multiple comparisons was made using the False Discovery Rate method [41].

## Results

Patients with a history of TBI and persistent symptoms generally had one or more abnormal perfusion findings on their brain scans (see Figures 1 and 2). In fact, TBI patients had an average of 6 brain regions with abnormal perfusion compared to controls who had an average of 2 abnormal regions out of 18 regions evaluated (see Table 2). In controls, all decreases in perfusion were mild whereas in the TBI group, 10 of 25 patients had regions graded as

**Table 1.** Demographic and clinical information for TBI patients.

| Subject # | Gender | AGE (at study) | Total Number of TBIs | Cause of TBI | Concurrent CNS Conditions |
|---|---|---|---|---|---|
| 1 | M | 76 | 1 | Sports | Memory loss, migraine headaches, |
| 2 | M | 61 | 2 | Sports | Memory loss, attention problems, anxiety, depression |
| 3 | M | 27 | 3 | Blast | Memory loss, attention deficits, anxiety, depression |
| 4 | F | 56 | 2 | Sports | Memory loss, headaches |
| 5 | F | 69 | 1 | Sports | Depression |
| 6 | F | 27 | 2 | Sports | Headaches |
| 7 | M | 64 | 4 | MVA | Depression, anxiety |
| 8 | M | 18 | 1 | Sports | Loss of concentration, apathy |
| 9 | F | 34 | 1 | Sports | Severe vertigo, memory loss, attention/concentration problems |
| 10 | M | 58 | 4 | Sports | Memory loss, headaches |
| 11 | F | 61 | 3 | MVA | Headaches, dizziness, memory loss, sleep disturbances |
| 12 | F | 50 | 1 | MVA | Memory loss, attention/visual problems |
| 13 | M | 58 | 1 | Accident | Vertigo, sleep problems, memory loss |
| 14 | M | 36 | 1 | Accident | Memory loss, attention deficits |
| 15 | F | 39 | 5 | Accident | Memory loss, attention deficits, language problems, anxiety, depression |
| 16 | F | 25 | 3 | Sports | Memory loss, attention deficits, depression, anxiety, apathy |
| 17 | F | 65 | 2 | | Memory loss, anxiety |
| 18 | M | 68 | 1 | MVA | Memory loss, tremors, agitation, disinhibition |
| 19 | M | 61 | 8 | MVA | Headaches, memory loss, language problems, attention deficits |
| 20 | M | 62 | 2 | MVA | Severe headaches, depression |
| 21 | F | 58 | 1 | MVA | Visual problems, headaches, tinnitus, memory loss |
| 22 | F | 70 | 3 | MVA | Memory loss, anxiety |
| 23 | M | 46 | 1 | MVA | Memory loss, attention deficits, depression |
| 24 | M | 42 | 3 | MVA | Memory loss, balance problems, falls |
| 25 | M | 52 | 1 | MVA | Visual problems, memory loss, headaches, vestibular problems |

MVA = motor vehicle accident; Accident = other type of accidental trauma.

moderate or severely decreased. Given the sample size, a sensitivity and specificity between the groups could not be performed, however, the number of abnormal regions was significantly higher in the TBI group compared to the control group (p<0.001). On the [123]I Ioflupane SPECT, 72% of TBI patients had abnormal DAT binding compared to 20% of controls (p = 0.01). However, the findings in the controls were typically mild and restricted to a single putamen, which may have even been related to artifact, whereas the TBI patients were more likely to have involvement of the caudate or both putamen. Interestingly, the TBI patients in this cohort had the abnormalities more in the left striatum with significantly lower (by Wilcoxon Two Sample Test) binding in the left caudate and left putamen compared to controls (left caudate mean of 3.6±0.6 in TBI and 4.0±0.0 in controls, p = 0.02; left putamen mean of 3.3±0.7 in TBI and 3.8±0.3 in controls, p = 0.01).

When CBF was compared to DAT binding, there were no clear associations between findings. Abnormal CBF in the caudate or basal ganglia did not appear to predict or correspond to abnormal DAT binding. Even asymmetries were not comparable with 10 patients having asymmetric CBF and 11 patients having asymmetric DAT binding, but concordance in only 2 patients.

We performed a limited set of comparisons between clinical symptoms, neuropsychological test scores, and CBF or DAT binding based upon expected associations observed in prior

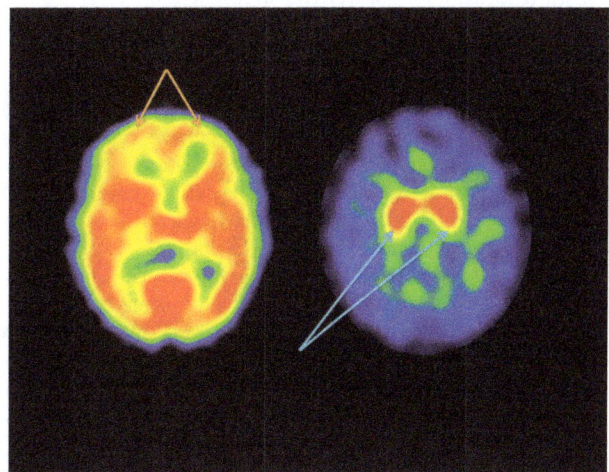

**Figure 1. [99m]Tc Exametazime and [123]I Ioflupane SPECT studies in a 61 year old male subject with multiple prior TBIs presenting with headache and memory loss.** Note the markedly decreased CBF primarily in the frontal lobes bilaterally (yellow arrows). However, this same patient had robust DAT binding in the striatum (blue arrows) with no significant abnormalities.

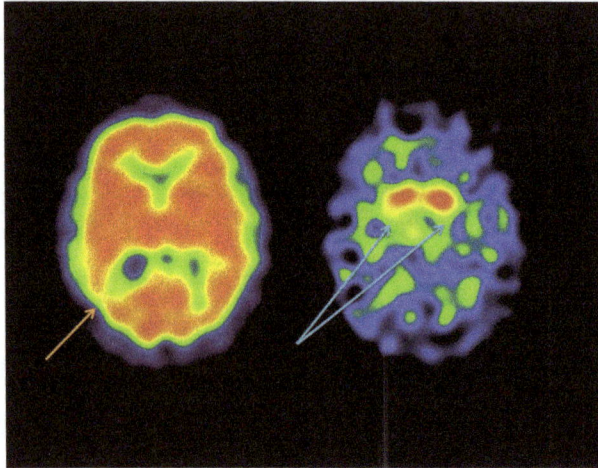

**Figure 2. $^{99m}$Tc Exametazime and $^{123}$I Ioflupane SPECT studies in a 58 year old male subject with a history of a single TBI with clinically presenting with problems with memory, sleep, and vertigo and no clear parkinsonian features.** The CBF shows only a mild decrease in the right temporo-parietal region. However, DAT binding is markedly abnormal with preserved uptake primarily in the caudate (R>L) and minimal uptake in the putamen bilaterally.

scores on the Spielberger trait anxiety scale versus those who were in the lowest quartile ($3.8\pm0.1$ versus $3.2\pm0.7$, p = 0.02 by Wilcoxon Two Sample Test).

## Discussion

The overall purpose of this study was to compare CBF using $^{99m}$Tc Exametazime SPECT and DAT binding using $^{123}$I Ioflupane SPECT in patients with persistent symptoms associated with a history of mild TBI. As described below, several studies have evaluated CBF or DAT binding alone in similar cohorts of patients, but not together [44,45,46]. For example, prior research studies have explored the relationship between CBF findings on SPECT imaging and TBI both in terms of diagnosis and clinical symptoms.

Some early studies compared the value of CBF SPECT imaging to anatomical findings on MRI or CT in TBI patients. Ichise et al. [19] studied 29 patients with chronic symptoms after either mild or major head injury. SPECT imaging detected abnormalities in 66% patients whereas MRI detected abnormalities in 45% and CT in 34% of patients. The SPECT scans also correlated better with tests of memory, attention and executive function than did structural imaging. A study of 43 patients with persistent post-concussive symptoms demonstrated abnormal SPECT scans in 53% of patients while MRI was read as abnormal in 9% and CT scan in only 5% of patients [44]. Although the SPECT scan results appeared to be more sensitive in detecting cerebral abnormalities in these patients, current neuropsychiatric symptoms did not seem to correlate with the SPECT scan findings. A more recent study of patients with acute mild TBI demonstrated CT abnormalities in 34% of patients while SPECT showed abnormal CBF in 63% corroborating earlier findings [45]. As in our study, the most common abnormality on many of these previous studies was hypoperfusion in the frontal lobes. We also found on average 6 regional abnormalities in CBF in the TBI group suggesting a more widespread pathophysiological process similar to other studies [20].

In the current study, we found a number of correlations between CBF and various clinical or neuropsychological parameters. For example, patients reporting headaches as part of their post-TBI symptoms had significant differences in the CBF in their right frontal lobe, and left parietal lobe. Such findings, which may reflect diffuse axonal injury and inflammation, are also consistent with several other studies of headache and pain syndromes [47,48,49]. An early study reported decreased cerebral blood flow is associated with common migraines suggesting that migraine attacks occur in connection with exacerbations of preexisting changes of neuronal activities, cerebral perfusion and metabolism [50]. In addition, in our study, low CBF in the left frontal lobe and right temporal lobe correlated with poorer reported physical health. The finding of decreased left frontal CBF is consistent with the well-known association of left dorsolateral prefrontal cortical dysfunction and depressed mood. Just as ischemic stroke, arteriovenous malformations, and neoplastic mass lesions in this area are often associated with depressed mood, this study suggests that TBI induces a 'functional lesion' of this area altering self-perception of health in a manner consistent with depressive thinking (anhedonia and despair) [51,52,53].

Other studies have evaluated the correlation between SPECT CBF findings and clinical findings as well as prognosis. For example, one study evaluated the results of neuropsychological tests in 12 alert, responsive patients aged 18–26 years, who were 2–13 months after head injury and found that global CBF was significantly decreased in patients with head injury relative to age-

studies. There were some interesting findings in the current cohort. For patients reporting headaches, there were significant findings compared to those patients without headaches. Patients with headaches had lower right frontal ($3.8\pm0.4$ without vs. $3.1\pm0.7$ with headaches, p = 0.02) and increased left parietal CBF ($3.4\pm0.6$ without vs. $4.0\pm0.0$ with headaches, p = 0.03 by Wilcoxon Two Sample Test). Please note that the findings for the right frontal lobe and left parietal lobe survived correction for multiple comparisons. Interestingly, there was no clear association between those reporting cognitive impairment or the type of impairment (i.e. loss of concentration, loss of memory, etc.) and either CBF or DAT binding. However, this lack of a finding might be due in part to so many patients reporting symptoms (only 3 patients reported no cognitive symptoms).

With regard to specific neuropsychological measures, there were also several interesting findings related to CBF and DAT binding. For the SF-12 PCS, there was a significant correlation between low CBF in the left frontal lobe and reports of lower physical health (r = 0.50, p = 0.01 corrected). Similarly, there was a significant correlation (Spearman rank correlation) between low CBF in the right temporal lobe and reports of lower physical health (r = 0.54, p = 0.005 corrected). The implication is that those patients with worse perceived physical health have lower CBF in these regions. Total CBF score for all regions correlated negatively with fatigue (r = 0.44, p = 0.03) but did not correlate with any other measures on the POMS. Furthermore, there were no significant findings between the MCS and CBF values.

For DAT binding, those patients in the lowest quartile for depression compared to the highest quartile had significantly higher binding in the total striatum ($3.3\pm0.7$ and $3.7\pm0.2$ respectively, p = 0.01 by Wilcoxon Two Sample Test). This is consistent with our prior depression data which demonstrated increased DAT binding in patients with depression and also in controls with depressive symptoms [42,43]. For the SF-12 MCS, the results for those with scores in the lowest quartile versus the highest quartile showed DAT binding of $3.8\pm0.2$ and $3.3\pm0.6$ respectively (p = 0.02 by Wilcoxon Two Sample Test). Finally, there was higher DAT binding in patients with the highest quartile

**Table 2.** General evaluation results of the 99mTc Exametazime and 123I Ioflupane SPECT scans (note that several additional regions were evaluated but not listed).

| TBI Subject | 99mTc Exametazime Results | | | | | | | 123I Ioflupane SPECT Results | | | | | | |
|---|---|---|---|---|---|---|---|---|---|---|---|---|---|---|
| | R Front | L Front | R Par | L Par | R Temp | L Temp | R Striat | L Striat | R Thal | L Thal | R Caud | L Caud | R Put | L Put |
| 1 | ABN | ABN | N | N | N | N | N | ABN | ABN | ABN | N | ABN | ABN | ABN |
| 2 | N | N | ABN | N | N | N | N | ABN | N | N | N | N | N | ABN |
| 3 | N | N | ABN | N | N | ABN | N | ABN | N | N | N | N | N | N |
| 4 | N | ABN | N | N | N | ABN | N | ABN | N | ABN | ABN | N | ABN | N |
| 5 | N | ABN | N | ABN | N | ABN | ABN | ABN | N | ABN | N | N | N | N |
| 6 | ABN | ABN | N | N | N | ABN | N | ABN | N | ABN | N | N | N | ABN |
| 7 | ABN | ABN | N | N | N | N | N | ABN | N | ABN | N | ABN | N | ABN |
| 8 | ABN | N | N | ABN | N | ABN | N | ABN | N | N | N | ABN | N | ABN |
| 9 | ABN | ABN | ABN | N | ABN | N | ABN | ABN | N | N | N | N | N | N |
| 10 | N | N | ABN | N | ABN | N | N | N | ABN | N | N | ABN | N | N |
| 11 | ABN | N | ABN | N | N | N | N | ABN | N | ABN | N | N | N | ABN |
| 12 | N | ABN | N | N | ABN | N | ABN | N | N | N | N | ABN | N | ABN |
| 13 | N | N | ABN | ABN | ABN | N | N | N | N | N | ABN | N | ABN | ABN |
| 14 | ABN | N | ABN | N | N | N | ABN | N | N | N | N | N | ABN | N |
| 15 | N | ABN | N | ABN | N | ABN | N | ABN | N | ABN | N | N | ABN | N |
| 16 | N | ABN | ABN | N | ABN | N | N | ABN | N | ABN | N | ABN | N | ABN |
| 17 | N | ABN | N | N | N | ABN | N | N | N | N | ABN | N | ABN | N |
| 18 | N | ABN | N | ABN | N | ABN | ABN | N | N | N | N | N | N | N |
| 19 | ABN | ABN | N | N | ABN | ABN | N | N | ABN | ABN | N | ABN | N | ABN |
| 20 | ABN | ABN | N | N | ABN | ABN | N | ABN | N | ABN | N | N | N | N |
| 21 | ABN | ABN | N | N | ABN | ABN | ABN | ABN | ABN | ABN | N | ABN | N | ABN |
| 22 | N | N | N | N | N | N | N | N | ABN | ABN | N | N | N | N |
| 23 | N | ABN | N | ABN | ABN | ABN | N | ABN | N | N | N | N | N | ABN |
| 24 | N | ABN | N | ABN | N | N | ABN | ABN | N | ABN | N | N | N | N |
| 25 | ABN | ABN | N | N | N | N | ABN | ABN | ABN | ABN | N | ABN | N | ABN |
| **Control** | | | | | | | | | | | | | | |
| 1 | ABN | N | N | N | N | N | N | N | N | N | N | N | ABN | N |
| 2 | N | ABN | N | N | N | N | ABN | ABN | N | N | N | N | N | N |
| 3 | ABN | ABN | ABN | ABN | N | N | N | N | N | N | N | N | N | N |
| 4 | N | N | N | N | N | N | ABN | N | ABN | N | N | N | N | N |
| 5 | N | N | N | N | N | ABN | N | N | N | N | N | N | N | N |
| 6 | N | N | N | N | N | N | N | N | N | N | N | N | N | N |
| 7 | N | N | N | N | N | N | N | ABN | N | ABN | N | N | ABN | N |
| 8 | N | ABN | N | N | N | N | N | N | N | N | N | N | N | N |
| 9 | N | N | ABN | ABN | N | ABN | N | N | N | N | N | N | N | N |
| 10 | N | ABN | N | N | N | ABN | N | N | N | N | N | N | N | N |

N = Normal; ABN = abnormal; R Front = Right Frontal; L Front = Left Frontal; R Par = Right Parietal; L Par = Left Parietal; R Temp = Right Temporal; L Temp = Left Temporal; R Striat = Right Striatum; L Striat = Left Striatum; R Thal = Right Thalamus; L Thal = Left Thalamus; R Caud = Right Caudate; L Caud = Left Caudate; R Put = Right Putamen; L Put = Left Putamen.

matched controls [54]. In that study, 3 of 4 patients with a well-localized injury had focally decreased CBF over the affected region. Also in that cohort, 2 of 3 patients with diffuse injury who underwent repeat studies 5–14 weeks after their initial study had improvement on both their psychological tests and CBF. These results suggested that the chronic sequelae of head injury include decreased CBF, presumably reflecting decreased cerebral metabolism related to diffuse axonal injury or continued inflammatory response, which correlates with the neuropsychological impairment. Our current study supports this overall hypothesis given the generally reduced CBF in patients with chronic symptoms related to prior TBI.

A more thorough evaluation of the correlation between SPECT findings and prognosis was found in a study by Jacobs et al. which prospectively evaluated 67 mild-to-moderate brain injured patients [55]. Each patient had a clinical evaluation and SPECT scan within four weeks of the initial injury and three months after the first scan. This study reported that of the 33 patients who showed no significant abnormalities on their initial SPECT scan, 97% experienced resolution in their clinical symptoms within three months. However, of the 34 patients with abnormalities on their initial SPECT scans, 59% continued to experience significant clinical symptoms three months later. The authors reported a positive predictive value of an abnormal initial scan of only 59%, but if the 12 month follow up scan was also abnormal, the sensitivity for the repeat SPECT was 95%. These authors suggested that negative initial SPECT studies are a reliable predictor of a favorable clinical outcome. The results showed that SPECT alterations correlated well with the severity of the trauma and a negative initial SPECT study was a reliable predictor of a favorable clinical outcome. The authors suggested that in cases with a positive initial SPECT scan, a follow-up consisting of a combination of SPECT and clinical evaluation is necessary especially in patients suffering from post-conclusive symptoms. Our current study would corroborate the notion that positive SPECT scans are associated with chronic symptoms in TBI patients.

Another prospective study evaluated 136 patients with mild head injury who underwent initial SPECT imaging within 4 weeks after the trauma and again up to 12 months post injury [56]. That study revealed that clinical normalization occurred earlier than normalization of CBF. However, at 12 months post injury, the investigators observed considerable improvement in the specificity and positive predictive value of SPECT (85% and 83%, respectively). Furthermore, persistent lesions on the SPECT scan were correlated with severity and to localization in the frontal cortex. The authors suggested that a normal 99mTc-HMPAO SPECT scan early in the post TBI course may be a reliable tool for predicting improvement. As with our study, patients with persistent symptoms frequently have a variety of CBF abnormalities even a year or more after TBI.

A study by Bonne et al. [57] studied 28 clinically symptomatic male subjects with mild TBI and twenty matched controls with neuropsychological testing and brain SPECT imaging. Similar to our study, mild TBI patients demonstrated regions of hypoperfusion in the frontal lobes, temporal lobes, and sub-cortical structures which was generally concordant with neuropsychological localization. The results from these CBF SPECT studies, in addition to the results from the current study support using SPECT to help assess the diagnosis, prognosis, and treatment of TBI patients.

In addition to alterations in CBF, a growing amount of evidence implicates damage to the dopaminergic nervous system in association with TBI. Additional evidence of dopamine system dysfunction after TBI is based upon data showing altered DAT binding after TBI. One study of only 10 subjects used single photon emission computed tomography (SPECT) with beta-CIT to show that striatal DAT binding was decreased in patients up to 4–5 months after severe TBI, even in cases where there was no evidence of structural striatal injury [46]. Patients with TBI also had significantly lower D2 post-synaptic receptor binding as measured by IBZM SPECT. However, the DAT deficit was more marked than the D2 receptor loss. The findings suggested that nigrostriatal dysfunction could be detected using SPECT following TBI despite relative structural preservation of the striatum. However, there still have been no studies that explored the comparison between dopamine function and cerebral blood flow as measured by SPECT.

The current study provides unique data by being able to directly compare CBF and DAT binding in the same TBI patients. Our SPECT results show that both CBF and DAT binding are abnormal in TBI patients with chronic symptoms. Furthermore, both CBF and DAT abnormalities appear to correlate with clinical symptoms. However, there does not seem to be a good correlation between CBF and DAT SPECT scan findings.

There are several limitations with regard to interpreting the findings in this study. One limitation is that the SPECT scans were all interpreted together by two expert reviewers. Thus, this study does not provide information on inter-rater or intra-rater reliability for the scans. However, the purpose of this study was to determine how these scans might be utilized in the traditional clinical setting in TBI patients so we sought to interpret the scans under optimal conditions. Given the potential importance of utilizing these scans for the clinical evaluation of chronic TBI patients suggested by the current data, future studies with larger numbers of subjects will be needed to better assess how well these scans can be evaluated by different readers under more complex conditions. However, such a study can potentially yield data to support the broader use of SPECT imaging in this population. In addition, it will be important to perform additional quantitative analyses in the future. Again though, since quantitative analysis with tools such as region of interest analysis or statistical parametric mapping is not typically used in the clinical setting, they were not performed as part of the current study. Another limitation for SPECT's use in TBI is that typically no pre-trauma SPECT study is available for comparison. Thus, it is often not possible to determine the date of trauma with functional neuroimaging. Even remote trauma from childhood can present with neuroimaging findings similar to those seen in more recent trauma.

## Conclusion

Overall, this study provides the first data on CBF and DAT binding in the same patients with a history of TBI and chronic symptoms. The results demonstrate that such TBI patients frequently have a number of perfusion and DAT binding abnormalities. Such abnormalities appear to correlate with specific symptoms or clinical measures. But, interestingly, the scans do not appear to correlate well with each other. The implication of this last finding is that the scans appear to provide insight into two separate pathophysiological processes associated with TBI symptoms. Thus, both scans might ultimately have utility in the setting of patients with TBI and persistent symptoms.

## Acknowledgments

Some of the data used in the preparation of this article were obtained from the Parkinson's Progression Markers Initiative (PPMI) database (www.ppmi-info.org/data). For up-to-date information on the study, visit www.ppmi-info.org. PPMI – a public-private partnership – is funded by the Michael J. Fox Foundation for Parkinson's Research and funding partners. A full list of PPMI funding partners can be found at www.ppmi-info.org/fundingpartners.

## Author Contributions

Conceived and designed the experiments: ABN MS CI TL DA DR NW. Performed the experiments: ABN MS AG CI TL DA DR NW. Analyzed the data: ABN MS AG CI TL DA DR NW. Contributed reagents/materials/analysis tools: ABN MS AG CI TL DA DR NW. Wrote the paper: ABN MS AG CI TL DA DR NW.

# References

1. Corsellis JA (1989) Boxing and the brain. British Med J 298 (6666): 105–109.
2. Jean-Bay E (2000) The biobehavioral correlates of post-traumatic brain injury depression. J Neurosci Nurs 32(3): 169–176.
3. Fayol P, Carrière H, Habonimana D, Dumond JJ (2009) Preliminary questions before studying mild traumatic brain injury outcome. Ann Phys Rehabil Med 52(6): 497–509.
4. Blostein P, Jones SJ (2003) Identification and evaluation of patients with mild traumatic brain injury: results of a national survey of level I trauma centers. J Trauma 55: 450–453.
5. Lippa SM, Pastorek NJ, Benge JF, Thornton GM (2010) Postconcussive symptoms after blast and nonblast-related mild traumatic brain injuries in Afghanistan and Iraq war veterans. J Int Neuropsychol Soc 16(5): 856–866.
6. Jordan BD (2013) The clinical spectrum of sport-related traumatic brain injury. Nat Rev Neurol 9(4): 222–230.
7. Lin AP, Liao HJ, Merugumala SK, Prabhu SP, Meehan WP 3rd, Ross BD (2012) Metabolic imaging of mild traumatic brain injury. Brain Imaging Behav 6(2): 208–223.
8. Slobounov S, Gay M, Johnson B, Zhang K (2012) Concussion in athletics: ongoing clinical and brain imaging research controversies. Brain Imaging Behav 6(2): 224–243.
9. Amen DG, Newberg A, Thatcher R, Jin Y, Wu J, et al. (2010) Impact of playing American professional football on long-term brain function. J Neuropsychiatry Clin Neurosci 23(1): 98–106.
10. Halbauer JD, Ashford JW, Zeitzer JM, Adamson MM, Lew HL, et al. (2009) Neuropsychiatric diagnosis and management of chronic sequelae of war-related mild to moderate traumatic brain injury. J Rehabil Res Dev 46(6): 757–796.
11. Hoffman JM, Lucas S, Dikmen S, Braden CA, Brown AW, et al. (2011) Natural history of headache after traumatic brain injury. J Neurotrauma 28(9): 1719–1725.
12. Obermann M, Keidel M, Diener HC (2010) Post-traumatic headache: is it for real? Crossfire debates on headache: pro. Headache 50(4): 710–715.
13. Bernstein C, Burstein R (2012) Sensitization of the trigeminovascular pathway: Perspective and implications to migraine pathophysiology. J Clin Neurol 8: 89–99.
14. Mayer CL, Huber BR, Peskind E (2013) Traumatic brain injury, neuroinflammation, and post-traumatic headaches. Headache.53(9): 1523–1530.
15. Amen DG, Trujillo M, Newberg A, Willeumier K, Tarzwell R, et al. (2011) Brain SPECT imaging in complex psychiatric cases: An evidence-based, underutilized tool. Open Neuroimag J 5: 40–48.
16. Moss A, Newberg A, Monti D, Alavi A (in press) Patterns associated with neurodegenerative disorders. In Papanicolaou AC. Functional Brain Imaging in Cognitive Neurosciences and Neuropsychology. New York: Oxford.
17. Moss A, Newberg A, Monti D, Alavi A (in press) Patterns associated with affective and cognitive disorders. In Papanicolaou AC. Functional Brain Imaging in Cognitive Neurosciences and Neuropsychology. New York: Oxford.
18. Dubroff JG, Newberg A (2008) Neuroimaging of traumatic brain injury. Semin Neurol 28(4): 548–557.
19. Ichise M, Chung DG, Wang P, Wortzman G, Gray BG, et al. (1994) Technetium-99m-HMPAO SPECT, CT and MRI in the evaluation of patients with chronic traumatic brain injury: a correlation with neuropsychological performance. J Nucl Med 35(2): 217–26.
20. Abdel-Dayem HM, Abu-Judeh H, Kumar M, Atay S, Naddaf S, et al. (1998) SPECT brain perfusion abnormalities in mild or moderate traumatic brain injury. Clin Nucl Med 23(5): 309–317.
21. Jacobs A, Put E, Ingels M, Bossuyt A (1994) Prospective evaluation of technetium-99m-HMPAO SPECT in mild and moderate traumatic brain injury. J Nucl Med 35: 942–947.
22. Baulieu F, Fournier P, Baulieu JL, Dalonneau M, Chiaroni P, et al. (2001) Technetium-99m ECD single photon emission computed tomography in brain trauma: comparison of early scintigraphic findings with long-term neuropsychological outcome. J Neuroimaging 11(2): 112–120.
23. Zafonte RD, Lexell J, Cullen N (2001) Possible applications for dopaminergic agents following traumatic brain injury: part 2. J Head Trauma Rehabil 16(1): 112–116.
24. Sivan M, Neumann V, Kent R, Stroud A, Bhakta BB (2010) Pharmacotherapy for treatment of attention deficits after non-progressive acquired brain injury. A systematic review. Clin Rehabil 24(2): 110–121.
25. Wroblewski BA, Joseph AB, Kupfer J, Kalliel K (1997) Effectiveness of valproic acid on destructive and aggressive behaviours in patients with acquired brain injury. Brain Inj 11(1): 37–47.
26. Lee H, Kim SW, Kim JM, Shin IS, Yang SJ, et al. (2005) Comparing effects of methylphenidate, sertraline and placebo on neuropsychiatric sequelae in patients with traumatic brain injury. Hum Psychopharmacol 20(2): 97–104.
27. Kant R, Smith-Seemiller L, Isaac G, Duffy J (1997) Tc-HMPAO SPECT in persistent post-concussion syndrome after mild head injury: comparison with MRI/CT. Brain Inj 11: 115–124.
28. Packard RC (2008) Chronic post-traumatic headache: associations with mild traumatic brain injury, concussion, and post-concussive disorder. Curr Pain Headache Rep 12(1): 67–73.
29. Kjeldgaard D, Forchhammer H, Teasdale T, Jensen RH (2013) Chronic post-traumatic headache after mild head injury: A descriptive study. Cephalalgia. 2013 Sep 17. [Epub ahead of print].
30. Faux S, Sheedy J (2008) A prospective controlled study in the prevalence of posttraumatic headache following mild traumatic brain injury. Pain Med 9(8): 1001–1011.
31. Goshen E, Zwas ST, Shahar E, Tadmor R (1996) The role of 99m Tc-HMPAO brain SPET in paediatric traumatic brain injury. Nucl Med Commun 17: 418–422.
32. Bales JW, Wagner AK, Kline AE, Dixon CE (2009) Persistent cognitive dysfunction after traumatic brain injury: A dopamine hypothesis. Neurosci Biobehav Rev 33(7): 981–1003.
33. Huger F, Patrick G (1979) Effect of concussive head injury on central catecholamine levels and synthesis rates in rat brain regions. J Neurochem 33: 89–95.
34. McIntosh TK, Yu T, Gennarelli TA (1994) Alterations in regional brain catecholamine concentrations after experimental brain injury in the rat. J Neurochem 63: 1426–1433.
35. Newberg AB, Arnold SE, Wintering N, Rovner BW, Alavi A (2012) Initial clinical comparison of 18F-Florbetapir and 18F-FDG PET in patients with Alzheimer disease and controls J Nucl Med 53(6): 902–907.
36. Musiek ES, Chen Y, Korczykowski M, Saboury B, Martinez PM, et al. (2012) Direct comparison of FDG-PET and ASL-MRI in Alzheimer's disease. Alzheimers Dement 8(1): 51–59.
37. McNair DM, Lorr M, Droppleman LF (1992) Manual for the Profile of Mood States. San Diego, CA: EdITS/Educational and Industrial Testing Service.
38. Spielberger CD, Gorsuch RL, Lushene R, Vagg PR, Jacobs GA (1983). Manual for the State-Trait Anxiety Inventory. Palo Alto, CA: Consulting Psychologists Press.
39. Beck AT, Beck AW (1972) Screening depressed patients in family practice. Postgrad Med 52: 81–85.
40. Ware JE, Jr., Kosinski M, Keller SD (1996) A 12 Item Short Form Health Survey: Construction of scales and preliminary tests of reliability and validity. Med Care 34: 220–233.
41. Benjamini Y, Hochberg Y (1995) Controlling the false discovery rate: a practical and powerful approach to multiple testing. J Royal Stat Soc, Series B (Methodological) 57: 289–300.
42. Newberg A, Amsterdam J, Shults J (2007) Dopamine transporter density may be associated with the depressed affect in healthy subjects. Nucl Med Commun 28(1): 3–6.
43. Amsterdam JD, Newberg AB, Soeller I, Shults J (2012) Greater striatal dopamine transporter density may be associated with major depressive episode. J Affect Dis 141(2–3): 425–431.
44. Kant R, Smith-Seemiller L, Isaac G, Duffy J (1997) Tc-HMPAO SPECT in persistent post-concussion syndrome after mild head injury: Comparison with MRI/CT. Brain Inj 11(2): 115–124.
45. Gowda NK, Agrawal D, Bal C, Chandrashekar N, Tripati M, et al. (2006) Technetium Tc-99m ethyl cysteinate dimer brain single-photon emission CT in mild traumatic brain injury: a prospective study. Am J Neuroradiol 27(2): 447–451.
46. Donnemiller E, Brenneis C, Wissel J, Scherfler C, Poewe W, et al. (2000) Impaired dopaminergic neurotransmission in patients with traumatic brain injury: a SPECT study using 123I-beta-CIT and 123I-IBZM. Eur J Nucl Med 27(9): 1410–1414.
47. Başoglu T, Ozbenli T, Bernay I, Sahin M, Onur A, et al. (1996) Demonstration of frontal hypoperfusion in benign exertional headache by Technetium-99m-HMPAO SPECT. J Nucl Med 37(7): 1172–1174.
48. Di Piero V, Fiacco F, Tombari D, Pantano P (1997) Tonic pain: a SPET study in normal subjects and cluster headache patients. Pain 70(2–3): 185–191.
49. Olesen J, Friberg L, Olsen TS, Iversen HK, Lassen NA, et al. (1990) Timing and topography of cerebral blood flow, aura, and headache during migraine attacks. Ann Neurol 28(6): 791–798.
50. Schlake HP, Böttger IG, Grotemeyer KH, Husstedt IW, Vollet B, et al. (1990) Single photon emission computed tomography with technetium-99m hexamethyl propylenamino oxime in the pain-free interval of migraine and cluster headache. Eur Neurol 30(3): 153–156.
51. Murakami T, Hama S, Yamashita H, Onoda K, Kobayashi M, et al. (2013) Neuroanatomic pathways associated with poststroke affective and apathetic depression. Am J Geriatr Psychiatry 21(9): 840–847.
52. Robinson RG, Boston JD, Starkstein SE, Price TR (1988) Comparison of mania and depression after brain injury: causal factors. Am J Psychiatry 145(2): 172–178.
53. Belyi BI (1987) Mental impairment in unilateral frontal tumours: role of the laterality of the lesion. Int J Neurosci 32(3–4): 799–810.
54. Barclay L, Zemcov A, Reichert W, Blass JP (1985) Cerebral blood flow decrements in chronic head injury syndrome. Biol Psychiatry 20(2): 146–157.
55. Jacobs A, Put E, Ingels M, Bossuyt A (1994) Prospective evaluation of technetium-99m-HMPAO SPECT in mild and moderate traumatic brain injury. J Nucl Med 35: 942–947.

# 8

# Assessment of Olfactory Nerve by SPECT-MRI Image with Nasal Thallium-201 Administration in Patients with Olfactory Impairments in Comparison to Healthy Volunteers

**Hideaki Shiga**[1,2]\*, **Junichi Taki**[3], **Kohshin Washiyama**[2], **Junpei Yamamoto**[1], **Sakae Kinase**[4], **Koichi Okuda**[3], **Seigo Kinuya**[3], **Naoto Watanabe**[5], **Hisao Tonami**[5], **Kichiro Koshida**[2], **Ryohei Amano**[2], **Mitsuru Furukawa**[6], **Takaki Miwa**[1]

1 Department of Otorhinolaryngology, Kanazawa Medical University, Ishikawa, Japan, 2 Department of Quantum Medical Technology, Graduate School of Medical Science, Kanazawa University, Ishikawa, Japan, 3 Department of Biotracer Medicine, Graduate School of Medical Science, Kanazawa University, Ishikawa, Japan, 4 Risk Analysis and Applications Research Group, Nuclear Safety Research Center, Japan Atomic Energy Agency, Ibaraki, Japan, 5 Department of Diagnostic and Therapeutic Radiology, Kanazawa Medical University, Ishikawa, Japan, 6 Headquarter, Kanazawa University, Ishikawa, Japan

## Abstract

***Purpose:*** The aim of this study was to assess whether migration of thallium-201 ($^{201}$Tl) to the olfactory bulb were reduced in patients with olfactory impairments in comparison to healthy volunteers after nasal administration of $^{201}$Tl.

***Procedures:*** 10 healthy volunteers and 21 patients enrolled in the study (19 males and 12 females; 26–71 years old). The causes of olfactory dysfunction in the patients were head trauma (n = 7), upper respiratory tract infection (n = 7), and chronic rhinosinusitis (n = 7). $^{201}$TlCl was administered unilaterally to the olfactory cleft, and SPECT-CT was conducted 24 h later. Separate MRI images were merged with the SPECT images. $^{201}$Tl olfactory migration was also correlated with the volume of the olfactory bulb determined from MRI images, as well as with odor recognition thresholds measured by using T&T olfactometry.

***Results:*** Nasal $^{201}$Tl migration to the olfactory bulb was significantly lower in the olfactory-impaired patients than in healthy volunteers. The migration of $^{201}$Tl to the olfactory bulb was significantly correlated with odor recognition thresholds obtained with T&T olfactometry and correlated with the volume of the olfactory bulb determined from MRI images when all subjects were included.

***Conclusions:*** Assessment of the $^{201}$Tl migration to the olfactory bulb was the new method for the evaluation of the olfactory nerve connectivity in patients with impaired olfaction.

**Editor:** Thomas Hummel, Technical University of Dresden Medical School, Germany

**Funding:** This study was funded in part by a Grant-in-Aid for Scientific Research from the Ministry of Education, Science and Culture of Japan (C21592174 to H.S.). No additional external funding received for this study. The funders had no role in study design, data collection and analysis, decision to publish, or preparation of the manuscript.

**Competing Interests:** The authors have declared that no competing interests exist.

\* E-mail: shigah@kanazawa-med.ac.jp

## Introduction

Many physicians find it difficult to detect malingering among olfaction-impaired patients. Current olfactory function tests (the University of Pennsylvania Smell Identification Test [1], the Connecticut Chemosensory Clinical Research Center Test [2], Sniffin sticks [3], and T&T olfactometry [4]) are useful for the analysis of olfactory function in olfaction-impaired patients. However, an abnormality in the olfactory function tests has not been used as an index for the connectivity of olfactory nerve axons passing through the cribriform plate of the ethmoid bone to enter glomeruli within the olfactory bulb in patients because it is difficult to directly view the connectivity of the peripheral olfactory nerve

with current magnetic resonance imaging. On the other hand, it has previously been shown that olfactory bulb volume is correlated with odor threshold determined by using Sniffin sticks in patients with postinfectious olfactory loss [5].

The radioisotope thallium-201 ($^{201}$Tl) migrates to the olfactory bulb after nasal administration in rodents [6], and this migration is significantly decreased by the transection of olfactory nerve fibers in mice [7]. Furthermore, The ability to detect odors and the rate of migration of $^{201}$Tl in the olfactory nerve are correlated in mice [8].

Nasally administered thallium-201 ($^{201}$Tl) migrates to the olfactory bulb 24 h after $^{201}$Tl administration in subjects, as has been shown in healthy volunteers using a combination of single photon emission computed tomography (SPECT), X-ray computed tomography (CT), and magnetic resonance imaging (MRI) [9]. The biological safety of nasal $^{201}$Tl administration has also previously been shown [10].

In this study, we applied the technique of nasal administration of $^{201}$Tl followed by SPECT-CT and MRI imaging to patients with hyposmia due to head trauma, upper respiratory tract infection, or chronic rhinosinusitis, which are major causes of olfactory dysfunction [11], and to healthy volunteers. $^{201}$Tl olfactory migration in patients with impaired olfaction was compared to that in healthy volunteers. $^{201}$Tl olfactory migration was also correlated with the volume of the olfactory bulb determined from MRI images, as well as with odor recognition thresholds measured by using T&T olfactometry.

## Methods

### Subjects

Participants were 10 healthy volunteers (7 males and 3 females, 30–66 years old; Table 1) recruited from medical workers in the Kanazawa Medical University Hospital and Kanazawa University Hospital with normal olfactory thresholds as determined with T&T olfactometry (i.e., the odor recognition threshold score of each nostril was less than 2.0) and 21 patients with olfactory disorders receiving treatment at the smell clinic in the Kanazawa Medical University Hospital (26–71 years old; 12 males and 9 females; odor recognition threshold score: 4.2±1.4 [mean ± S.D.]; Table 1; i.e., the odor recognition threshold score of each nostril was 2.0 or more than 2.0 with self-reported olfactory disturbance). The mean age was not significantly different in the patients with head trauma, upper respiratory infection, or chronic sinusitis than in the healthy volunteers (Table 1). The numbers of smokers were not significantly different among healthy volunteer group and each patient group (Table 1).

Causes of olfactory dysfunction in the patients were head trauma (n = 7), upper respiratory tract infection (n = 7), and chronic rhinosinusitis (n = 7). For head trauma subjects, types of head trauma were concussion (n = 2), cerebral contusion (n = 2), and cerebral contusion with intracranial hemorrhage (n = 3). One patient with hyposmia due to head trauma showed a shallow olfactory sulcus. Another patients with hyposmia due to head trauma showed no abnormal frontal lobe findings on MRI.

The duration of olfactory deficits at the time of the examination ranged from 4 weeks to 10 years (58 months ±53 months [mean ± S.D.]). Patients with chronic rhinosinusitis were assessed in this trial if they continued to suffer olfactory impairments even though receiving medical and/or surgical treatment. Olfactory clefts were open in all subjects.

All participants were informed of the objectives of the study and possible side effects (allergic reactions to $^{201}$TlCl, irritation of the digestive system, blood pressure fluctuation, or asthmatic crisis), and have given written informed consent. Subjects were excluded if they were pregnant or lactating. Exclusion criteria also included a history of kidney disease, liver injury, or other serious illness. Healthy volunteers who might have olfactory dysfunction due to head trauma, upper respiratory tract infection, or chronic rhinosinusitis were excluded in this study. Both groups of healthy volunteers (medical workers) and patients did not include nuclear medicine specialists. Therefore, their knowledge about $^{201}$Tl imaging may be same. The Medical Ethics Committees of Kanazawa Medical University and Kanazawa University approved this trial in advance.

### T&T Olfactometry

Each odorant was dissolved in mineral oil to form a graded series of concentrations, and then applied liberally to blotting paper and presented to subjects by using T&T olfactometry (Daiichi Yakuhin Sangyo, Tokyo, Japan). In Japan, T&T olfactometry is now a standard means of measuring olfactory thresholds. The normal odor recognition threshold score of each nostril is less than 2.0. The recognition threshold was obtained with T&T olfactometry on the side $^{201}$Tl nasally administered in this study.

### Merging of $^{201}$Tl SPECT Images with MRI Images and Analysis of Olfactory Bulb Volume

All procedures involving the handling of radioisotopic materials were performed in the Division of Radiology at Kanazawa Medical University or the Division of Radioisotopes at Kanazawa University Hospital. A solution of $^{201}$TlCl in saline (74 MBq/mL) was obtained from Nihon Medi-Physics (Tokyo, Japan). For each subject, 0.3 mL $^{201}$TlCl saline solution (22 MBq) was instilled via syringe into the olfactory cleft in the right or left larger nasal cavity. The unilateral $^{201}$Tl nasal administration was performed in this study, because uptake of $^{201}$Tl in the right or left distinction may be unclear in the case of bilateral $^{201}$Tl nasal administration. Under endoscopic findings, we choose the side of larger olfactory cleft to be assessed for the certain nasal administration to the olfactory cleft. After $^{201}$Tl nasal administration, subjects laid on their sides for 30 min. Uptake of $^{201}$Tl was assessed from SPECT scans performed 24 h after $^{201}$Tl administration. It has been shown that $^{201}$Tl migration from the olfactory epithelium to the olfactory bulb is visible 24 h after $^{201}$Tl nasal administration in healthy volunteers [9]. Each SPECT scan was 30 min in duration and was followed by an X-ray CT scan to localize the nasal cavity and olfactory bulb. The data acquisition was started using a dual-headed SPECT-CT hybrid system (Symbia T6; Siemens Japan Healthcare, Japan) equipped with low-energy, high-resolution collimators. Data were acquired over 360 degrees, with 90

**Table 1.** Odor recognition thresholds measured by using T&T olfactometry.

| Subject Group | Age, years (Mean ± S.D.) | Gender (Male/Female) | Non-smokers/Smokers or ex-smokers | Odor recognition threshold (Mean ± S.D.) |
|---|---|---|---|---|
| Healthy volunteer (n = 10) | 44.7±11.9 | 7/3 | 7/3 | 0.9±0.6 |
| Head trauma (n = 7) | 43.0±13.3 | 3/4 | 3/4 | 4.9±0.9* |
| Upper respiratory tract infection (n = 7) | 50.4±10.0 | 4/3 | 6/1 | 3.4±1.5* |
| Chronic rhinosinusitis (n = 7) | 54.7±15.1 | 5/2 | 4/3 | 4.4±1.4* |

*P<0.05 (unpaired t-tests: comparison with healthy volunteers).

projections (30 s per projection in continuous rotation), $128 \times 128$ matrix (with 2.29-times zoom, pixel size 2.1 mm), and 72 KeV photopeak with a 30% main window and 7% subwindow on both sides. Data reconstruction underwent by using ordered subsets expectation maximization (9 subsets and 8 iterations) with 3-dimensional resolution recovery, CT-based attenuation correction, and scatter correction [12,13] (Flash 3D, Siemens Japan Healthcare, Japan).

For each subject, MRI T2 weighted images (Syngo MR B17 3.0T; Siemens Japan Healthcare, Japan, or Signa HDx 3.0T; GE Healthcare-Japan, Japan) were collected separately from the SPECT scan, one day before. Each MRI image was merged with the corresponding SPECT image through fusion with the CT part of the SPECT-CT by using the mutual information–based registration method [14]. Experienced radiologists, (N.W. and H.T.) who were blind to the olfactory test data, separately determined the volume of the olfactory bulb by manual segmentation of MRI coronal slices (2-mm slice thickness) through the olfactory bulb on the side of nasal administration. The change of diameter at the beginning of the olfactory tract was used as the proximal demarcation of the olfactory bulb. The average scores of those were used for the statistical analysis. Olfactory bulb volume was not regarded as criteria for the selection of patients.

## Analysis of $^{201}$Tl Counts on the SPECT-MRI Image

Two regions of interest for the nasal turbinate area and the anterior skull base (olfactory bulb area) were set on the $^{201}$Tl SPECT–MRI fusion image. On 3 sequential fused images in both sagittal and coronal planes, large regions of interest were tentatively set manually on the nasal turbinate area to cover all of the residual $^{201}$Tl activity in the nasal cavity. The nasal cavity region of interest was defined as the area bounded by the 50% threshold of the peak $^{201}$Tl count and delineated. Then, oval regions of interest were set manually to delineate the olfactory bulb on the side of nasal administration of the tracer by referencing the MRI T2 weighted images. The size of the oval olfactory bulb region of interest was approximately 8 to 9 pixels on the long axis and 3 to 4 pixels on the short axis in the sagittal image and 5 to 6 pixels by 2 to 3 pixels in the coronal image. The regions of interest were set excluding the sphenoidal sinus area and the nasopharyngeal area.

The index of $^{201}$Tl migration from the olfactory epithelium to the olfactory bulb was determined as the ratio of the total $^{201}$Tl counts in the olfactory bulb region of interest to the total $^{201}$Tl counts in the nasal turbinate region of interest, expressed as a mean percentage of the values calculated from both sagittal and coronal images. Experienced nuclear radiologists (J.T. and K.O.) who were blind to the olfactory test data determined separately the two regions of interest on the SPECT-MRI image. The average scores of those were used for the statistical analysis.

## Phantom Study

A phantom study was performed with the same data acquisition and reconstruction method used in the clinical study. In a cylindrical phantom (20 cm in diameter) filled with water, a $^{201}$Tl (40 µCi) spherical source (4 mm in diameter) was positioned on the center of the rotation. Then the counts of pixels on the line passing through the center of the source and at a right angle to the axis of camera rotation were measured. Full width at half maximum (FWHM) was 7.0 mm. When normalized by the maximum pixel count (7972 counts) of the spherical source, pixel counts at 1 (2.1 mm), 2 (4.2 mm), 3 (6.3 mm), 4 (8.4 mm), and 5 (10.5 mm) pixels from the center of the source were 0.76, 0.34, 0.09, 0.016, 0.001, respectively. Thus, when the olfactory bulb is

located more than 4 pixels (8.4 mm) from the high radioactivity in the nasal cavity, the count contamination to the olfactory bulb will be less than 2% of the activity of the nasal cavity.

## Statistical Analysis

Two-tailed Spearman correlations, unpaired t-tests, Bonferroni's multiple comparison test, and Kruskal-Wallis tests were performed using Prism 5 software (GraphPad, San Diego, CA, USA). $P$ values less than 0.05 were considered significant. A sample size of 31 subjects gave 99.9% power (alpha = .05, two-tailed) for comparing nasal $^{201}$Tl migration to the olfactory bulb in 4 groups (JMP software, Cary, NC, USA).

## Results

### Reductions in Nasal $^{201}$Tl Migration to the Olfactory Bulb in Patients

To determine whether the viability or function of the peripheral olfactory nerve was reduced in the patients with impaired olfaction, we assessed migration of nasally administered $^{201}$Tl to the olfactory bulb in the patients and healthy volunteers. Migration of nasal $^{201}$Tl to the olfactory bulb was significantly lower in the patients with head trauma, upper respiratory infection, or chronic sinusitis than in the healthy volunteers (Fig. 1; Kruskal-Wallis test for comparing 4 groups, $P = 0.0004$; unpaired t-tests for comparing 2 groups: head trauma, $P = 0.0005$; upper respiratory tract infection, $P = 0.0001$; chronic sinusitis, $P = 0.0003$; Bonferroni's multiple comparison test for comparing 2 groups: head trauma, $P < 0.0001$; upper respiratory tract infection, $P < 0.0001$; chronic sinusitis, $P < 0.0001$). There were no significant differences between each patient group in migration of nasally administered $^{201}$Tl to the olfactory bulb.

Representative cases are shown in Fig. 2 and summarized in Table 2. A 60-year-old healthy male volunteer showed good olfactory function and a high level of nasal $^{201}$Tl migration to the olfactory bulb (Fig. 2A, Table 2), a 44-year-old female with hyposmia after head trauma showed severe olfactory dysfunction and a low level of nasal $^{201}$Tl migration to the olfactory bulb (Fig. 2B, Table 2), a 42-year-old female with hyposmia after upper respiratory tract infection showed moderate olfactory dysfunction and a low level of nasal $^{201}$Tl migration to the olfactory bulb (Fig. 2C, Table 2), and a 67-year-old female with hyposmia from chronic rhinosinusitis showed moderate olfactory dysfunction and a low level of nasal $^{201}$Tl migration to the olfactory bulb (Fig. 2D, Table 2). MRI images of the representative cases are shown in Fig. 3.

### Nasal $^{201}$Tl Migration to the Olfactory Bulb and Olfactory Function Assessed by T&T Olfactometry

To assess whether nasal $^{201}$Tl migration to the olfactory bulb reflects olfactory function, we examined the relationships between the recognition threshold obtained with T&T olfactometry and the amount of nasal $^{201}$Tl that migrated to the olfactory bulb in the subjects.

Nasal $^{201}$Tl migration to the olfactory bulb was correlated with the odor recognition threshold obtained by T&T olfactometry (Spearman $r = -0.62$, $P = 0.0002$) in the healthy volunteers and the olfaction-impaired patients evaluated as a single group (Fig. 4). Nasal $^{201}$Tl migration to the olfactory bulb was not correlated with duration of olfactory deficits at the time of the examination in the patients with impaired olfaction (Spearman $r = 0.33$, $P = 0.15$).

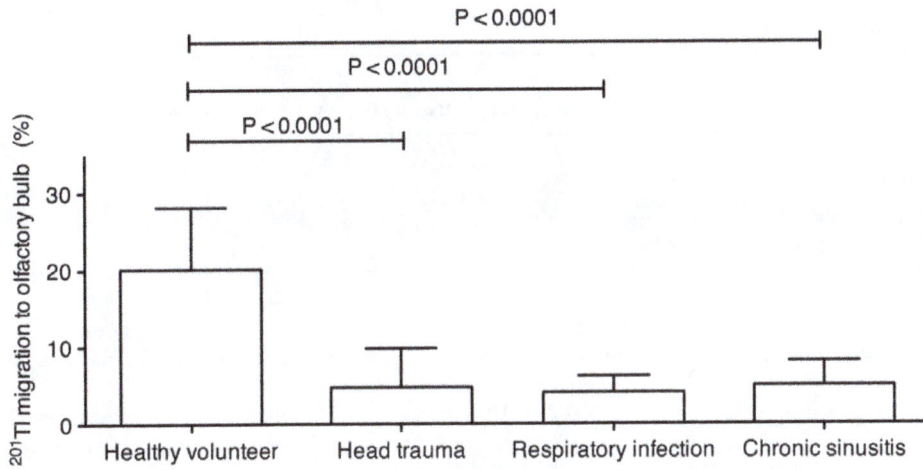

**Figure 1. $^{201}$Tl migration in patients with impaired olfaction in comparison to healthy volunteers.** Nasal $^{201}$Tl migration to the olfactory bulb in healthy volunteers (n = 10) and patients with impaired olfaction due to head trauma (n = 7), upper respiratory tract infection (respiratory infection; n = 7), or chronic rhinosinusitis (n = 7). *P* values were obtained with Bonferroni's multiple comparison test and the Kruskal-Wallis test. Bars: Mean ± S.D.

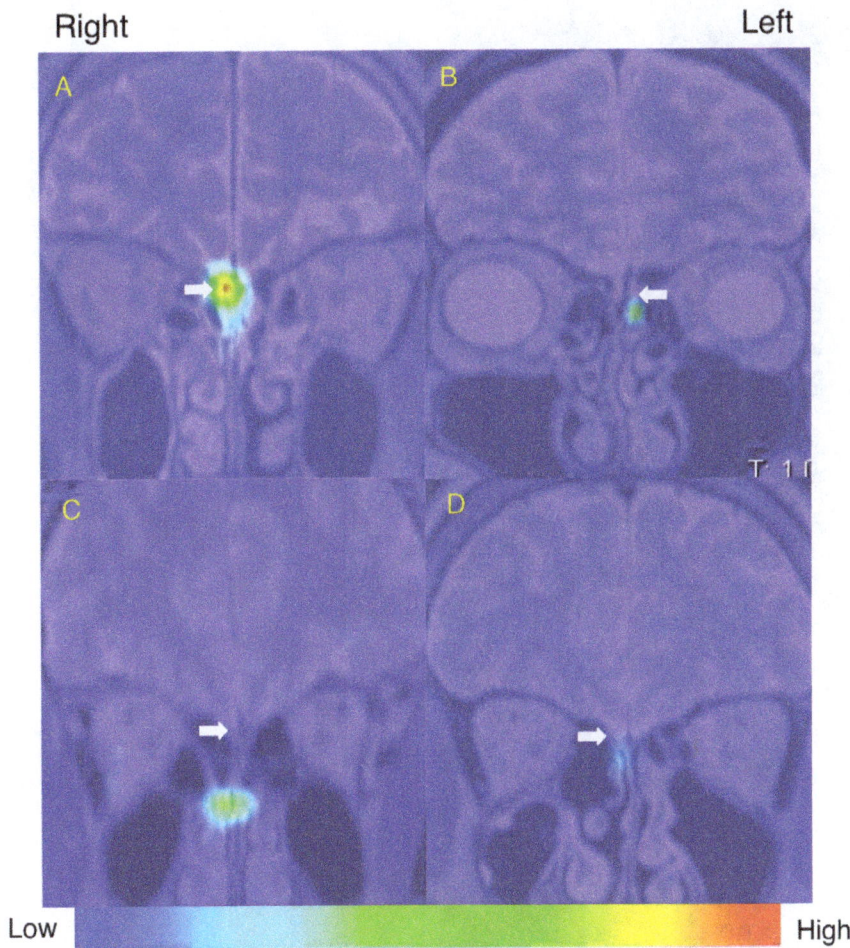

**Figure 2. SPECT-MRI fusion image (coronal view) of nasal $^{201}$Tl migration to the olfactory bulb.** White arrows indicate the olfactory bulb and olfactory nerve. (A) A 60-year-old healthy male volunteer. (B) A 44-year-old female with hyposmia after head trauma. (C) A 42-year-old female with hyposmia after upper respiratory tract infection. (D) A 67-year-old female with hyposmia due to chronic rhinosinusitis. The index of $^{201}$Tl migration from the olfactory epithelium to the olfactory bulb in the selected subjects was shown in Table 2.

**Table 2.** Functional olfactory measurements in selected subjects.

| Selected subjects | Nasal $^{201}$Tl migration to the olfactory bulb, % | Odor recognition threshold |
|---|---|---|
| 60-year-old healthy male volunteer | 29.0 | 1.4 |
| 44-year-old female with hyposmia after head trauma | 4.2 | 5.8 |
| 42-year-old female with hyposmia after upper respiratory tract infection | 4.5 | 4.8 |
| 67-year-old female with hyposmia due to chronic rhinosinusitis | 5.0 | 3.2 |

## Nasal $^{201}$Tl Migration to the Olfactory Bulb and Olfactory Bulb Volume Determined from MRI Images

To assess whether nasal $^{201}$Tl migration to the olfactory bulb reflects olfactory bulb size, we examined the relationships between the olfactory bulb volume determined from MRI images and the amount of nasal $^{201}$Tl that migrated to the olfactory bulb in the subjects. Olfactory bulb volume was significantly lower in the patients with head trauma, upper respiratory infection, or chronic sinusitis than in the healthy volunteers (Table 3).

Nasal $^{201}$Tl migration to the olfactory bulb was correlated with the olfactory bulb volume determined from MRI images (Spearman $r = 0.73$, $P < 0.0001$) in the healthy volunteers and the olfaction-impaired patients evaluated as a single group (Fig. 5).

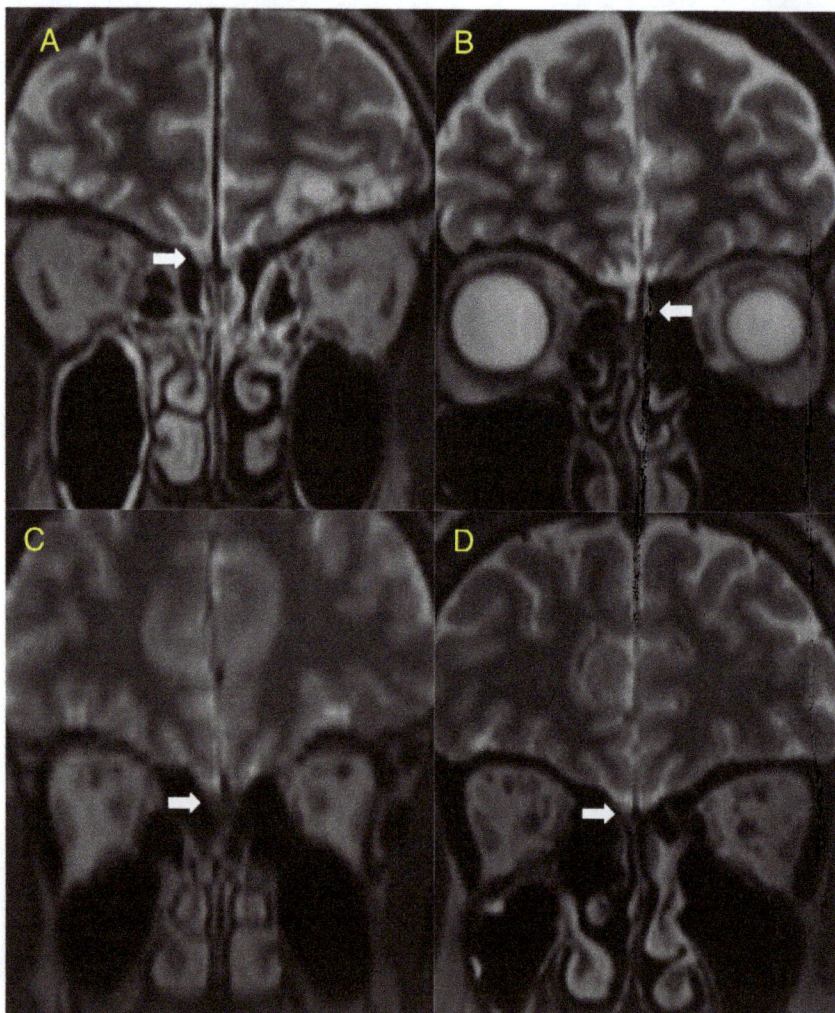

**Figure 3. MRI image (T2 weighted, coronal view).** White arrows indicate the olfactory bulb and olfactory nerve. (A) A 60-year-old healthy male volunteer. (B) A 44-year-old female with hyposmia after head trauma. (C) A 42-year-old female with hyposmia after upper respiratory tract infection. (D) A 67-year-old female with hyposmia due to chronic rhinosinusitis.

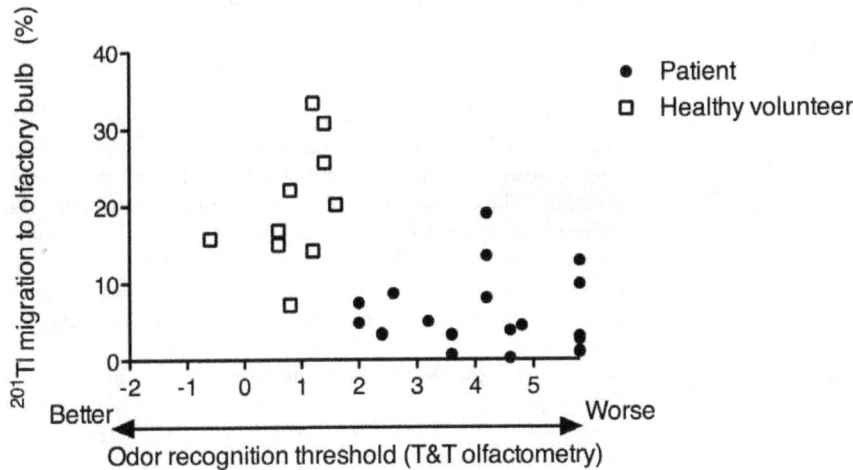

**Figure 4. Correlation between olfactory $^{201}$Tl migration and olfactory function as assessed by T&T olfactometry.** Nasal $^{201}$Tl migration to the olfactory bulb as a function of odor recognition threshold in patients and healthy volunteers (n = 31). Spearman $r = -0.62$, $P = 0.0002$. Closed circles, patients; Open squares, healthy volunteers.

## Discussion

Nasal $^{201}$Tl migration to the olfactory bulb was reduced in the patients with impaired olfaction due to head trauma, upper respiratory tract infection, and chronic rhinosinusitis, which are major causes of olfactory dysfunction [11] relative to the values in healthy volunteers. The assessment of olfactory nerve damage using our imaging method may be useful for scanning the lesion of the olfactory nerve connectivity in patients with impaired olfaction. Patients with impaired olfaction due to major causes of olfactory dysfunction would have damage of olfactory mucosa, because histological changes have been reported in the olfactory mucosa of patients with olfactory deficits due to head trauma [15,16], upper respiratory tract infection [17], or chronic sinusitis [18]. The degree of axon degeneration in human olfactory mucosa correlates with olfactory function [19]. Decreased peripheral olfactory neuron in olfactory mucosa of the patients with impaired olfaction may reduce the nasal $^{201}$Tl migration to the olfactory bulb.

The migration of $^{201}$Tl to the olfactory bulb was correlated with odor recognition thresholds obtained with T&T olfactometry when all subjects were included. Furthermore, the volume of the olfactory bulb determined by using MR images was positively correlated with the level of $^{201}$Tl migration from the nasal turbinate area to the olfactory bulb on SPECT-MRI fusion images in both the healthy volunteers and patients with impaired olfaction. Our results suggest that the connectivity of olfactory neurons between the olfactory bulb and olfactory mucosa reflect

the volume of the olfactory bulb. Increasing olfactory stimulation leads to decreased cell mortality in the olfactory bulb *in vivo* [20]. Reduced connectivity of olfactory neurons between the olfactory bulb and olfactory mucosa may effect on olfactory bulb volume with a decrease of olfactory stimulation in the patients with impaired olfaction.

The nasal $^{201}$Tl migration to the olfactory bulb was not significantly correlated with olfactory bulb volume determined by using MR images in the healthy volunteers or in the patients with impaired olfaction evaluated as separate groups (data not shown), likely because of the small number of subjects in each group. It has been shown that olfactory bulb volume is larger in men than in women [21]. It warrants further investigation whether gender would effect on the nasal $^{201}$Tl migration to the olfactory bulb.

In this study, the decrease of the migration of $^{201}$Tl to the olfactory bulb was not significantly different among the patients with head trauma, upper respiratory tract infection, or chronic sinusitis. The degree of peripheral olfactory nerve degeneration may be similar in the patient groups included in this study, because we observed no significant different olfactory thresholds among the patient groups.

In this study, we observed no adverse effects in the subjects. Unlike intravenous administration of radiopharmaceutical agents, which would deliver only small amounts of radiation to the nasal cavity, nasal administration of $^{201}$Tl delivers a high radiation dose to the nasal cavity. Therefore, the estimation of the absorbed dose in the nasal cavity and neighboring organ such as brain and lens are important. We calculated the absorbed dose of $^{201}$Tl in the

**Table 3.** Olfactory bulb volume measurements in subjects.

| Subject Group | Olfactory bulb volume, mm$^3$ (Mean ± S.D.) |
|---|---|
| Healthy volunteer (n = 10) | 83.2±25.5 |
| Head trauma (n = 7) | 22.4±7.5* |
| Upper respiratory tract infection (n = 7) | 35.8±12.3* |
| Chronic rhinosinusitis (n = 7) | 33.3±10.5* |

*$P<0.05$ (unpaired t-tests: comparison with healthy volunteers).

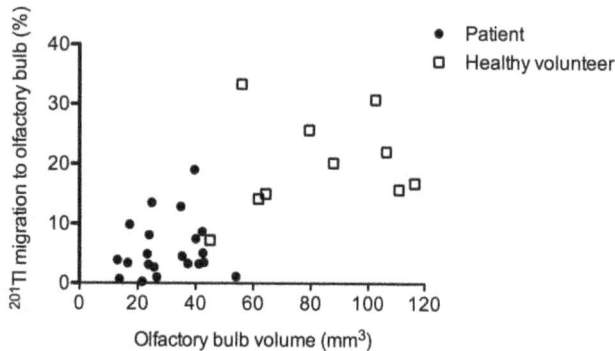

**Figure 5. Correlation between olfactory $^{201}$Tl migration and unilateral olfactory bulb volume as determined by using MRI images.** Nasal $^{201}$Tl migration to the olfactory bulb as a volume of olfactory bulb in patients and healthy volunteers (n = 31). Spearman r = 0.73, P<0.0001. Closed circles, patients; Open squares, healthy volunteers.

nasal cavity in a previous clinical study, and its dose was too low for acute radiation effects [9]. The brain and eyes are separated from the nasal cavity by the nasal bone, ethmoturbinals, and the sphenoidal bone. A Monte Carlo simulation using the ICRP reference adult male [22] showed that almost all conversion electrons and Auger electrons emitted from $^{201}$Tl in the nasal cavity were stopped in the nasal cavity and were not absorbed by neighboring organs (data not shown). Therefore, gamma-rays and X-rays from the $^{201}$Tl in the nasal cavity contributed the doses of $^{201}$Tl absorbed in the brain and lens. Our preliminary calculation showed that the absorbed doses in the brain and lens after nasal administration of 22 MBq $^{201}$Tl were 0.067 mGy and 0.59 mGy, respectively. Therefore, acute radiation effects in the brain and lens can be also avoided.

The majority of $^{201}$Tl administered intranasally in this study migrated to the nasopharyngeal region and then was swallowed. It has been shown that intravenously administered $^{201}$Tl is hardly absorbed by the central nervous system, including the olfactory bulb, in vivo [6]. Therefore, the potential systemic effects of swallowed $^{201}$Tl can be ignored. Residual activity in the olfactory epithelium may be independent from mucosal clearance of the administered $^{201}$Tl, because mature olfactory neurons have immotile cilia [23].

It will be important to study whether an increase in $^{201}$Tl migration to the olfactory bulb during treatment is correlated with a decrease in odor recognition thresholds in patients with olfactory disorders. The recovery rate of olfactory function in patients with traumatic olfactory dysfunction is less than 30% [24]. In this study, we did not assess follow-up data in the subjects, but $^{201}$Tl migration can be used to visualize olfactory nerve regeneration in vivo [25]. Our imaging method could be especially helpful for assessing the connectivity of the peripheral olfactory nerve in patients with olfactory disorders during treatment and predicting the course of olfactory impairment. Patients with intact olfactory nerve fibers may be well selected by means of a new isotope imaging technique for the long-term treatment of olfactory dysfunction.

## Conclusions

Nasal $^{201}$Tl migration to the olfactory bulb was reduced in patients with impaired olfaction due to head trauma, upper respiratory tract infection, and chronic rhinosinusitis, which are major causes of olfactory dysfunction when compared to the $^{201}$Tl migration in healthy volunteers. Assessment of the $^{201}$Tl migration to the olfactory bulb was the new method for the evaluation of the olfactory nerve connectivity in patients with olfactory disorders.

## Acknowledgments

We are grateful to the staff in the Division of Radioisotopes, Kanazawa University, and the Division of Radiology, Kanazawa Medical University, for their technical support.

## Author Contributions

Conceived and designed the experiments: HS JT TM. Performed the experiments: HS JT JY KW. Analyzed the data: HS JT S. Kinase KO NW HT. Contributed reagents/materials/analysis tools: TM S. Kinuya KK RA MF. Wrote the paper: HS JT KW TM.

## References

1. Doty RL, Shaman P, Kimmelman CP, Dann MS (1984) University of Pennsylvania Smell Identification Test: a rapid quantitative olfactory function test for the clinic. Laryngoscope 94: 176–178.
2. Cain WS, Gent JF, Goodspeed RB, Leonard G (1988) Evaluation of olfactory dysfunction in the Connecticut Chemosensory Clinical Research Center (CCCRC). Laryngoscope 98: 83–88.
3. Hummel T, Sekinger B, Wolf S, Pauli E, Kobal G (1997) 'Sniffin' sticks': olfactory performance assessed by the combined testing of odor identification, odor discrimination and olfactory threshold. Chem Senses 22: 39–52.
4. Takagi SF (1987) A standardized olfactometer in Japan. A review over ten years. Ann NY Acad Sci 510: 113–118.
5. Rombaux P, Mouraux A, Bertrand B, Nicolas G, Duprez T, et al. (2006) Olfactory function and olfactory bulb volume in patients with postinfectious olfactory loss. Laryngoscope 116: 436–439.
6. Kanayama Y, Enomoto S, Irie T, Amano R (2005) Axonal transport of rubidium and thallium in the olfactory nerve of mice. Nucl Med Biol 32: 505–512.
7. Kinoshita Y, Shiga H, Washiyama K, Ogawa D, Amano R, et al. (2008) Thallium transport and the evaluation of olfactory nerve connectivity between the nasal cavity and olfactory bulb. Chem Senses 33: 73–78.
8. Shiga H, Kinoshita Y, Washiyama K, Ogawa D, Amano R, et al. (2008) Odor detection ability and thallium-201 transport in the olfactory nerve of traumatic olfactory-impaired mice. Chem Senses 33: 633–637.
9. Shiga H, Taki J, Yamada M, Washiyama K, Amano R, et al. (2011) Evaluation of the olfactory nerve transport function by SPECT-MRI fusion image with nasal thallium-201 administration. Mol Imaging Biol 13: 1262–1266.

10. Washiyama K, Shiga H, Hirota K, Tsuchida A, Yamamoto J, et al. (2011) Biological safety of nasal thallium-201 administration: a preclinical study for olfacto-scintigraphy. J. Rad. Res. (Tokyo) 52: 450–455.
11. Holbrook EH, Leopold DA (2006) An updated review of clinical olfaction. Curr Opin Otolaryngol Head Neck Surg 14: 23–28.
12. Zeintl J, Vija AH, Yahil A, Hornegger J, Kuwert T (2010) Quantitative accuracy of clinical 99mTc SPECT/CT using ordered-subset expectation maximization with 3-dimensional resolution recovery, attenuation, and scatter correction. J Nucl Med 51: 921–928.
13. Stansfield EC, Sheehy N, Zurakowski D, Vija AH, Fahey FH, et al. (2010) Pediatric 99mTc-MDP bone SPECT with ordered subset expectation maximization iterative reconstruction with isotropic 3D resolution recovery. Radiology 257: 793–801.
14. Ken S, Di Gennaro G, Giulietti G, Sebastiano F, De Carli D, et al. (2007) Quantitative evaluation for brain CT/MRI coregistration based on maximization of mutual information in patients with focal epilepsy investigated with subdural electrodes. Magn Reson Imaging 25: 883–888.
15. Hasegawa S, Yamagishi M, Nakano Y (1986) Microscopic studies of human olfactory epithelia following traumatic anosmia. Arch Otorhinolaryngol 243: 112–116.
16. Jafek BW, Eller PM, Esses BA, Moran DT (1989) Post-traumatic anosmia. Ultrastructural correlates. Arch Neurol 46: 300–304.
17. Jafek BW, Hartman D, Eller PM, Johnson EW, Strahan RC, et al. (1990) Postviral olfactory dysfunction. Am J Rhinol 4: 91–100.
18. Kern RC (2000) Chronic sinusitis and anosmia: pathologic changes in the olfactory mucosa. Laryngoscope 110: 1071–1077.
19. Holbrook EH, Leopold DA, Schwob JE (2005) Abnormalities of axon growth in human olfactory mucosa. Laryngoscope 115: 2144–2154.

20. Rochefort C, Gheusi G, Vincent JD, Lledo PM (2002) Enriched odor exposure increases the number of newborn neurons in the adult olfactory bulb and improves odor memory. J Neurosci 22: 2679–2689.

21. Buschhuter M, Smitka S, Puschmann S, Gerber JC, Witt M, et al. (2008) Correlation between olfactory bulb volume and olfactory function. Neuroimage 42: 498–502.

22. Menzel HG, Clement C, DeLuca P (2009) ICRP Publication 110. Realistic reference phantoms: an ICRP/ICRU joint effort. A report of adult reference computational phantoms. Ann. ICRP 39: 1–164.

23. Mair RG, Gesteland RC, Blank DL (1982) Changes in morphology and physiology of olfactory receptor cilia during development. Neuroscience 7: 3091–3103.

24. Fujii M, Fukazawa K, Takayasu S, Sakagami M (2002) Olfactory dysfunction in patients with head trauma. Auris Nasus Larynx 29: 35–40.

25. Shiga H, Washiyama K, Hirota K, Amano R, Furukawa M, et al. (2009) Use of thallium transport to visualize functional olfactory nerve regeneration in vivo. Rhinology 47: 460–464.

# 9

# The Effects of Intracranial Pressure Monitoring in Patients with Traumatic Brain Injury

**Shao-Hua Su, Fei Wang\*, Jian Hai, Ning-Tao Liu, Fei Yu, Yi-Fang Wu, You-Hou Zhu**

The Department of Neurosurgery, Tongji Hospital, Tongji University School of Medicine, Shanghai, China

## Abstract

*Background:* Although international guideline recommended routine intracranial pressure (ICP) monitoring for patients with severe traumatic brain injury(TBI), there were conflicting outcomes attributable to ICP monitoring according to the published studies. Hence, we conducted a meta-analysis to evaluate the efficacy and safety of ICP monitoring in patients with TBI.

*Methods:* Based on previous reviews, PubMed and two Chinese databases (Wangfang and VIP) were further searched to identify eligible studies. The primary outcome was mortality. Secondary outcomes included unfavourable outcome, adverse events, length of ICU stay and length of hospital stay. Weighted mean difference (WMD), odds ratio (OR) and 95% confidence intervals (CIs) were calculated and pooled using fixed-effects or random-effects model.

*Results:* two randomized controlled trials (RCTs) and seven cohort studies involving 11,038 patients met the inclusion criteria. ICP monitoring was not associated with a significant reduction in mortality (OR, 1.16; 95% CI, 0.87–1.54), with substantial heterogeneity ($I^2 = 80\%$, P<0.00001), which was verified by the sensitivity analyses. No significant difference was found in the occurrence of unfavourable outcome (OR, 1.40; 95% CI, 0.99–1.98; $I^2 = 4\%$, P = 0.35) and advese events (OR, 1.04; 95% CI, 0.64–1.70; $I^2 = 78\%$, P = 0.03). However, we should be cautious to the result of adverse events because of the substantial heterogeneity in the comparison. Furthermore, longer ICU and hospital stay were the consistent tendency according to the pooled studies.

*Conclusions:* No benefit was found in patients with TBI who underwent ICP monitoring. Considering substantial clinical heterogeneity, further large sample size RCTs are needed to confirm the current findings.

**Editor:** Jorge I. F. Salluh, D'or Institute of Research and Education, Brazil

**Funding:** The authors have no support or funding to report.

**Competing Interests:** The authors have declared that no competing interests exist.

\* E-mail: wangfeidoc@163.com

## Introduction

Traumatic brain injury (TBI) is the leading cause of death and disability after serious injury, an average of 235,000 hospitalizations and 50,000 deaths occurring each year in United States [1]. The damage in patients with TBI is not just due to direct consequences of the primary injury. Subsequently, traumatic space occupying lesions and cerebral edema accompanied by raised intracranial pressure (ICP) may lead to the hypoxic -ischaemic damage, which might result in herniation of brain tissue, inadequate cerebral perfusion, ischemia and death [2,3]. Theoretically, the management of patients with TBI would benefit from ICP monitoring [4]. The guideline from Brain Trauma Foundation (BTF) recommended ICP monitoring for patients with severe TBI (Glasgow Coma Scale (GCS) score ≤8 ) and an abnormal brain computerized tomography (CT) scan. Furthermore, ICP monitoring was also recommended for patients with severe TBI without CT abnormalities but with at least two of the following criteria: age >40 years, motor posturing, or systolic blood pressure < 90 mm Hg [5]. Lane et al. [6], Stocchetti et al. [7] and

Mauritz et al. [8,9] confirmed the benefit of ICP monitoring. Conversely, Shafi et al. [10] and Griesdale et al. [11] reported ICP monitoring was associated with increased mortality. Biersteker et al. [12] and Thompson et al. [13] presented that ICP monitoring was not associated with mortality and unfavorable outcome, which was consistent with Cremer and colleagues [14]. Based on the published two randomized controlled trials (RCTs) [15,16], no significant difference was observed in the survival rate between ICP monitoring group and no ICP monitoring group. Up to date, the efficacy and safety of ICP monitoring following TBI still remains controversial.

Owning to the sample size (324 and 61 patients respectively) included in the two RCTs, the evidences from RCTs were not enough for the definite conclusion. Given no results from registered cochrane database systematic review [17], in our opinion, it would be interesting for us to conduct the first meta-analysis with respect to the efficacy and safety of ICP monitoring in the patients with TBI, which might be a beneficial complement to the present results from RCTs.

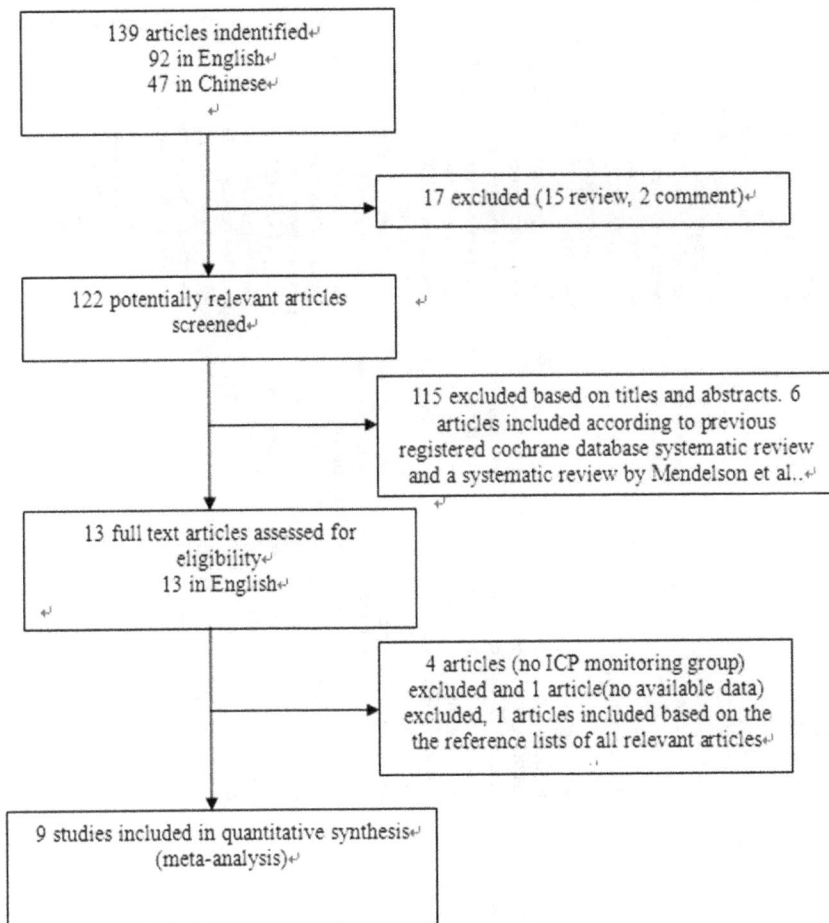

**Figure 1. Selection process for studies included in the meta-analysis.**

## Methods

### Search Strategy and Inclusion Criteria

Based on the previous registered cochrane database systematic review [17] and Mendelson et al. [18], two authors (S.-H.S and F. Y) further searched PubMed and two Chinese databases (Wangfang and VIP) for the relevant articles published up to March, 2013. Research works were examined with language restricted to English and Chinese, and were identified by using the following keywords: "intracranial pressure monitoring" or "intra-cranial pressure monitor*", and "random" or "random*" or "case control" or "cohort" or "observational". The references of all publications and reviews were then reviewed and re-searched to prevent missing any relevant publications.

The following inclusion criteria in PICOS order included: (i) population: patients with diagnosed TBI; (ii) intervention: ICP monitoring; (iii) comparisons: ICP monitoring group versus no ICP monitoring group (imaging or clinical examination); (iv) outcome measures: mortality, unfavourable outcome, length of ICU stay, length of hospital stay and adverse events, one of which should be mentioned in the studies; (v) study design: RCT, case control study and cohort study.

### Data Extraction and Outcome Measures

Two authors (S.-H.S and Y.-F.W) independently screened studies. For each study, we recorded the first author, year of publication, the sample size of population, patients characteristics, patients selection criteria, definitions of outcomes, etc. Any disagreements were resolved by discussion and consensus. A third investigator (F.W) was consulted in case of disagreement to improve accuracy. The analytical data missing from the primary reports were requested from their authors. When the same population was reported in several publications, we retained only the most informative article or complete study to avoid duplication of information.

The primary outcome was mortality. Secondary outcomes included unfavourable outcome, adverse events, length of ICU stay and length of hospital stay.

### Quality Assessment

Cochrane risk of bias assessment [19], which consists of seven items including random sequence generation, allocation conceal-ment, blinding of participants and personnel, blinding of outcome assessment, incomplete outcome data, selective reporting and other bias, was used to evaluate the methodologic quality of RCTs. Newcastle-Ottawa quality assessment scale (NOS) [20], which includes three questions in selection, one question in comparability and three questions in outcome, was applied to assess the methodologic quality of cohort studies. Two authors (J. H and Y.-H. Z) subjectively reviewed all studies and assigned a value of low risk, high risk and unclear risk to the RCTs, and awarding

**Table 1.** Characteristics of patients with TBI.

| Study ID | Design | Number of patients (ICP+/ICP-) | Patients age (years, range or mean±SD) | Male | Diffuse injury II-IV and evacuated mass lesion (ICP+/ICP-) | Midline shift ≥5 mm (ICP+/ICP-) | ICU and hospital stay(ICP+/ICP-) (mean, days) | Neurosurgical Treatment (ICP+/ICP-) | Patients selection criteria | Criteria for ICP+ | Definitons of outcomes | Therapeutic strategies | Studies quality assessed by NOS† |
|---|---|---|---|---|---|---|---|---|---|---|---|---|---|
| Chesnut 2012 | multicenter RCT | 157/167 | >13(22-44) | 87%(283/324) | 97% (152/157) /95% (159/167) | 34% (53/157) /39% (64/164) | (12 and 26) /(9 and 7) | 68% (107/157) /74% (123/166) | Inclusion: Patients with 3< GCS <8 (with a score on the GCS motor component of 1 to 5 if the patient was intubated) or a higher score on admission that dropped to the specified range within 48 hours after injury. Exclusion: Patients with a GCS of 3 and bilateral fixed and dilated pupils and those with an injury believed to be unsurvivable | randomized allocation | GOSE ranges from 1 to 8, with 1 indicating death and 8 indicating the most favorable recovery. Patients with scores ranging from 2 to 4 were classified as having an unfavorable outcome, andthose with scores ranging from 5 to 8 were classified as having a favorable outcome at 6 months | Standard supportive care for each patient, including mechanical ventilation, sedation, and analgesia. Non-neurologic problems were managed aggressively in both groups.Individual treatments: mannitol, hypertonic saline, furosemide,hyperventilation, CSF drainage, barbiturates Neurosurgical procedures: craniotomy for mass lesion, craniectomy with other neurosurgical procedureICP-: more hypertonic saline and hyperventilationICP treatment thresholds: 20 mmHg | NA |
| Biersteker 2012 | prospective observational multicenter cohort study | 123/142 | ≥16(26-69) | 68%(180/265) | 85% (105/123) /70% (99/142) | 34% (42/123) /24% (34/142) | (10.8 and 22) /(2.7 and 7.5) | 69% (85/123) /39% (56/142) | Inclusion: GCS ≤13(GCS ≤13 before intubation if the patient was intubated). Exclusion: Patients'age <16 years, and hospital admission >72 hours zafter the injury was sustained or gunshot injury | 1) patients with severe TBI (GCS ≤8 on ED admission) and an abnormal CT scan; 2) patients with severe TBI without CT abnormalities but with at least two of the following criteria: age >40 yrs, unilateral or bilateral motor posturing (ED GCS motor score ≤3), or systolic blood pressure <90 mm Hg before hospital arrival or at the ED. | GOSE ranges from 1 to 8, with 1 indicating death and 8 indicating the most favorable recovery. Patients with scores ranging from 2 to 4 were classified as having an unfavorable outcome at 6 months | Standard supportive care for each patient, including mechanical ventilation, sedation, intra- and extracranial surgery.Brain-specific treatment included osmotherapy (mannitol or hypertonic saline), vasopressor medication to maintain cerebral perfusion pressure, hyperventilation (Paco$_2$≤4 kPa), CSF drainage, hypothermia (body temperature <35°C), and use of barbiturates. ICP+: more osmotherapy, vasopressors, hypothermia, CSF drainage, hyperventilation, and acute craniotomyICP treatment thresholds: 20 mmHg | 8 |

**Table 1.** Cont.

| Study ID | Design | Number of patients (ICP+/ICP -) | Patients age (years, range or mean±SD) | Male | Diffuse injury II-IV and evacuated mass lesion (ICP+/ICP -) | Midline shift ≥5 mm (ICP+/ICP -) | ICU and hospital stay(ICP+/ICP -) (mean, days) | Neurosurgical Treatment (ICP+/ICP -) | Paitents selection criteria | Criteria for ICP+ | Definitons of outcomes | Therapeutic strategies | Studies quality assessed by NOS [†] |
|---|---|---|---|---|---|---|---|---|---|---|---|---|---|
| Kostic2011 | RCT | 32/29 | 42.2±22 | 87%(53/61) | NA | NA | NA | Total 36% (22/61) | Inclusion: patients with brain trauma and with: GCS≤8 or abnormal CT scan of the brain in terms of present mass lesions. | randomized allocation | GCS at 21st days | Appropriate nutritional support, glycemia control,and peptic ulcer prophylaxis was provided to all ofthe patients. General treatment: 1. headboard at 30°,2. avoidance of the neck flexion, 3. avoidance of hypotension (SAP<90 mm Hg), 4. controlling hypertension (nitroprusside, beta blockers), ventilation to normocarbia (pCO$_2$= 35–40 mmHg), light sedation (e.g.codeine).Specific treatment: 1. deep sedation and/or relaxation (fentanyl, vecuronium), 2.drainage of 3 to 5 ml of CSF (in cases of intraventricularly placed systems), 3. mannitol bolus at first and then application intravenously for 6 hours, 4. hyperventilation to pCO$_2$= 30–35 mmHg. Ultimate treatments: 1. high doses of barbiturates (barbituric coma), 2. hyperventilation to pCO2= 25–30 mmHg, 3. internal or external decompression.ICP treatment thresholds: 20 mmHg | NA |

**Table 1.** Cont.

| Study ID | Design | Number of patients (ICP+/ICP -) | Patients age (years, range or mean±SD) | Male | Diffuse injury II-IV and evacuated mass lesion (ICP+/ICP -) | Midline shift ≥5 mm (ICP+/ICP -) | ICU and hospital stay(ICP+/ICP -) (mean, days) | Neurosurgical Treatment (ICP+/ICP -) | Paitents selection criteria | Criteria for ICP+ | Definitons of outcomes | Therapeutic strategies | Studies quality assessed by NOS † |
|---|---|---|---|---|---|---|---|---|---|---|---|---|---|
| Griesdale 2010 | observational cohort study | 98/73 | NA | 77%(132/ 171) | NA | NA | (14 and ?) /(6 and ?) | NA | Inclusion: GCS ≤8. Exclusion: non-severe TBI, patients who died within 12 hours of ICU admission, and patients with concomitant high cervical spine injury or obvious non-traumatic causes of their decreased level of consciousness | NA | GCS at hospital discharge and 28 th days | All patients are maintained with: 1.head of bed elevated above 30° with their neck in a neutral position. 2. mean arterial pressure≥70 mmHg and $PaO_2$≥70 mmHg. 3. If ICP increases >20 mmHg for greater than five minutes without stimulation, the EVD is opened to 26 cm $H_2O$ and CSF is drained. 4. Cerebral oxygen extraction ratio is maintained <40% by ensuring adequate cerebral perfusion pressure, sedation and paralysisand careful titration of arterial $CO_2$ tension to modify cerebral blood flow. 5. hyperthermia is avoided by using acetaminophen 650 mg every four hours and cooling blankets if required to keep the core temperature <38°. ICP+: more mannitol use and craniotomy.ICP treatment thresholds: 20 mmHg | 7 |

**Table 1.** Cont.

| Study ID | Design | Number of patients (ICP+/ICP-) | Patients age (years, range or mean±SD) | Male | Diffuse injury II-IV and evacuated mass lesion (ICP+/ICP-) | Midline shift ≥5 mm (ICP+/ICP-) | ICU and hospital stay (ICP+/ICP-) (mean, days) | Neurosurgical Treatment (ICP+/ICP-) | Patients selection criteria | Criteria for ICP+ | Definitions of outcomes | Therapeutic strategies | Studies quality assessed by NOS[†] |
|---|---|---|---|---|---|---|---|---|---|---|---|---|---|
| Shafi 2008 | observational multicenter cohort study | 708/938 | 33±8.4 | 76%(1248/1646) | NA | NA | (? and 22) /(? and 25) | 59% (419/708) /39% (248/938) | Inclusion: AIS head scores 3-6, GCS≤8, blunt mechanism, age 20 to 50 years, admission to an ICU for at least 3 days. Exclusion: Early deaths (<48 hours) and delayed admissions (>24 hours after injury) | GCS≤8 in the ED, and CT scan demonstrating a TBI | modified FIM scores range from 1 (completely dependent) to 4 (completely independent) for each of the three functions assessed for a total ranging from 3 to 12 at discharge | NA | 8 |
| Mauritz 2008 | multicenter cohort study | 1031/825 | 29-74 | 73%(1363/1856) | NA | NA | (18 and ?) /(9 and ?) | NA | Inclusion: AIS head >2,GCS<9, TBI Exclusion: discharged alive after <4 days of intensive care, without a documented GCS | NA | AIS and GCS at discharge | Standard supportive care for each patient, including mechanical ventilation, sedation, analgesia, intra- and extracranial surgery. Brain-specific treatment: barbiturates, steroids, mannitol, hypertonic saline, hyperventilation, hypothermia, catecholamines,and fluid balance ICP-: more mechanical ventilation,catecholamines use at first week.ICP treatment thresholds: 20 mm Hg | 8 |

**Table 1.** Cont.

| Study ID | Design | Number of patients (ICP+/ICP-) | Patients age (years, range or mean±SD) | Male | Diffuse injury II-IV and evacuated mass lesion (ICP+/ICP-) | Midline shift ≥5 mm (ICP+/ICP-) | ICU and hospital stay(ICP+/ICP-) (mean, days) | Neurosurgical Treatment (ICP+/ICP-) | Paitents selection criteria | Criteria for ICP+ | Definitons of outcomes | Therapeutic strategies | Studies quality assessed by NOS† |
|---|---|---|---|---|---|---|---|---|---|---|---|---|---|
| Mauritz 2007 * | multicenter cohort study | 248/152 | 50±21 | 72%(286/400) | NA | 28% (69/247) /30% (45/152) | NA | 91% (224/247) /38% (57/152) | Inclusion: patients fulfilled the criteria for severe TBI, GCS,AIS head, ISSExclusion: died at the scene, during transport to the hospital, or immediately after admission to the emergency room | NA | GOS at 6 months. vegetative state and severe disability as unfavourable outcome; good recovery, moderate disability as favourable outcome | Standard supportive care for each patient, including mechanical ventilation, sedation, analgesia, intra- and extracranial surgery. Brain-specific treatment: barbiturates, steroids, mannitol, hypertonic saline, hyperventilation, hypothermia, catecholamines, and fluid balance.ICP+: more craniectomy and craniotomy.ICP treatment thresholds: 20 mm Hg | 8 |
| Stocchetti 2001 | observational multicenter cohort study | 344/589 | >16 42±21 | 74%(738/1000) | Total 86% (862/1000) | NA | NA | NA | Inclusion: all adults(>16 yrs) with GCS≤12 admitted to their care within 24 hours of injury. | NA | GOS at 6 months. death; vegetative state, severe disability as unfavourable outcome; moderate disability, good recovery as favourable outcome. | NA | 7 |
| Lane2000 | observational multicenter cohort study | 541/4946 | 40±24 | 72%(8681/ 12058) | NA | NA | (9.7 and 44) /(4.3 and 22.8) | NA | Inclusion: TBI and a maximum AIS score in the head region (MAIS head) >3, ISS | NA | FIM at discharge | NA | 7 |

TBI: trauma brain injury; ED:emergence department; RCTs: randomized controlled trials; ICP-: no intracranial pressure monitoring; ICP+: intracranial pressure monitoring; AIS: abbreviated injury score; GCS: glasgow coma scale; GOSE: the extended glasgow outcome scale; FIM: functional independence measure; GOS: glasgow outcome scale; ISS: injury severity score; AIS: abbreviated injury scale; CSF: cerebrospinal fluid; EVD: external ventricular drain; NOS: newcastle - ottawa quality assessment scale; NA: not available.

* Data from correspondence author.

† A paper with NOS score ≥7 points was regarded as the paper with high-quality study.

**Table 2.** Quality of RCTs accessed by Cochrane risk of bias assessment.

| Study ID | Random sequence generation | Allocation concealment | Blinding of participants and personnel | Blinding of outcome assessment | Incomplete outcome data | Selective reporting | Other bias |
|---|---|---|---|---|---|---|---|
| Chesnut 2012 | low risk | unclear risk | unclear risk | unclear risk | low risk | unclear risk | unclear risk |
| Kostic 2011 | high risk | unclear risk | unclear risk | unclear risk | low risk | unclear risk | unclear risk |

RCTs: randomized controlled trials.

points for cohort studies (points were then added up and used to compare quality of each study).

## Statistical Analysis

Meta-analysis was carried out by using Cochrane RevMan (version 5.1) software. Continuous data presented as median and interquartile range were transformed to the data with mean ± standard deviation (SD) [21]. For continuous and dichotomous outcomes, differences were calculated using weighted mean difference (WMD) or odds ratio (OR), 95% Confidence Interval (CI) respectively. Heterogeneity for each pooled summary was estimated using Cochran's Q statistic and the $I^2$ statistic. Substantial heterogeneity will be considered to exist with $I^2 > 50\%$ and Chi square test P<0.1. Fixed-effects model was used if the number of studies included in the meta-analysis was less than 5, while random-effects model were used if the number of studies included in the meta-analysis was more than 5. Because patients characteristics, clinical center, types of ICP monitoring used, definitions of outcomes, and other confounding factors were not consistent among studies, we further conducted sensitivity analyses to verify the results or explore possible explanations for heterogeneity or examine the influence of various inconsistent criteria on the overall pooled estimate. We also investigated the influence of a single study on the overall pooled estimate by omitting one study in each turn. If the same directional tendency of outcome was found among studies, meta-analysis would not be applied. Potential publication bias was assessed visually with funnel plot.

## Results

### Study Identification and Selection

The combined search strategy identified 139 papers (92 in English, 47 in Chinese). After careful screening, two RCTs and seven cohort studies satisfied all the inclusion criteria. An additional cohort study was identified by hand searching. One article was excluded for no available data. Thus, eventually nine studies were included in the present meta-analysis. We only received the missing analytical data for meta-analysis from one correspondence author of the included studies [9]. The selection process for studies included in the meta-analysis is shown in Figure 1.

### Characteristics of the Included Studies

Characteristics of patients with TBI present in Table 1. Studies included in our meta-analysis enrolled a total of 11,038 adult patients [6–12,15,16]. Most of patients were male. Glasgow coma scale (GCS) score was used as the patients inclusion criteria in eight studies (GCS≤8 [8–11,15,16], GCS≤12 [7], GCS≤13 [12] ), whereas abbreviated injury score (AIS) head was applied in four studies (AIS head >3 [6,10], AIS head >2 [8,9]) and injury severity score (ISS) was used in two studies [6,9]. Marshall classification on initial CT was described in three studies [7,12,16]. Neurosurgical treatment was mentioned in five studies [9,10,12,15,16]. Criteria for ICP monitoring was presented in two RCTs and two cohort studies [10,12,15,16], which met the BTF guideline. The therapeutic strategies and ICP treatment thresholds were mentioned in two RCTs and four cohort studies [8,9,11,12,15,16]. Baseline of patients characteristics was inconsistent among each studies.

The quality of the included RCTs was assessed by Cochrane risk of bias assessment. If no specific descriptions were found in studies, we tended to choose the answer of unclear risk (Table 2).

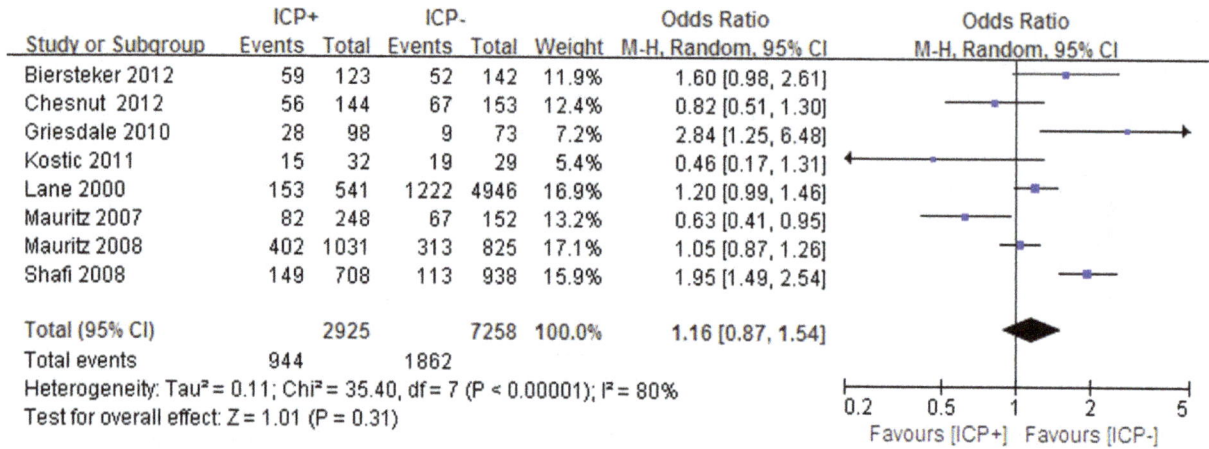

|  | ICP+ | | ICP- | | | Odds Ratio | |
| Study or Subgroup | Events | Total | Events | Total | Weight | M-H, Random, 95% CI | |
| Biersteker 2012 | 59 | 123 | 52 | 142 | 11.9% | 1.60 [0.98, 2.61] |
| Chesnut 2012 | 56 | 144 | 67 | 153 | 12.4% | 0.82 [0.51, 1.30] |
| Griesdale 2010 | 28 | 98 | 9 | 73 | 7.2% | 2.84 [1.25, 6.48] |
| Kostic 2011 | 15 | 32 | 19 | 29 | 5.4% | 0.46 [0.17, 1.31] |
| Lane 2000 | 153 | 541 | 1222 | 4946 | 16.9% | 1.20 [0.99, 1.46] |
| Mauritz 2007 | 82 | 248 | 67 | 152 | 13.2% | 0.63 [0.41, 0.95] |
| Mauritz 2008 | 402 | 1031 | 313 | 825 | 17.1% | 1.05 [0.87, 1.26] |
| Shafi 2008 | 149 | 708 | 113 | 938 | 15.9% | 1.95 [1.49, 2.54] |
| | | | | | | |
| Total (95% CI) | | 2925 | | 7258 | 100.0% | 1.16 [0.87, 1.54] |
| Total events | 944 | | 1862 | | | |

Heterogeneity: Tau² = 0.11; Chi² = 35.40, df = 7 (P < 0.00001); I² = 80%
Test for overall effect: Z = 1.01 (P = 0.31)

**Figure 2. Efficacy of ICP monitoring in the prevention of mortality.** According to Chesnut 2012, the clinical outcomes were evaluated by GOSE at 6 months. Although 157 patients and 167 patients in the ICP(+) group and ICP(−) group respectively, actually only 144 patients in ICP(+) group and 153 patients in ICP(−) group had been assessed at 6 months. ICP: intracranial pressure; GOSE: the extended glasgow outcome scale.

The quality of the included cohort studies was evaluated by NOS (Table 1). The results only reflected our views.

### Primary Outcome

Mortality was observed in eight studies [6,8–12,15,16], which occurred in 944/2925 (32%) patients with ICP monitoring and 1862/7258 (26%) patients with no ICP monitoring respectively. Six-months mortality was shown in two RCTs and one cohort study [12,15,16] and hospital mortality was used in three cohort studies [8,9,11], while no specific time of mortality evaluation was found in two cohort studies [6,10]. ICP monitoring was not associated with a significant reduction in mortality (OR, 1.16; 95% CI, 0.87–1.54) (Figure 2). However, there was evidence of substantial heterogeneity ($I^2 = 80\%$, P<0.00001). Further exclusion of any single study was used to verify the result, which did not materially alter the overall combined OR, with a range from 1.05 (95% CI, 0.81–1.37) to 1.27 (95% CI, 0.96–1.68). Moreover, the sensitivity analyses were also performed to examine the influence of various criteria on the combined estimates, which also showed

that our result was reliable (Table 3).

### Secondary Outcomes

The prognosis of patients with ICP monitoring was evaluated in eight studies [6,8–12,15,16]. However, three studies [8,11,15] presented no detailed data for comparison, whereas two studies [6,10] reported only FIM scores [6] (ICP: 62.1 points, no ICP: 86.8 points) and modified FIM scores [10] (ICP: 5.9 points, no ICP: 7.9 points), which may not be appropriate to be used in meta-analysis because of completely inconsistent scores. Thus, the unfavourable outcome in our meta-analysis was defined as the extended glasgow outcome scale (GOSE) scores ranging from 2 to 4 or glasgow outcome scale (GOS) scores ranging from 2 to 3, which was consistent in three studies [9,12,16]. Figure 3 outlines secondary outcomes from meta-analysis. Unfavorable outcome was confirmed in three studies [9,12,16], which was found in 100/515 (19%) ICP monitoring patients and 64/447 (14%) no ICP monitoring patients respectively. ICP monitoring demonstrated no significant reduction in the occurrence of unfavorable outcome

**Table 3.** Sensitivity analyses based on various criteria for mortality.

| | No. patients | ICP monitoring | No ICPmonitoring | OR (95%CI) | $I^2$ | P Value forHeterogeneity |
|---|---|---|---|---|---|---|
| All studies[6,8–12,15,16] | 10,183 | 944 of 2925 | 1862 of 7258 | 1.16(0.87–1.54) | 80% | <0.00001 |
| Only RCTs [15,16] | 358 | 71 of 176 | 86 of 182 | 0.74(0.49–1.13) | 0% | 0.33 |
| Only cohort studies[6,8–12] | 9,825 | 873 of 2749 | 1776 of 7076 | 1.30(0.95–1.77) | 83% | <0.0001 |
| Cohort studies and pseudo RCT[6–12,15] | 9,886 | 888 of 2781 | 1795 of 7105 | 1.22(0.89–1.66) | 82% | <0.0001 |
| Studies with 6-months mortality [12,15,16] | 623 | 130 of 299 | 138 of 324 | 1.03(0.75–1.41) | 68% | 0.04 |
| Studies with hospital mortality [8,9,11] | 2,427 | 512 of 1377 | 389 of 1050 | 1.01(0.85–1.19) | 82% | 0.0004 |
| Studies with same ICP treatment thresholds (20 mmHg) [8,9,11,12,15,16] | 3,050 | 645 of 1676 | 527 of 1374 | 1.02(0.71–1.46) | 72% | 0.004 |
| Studies with same patients inclusion criteria (GCS≤8) [8–11,15,16] | 4,431 | 732 of 2261 | 588 of 2170 | 1.08(0.71–1.65) | 85% | <0.00001 |

RCTs: randomized controlled trials; ICP: intracranial pressure; GCS: glasgow coma scale.

| Study or Subgroup | ICP+ Events | ICP+ Total | ICP- Events | ICP- Total | Weight | Odds Ratio M-H, Fixed, 95% CI | Odds Ratio M-H, Fixed, 95% CI |
|---|---|---|---|---|---|---|---|
| Biersteker 2012 | 22 | 123 | 15 | 142 | 20.9% | 1.84 [0.91, 3.74] | |
| Chesnut 2012 | 24 | 144 | 26 | 153 | 38.4% | 0.98 [0.53, 1.79] | |
| Mauritz 2007 | 54 | 248 | 23 | 152 | 40.7% | 1.56 [0.91, 2.67] | |
| Total (95% CI) | | 515 | | 447 | 100.0% | 1.40 [0.99, 1.98] | |
| Total events | 100 | | 64 | | | | |

Heterogeneity: Chi² = 2.09, df = 2 (P = 0.35); I² = 4%
Test for overall effect: Z = 1.88 (P = 0.06)

0.2 0.5 1 2 5
Favours [ICP+] Favours [ICP-]

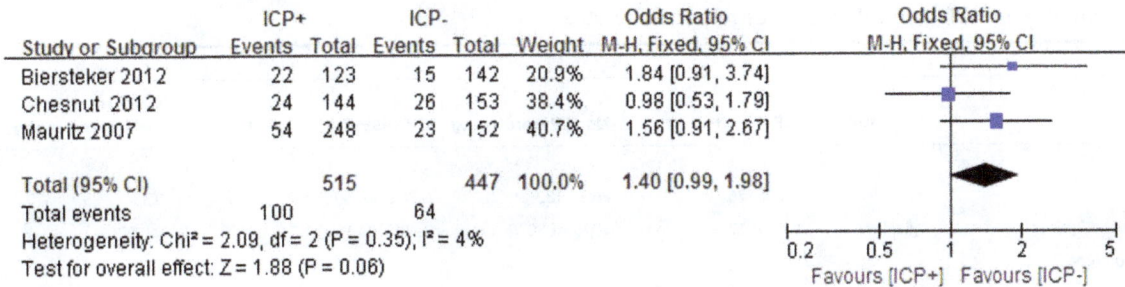

Efficacy of ICP monitoring in the prevention of unfavourable outcome

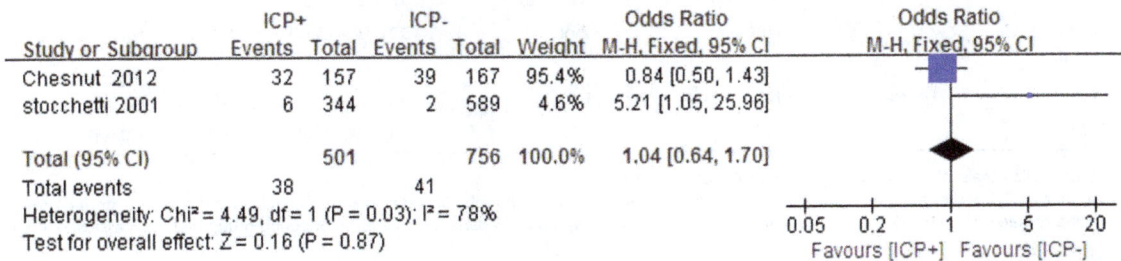

| Study or Subgroup | ICP+ Events | ICP+ Total | ICP- Events | ICP- Total | Weight | Odds Ratio M-H, Fixed, 95% CI | Odds Ratio M-H, Fixed, 95% CI |
|---|---|---|---|---|---|---|---|
| Chesnut 2012 | 32 | 157 | 39 | 167 | 95.4% | 0.84 [0.50, 1.43] | |
| stocchetti 2001 | 6 | 344 | 2 | 589 | 4.6% | 5.21 [1.05, 25.96] | |
| Total (95% CI) | | 501 | | 756 | 100.0% | 1.04 [0.64, 1.70] | |
| Total events | 38 | | 41 | | | | |

Heterogeneity: Chi² = 4.49, df = 1 (P = 0.03); I² = 78%
Test for overall effect: Z = 0.16 (P = 0.87)

0.05 0.2 1 5 20
Favours [ICP+] Favours [ICP-]

Efficacy of ICP monitoring in the prevention of adverse events

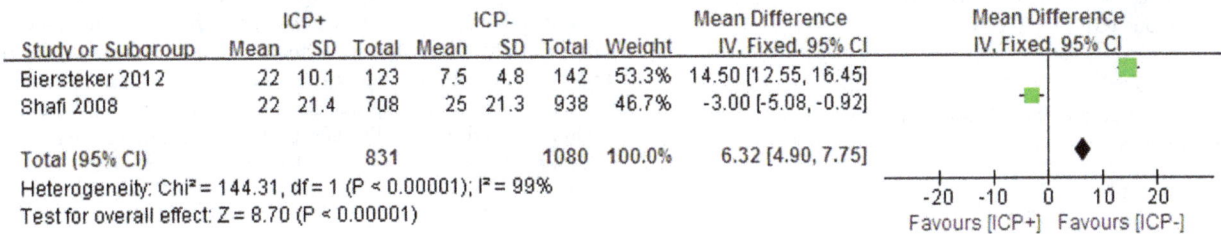

| Study or Subgroup | ICP+ Mean | ICP+ SD | ICP+ Total | ICP- Mean | ICP- SD | ICP- Total | Weight | Mean Difference IV, Fixed, 95% CI | Mean Difference IV, Fixed, 95% CI |
|---|---|---|---|---|---|---|---|---|---|
| Biersteker 2012 | 22 | 10.1 | 123 | 7.5 | 4.8 | 142 | 53.3% | 14.50 [12.55, 16.45] | |
| Shafi 2008 | 22 | 21.4 | 708 | 25 | 21.3 | 938 | 46.7% | -3.00 [-5.08, -0.92] | |
| Total (95% CI) | | | 831 | | | 1080 | 100.0% | 6.32 [4.90, 7.75] | |

Heterogeneity: Chi² = 144.31, df = 1 (P < 0.00001); I² = 99%
Test for overall effect: Z = 8.70 (P < 0.00001)

-20 -10 0 10 20
Favours [ICP+] Favours [ICP-]

Length of hospital stay

**Figure 3. Efficacy of ICP monitoring in the prevention of unfavourable outcome, adverse events and hospital stay.** ICP: intracranial pressure.

(OR, 1.40; 95% CI, 0.99–1.98), with no substantial heterogeneity ($I^2 = 4\%$, P = 0.35). Moreover, unfavorable outcome was assessed by GOSE scores ranging from 2 to 4 at 6 months after hospital discharge, which was completely consistent in two studies [12,16]. The further meta-analysis using the two studies [12,16] confirmed ICP monitoring demonstrated no significant reduction in the occurrence of unfavorable outcome (OR, 1.28; 95% CI, 0.81–2.03), with no substantial heterogeneity ($I^2 = 44\%$, P = 0.18).

Two studies [7,16] reported the adverse events, which included infections, nervous system events, respiratory system events, cardiovascular system events, death from an unspecified cause,etc. The definition of adverse events in our study was infections and nervous system events, which was consistent in two studies [7,16]. Infections and nervous system events as the adverse events occurred in 38/501 (8%) ICP monitoring patients and 41/756 (6%) no ICP monitoring patients respectively. No significant difference (OR, 1.04; 95% CI, 0.64–1.70), with substantial heterogeneity ($I^2 = 78\%$, P = 0.03), was found between two groups.

Length of ICU stay was observed in five studies [6,8,11,12,16]. The same directional tendency was found in all the studies that the days of ICU stay were longer in ICP monitoring patients.

Length of hospital stay was presented in four studies [6,10,12,16]. Due to no data for comparison in one RCT [16] and data only presented as mean in one cohort study [6], hence, two cohort studies included in the final meta-analysis. ICP monitoring had significant impact on length of hospital stay (WMD, 6.32 days; 95% CI, 4.90–7.75), with substantial heterogeneity ($I^2 = 99\%$, P<0.00001).

## Outcomes from RCTs or Cohort Studies

RCTs and cohort studies are two different types of studies, which may enhance the methodological heterogeneity if they were used together in the meta-analysis. Thus, we further conducted the meta-analysis using RCTs or cohort studies respectively. Outcomes from RCTs or cohort studies are shown in Table 4. According to meta-analysis using cohort studies, the incidence of unfavourable outcome, adverse events and longer hospital stay were significant higher in patients with ICP

**Table 4.** Outcomes from RCTs and cohort studies respectively.

| outcomes | No. patients | ICP monitoring | No ICPmonitoring | OR (95%CI) | I² | P Value forHeterogeneity |
|---|---|---|---|---|---|---|
| Mortality | | | | | | |
| RCTs[15,16 *] | 358 | 71 of 176 | 86 of 182 | 0.74(0.49–1.13) | 0% | 0.33 |
| Cohort studies[6,8–12] | 9,825 | 873 of 2749 | 1776 of 7076 | 1.30(0.95–1.77) | 83% | <0.0001 |
| Unfavourable outcome | | | | | | |
| RCTs[16 *] | 297 | 24 of 144 | 26 of 153 | 0.98(0.53–1.79) | NA | NA |
| Cohort studies [9,12] | 665 | 76 of 371 | 38 of 297 | 1.66(1.08–2.54) | 0% | 0.71 |
| Adverse events | | | | | | |
| RCTs [16] | 324 | 32 of 157 | 39 of 167 | 0.84(0.50–1.43) | NA | NA |
| Cohort studies [7] | 933 | 6 of 344 | 2 of 589 | 5.21(1.05–25.96) | NA | NA |
| Length of hospital stay | | | | | | |
| RCTs | NA | NA | NA | NA | NA | NA |
| Cohort studies [10,12] | 1,911 | 831 | 1080 | 6.32(4.90–7.75) | 99% | <0.00001 |

RCTs: randomized controlled trials; ICP: intracranial pressure; NA: not available.

* According to Chesnut 2012, the clinical outcomes were evaluated by GOSE at 6 months. Although 157 patients and 167 patients in the ICP monitoring group and no ICP monitoring group respectively, actually only 144 patients in ICP monitoring group and 153 patients in no ICP monitoring group had been assessed at 6 months.

monitoring, while mortality were not associated with ICP monitoring. Based on the meta-analysis using RCTs, no difference was found for mortality, unfavourable outcomes and adverse events between patients with ICP monitoring and patients without ICP monitoring.

## Publication Bias

No obvious evidence of publication bias was found from funnel plots (Figure 4).

## Discussion

ICP monitoring allows early detection of pressure changes and can guide treatment of elevated ICP [22,23], which has been recommended by international guideline in the treatment of severe TBI [5,24,25]. Nevertheless, owing to the definitions of severe TBI, the types of ICP monitor used, and the levels of intervention, etc, there were conflicting outcomes attributable to ICP monitoring in published studies. The effects of ICP monitoring still remain controversial. In our study, two RCTs and seven obersevational

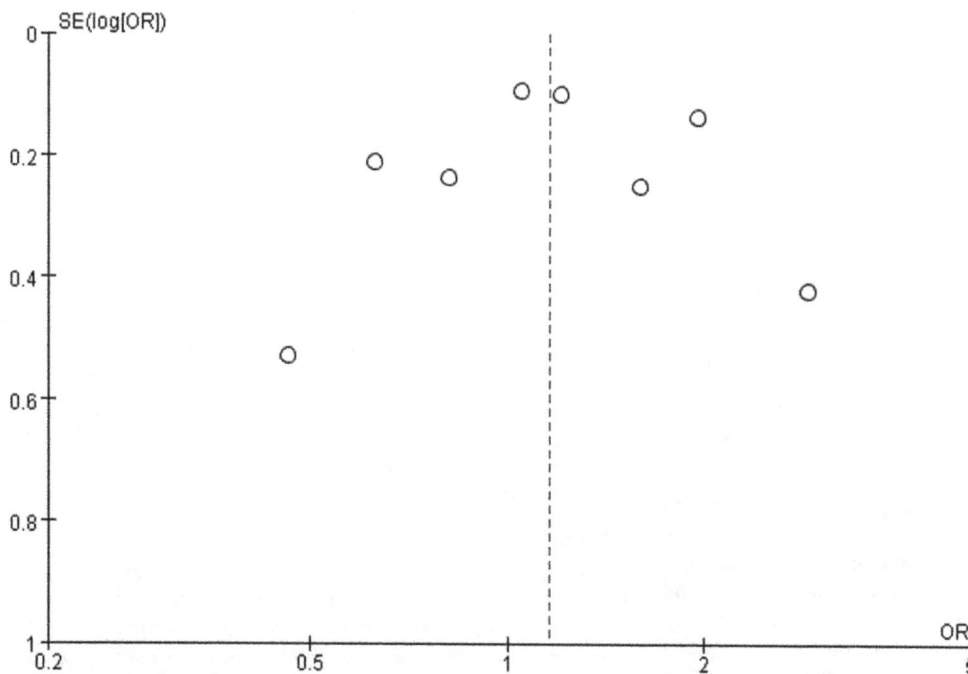

**Figure 4. Publication bias was assessed by inspection of funnel plots for mortality.** Dots was basically symmetrical distribution on both sides of dashed line, indicating that there was no obvious evidence of significant publication bias.

cohort studies with available crude data were firstly pooled to evaluate the efficacy and safety of ICP monitoring in adult patients with TBI. Restricting meta-analysis only to RCTs, which could ensure that confounders are balanced between different treatment groups, would be more accurate to speculate the effects of treatment. However, case control studies or cohort studies are also used for meta-anlysis in recent years. Heterogeneity, which consists of clinical heterogeneity, methodological heterogeneity and statistical heterogeneity, can not be actually eliminated in the process of meta-analysis. If substantial heterogeneity is found in the meta-analysis, sensitivity analysis or stratified analysis could be used to verify the results reliable or find the probable explanations of heterogeneity. Hence, it may be a deserved choice to conduct this meta-analysis to investigate the effects of ICP monitoring in patients with TBI under the current studies.

In our study, we found ICP monitoring did not significantly decrease mortality. Due to the inconsistent baseline of patients characteristics and various clinical interventions, substantial heterogeneity was presented in the analysis. Nevertheless, exclusion of any single study did not materially alter the pooled results. In addition, sensitivity analyses based on different categories of included studies were used to verify the pooled results, suggestive of reliable result. Moreover, the subgroup meta-analysis using RCTs or cohort studies also showed that ICP monitoring was not associated with mortality. With respects to unfavourable outcome and advese events, we only chose the data with consistent inclusion criteria for meta-analysis to reduce the clinical heterogeneity. No significant difference was found in the occurrence of unfavourable outcome and advese events. However, We should be cautious to the result of adverse events because of the substantial heterogeneity in the comparison. Meta-analysis using RCTs confirmed the above results, whereas the meta-analysis with only cohort studies found ICP monitoring was related to the higher incidence of unfavourable outcome and advese events. More aggressive interventions (osmotherapy, hypothermia, cerebrospinal fluid [CSF] drainage, hyperventilation, craniotomy, etc) were found in the patients with ICP monitoring in the cohort studies [9,11,12], in which two studies [9,12] were included in the meta-analysis of unfavourable outcome using only cohort studies. Hence, more aggressive interventions might be responsible for the unfavourable outcome following TBI. Huge difference in the number of patients (1646 patient in Shafi 2008, 265 patients in Biersteker 2012) exactly existed, which may be the reason of substantial heterogeneity in the meta-analysis of the length of hospital stay. Although no futher meta-analysis could be conducted because of the missing data from the included studies, we could speculate longer days in hospital for patients underwent ICP monitoring through these incomplete data.

ICP monitoring is only the first step in ICP/cerebral perfusion pressure (CPP) -based therapy, subsequent therapeutic strategies including efficient interventions (analgesia, sedation, barbiturates, steroids, mannitol, hypertonic saline, hyperventilation, hypothermia, CSF drainage, etc), mechanical ventilation strategies (peak inspiratory pressure, positive end-expiratory pressure, and $pO_2/FiO_2$ ratio), neurosurgical procedures (intra- and extracranial surgery), and ICP treatment thresholds also played important roles in the management of TBI [9]. Different cut-off point of ICP (18 mmHg or 20 mmHg) oriented therapy, different types of ICP monitor used (intraventricular, intraparenchymal or non-invasive) and different therapeutic strategies following ICP monitoring might result in different outcomes, which did not achieve consensus at present. Nevertheless, the articles comparing the above aspects were scarce. Furthermore, we found adverse events (such as infection, nervous system events, cardiovascular system events,etc) seldom mentioned in the published studies, which could be the important risk factor of mortality and poor prognosis in TBI patients who underwent ICP monitoring. Apparently, the need for such further studies should be stressed.

One potential limitation of the present meta-analysis is the various diagnostic or inclusion criteria for ICP monitoring and different levels of interventions used among each studies. With special respect to mortality, the data without scaling the mortality into the same time interval were pooled together for the meta-analysis. Although sensitivity analyses and further exclusion of any single study were used to verify that our result was reliable, we should be very cautious to treat this result. Another limitation is that RCTs and cohort studies were used together in this meta-analysis, which could enlarge potential methodological heterogeneity. The clinical and methodological heterogeneity in the discussed studies may be resposible for the lack of clear evidence to support our results. Finally, missing data in these studies might influence the overall results and should be taken into account. Therefore, our current data need to be substantiated by adequate prospective studies.

In summary, our meta-analysis suggested that no benefit was found in patients with TBI who underwent ICP monitoring. Considering substantial clinical heterogeneity, further large sample size RCTs are needed to confirm our current findings. Hopefully, clinicians may be able to elicit indications and benefit from ICP monitoring by refining and optimizing the use of ICP monitors in the future.

## Acknowledgments

We thank professor Walter Mauritz for sharing unpublished data.

## Author Contributions

Conceived and designed the experiments: SHS FW JH. Performed the experiments: SHS FW YFW FY YHZ JH. Analyzed the data: SHS FW YFW FY YHZ. Contributed reagents/materials/analysis tools: NTL. Wrote the paper: SHS FW JH.

## References

1. Langlois JA, Rutland-Brown W, Wald MM (2006) The epidemiology and impact of traumatic brain injury: a brief overview. J Head Trauma Rehabil 21: 375–378.
2. Padayachy LC, Figaji AA, Bullock MR (2010) Intracranial pressure monitoring for traumatic brain injury in the modern era. Childs Nerv Syst 26: 441–452.
3. Miller JD, Becker DP, Ward JD, Sullivan HG, Adams WE, et al. (1977) Significance of intracranial hypertension in severe head injury. J Neurosurg 47: 503–516.
4. Enblad P, Nilsson P, Chambers I, Citerio G, Fiddes H, et al. (2004) R3-survey of traumatic brain injury management in European Brain IT centres year 2001. Intensive Care Med 30: 1058–1065.
5. Brain Trauma Foundation, American Association of Neurological Surgeons, Congress of Neurological Surgeons, Joint Section on Neurotrauma and Critical Care, AANS/CNS, et al. (2007) Guidelines for the management of severe traumatic brain injury. VI. Indications for intracranial pressure monitoring. J Neurotrauma 24 Suppl 1: S37–S44.
6. Lane PL, Skoretz TG, Doig G, Girotti MJ (2000) Intracranial pressure monitoring and outcomes after traumatic brain injury. Can J Surg 43: 442–448.
7. Stocchetti N, Penny KI, Dearden M, Braakman R, Cohadon F, et al. (2001) Intensive care management of head-injured patients in Europe: a survey from the European brain injury consortium. Intensive Care Med 27: 400–406.

8. Mauritz W, Steltzer H, Bauer P, Dolanski-Aghamanoukjan L, Metnitz P (2008) Monitoring of intracranial pressure in patients with severe traumatic brain injury: an Austrian prospective multicenter study. Intensive Care Med 34: 1208–1215.

9. Mauritz W, Janciak I, Wilbacher I, Rusnak M, Australian Severe TBI Study Investigators (2007) Severe traumatic brain injury in Austria IV: intensive care management. Wien Klin Wochenschr 119: 46–55.

10. Shafi S, Diaz-Arrastia R, Madden C, Gentilello L (2008) Intracranial pressure monitoring in brain-injured patients is associated with worsening of survival. J Trauma 64: 335–340.

11. Griesdale DE, McEwen J, Kurth T, Chittock DR (2010) External ventricular drains and mortality in patients with severe traumatic brain injury. Can J Neurol Sci 37: 43–48.

12. Biersteker HA, Andriessen TM, Horn J, Franschman G, van der Naalt J, et al. (2012) Factors influencing intracranial pressure monitoring guideline compliance and outcome after severe traumatic brain injury. Crit Care Med 40: 1914–1922.

13. Thompson HJ, Rivara FP, Jurkovich GJ, Wang J, Nathens AB, et al. (2008) Evaluation of the effect of intensity of care on mortality after traumatic brain injury. Crit Care Med 36: 282–290.

14. Cremer OL, van Dijk GW, van Wensen E, Brekelmans GJ, Moons KG, et al. (2005) Effect of intracranial pressure monitoring and targeted intensive care on functional outcome after severe head injury. Crit Care Med 33: 2207–2213.

15. Kostić A, Stefanović I, Novak V, Veselinović D, Ivanov G, et al. (2011) Prognostic significance of intracranial pressure monitoring and intracranial hypertension in severe brain trauma patients. Med Pregl 64: 461–465.

16. Chesnut RM, Temkin N, Carney N, Dikmen S, Rondina C, et al. (2012) A trial of intracranial-pressure monitoring in traumatic brain injury. N Engl J Med 367: 2471–2481.

17. Forsyth RJ, Wolny S, Rodrigues B (2010) Routine intracranial pressure monitoring in acute coma. Cochrane Database Syst Rev 17:CD002043.

18. Mendelson AA, Gillis C, Henderson WR, Ronco JJ, Dhingra V, et al. (2012) Intracranial pressure monitors in traumatic brain injury: a systematic review. Can J Neurol Sci 39: 571–576.

19. Higgins JPT, Green S, editors (2013) Cochrane handbook for systematic reviews of interventions. Version 5.1.0. The Cochrane Collaboration. Available: http://www.cochrane-handbook.org.

20. Wells GA, Shea B, O'Connell D, Peterson J, Welch V, et al. (2011) The Newcastle-Ottawa Scale (NOS) for assessing the quality if nonrandomized studies in meta-analyses. Available: http://www.ohri.ca/programs/clinical_epidemiology/oxford.asp.

21. Hozo SP, Djulbegovic B, Hozo I (2005) Estimating the mean and variance from the median, range, and the size of a sample. BMC Med Res Methodo 5: 13.

22. Bulger EM, Nathens AB, Rivara FP, Moore M, MacKenzie EJ, et al. (2002) Management of severe head injury: institutional variations in care and effect on outcome. Crit Care Med 30: 1870–1876.

23. Kristiansson H, Nissborg E, Bartek J Jr, Andresen M, Reinstrup P, et al.(2013) Measuring Elevated Intracranial Pressure through Noninvasive Methods: A Review of the Literature. J Neurosurg Anesthesiol 25: 372–385.

24. Maas AI, Dearden M, Teasdale GM, Braakman R, Cohadon F, et al. (1997) EBIC-guidelines for management of severe head injury in adults. European Brain Injury Consortium. Acta Neurochir (Wien) 139: 286–294.

25. Andrews PJ, Citerio G, Longhi L, Polderman K, Sahuquillo J, et al. (2008) Neuro-Intensive Care and Emergency Medicine (NICEM) Section of the European Society of Intensive Care Medicine: NICEM consensus on neurological monitoring in acute neurological disease. Intensive Care Med 34: 1362–1370.

# 10

# Pre-Bout Standing Body Sway Differs between Adult Boxers Who do and do not Report Post-Bout Motion Sickness

Yi-Chou Chen[1], Ting-Hsuan Hung[2], Tzu-Chiang Tseng[3], City C. Hsieh[4], Fu-Chen Chen[5], Thomas A. Stoffregen[1]*

[1] School of Kinesiology, University of Minnesota, Minneapolis, Minnesota, United States of America, [2] Office of Institutional Research, Edgewood College, Madison, Wisconsin, United States of America, [3] Graduate Institute of Sport Coaching Science, Chinese Cultural University, Taipei, Taiwan, [4] College of Well Being, YuanPei University, HsinChu, Taiwan, [5] Department of Recreation Sport and Health Promotion, National Pingtung University of Science and Technology, Pingtung, Taiwan

## Abstract

*Background:* Motion sickness is characterized by subjective symptoms that include dizziness and nausea. Studies have shown that subjective symptoms of motion sickness are preceded by differences in standing body sway between those who experience the symptoms and those who are not. Boxers often report dizziness and nausea immediately after bouts. We predicted that pre-bout standing body sway would differ between boxers who experienced post-bout motion sickness and those who did not.

*Methodology/Principal Findings:* We collected data on standing body sway before bouts. During measurement of body sway participants performed two visual tasks. In addition, we varied stance width (the distance between the heels). Postural testing was conducted separately before and after participants' regular warm-up routines. After bouts, we collected self-reports of motion sickness incidence and symptoms. Results revealed that standing body sway was greater after warm-up than before warm-up, and that wider stance width was associated with reduced sway. Eight of 15 amateur boxers reported motion sickness after a bout. Two statistically significant interactions revealed that standing body sway before bouts differed between participants who reported post-bout motion sickness and those who did not.

*Conclusions/Significance:* The results suggest that susceptibility to motion sickness in boxers may be manifested in characteristic patterns of body sway. It may be possible to use pre-bout data on postural sway to predict susceptibility to post-bout motion sickness.

**Editor:** Stephen D. Ginsberg, Nathan Kline Institute and New York University School of Medicine, United States of America

**Funding:** There was no external funding for this research.

**Competing Interests:** The authors have declared that no competing interests exist.

* E-mail: tas@umn.edu

## Introduction

Boxing is characterized by high intensity cardiovascular activity, by intense concentration and, in many cases, by blows to the head. After bouts, boxers often experience headache, confusion, memory difficulties, fatigue, attention and concentration difficulties, and sleep disturbances that can persist for hours, days, weeks, or months [1]. Immediately after bouts, boxers often experience dizziness and nausea [2]. These latter symptoms classically are associated with motion sickness and, indeed, boxers often refer to their acute post-bout symptoms as *motion sickness*. In the present study, our focus was on relations between motion sickness and standing body sway in adult boxers.

### Postural sway and motion sickness

People often experience motion sickness when exposed to simulation and virtual environment systems. Examples include video games [3–5], video projection systems [6–7], head-mounted displays [8–9] and flight simulators [10–12]. Exposure to

simulators and virtual environments is associated with generalized increases in postural sway [6,10–11,13]. That is, postural sway measured after using one of these systems differs from sway measured before exposure to the system. Typically, it is assumed that both motion sickness and postural sway effects are caused by the fact of being exposed to a virtual environment. However, several studies have revealed differences in postural activity between participants who (later) reported motion sickness and those who did not. Differences have been observed in the spatial magnitude of postural sway [12,14], with greater movement magnitude among participants who later reported motion sickness. Differences have also been observed in the temporal dynamics of postural sway, with greater temporal structure or self-similarity among participants who later reported motion sickness [15]. These effects are not limited to virtual environments. Nachum et al. [16] measured participants' standing sway before and after a sea voyage and related these data to the incidence of mal de debarquement (motion sickness that occurs after returning to land from a ship). Prior to a sea voyage, postural activity differed between sailors who reported mal de debarquement after sailing and those who did not. These effects provide the empirical motivation for the present study.

Motion sickness-like symptoms, such as nausea and dizziness, characterize many conditions that typically are not considered to be related to motion sickness, such as altitude sickness [17], vertigo [18–19], and morning sickness in pregnancy [20], as well as boxing. Stoffregen [21] argued that there might be differences in postural sway between persons who are susceptible to these maladies and persons who are not susceptible. The documented relation between postural sway and the subsequent experience of visually induced motion sickness suggests that data on body sway might be used to predict susceptibility to motion sickness in individuals [21]. In the present study our primary aim was to test the hypothesis that postural sway before a bout would differ between boxers who experienced post-bout motion sickness and those who did not.

## Modulating factors

Under controlled manipulations of stance width (the distance between the heels) body sway tends to be greater when the feet are close together, and less when the feet are farther apart [22–23]. Variations in stance width can also alter the temporal dynamics of sway [24,25]. When asked to stand comfortably, healthy adults typically place their heels about 17 cm apart [26]. However, self-selected stance width can change according to circumstances. During pregnancy women tend to select wider stance, that is, they increase the distance between the feet [27]. We also vary stance width rapidly in different situations. For example, mariners adopt wider stance width at sea than they do on land [28], and baseball players typically adopt a wide stance when batting. Of greater relevance to the present study, boxers typically adopt a wide stance in the ring. This habitual, task-specific choice may influence relations between stance width and standing body sway. An important additional factor is the experimental finding that wider stance reduces susceptibility to visually induced motion sickness [15]. In light of these factors we elected to manipulate stance width, and we predicted that wider stance would lead to reduced sway in boxers.

In the general population, standing body sway is influenced by variations in visual and cognitive tasks such as auditory reaction time, or visual task difficulty [29]. For example, sway magnitude is often reduced during performance of demanding tasks, such as reading, relative to sway during less demanding tasks, such as looking at a blank target [24,30–32]. Studies of standing body sway in athletes have evaluated eyes open and eyes closed conditions but have not included variations in visual tasks [33–36]. We hypothesized that the magnitude and self-similarity of postural sway would be reduced during performance of a demanding visual task in boxers when tested before a bout.

## The present study

In the present study, our primary objective was to determine whether standing body sway measured before a bout would differ between boxers who reported post-bout motion sickness and those who did not. We measured standing body sway before boxers entered the ring. After boxers completed their bout, we evaluated subjective symptoms that typically are associated with motion sickness. We predicted that patterns of pre-bout postural sway would differ between boxers who later experienced motion sickness and those that did not.

We measured body sway in the absence of any external source of motion (i.e., there was no mechanical perturbation, such as occurs in moving platform posturography [33–34]). In addition,

unlike many previous studies we did not ask participants to stand "as still as possible" [36–37]; rather, we instructed participants to stand comfortably.

## Methods

### Ethics statement

The research protocol was approved in advance by the YuanPei University IRB. Prior to data collection, we obtained informed consent from each participant.

Testing was conducted at the Contender Fitness Boxing Club, New Taipei City, Taiwan during a national boxing competition for club level boxers. In Taiwan, *club level* refers to amateur boxers whose age and training background are compatible with rules of the World Series of Boxing of the International Boxing Association (known as AIBA).

### Participants

Seventeen boxers participated. Due to time pressure relating to the schedule of bouts, two participants were not able to participate in postural testing and, for this reason, were deleted from our analyses. Accordingly, our sample included 15 individuals. All were male. They varied in age from 18–34 years (mean = 25.6 years, SD = 5.1 years), in height from 160–186 cm (mean = 173.5 cm, SD = 7.9 cm), and in weight from 53–106 kg (mean = 72.8 kg, SD = 15.7 kg).

### Apparatus

Data on postural activity were collected using a force plate (AccuswayPlus, AMTI). We collected data on the kinematics of the center of pressure, sampled at 60 Hz in the AP and ML axes.

### Procedure

We evaluated motion sickness incidence and symptoms using the Simulator Sickness Questionnaire, or SSQ [38]. We used a modified version of the SSQ. The modification consisted of the addition of one question: *Are you motion sick?* In responding to this question, participants were required to circle either *yes* or *no*. For this study the SSQ was translated into Chinese.

Data were collected in relation to each individual's first bout in the national competition. All data were collected on the day of the bout. Prior to their bout, boxers went through a warm-up routine, usually consisting of 5 minutes of light jogging, extensive stretching, and "mitten drills" in which they practiced different types of punches. The total duration of the warm-up was approximately 30 minutes. The warm-up increased heart rate and respiration and for this reason might influence postural sway which, in turn, might influence relations between pre-bout sway and post-bout subjective symptoms. To account for this possibility we measured postural sway before warm-up and again after warm-up.

Before each participant went through his regular warm-up routine he completed the informed consent procedure, the first SSQ and the first session of postural testing. After completing the warm-up each participant completed the second SSQ and the second session of postural testing.

Postural testing consisted of 6 trials, each 60 s in duration, standing on the force plate. We used a 2 (Inspection vs. Search)×3 (Stance Width = 5 cm vs. 17 cm vs. 30 cm) design with one trial per session (before vs. after warm-up) in each of six conditions for a total of 12 trials per participant. Within each session the order of conditions was counterbalanced across participants.

Visual targets used during postural testing were identical to those used by Stoffregen et al. [31], and consisted of sheets of white paper 13.5 cm×17 cm mounted on rigid cardboard. In the Search task the target was one of four blocks of English text, each consisting of 13 or 14 lines of text printed in a 12-point sans serif font. Before each trial the participant was given a target letter (A, R, N, or S) and asked to count the number of times the target letter appeared in the block of text. At the end of each trial, the participant reported the number of letters counted. The Search task resembled the King-Devick test, which has been used to assess cognitive consequences of head trauma in boxers [39]. In the Inspection task, the target consisted of a blank sheet of white paper; participants were instructed to keep their gaze within the borders of the target. The Inspection task was similar to "quiet stance" conditions used in previous studies [29] and can be considered a control condition for the Search task.

Bouts consisted of three rounds (3 minutes per round), and could be terminated early in the event of knockout (KO) or technical knockout (TKO). The third SSQ was administered during the "cool down" period, 10 to 20 minutes after the bout.

## Analysis of Postural Data

We separately evaluated the magnitude and temporal dynamics of postural activity. Magnitude measures, such as positional variability, velocity, and range, provide information about the size or spatial extent of movement (e.g., "by how many centimeters do COP data points tend to differ from each other?"). Magnitude measures, by their nature, tend to eliminate or discard the temporal structure of movement data, that is, how the measured quantity varies in time (e.g., "to what extent does COP displacement at time A resemble displacement at time B?"). Analyses that preserve information about the temporal structure of data on human movement (that is, analyses of the temporal dynamics of movement) are increasingly common [40–41], and can reveal changes in the temporal structure of postural activity in response to variations in visual tasks [42]. We assessed movement dynamics using detrended fluctuation analysis, or *DFA*. DFA describes the relation between the magnitude of fluctuations in postural motion and the time scale over which those fluctuations are measured [43]. DFA has been used in several studies of the control of stance [35], and in our own research on visually induced motion sickness [4,7,15]. We did not integrate the time series before performing DFA. We conducted inferential tests on $\alpha$, the scaling exponent of DFA, as derived from the COP data. The scaling exponent is an index of long-range autocorrelation in the data, that is, the extent to which the data are self-similar over different time-scales. Postural sway in healthy adults tends to be non-stationary, typically yielding $1.0 > \alpha > 1.5$ [41].

We conducted 2×2×2×3 repeated measures ANOVAs on factors Group (Sick vs. Well), Task (Inspection vs. Search), Warm-up (Before warm-up vs. After warm-up), and Stance Width (5 cm vs. 17 cm vs. 30 cm). The dependent variables were the positional variability of the center of pressure, and $\alpha$ of DFA. Separate analyses were conducted for postural activity in the AP and ML axes. To accommodate any violations of the ANOVA sphericity assumption, we used the Greenhouse-Giesser correction [44], which adjusts the number of degrees of freedom used for individual comparisons in the ANOVA in response to violations of sphericity. Where appropriate we report the fractional degrees of freedom that characterize this correction. For statistically significant effects we used the partial $\eta^2$ statistic as a measure of effect size.

## Results

Participants (and their coaches) indicated that they regularly trained and sparred at their local boxing clubs and participated in local, club level competitions. None of the participants had competed in any boxing tournament in the previous month. In the two weeks preceding the national competition all competitors had reduced schedules of sparring. This less intensive level of practice was maintained until the day of the competition. Thus, none of the participants had experienced a concussion or loss of consciousness during the two weeks prior to their participation in our study.

None of the participants were diagnosed with a concussion following their participation in the study.

### Visual performance

There was no measure of performance for the Inspection task. Following previous studies, we took for granted that participants maintained their gaze within the boundaries of the blank target [31]. For the Search task, the dependent variable was the number of target letters that S reported at the end of each trial. We conducted a 2×2×3 repeated measures ANOVA on factors Group (Sick vs. Well), Time (Before warm-up vs. After warm-up), and Stance Width (5 cm vs. 17 cm vs. 30 cm). Visual performance was influenced by stance width, $F(2,26) = 3.64$, $p = .04$. As shown in Figure 1, the number of letters counted was positively associated with greater stance width. There were no other significant effects.

### Subjective symptoms

Before and after warm-up, each participant stated that they were not motion sick. After their bout, 8 participants stated that they were not motion sick. Seven of 15 (47%) stated that they were motion sick (should sum. Data on wins and losses are presented in Table 1.

Data on symptom severity are summarized in Figure 2. In evaluating the severity of symptoms we used the Total Severity Score, which we computed in the recommended manner [38]. The third SSQ was completed approximately 15 minutes after each participant's bout. Before warm-up, SSQ scores did not differ between participants who later reported motion sickness and participants who did not, $U = 31$, $p = .340$. After warm-up, SSQ scores did not differ between participants who later reported motion sickness and participants who did not, $U = 30$, $p = .386$. After their bouts, SSQ scores were higher among participants in the Sick group than in the Well group, $U = 42$, $p < .05$.

### Postural activity

For positional variability in the ML axis we found a significant main effect of Warm-up, $F(1,13) = 51.87$, $p < .001$, partial $\eta^2 = 0.800$. Positional variability after warm-up (mean = 0.323, SD = 0.019) was greater than before warm-up (mean = 0.223, SD = 0.023). The main effect of Stance Width was also significant, $F(1.22,26) = 22.98$, $p < .001$, partial $\eta^2 = 0.639$ (Figure 3a). Post-hoc tests revealed that each stance width differed from each of the other two stance widths, each $p < .008$. There was a significant Group×Warm-up interaction, $F(1,6) = 14.94$, $p = .002$, partial $\eta^2 = 0.535$ (Figure 4). Post-hoc comparisons revealed that, after warm-up, positional variability was greater for the Sick group than for the Well group, $p < .001$. Finally, the Warm-up×Stance Width interaction was significant, $F(1.55,20.13) = 7.42$, $p = .006$, partial $\eta^2 = 0.363$ (Figure 5). Post-hoc comparisons revealed that stance width had a significant influence on sway after warm-up but not before warm-up, $p < .05$, confirming our prediction.

For positional variability in the AP axis we found no significant main effects. There was a significant interaction between Group

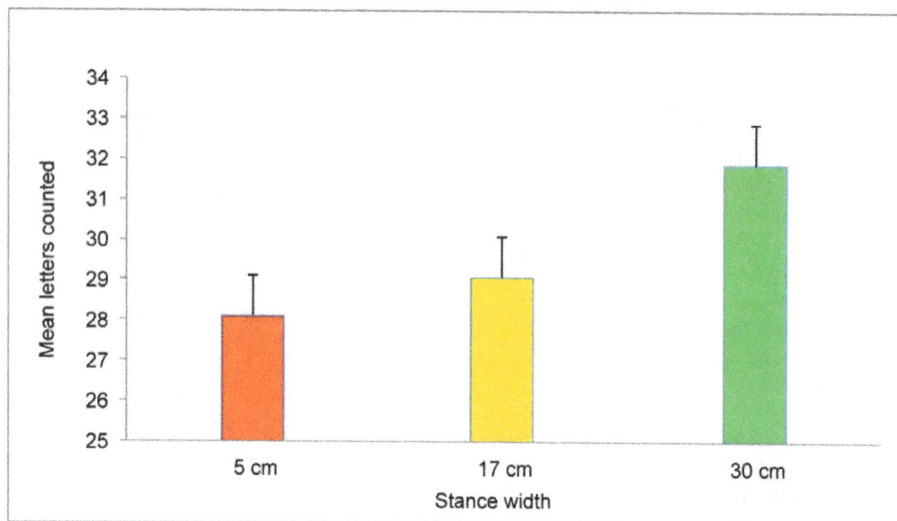

**Figure 1. Performance on the Search task (mean letters counted per trial) as a function of stance width.** The error bars represent standard error of the mean.

and Task, $F_{(1,13)} = 6.69$, $p = .023$, partial $\eta^2 = 0.340$, which is illustrated in Figure 6. Post-hoc tests revealed that for boxers in the Sick group sway was reduced during the Search task, relative to sway during the Inspection task, $p<.05$, whereas for boxers in the Well group sway did not differ as a function of visual task. In addition, there was a significant 3-way interaction between Task, Warm-up, and Stance Width, $F_{(1.75,22.69)} = 4.69$, $p = .023$, partial $\eta^2 = 0.265$, which is illustrated in Figure 7. Post-hoc tests revealed that before the warm-up (Figure 7A) positional variability was reduced during performance of the Search task (relative to sway during performance of the Inspection task) when stance width was 17 cm, $p = .018$.

For $\alpha$ of DFA in the ML axis we found a significant main effect of stance width, $F_{(1,1.351)} = 77.13$, $p<.001$, partial $\eta^2 = .847$ (Figure 3b). Post-hoc tests revealed that each condition differed from both of the others. The effect of stance width on $\alpha$ in the ML axis resembled that reported by Stoffregen et al. ([15], their figure 7) for healthy undergraduates (mean age = 20 years). For $\alpha$ of DFA in the AP axis there were no significant effects.

## Discussion

Using a simple, non-invasive testing protocol, we measured the standing body sway of amateur boxers before they entered the ring for a competitive bout. After completing the bout boxers reported the presence and severity of motion sickness. Measures of standing body sway taken before the bout differed significantly between boxers who did and did not report motion sickness after the bout as a function of time (before warm-up versus after warm-up) and as a function of visual task (Inspection vs. Search). The present study appears to be the first to document relationships between pre-bout postural sway and post-bout motion sickness.

### Boxers relative to the general population

Postural sway often is reduced during performance of difficult visual tasks, relative to sway during performance of easy visual tasks [29,31]. In previous studies body sway has been measured in the absence of any physical exertion and with participants adopting their preferred stance width. In the present study we found the same effect under comparable conditions (i.e., before warm-up, with stance width = 17 cm; Figure 7A). In the general population, the positional variability of postural sway is inversely related to stance width [22–23]. In the present study we found the same effect in the body's ML axis (Figure 3). In these two ways the body sway of boxers in the present study resembled effects documented in the general population. While stance width influenced postural sway, it also influenced performance on the visual search task: Wider stance was associated with increases in the reported count of target letters (Figure 1). Yu et al. [24] observed a similar effect in the context of visual performance among mariners on a ship at sea.

**Table 1.** Bout outcomes for boxers in the Well and Sick groups.

|  | Total | Unanimous | Split | TKO-1 | TKO-2 | TKO-3 |
|---|---|---|---|---|---|---|
| Well wins | 6 | 3 | 1 | 1 | 0 | 1 |
| Well losses | 2 | 2 | 0 | 0 | 0 | 0 |
| Sick wins | 3 | 0 | 1 | 0 | 1 | 1 |
| Sick losses | 4 | 2 | 0 | 0 | 1 | 1 |

Bouts were evaluated by three judges. Unanimous: All three judges concurred on the winner. Split: Two judges agreed on the winner. Some bouts ended with a technical knockout, or TKO. In these bouts no judges' decision was needed. TKO-1,2,3 indicates the TKOs that occurred in the first, second, or third round.

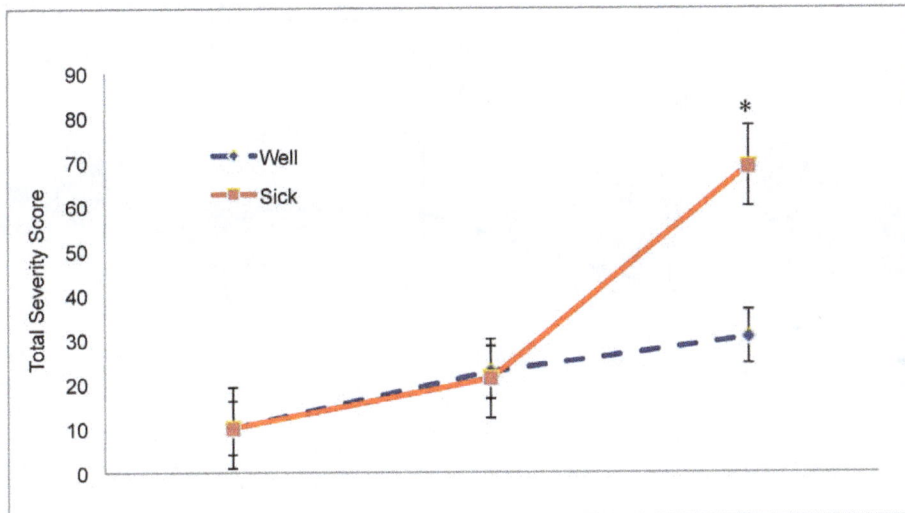

**Figure 2. Severity of motion sickness symptoms as measured using the Total Severity Score of the Simulator Sickness Questionnaire.** *, post-hoc difference between Well and Sick groups after completion of bouts, $p<.05$. The error bars represent standard error of the mean.

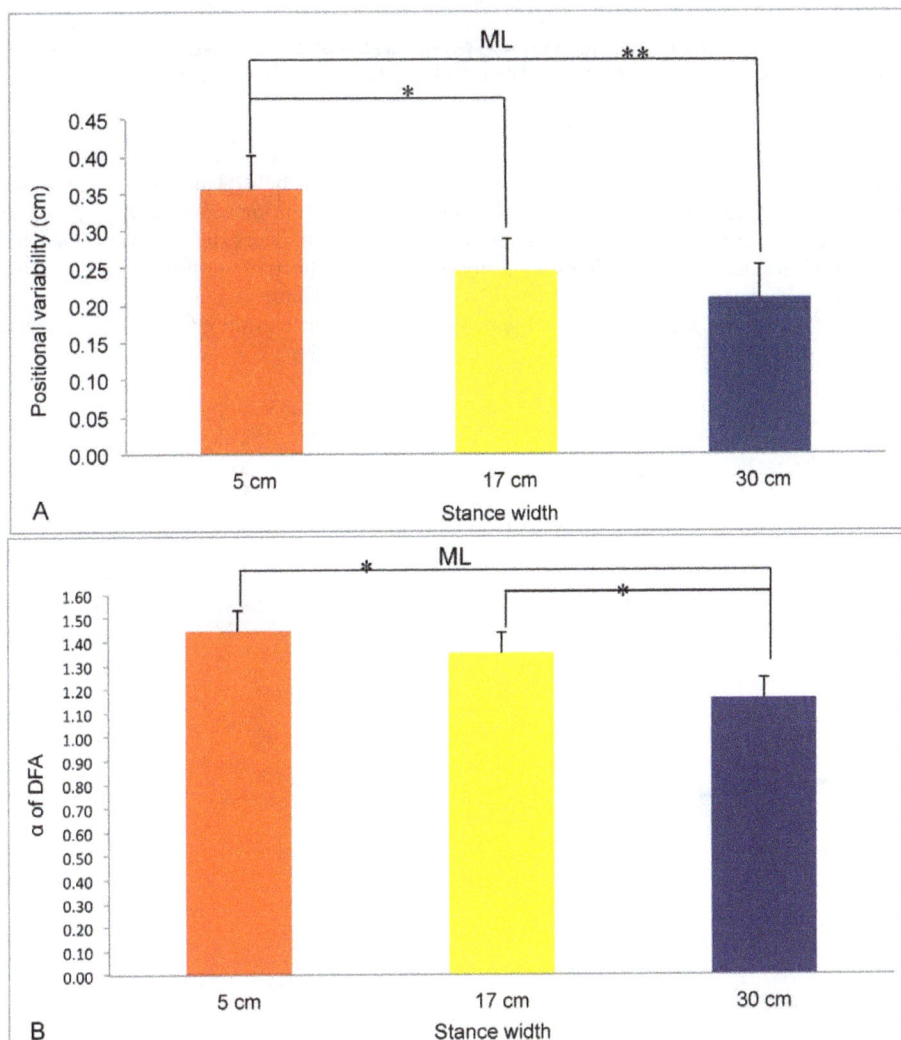

**Figure 3. Postural activity in the ML axis as a function of stance width.** A. Positional variability of the COP. B. Self-similarity of COP positions as quantified by $\alpha$, the scaling exponent of detrended fluctuation analysis. *, $p<.05$; ** $p<.01$. The error bars represent standard error of the mean.

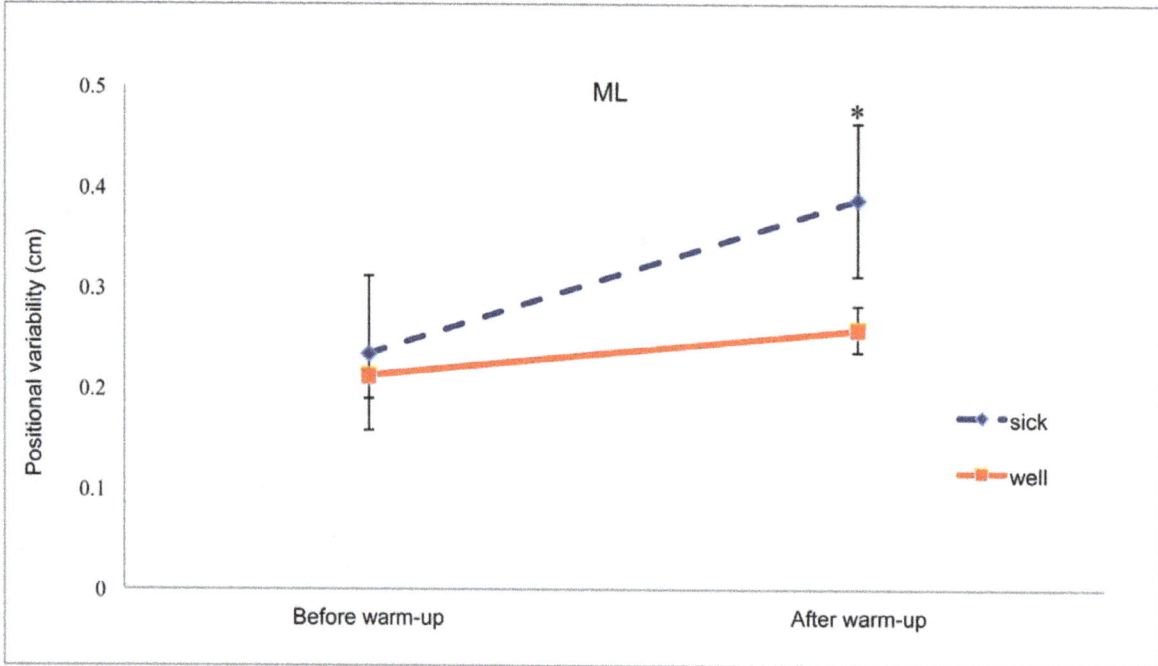

**Figure 4. Positional variability of the COP in the ML axis before and after warm-up for the Well and Sick groups.** *, post-hoc difference between Well and Sick groups after boxers completed their warm-up routine, $p<.05$. The error bars represent standard error of the mean.

## Postural effects of pre-bout warm-up routine

Body sway differed before and after the pre-bout warm-up routine. As expected, the positional variability of the COP was greater after warm-up than before warm-up, but this was true only for sway in the ML axis. Warm-up also increased the influence of stance width on the positional variability of the COP in the ML axis (Figure 5). These effects can be explained by the increased physiological arousal that occurs during warm-up. By contrast, in the AP axis positional variability did not exhibit an overall increase following warm-up; rather, the effects of warm-up were modulated by stance width and visual task (Figure 7). Warm-up influenced the positional variability of sway but had no effect on the temporal

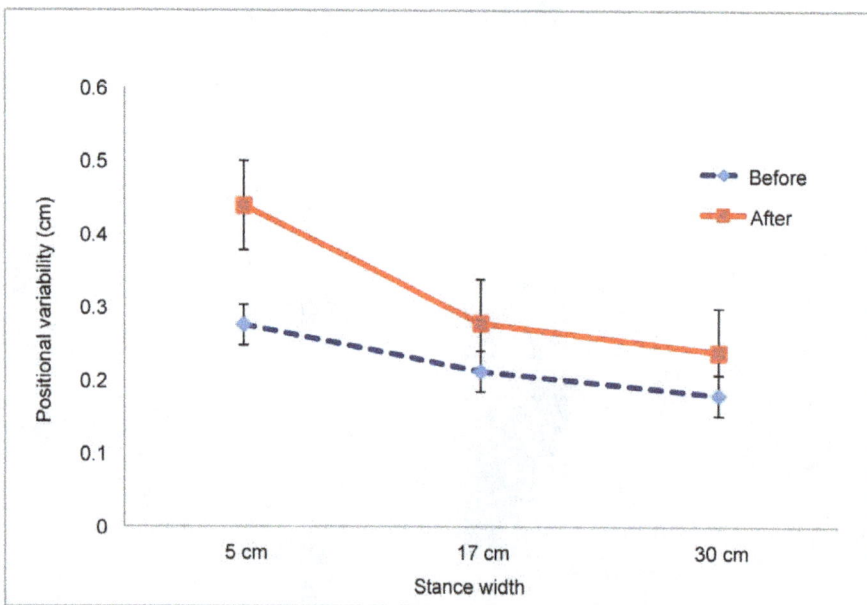

**Figure 5. Positional variability of the COP in the ML axis before and after warm-up as a function of stance width.** The error bars represent standard error of the mean.

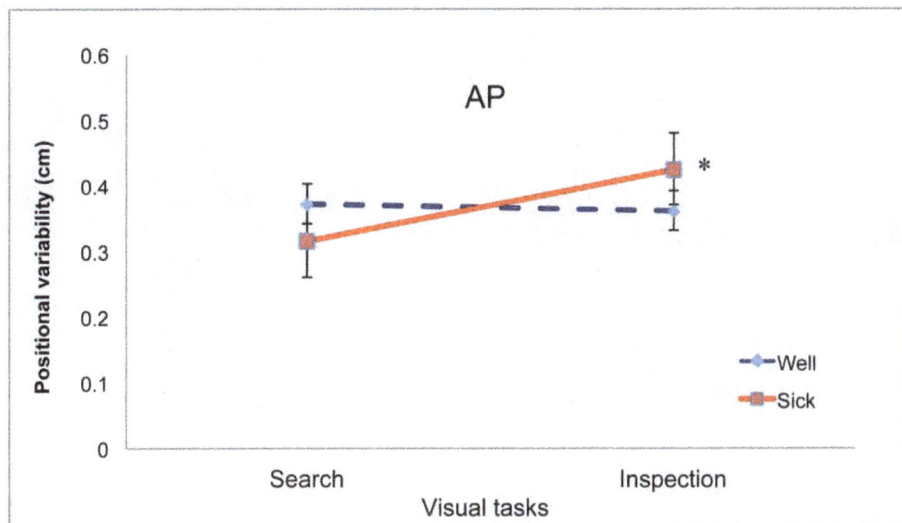

**Figure 6. Positional variability of the COP in the AP axis during performance of the Inspection and Search tasks for the Well and Sick groups.** *, post-hoc effect for the Sick group, sway was reduced during performance of the Search task, relative to sway during performance of the Inspection task, $p<.05$. The error bars represent standard error of the mean.

dynamics of sway; that is, warm-up increased the magnitude of sway not its temporal structure.

## Pre-bout postural sway and post-bout motion sickness

Our principal hypothesis was that postural sway before a bout would differ between boxers who reported motion sickness after the bout those who did not. This prediction was confirmed for the positional variability of the COP. In previous research on the general population of healthy adults we have examined relations between visual motion, postural sway, and motion sickness [12,15]. In those studies, we found that changes in postural sway occurred among individuals who reported visual motion sickness, and that these changes began before the onset of subjective symptoms of visual motion sickness. In the present study we found similar effects: Postural sway differed between boxers who did and did not report motion sickness, and these changes existed before boxers entered the ring.

After warm-up, the positional variability of the COP in the ML axis was greater for boxers who reported post-bout motion sickness than for boxers who did not (Figure 4). One possible interpretation of this effect is that participants in the Sick group were less able than their Well peers to compensate for postural effects of physiological arousal. An alternative interpretation is that, after warm-up, participants in the Sick group relaxed their criterion for "comfortable" stance.

We also found that our manipulation of visual tasks influenced the positional variability of the COP in the AP axis for Sick boxers, but not for Well boxers (Figure 6). Participants in the Sick group tended to reduce their sway during performance of the Search task, relative to sway during performance of the Inspection task. Modulation of postural sway in response to different visual tasks has been reported in many studies [29,45]. Separately, the control of standing body sway can be affected by clinical conditions such as aging [32] and Parkinson's disease [46]. Clinical conditions can also influence the task specific modulation of standing body sway. For example, children with autism spectrum disorder modulate their sway in response to variations in visual tasks [30], but children at risk for developmental coordination disorder do not

[47]. The present study provides the first evidence that task-specific variation in postural sway may be related to individual differences in susceptibility to motion sickness.

## Causal factors

Dizziness, nausea and vomiting are common acute symptoms of concussion [2,48]. In addition to these subjective symptoms concussion also is associated with changes in standing body sway, both in the immediate aftermath of head trauma [2] and up to several months later [33–35,49]. Boxing is widely associated with concussion [39,50]. Given the results of the present study these facts suggest that pre-bout postural sway may be related to an individual's susceptibility to concussion. In future research it will be important to examine possible relations between pre-bout postural sway, post-bout motion sickness, and concussion. It may be possible to use pre-bout data on postural sway as a predictor of susceptibility to boxing-related concussion.

We were not able to record the number or severity of blows to the head during bouts. It is possible that participants in the Sick group sustained more blows to the head, or more severe blows to the head, than participants in the Well group. Such a relation would be expected if post-bout motion sickness were causally related to head trauma (either concussive or sub-concussive) experienced during individual bouts. We predict that pre-bout postural sway would differ between boxers who did and did not experience post-bout motion sickness when controlling for the number and severity of blows to the head experienced by each boxer. Similarly, a person's experience of post-bout motion sickness might vary from bout to bout, that is, a person who did not experience motion sickness after one bout might experience it after a subsequent bout, and vice versa (as one example, if participants who did not experience motion sickness in the present study were paired to fight each other, then they might experience motion sickness in this second bout). In particular, known long-term effects of concussion on body sway [33–35,49] indicate lingering effects of concussion on motor control which, in turn, might increase susceptibility to motion sickness-like symptoms in subsequent bouts. It would be interesting to conduct a longitudinal

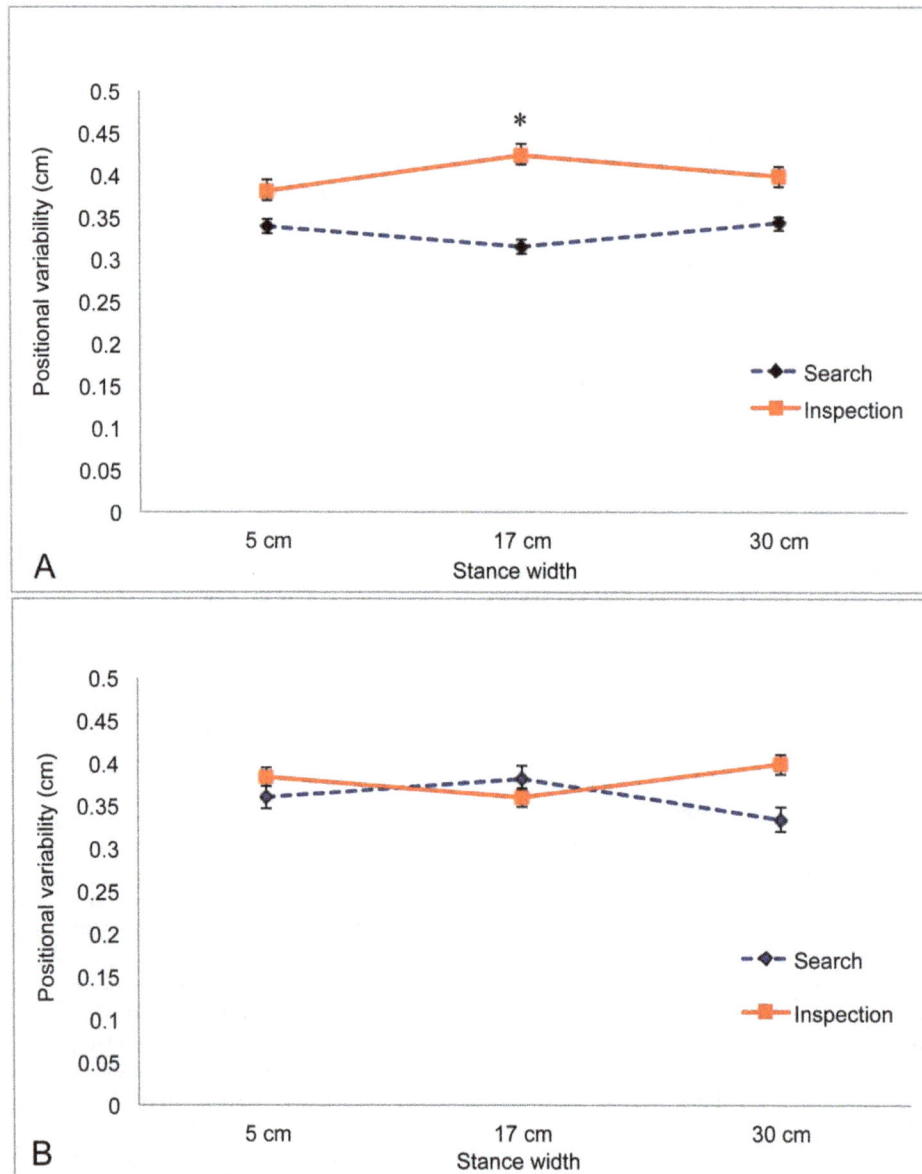

**Figure 7. Positional variability of the COP in the AP axis as a function of stance width during performance of the Inspection and Search tasks.** A. Before warm-up. B. After warm-up. *, post-hoc effect showing that before warm-up sway was reduced during performance of the Search task, relative to sway during performance of the Inspection task, when stance width was 17 cm, $p<.05$. The error bars represent standard error of the mean.

study evaluating pre-bout postural sway and post-bout motion sickness in the same individuals over a succession of bouts. Such a study would make it possible to determine whether relations between pre-bout postural sway and post-bout motion sickness persist across bouts.

It is important to recall, however, that in the present study none of the participants were diagnosed with a concussion following their participation. Motion sickness is a common consequence of athletic concussion [2,48]; however, athletes sometimes experience motion sickness in the absence of concussion, and in the absence of any head trauma [51,52]. Thus, in the present study it is possible that post-bout motion sickness occurred in the absence of significant head trauma. The preceding possibilities are not mutually exclusive; that is, it may be that post-bout motion

sickness has multiple causal factors, including but not limited to head trauma sustained during the bout. This is an area for future research.

## Conclusion

We conducted the first assessment of the quantitative kinematics of standing body sway in boxers. We used data on pre-bout postural sway in a prospective manner. We showed that before entering the ring there were differences in standing body sway between boxers who experienced post-bout motion sickness and those who did not. These effects suggest the possibility that objective, non-invasive measures of postural control might be helpful in evaluating susceptibility to boxing-related concussion.

## Acknowledgments

We thank Coach Hsu Hua-Yen, owner of the Contender Fitness Boxing Club, New Taipei City, Taiwan.

## Author Contributions

Conceived and designed the experiments: Y-CC TAS CCH. Performed the experiments: T-HH T-CT. Analyzed the data: Y-CC F-CC TAS. Wrote the paper: TAS Y-CC F-CC.

## References

1.  Ohhashi G, Tani S, Murakami S, Kamio M, Abe T, et al. (2002) Problems in health management of professional boxers in Japan. Br J Sports Med 36: 346–353.
2.  Erlanger D, Kaushik T, Cantu R, Barth JT, Broshek DK, et al. (2003) Symptom-based measurement of the severity of a concussion. J Neurosurg 98: 477–484.
3.  Chang C-H, Pan W-W, Tseng L-Y, Stoffregen TA (2012) Postural activity and motion sickness during video game play in children and adults. Exp Brain Res 217: 299–309.
4.  Dong X, Yoshida K, Stoffregen TA (2011) Control of a virtual vehicle influences postural activity and motion sickness. J Exp Psychol Appl 17: 128–138.
5.  Stoffregen TA, Faugloire E, Yoshida K, Flanagan M, Merhi O (2008) Motion sickness and postural sway in console video games. Hum Factors 50: 322–331.
6.  Akiduki H, Nishiike S, Watanabe H, Matsuoka K, Kubo T et al. (2005) Visual-vestibular conflict induced by virtual reality in humans. Neurosci Lett 340: 197–200.
7.  Villard S, Flanagan MB, Albanese G, Stoffregen TA (2008) Postural instability and motion sickness in a virtual moving room. Hum Factors 50: 332–345.
8.  Draper MH, Viirre ES, Gawron VJ, Furness TA (2001) The effects of image scale and system delay on simulator sickness within head-coupled virtual environments. Hum Factors 43: 129–146.
9.  Merhi O, Faugloire E, Flanagan M, Stoffregen TA (2007) Motion sickness, console video games, and head mounted displays. Hum Factors 49: 920–934.
10. Kennedy RS, Berbaum KS, Lilienthal MG (1997) Disorientation and postural ataxia following flight simulation. Aviat Space Environ Med 68: 13–17.
11. Kennedy RS, Fowlkes JE, Lilienthal MG (1993) Postural and performance changes following exposure to flight simulators. Aviat Space Environ Med 64: 912–920.
12. Stoffregen TA, Hettinger LJ, Haas MW, Roe M, Smart LJ, 2000 Postural instability and motion sickness in a fixed-base flight simulator. Hum Factors 42: 458–469.
13. Kennedy RS, Stanney KM (1996) Postural instability induced by virtual reality exposure: Development of a certification protocol. Int J Hum Comput Interact 8: 25–47.
14. Stoffregen TA, Smart LJ (1998) Postural instability precedes motion sickness. Brain Res Bull 47: 437–448.
15. Stoffregen TA, Yoshida K, Villard S, Scibora L, Bardy BG (2010) Stance width influences postural stability and motion sickness. Ecol Psychol 22: 169–191.
16. Nachum Z, Shupak A, Letichevsky V, Ben-David J, Tal D et al. (2004) Mal de debarquement and posture: Reduced reliance on vestibular and visual cures. Laryngoscope 114: 581–586.
17. Singh I, Khanna PK, Srivastava MC, Lal M, Roy SB et al. (1969) Acute mountain sickness. N Engl J Med 280: 175–184.
18. Lempert T, Neuhausser H (2009) Epidemiology of vertigo, migraine, and vestibular migraine. J Neurol 256: 333–338.
19. Troost BT (2004) Vestibular migraine. Curr Pain Headache Rep 8: 310–314.
20. Gadsby R, Barnie-Adshead AM, Jagger C (1993) A prospective study of nausea and vomiting during pregnancy. Br J Gen Pract 43: 245–248.
21. Stoffregen TA (2011) Motion sickness considered as a movement disorder. Science & Motricité 74: 19–30.
22. Day BL, Steiger MJ, Thompson PD, Marsen CD (1993) Effects of vision and stance width on human body motion when standing: implications for afferent control of lateral sway. J Physiol 469: 479–499.
23. Stoffregen TA, Villard S, Chen F-C, Yu Y (2011) Standing body sway on land and at sea. Ecol Psychol 23: 19–36.
24. Yu Y, Yank JR, Katsumata Y, Villard S, Kennedy RS et al. (2010) Visual vigilance performance and standing posture at sea. Aviat Space Environ Med 81: 375–382.
25. Yu Y, Chung H-C, Hemingway L, Stoffregen TA (2012) Standing body sway in women with and without morning sickness in pregnancy. Gait Posture, in press.
26. McIlroy WE, Maki BE (1997) Preferred placement of the feet during quiet stance: development of a standardized foot placement for balance testing. Clin Biomech 12: 66–70.
27. Jang J, Hsiao KT, Hsiao-Wecksler ET (2008) Balance (perceived and actual) and preferred stance width during pregnancy. Clin Biomech 23: 468–476.
28. Stoffregen TA, Chen F-C, Yu Y, Villard S (2009) Stance width and angle at sea: Effects of sea state and body orientation. Aviat Space Environ Med 80: 845–849.
29. Woollacott M, Shumway-Cook A (2002) Attention and the control of posture and gait: A review of an emerging area of research. Gait Posture 16: 1–14.
30. Chang C-H, Wade MG, Stoffregen TA, Hsu C-Y, Pan C-Y (2010) Visual tasks and postural sway in children with and without Autism Spectrum Disorder. Res Dev Disabil 31: 1536–1542.
31. Stoffregen TA, Pagulayan RJ, Bardy BG, Hettinger L J (2000) Modulating postural control to facilitate visual performance. Hum Mov Sci 19: 203–220.
32. Prado JM, Stoffregen TA, Duarte M (2007) Postural sway during dual tasks in young and elderly adults. Geront 53: 274–281.
33. Cavanaugh JT, Guskiewicz KM, Giuliani C, Marshall S, Mercer VS et al. (2005) Detecting altered postural control after cerebral concussion in athletes without postural instability. Br J Sports Med 39(11): 805–11.
34. Cavanaugh JT, Guskiewicz KM, Giuliani C, Marshall S, Mercer VS et al. (2006) Recovery of postural control after cerebral concussion: New insights using Approximate Entropy. J Athl Train 41(3): 305–13.
35. Slobounov S, Cao C, Sebastianelli W, Slobounov E, Newell K (2008) Residual deficits from concussion as revealed by virtual time to contact measures of postural stability. Clin Neurophys 119: 281–289.
36. Gao J, Hu J, Buckley T, White K, Hass C (2011) Shannon and Renyi entropies to classify effects of mild traumatic brain injury on postural sway. PLoS One, 6(9): e24446. doi:10.1371/journal.pone.0024446
37. Mackey DC, Rabinovitch SN (2005) Postural steadiness during quiet stance does not associate with ability to recover balance in older women. Clin Biomech 20: 776–783.
38. Kennedy RS, Lane NE, Berbaum KS, Lilienthal MG (1993) Simulator sickness questionnaire: An enhanced method for quantifying simulator sickness. Int J Aviat Psychol 3: 203–220.
39. Galetta KM, Barrett J, Allen M, Madda F, Delicata D et al. (2011) The King-Device test as a determinant of head trauma and concussion in boxers and MMA fighters. Neurol 76(17): 1456–1462.
40. Kinsella–Shaw JM, Harrison SJ, Colon–Semenza C, Turvey MT (2006) Effects of visual environment on quiet standing by young and old adults. J Mot Behav 38: 251–264. doi:10.3200/JMBR.38.4.251–264
41. Lin D, Seol H, Nussbaum MA, Madigan ML (2008) Reliability of COP-based postural sway measures and age-related differences. Gait Posture 28: 337–342.
42. Chen F-C, Stoffregen TA (2012) Specificity of postural sway to the demands of a precision task at sea. J Exp Psychol Appl 18: 203–212.
43. Chen Z, Ivanov PCh, Hu K, Stanley HE (2002) Effect of nonstationarities on detrended fluctuation analysis. Phys Rev E Stat Nonlin Soft Matter Phys 65(4, Pt. 1): 041017-1-15.
44. Winer BJ (1971) Statistical principles in experimental design. New York: McGraw-Hill. 907 p.
45. Stoffregen TA, Hove P, Bardy BG, Riley MA, Bonnet CT (2007) Postural stabilization of perceptual but not cognitive performance. J Mot Behav 39: 126–138.
46. Schmit JM, Riley MA, Dalvi A, Sahay A, Shear PK et al. (2006). Deterministic center of pressure patterns characterize postural instability in Parkinson's disease. Exp Brain Res 168: 357–367.
47. Chen F-C, Stoffregen TA, Wade MG (2011) Postural responses to a suprapostural visual task among children with and without Developmental Coordination Disorder. Res Dev Disabil 32: 1948–1956.
48. McRrea M, Guskiewicz KM, Marshall SW, Barr W, Randolph C, et al. (2003) Acute effects and recovery time following concussion in collegiate football players: The NCAA concussion study. JAMA 290: 2556–2563.
49. Peterson CL, Ferrara MS, Mrazik M, Piland S, Elliott R (2003) Evaluation of neuropsychological domain scores and postural stability following cerebral concussion in sports. Clin J Sport Med 13: 230–237.
50. Moriarity JM, Pietrzak RH, Kutcher JS, Clausen MH, McAward K, et al. (2012) Unrecognized ringside concussive injury in amateur boxers. Br J Sports Med 10.1136/bjsports-2011-090893.
51. Kondo T, Nakae T, Mitsui T, Kagaya M, Matsutani Y, et al. (2001) Exercise-induced nausea is exaggerated by eating. Appetite 36: 119–125.
52. Kraemer WJ, Noble BJ, Clark MJ, Culver BW (1987) Physiologic responses to heavy-resistance exercise with very short rest periods. Int J Sports Med 8: 247–252.

# 11

# Hospital based Emergency Department Visits Attributed to Child Physical Abuse in United States: Predictors of In-Hospital Mortality

**Veerajalandhar Allareddy**[1]*, **Rahimullah Asad**[1], **Min Kyeong Lee**[2], **Romesh P. Nalliah**[2], **Sankeerth Rampa**[3], **David G. Speicher**[1], **Alexandre T. Rotta**[1], **Veerasathpurush Allareddy**[4]

1 Department of Pediatric Critical Care, Rainbow Babies and Children's Hospital, Case Western Reserve University School of Medicine, Cleveland, Ohio, United States of America, 2 Department of Dental Medicine, Harvard University, Boston, Massachusetts, United States of America, 3 Department of Public Health, Texas A & M University, College Station, Texas, United States of America, 4 Department of Dentistry, University of Iowa, Iowa City, Iowa, United States of America

## Abstract

*Objectives:* To describe nationally representative outcomes of physical abuse injuries in children necessitating Emergency Department (ED) visits in United States. The impact of various injuries on mortality is examined. We hypothesize that physical abuse resulting in intracranial injuries are associated with worse outcome.

*Materials and Methods:* We performed a retrospective analysis of the Nationwide Emergency Department Sample (NEDS), the largest all payer hospital based ED database, for the years 2008–2010. All ED visits and subsequent hospitalizations with a diagnosis of "Child physical abuse" (Battered baby or child syndrome) due to various injuries were identified using ICD-9-CM (International Classification of Diseases, 9th Revision, Clinical Modification) codes. In addition, we also examined the prevalence of sexual abuse in this cohort. A multivariable logistic regression model was used to examine the association between mortality and types of injuries after adjusting for a multitude of patient and hospital level factors.

*Results:* Of the 16897 ED visits that were attributed to child physical abuse, 5182 (30.7%) required hospitalization. Hospitalized children were younger than those released treated and released from the ED (1.9 years vs. 6.4 years). Male or female partner of the child's parent/guardian accounted for >45% of perpetrators. Common injuries in hospitalized children include- any fractures (63.5%), intracranial injuries (32.3%) and crushing/internal injuries (9.1%). Death occurred in 246 patients (13 in ED and 233 following hospitalization). Amongst the 16897 ED visits, 1.3% also had sexual abuse. Multivariable analyses revealed each 1 year increase in age was associated with a lower odds of mortality (OR = 0.88, 95% CI = 0.81–0.96, p<0.0001). Females (OR = 2.39, 1.07–5.34, p = 0.03), those with intracranial injuries (OR = 65.24, 27.57–154.41, p<0.0001), or crushing/internal injury (OR = 4.98, 2.24–11.07, p<0.0001) had higher odds of mortality compared to their male counterparts.

*Conclusions:* In this large cohort of physically abused children, younger age, females and intracranial or crushing/internal injuries were independent predictors of mortality. Identification of high risk cohorts in the ED may enable strengthening of existing screening programs and optimization of outcomes.

**Editor:** James G. Scott, The University of Queensland, Australia

**Funding:** The authors have no support or funding to report.

**Competing Interests:** The authors have declared that no competing interests exist.

* E-mail: Veerajalandhar.Allareddy@UHhospitals.org

## Introduction

Child maltreatment occurs worldwide and is an important cause of morbidity and mortality. [1,10] In United States, child maltreatment includes any act which results in physical, emotional or sexual abuse; or failure to act (neglect) resulting in imminent risk of harm, usually by a parent, caregiver or, occasionally, by an unknown perpetrator [2,3].

Available estimates indicate that approximately 700,000 to 1.25 million children are abused or neglected annually in the United States [4,5,6] and about 18 percent of these cases involve physical abuse [7]. An estimated 1.3% to 15% of injuries in children that result in emergency department visits are actually caused by

physical abuse [8]. Physical abuse is often an underreported problem due to a variety of reasons including misdiagnosis. In fact, a study revealed that 31% of infants and children with abusive head trauma were initially misdiagnosed [9].

Although early detection rate of child abuse in emergency departments varies among different countries (Netherlands: 0.2%, Italy 2%, the United Kingdom: 4%–6.4%, United States: 10%) [16,17,18,19,20,21] due to varied screening tools, emergency departments are important in the initial evaluation of suspected physical abuse in children [11,12,13,14,15]. Current national estimates and outcomes of physical abuse in children necessitating emergency department visit in United States are unclear.

The objective of our study is to describe nationally representative outcomes of physical abuse injuries in children necessitating hospital based emergency department (ED) visits in United States. The impact of facial and intracranial injuries on hospital mortality is also examined. We hypothesize that those with intracranial injuries are more likely to have higher in-hospital mortality compared to their counterparts.

## Materials and Methods

### Design, Database Description, Institutional Review Board and Data User Agreement

We performed a retrospective analysis of the Nationwide Emergency Department Sample (NEDS) for the years 2008 to 2010. The NEDS is a component database of the Healthcare Cost and Utilization Project (HCUP) sponsored by the Agency for Healthcare Research and Quality (AHRQ). [22] The NEDS is the largest all payer, nationally representative hospital based emergency department database in the United States. NEDS contains discharge data for ED visits from over 950 hospitals located in 30 States, approximating a 20-percent stratified sample of U.S. hospital-based EDs. The NEDS database has information on close to 100 different patient and hospital-related variables for each ED visit. Demographic data such as hospital and patient characteristics, geographic area, and the nature of ED visits (e.g., common reasons for ED visits, including injuries); and ED charge information for over 85 percent of patients, including individuals covered by Medicare, Medicaid, or private insurance, as well as those who are uninsured are available in NEDS [22].

As per University Hospitals Case Medical Center institutional review board (IRB) and in agreement with Federal Regulations 45 CFR 46.101 (b) which states "research involving the collection or study of existing data, documents, records, pathological specimens, or diagnostic specimens, if these sources are **publicly available** or if the information is recorded by the investigator in such a manner that **subjects cannot be identified**, directly or through identifiers linked to the subjects," such studies are permitted to be classified as research that is "exempt" from IRB full or expedited review. IRB was not consulted for approval since the current study was a retrospective analysis of hospital based discharge dataset that is **available publicly** for purchase from AHRQ. The first author (VJA) completed the data user agreement with HCUP-AHRQ and the obtained the pertinent datasets. As per the data user agreement, cell counts ≤10 cannot be reported to maintain patient privacy. In accordance with the agreement, low cell counts are not reported and the term "DS" (Discharge information suppressed) is used instead.

### Case Selection and Outcome Variables Examined

All hospital based ED visits with a diagnosis of *child physical abuse* were selected for analysis. The ICD-9-CM code of 995.54 (battered baby or child syndrome) was used to identify these cases. In addition, in this cohort we also examined if patients had sexual abuse. This was identified by using the ICD-9-CM code of 995.53. Injury types were classified by using Clinical Classification Software codes and included Joint disorders and dislocations due to trauma (Clinical Classification Software code 225), fracture of neck of femur [hip] (226), spinal cord injury (227), skull and facial fractures (228), fracture of upper limb (229), fracture of lower limb (230), other fractures (231), sprains and strains (232), intracranial injury (233), crushing injury or internal injury (234), open wounds of head, neck, and trunk (235), and open wounds of extremities (236). Perpetrators of physical abuse were identified by using external cause of injury codes. The primary outcome variable of

interest included hospital mortality (either in the emergency department or following hospitalization). The primary independent variables of interest included types of injuries.

The income quartiles varied by year. For 2008, the levels were $1–$38,999 (quartile 1), $39,000–$48,999 (quartile 2), $49,000–$63,999 (quartile 3), and > = $64,000 (quartile 4). For 2009, the levels were $1–$39,999 (quartile 1), $40,000–$49,999 (quartile 2), $50,000–$65,999 (quartile 3), and > = $66,000 (quartile 4). For 2010 the levels were $1–$40,999 (quartile 1), $41,000–$50,999 (quartile 2), $51,000–$66,999 (quartile 3), and > = $67,000 (quartile 4).

### Analytical Approach

A multivariable logistic regression model was used to examine the association between hospital mortality and types of injuries. Injuries that occurred in at least 1% of the ED visits were examined. The effects of age, sex, insurance status, and hospital region were adjusted in the multivariable logistic regression model. Odds ratios for hospital mortality and the associated 95% confidence intervals were computed. Each individual ED visit was the unit of analysis and the hospital stratum was the stratification unit. The effect of clustering of outcomes within hospitals was adjusted in the regression model. All statistical tests were two-sided a p-value of <0.05 was deemed to be statistically significant. Statistical analyses were conducted using SAS version 9.3 (SAS Institute, Cary, NC) and SUDAAN version 10.0.1 (Research Triangle Park, NC).

### Results

During the study period, there were a total of 16,897 ED visits due to physical abuse against children-refer to table 1. Amongst these, 1.3% also reported a sexual abuse. Characteristics of the sample are summarized in Table 1. Medicaid (58.9%) and private insurance plans (23.8%) were primary payers for most ED visits, while 14.1% of patients were uninsured. Most patients (71%) were found to reside in geographic areas with low annual household income levels The number of ED visits and the number of hospitalizations due to physical abuse decreased over the analyzed time period (Figure 1).

The types of injuries identified during the ED visit or subsequent hospitalization are summarized in Table 2, with intracranial injuries being the most prevalent. Commonly reported perpetrators of physical abuse included male partner of child's parent/guardian (28.5% of all ED visits) and female partner of child's parent/guardian (16.7%), unspecified person (14.4%) (Table 3).

Following an ED visit, 65.2% of patients were discharged routinely, 2.5% were transferred to another short term hospital, 0.7% to long term care facilities like skilled nursing facility, 0.2% to home health care, and 0.3% were discharged against medical advice. A total of 5,182 ED visits (30.7%) resulted in admission as in-patients into the same hospital. A total of 246 patients died in hospitals (13 patients died in the ED and 233 died following in-patient admission). 0.3% were discharged-transferred to court/law enforcement agency.

Characteristics of hospitalizations (ED visits that resulted in in-patient admission into the same hospital) are summarized in table 4. The mean age of hospitalizations was 1.9 years, which is lower compared to 6.4 years for those visiting the ED. Males comprised 61.3% of hospitalizations. Medicaid was the primary payer for 77.3% of hospitalizations. Close to 64.7% of hospitalizations occurred among the low income quartiles. Frequently occurring injuries among those hospitalized (Table 5) included

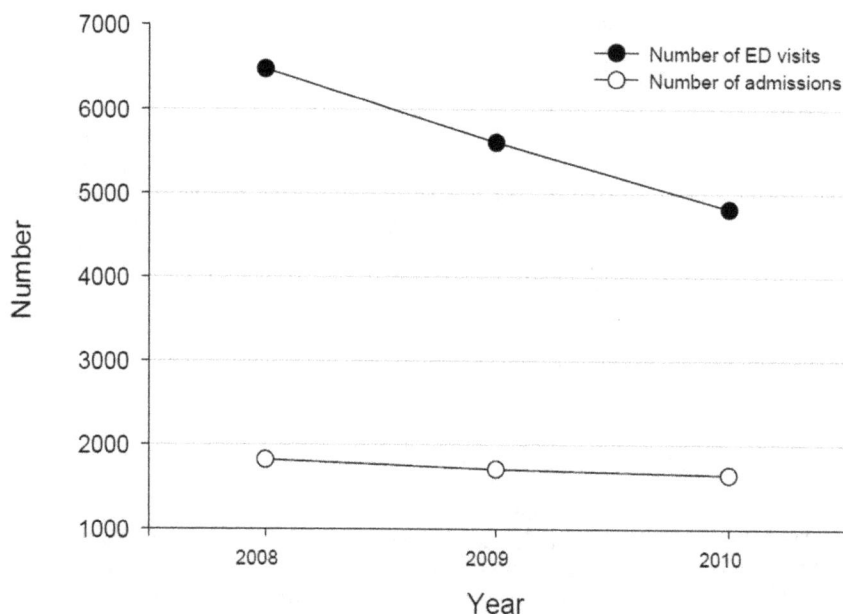

**Figure 1. The number of ED visits and the number of hospitalizations due to physical abuse decreased over the analyzed time period (2008 to 2010).**

intracranial injuries (32.3% of hospitalizations), fracture of lower limb (20.7%), and fracture of upper limb (16.5%). Skull and facial fractures occurred in 9% of hospitalizations. Figure 2 illustrates the common types of injuries in hospitalized children on a yearly basis. Intracranial injures were present in more than 30% of hospitalizations/year. Any type of fracture was present in >65% of hospitalizations/year and crushing/internal injuries were present in 5.4% to 13.2% hospitalizations/year. The in-hospital mortality was consistently 1.4 to 1.6% of hospitalizations/year. Figure 3 illustrates the effect of age on ED visits and in-hospital mortality. Younger age group children were more likely to visit the ED due to physical injury and had higher in-hospital mortality than their counterparts. Infants ($\leq 1$ year) had the highest in-hospital mortality rate of 7.5%.

**Table 1.** Characteristics of ED Visits due to Child Physical Abuse (Total N = 16,897).

| Characteristic | Response | % of ED Visits |
|---|---|---|
| Sex | Male | 55.9% |
| | Female | 44.1% |
| Insurance status | Medicare | 0.1% |
| | Medicaid | 58.9% |
| | Private insurance | 23.8% |
| | Uninsured | 14.1% |
| | Other insurance | 3.1% |
| ED visit | Weekday | 75.6% |
| | Weekend | 23.4% |
| Income quartile based on zip code* | Quartile 1 | 41.6% |
| | Quartile 2 | 29.4% |
| | Quartile 3 | 18.7% |
| | Quartile 4 | 10.3% |
| Hospital region | Northeast | 24.5% |
| | Midwest | 28.5% |
| | South | 28.8% |
| | West | 18.2% |
| Age in years | Mean | 6.4 years |
| | Standard error | 0.34 |

*Income quartile varied per year (see methods).

**Table 2.** Types of Injuries in patients visiting the Emergency Department.

| Type of injury (CCS Code) | % of all ED visits (N = 16,897) | % of ED visits in year 2008 (N = 6,477) | % of ED visits in year 2009 (N = 5,605) | % of ED visits in year 2010 (N = 4,815) |
|---|---|---|---|---|
| Joint disorders and dislocations; trauma-related (225) | 0.2% | 0.3% | DS | 0.3% |
| Fracture of neck of femur [hip] (226) | 0.4% | 0.4% | 0.3% | 0.4% |
| Spinal cord injury (227) | DS | DS | DS | DS |
| Skull and facial fractures (228) | 3.4% | 2.9% | 3.7% | 3.7% |
| Fracture of upper limb (229) | 6.3% | 6% | 6.4% | 6.6% |
| Fracture of lower limb (230) | 6.8% | 6.7% | 6% | 7.9% |
| Other fractures (231) | 5.4% | 5.6% | 4.8% | 5.7% |
| Sprains and strains (232) | 1.4% | 1.4% | 0.9% | 2.1% |
| Intracranial injury (233) | 11% | 10.6% | 10.5% | 12% |
| Crushing injury or internal injury (234) | 3% | 2.8% | 1.9% | 4.7% |
| Open wounds of head, neck, and trunk (235) | 5.6% | 4.5% | 6.7% | 5.6% |
| Open wounds of extremities (236) | 1.6% | 1.5% | 1.8% | 1.6% |

Results of the multivariable analyses examining the odds of hospital mortality (n = 246 deaths) are summarized in table 6. Each 1 year increase in age was associated with lower odds for mortality. Females were associated with higher odds for mortality compared to males. Patients with intracranial and those with crushing injury or internal injury had higher odds of mortality compared to those without these respective injuries. Hospitals located in the Southern regions of the country had lower odds for mortality compared to those located in the western regions.

## Discussion

Child physical abuse affects all ages, genders, races, ethnicities and socioeconomic groups. [1,3,10]. To our knowledge this study is the largest and most recent cohort of children visiting the emergency department due to physical abuse whose risk of in-hospital mortality was assessed using a multitude of patient and hospital level characteristics at a national level. Using a large all payer national emergency department dataset, we show that younger age group, female gender, and intracranial or crushing/internal injuries are independent predictors of in-hospital mortality in those children admitted from the emergency department due to physical abuse.

In the present study nearly two-thirds of the patients presenting with physical abuse were routinely discharged from the ED. It is likely that these physical abuse injuries were in the less severe end of the spectrum. Such injuries could include bruises and abrasions due to slapping, beating or kicking. In addition, minor burns are a common cause of physical abuse in children. Although, any form of physical abuse is a concern and may require mandatory reporting to authorities in certain countries, in this study we sought to specifically describe the outcomes of physically abused children needing hospitalization. Hospitalized children are likely to have multiple injuries, higher severity of injuries or ongoing risk of exposure to perpetrator which requires hospitalization. Identification of certain types of injuries in high risk population groups in the emergency department may enable optimization of outcomes.

**Table 3.** Perpetrators of Physical Abuse.

| Perpetrator | % of ED Visits* |
|---|---|
| Male partner of child's parent or guardian | 28.5% |
| Other specified person | 5.5% |
| Female partner of child's parent or guardian | 16.7% |
| Abuse of spouse or partner by ex-spouse or ex-partner | 0.4% |
| Child | 0.4% |
| Sibling | 1.4% |
| Grand parent | 1.4% |
| Other relative | 2.4% |
| Non-related care giver | 1.4% |
| Unspecified person | 14.4% |

*Values do not add up to 100% due to missing or unreported data.

**Table 4.** Characteristics of Hospitalizations (admitted as inpatient into same hospital following ED visit) [N = 5,182).

| Characteristic | Response | % of Hospitalizations |
|---|---|---|
| Sex | Male | 61.3% |
| | Female | 38.7% |
| Insurance status | Medicare | 0.2% |
| | Medicaid | 77.3% |
| | Private insurance | 15.8% |
| | Uninsured | 3% |
| | Other insurance | 3.7% |
| Admission | Weekday | 75.5% |
| | Weekend | 24.5% |
| Income quartile based on zip code* | Quartile 1 | 33.3% |
| | Quartile 2 | 31.4% |
| | Quartile 3 | 21% |
| | Quartile 4 | 14.3% |
| Age in years | Mean | 1.9 years |
| | Standard error | 0.20 |

*Income quartiles varied per year (see methods).

In our study, although children in the older age group were likely to visit the ED for physical abuse, children in the younger age group were more likely to be admitted and the risk of in-hospital mortality significantly decreased with increasing age. This is consistent with prior findings that although the risk of physical abuse increases with age [34], fatal abuse is more common among

**Table 5.** Types of Injuries among those hospitalized.

| Type of injury (CCS Code) | % of all Hospitalizations (N = 5,182) | % of Hospitalizations in year 2008 (N = 1,826) | % of Hospitalizations in year 2009 (N = 1,710) | % of Hospitalizations in year 2010 (N = 1,646) |
|---|---|---|---|---|
| Joint disorders and dislocations; trauma-related (225) | 0.5% | 0.8% | DS | 0.6% |
| Fracture of neck of femur [hip] (226) | 1.1% | 1% | 0.9% | 1.3% |
| Spinal cord injury (227) | DS | DS | DS | DS |
| Skull and facial fractures (228) | 9% | 8.9% | 9.6% | 8.4% |
| Fracture of upper limb (229) | 16.5% | 17.6% | 16% | 15.9% |
| Fracture of lower limb (230) | 20.7% | 21.9% | 18.4% | 21.6% |
| Other fractures (231) | 16.3% | 18.4% | 14.8% | 15.5% |
| Sprains and strains (232) | 0.5% | DS | DS | 1.4% |
| Intracranial injury (233) | 32.3% | 35.2% | 29.9% | 31.7% |
| Crushing injury or internal injury (234) | 9.1% | 8.8% | 5.4% | 13.2% |
| Open wounds of head, neck, and trunk (235) | 8.8% | 9% | 9.8% | 7.8% |
| Open wounds of extremities (236) | 2.2% | 1.2% | 3.9% | 1.6% |

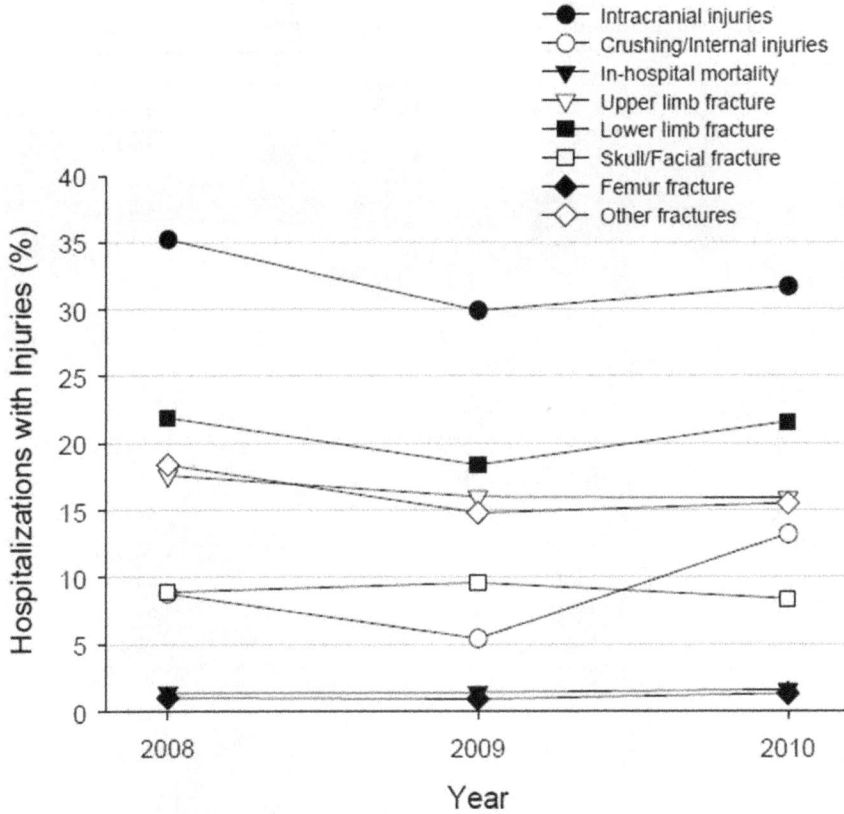

**Figure 2. Common types of Injuries in Hospitalized Children.**

infant and children younger than 2 years [35]. Infants had the highest risk of mortality. Possible explanations include higher severity of injuries, delay in seeking medical attention due to non-specific symptoms/signs, repeated abuse by perpetrator over a period of time before suspicion is confirmed, or multiple injuries that infants are at risk for (intracranial, abdominal organ lacerations, fractures). Also, older age group children are more likely to report and seek medical attention for physical abuse than younger age group children.

Further, in our study, males were more likely to visit ED and get admitted for physical abuse; however, females were associated with significantly higher risk of in-hospital mortality. This gender

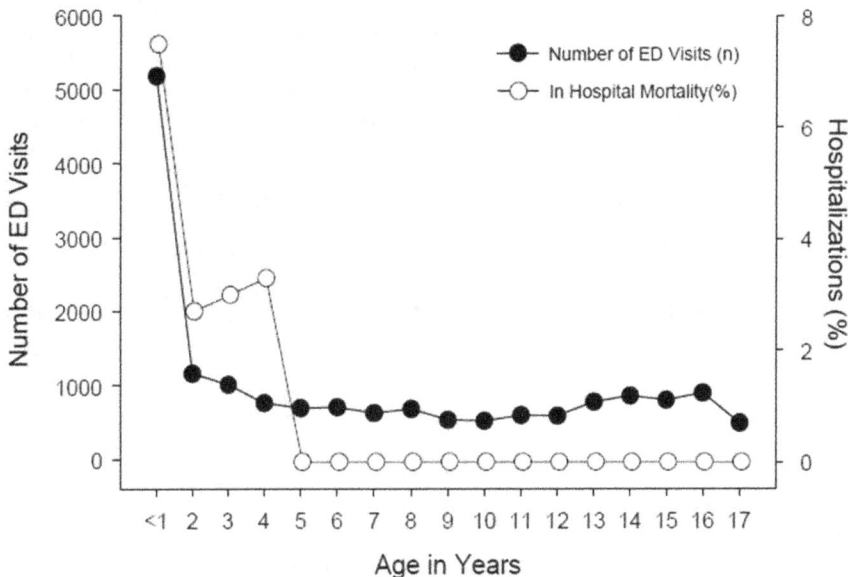

**Figure 3. Effect of age on ED visits and in-hospital mortality.** ED visits represented by left y axis and in-hospital mortality (%) by right y axis.

**Table 6.** Characteristics associated with hospital mortality (multivariable logistic regression analysis).

| Characteristic | Odds Ratio (95% CI) | p-value |
|---|---|---|
| Age (1 year increase) | 0.88 (0.81–0.96) | <0.0001 |
| **Sex** | | |
| Female | 2.39 (1.07–5.34) | 0.03 |
| Male | Reference | |
| **Insurance status** | | |
| Medicaid | 0.89 (0.41–1.92) | 0.76 |
| Medicare, private, uninsured, others | Reference | |
| **Type of injury** | | |
| Skull and facial fractures | 1.00 (0.18–5.55) | 0.99 |
| Intracranial injury | 65.24 (27.57–154.41) | <0.0001 |
| Open wounds of head, neck, and trunk | 2.56 (0.67–9.73) | 0.17 |
| Fracture of upper limb | 1.22 (0.58–2.55) | 0.60 |
| Fracture of lower limb | 0.35 (0.10–1.27) | 0.11 |
| Other fractures | 0.59 (0.24–1.41) | 0.23 |
| Sprains and strains | 2.77 (0.40–19.12) | 0.30 |
| Crushing injury or internal injury | 4.98 (2.24–11.07) | <0.0001 |
| **Hospital region** | | |
| Northeast | 0.61 (0.27–1.39) | 0.24 |
| Midwest | 0.73 (0.33–1.59) | 0.42 |
| South | 0.41 (0.18–0.93) | 0.03 |
| West | Reference | |

difference may be due to presence of other concomitant injuries such as sexual abuse in female children [40]. However, this premise merits empirical support through future studies. In the present study, amongst the 16897 ED visits 1.3% had associated sexual abuse. A prior study had revealed that children living in lower annual income households (<$15000 per year) had 3 times the number of fatalities, 7 times the number of serious inflicted injuries, and 5 times the number of moderate inflicted injuries when compared to their counterparts [36]. In our study, 70% of children who visited ED and more than 60% of those who were admitted following a physical abuse injury were from homes with lower income quartiles. Further studies are needed to explore the complex relationship between income levels and child abuse. In our study, the type of insurance did not influence the risk of mortality.

Head injury is the leading cause of child abuse fatalities [33]. In our study, abused children with intracranial injury or crushing/internal injury had a significantly higher risk of in-hospital mortality. This is consistent with prior studies which showed that infants or children with head or abdominal injuries due to physical abuse are more likely to die or become severely debilitated than are children with accidental head or abdominal injuries. [30,31,32,39]. In our study, although, more than 60% of hospitalized children with physical abuse had some form of fractures, their presence did not influence the in-hospital mortality. A significant association for increased risk of abusive head trauma by non-parental perpetrator in the older children was identified in a prior study [40]. In our study, male or female partner of child's parent or guardian was the most common perpetrator of physical abuse, which is consistent with prior findings [37].

There are methodological limitations to our study pertaining to the use of large administrative datasets. Although, the retrospective nature of the study precludes us from drawing a definite cause and effect relationship between the independent variables and occurrence of a specific event, we have shown associations between the type of physical abuse injury and outcomes which are consistent with prior research. In addition, though we used a multivariable logistic regression analysis to account for the confounding effects of patient- and hospital-level variables, the risk adjustment performed is not comprehensive due to the lack of adequate patient level clinical data (e.g. PRISM scores, GCS scores, retinal hemorrhages, intraparenchymal hemorrhage, and cerebral edema) in the NEDS dataset that have been shown to influence outcomes [39]. The use of ICD-9-CM codes for identification of physical child abuse cases may be prone to coding and or billing underestimates [24,25,26]. However, a recent study demonstrated the effective use of ICD-9-CM codes for child maltreatment conditions [23]. In addition, a recent study demonstrated very high specificity in identifying child physical abuse using ICD-9-CM codes. [24]. Our study is limited to children with injuries due to physical abuse visiting the emergency departments and hence does not capture hospitalizations from the primary care provider or inter-hospital transfers without emergency department triage. Victims of physical abuse are more likely to develop significant long-term medical and psycho-social morbidity [27,28,29,38]. The nature of the dataset precludes us from further evaluation of outcomes following discharge. Neglect or abuse due to sexual or emotional causes were not evaluated in this study and should be the focus in future studies.

Despite these limitations, our study findings are likely representative of practices beyond single center experiences, and hence generalizable. Identification of high risk cohorts in emergency department may enable strengthening of existing screening programs and optimization of outcomes. Given the unique position emergency care professionals hold in the health care system, opportunities exist for them to become a major stakeholder in the care of physically abused children.

## Conclusion

Physical abuse is not an uncommon cause of emergency department visits in children in United States. In this large cohort of hospitalized children with physical abuse, younger age group,

female gender and intracranial or crushing/internal injuries were independent predictors of in-hospital mortality.

## Author Contributions

Conceived and designed the experiments: VJA VSA ATR. Performed the experiments: VJA VSA SR RA MKL RPN. Analyzed the data: VJA VSA SR RA MKL RPN. Contributed reagents/materials/analysis tools: VJA VSA SR RA MKL RPN DGS ATR. Wrote the paper: VJA VSA SR RA MKL RPN DGS ATR.

## References

1. Dubowitz H, Bennett S (2007) Physical abuse and neglect of children. Lancet. 369(9576): 1891.
2. The Child Abuse Prevention and Treatment Act (CAPTA) amended in December 20th, 2010, by the CAPTA Reauthorization Act of 2010 (2010) (Public Law 111–320). The Child Abuse Prevention and Treatment Act (CAPTA). Available: http://www.acf.hhs.gov/sites/d, U.S. Department of Health and Human Services, 2010. Accessed 2013 Dec 1.
3. Kellogg ND (2007) American Academy of Pediatrics Committee on Child Abuse and Neglect. Evaluation of suspected child physical abuse. Pediatrics.119(6): 1232.
4. Sedlak AJ, Mettenburg J, Basena M, Petta I, McPherson K, et al. (2010) Fourth National Incidence Study of Child Abuse and Neglect (NIS–4): Report to Congress. Washington, DC: U.S. Department of Health and Human Services, Administration for Children and Families. http://www.acf.hhs.gov/sites/default/files/opre/nis4_report_congress_full_pdf_jan2010.pdf. Accessed 2013 Dec 4.
5. Child Maltreatment 2011 (2011) Report, Children's Bureau. U.S. Department of Health and Human Services, Washington, DC, 2011. Available: http://www.acf.hhs.gov/sites/default/files/cb/cm11.pdf. Accessed 2013 Dec 3.
6. Administration for Children & Families Child Maltreatment 2010 (2010) Annual Report, US Government Printing Office; US Department of Health and Human Services, Washington, DC 2010. Available: http://www.acf.hhs.gov/programs/cb/pubs/cm10/cm10.pdf. Accessed 2013 Dec 4.
7. US Department of Health and Human Services, Administration on Children, Youth, and Families (2004) Child Maltreatment. Washington, DC: US Government Printing Office; 2006. Accessed 2013 Nov 2.
8. Pless IB, Sibald AD, Smith MA, Russell MD (1987) A reappraisal of the frequency of child abuse seen in pediatric emergency rooms. Child Abuse Negl.11: 193–200.
9. Jenny C, Hymel KP, Ritzen A, Reinert SE, Hay TC (1999) Analysis of missed cases of abusive head trauma. JAMA.281: 621–626. [published correction appears in JAMA. 1999; 282: 29].
10. Gilbert R, Widom CS, Browne K, Fergusson D, Webb E, et al. (2009) Burden and consequences of child maltreatment in high-income countries. Lancet 373(9657): 68–81.
11. Sittig JS, Post ED, Russel IM, van Dijk IA, Nieuwenhuis EE, et al. (2013) Evaluation of suspected child abuse at the ED; implementation of American Academy of Pediatrics guidelines in the Netherlands. Am J Emerg Med. 2013 Oct 4. pii: S0735-6757(13)00545-7.
12. Smeekens AE, Broekhuijsen-van Henten DM, Sittig JS, Russel IM, ten Cate OT, et al. (2011) Successful e-learning programme on the detection of child abuse in emergency departments: a randomised controlled trial. Arch Dis Child 96. 330–334.
13. Louwers EC, Affourtit MJ, Moll HA, de Koning HJ, Korfage IJ (2010) Screening for child abuse at emergency departments: a systematic review. Arch Dis Child. Mar: 95(3): 214–218.
14. Clark KD, Tepper D, Jenny C (1997) Effect of a screening profile on the diagnosis of nonaccidental burns in children. Pediatr Emerg Care 13. 259–261.
15. Louwers EC, Korfage IJ, Affourtit MJ, Scheewe DJ, van de Merwe MH, et al. (2012) Effects of systematic screening and detection of child abuse in emergency departments. Pediatrics. Sep: 130(3): 457–64.
16. Bleeker G, Vet NJ, Haumann TJ, van Wijk IJ, Gemke RJ (2005) Increase in the number of reported cases of child abuse following adoption of a structured approach in the VU Medical Centre, Amsterdam, in the period 2001–2004. Ned Tijdschr Geneeskd. 149(29): 1620–1624.
17. Palazzi S, de Girolamo G, Liverani T, I ChilMa (2005) Italian Child Maltreatment study group. Observational study of suspected maltreatment in Italian paediatric emergency departments. Arch Dis Child. 90(4): 406–410.
18. González-Izquierdo A, Woodman J, Copley L, van der Meulen J, Brandon M, et al. (2010) Variation in recording of child maltreatment in administrative records of hospital admissions for injury in England, 1997–2009. Arch Dis Child. 95(11): 918–925.
19. Benger JR, Pearce V (2002) Simple intervention to improve detection of child abuse in emergency departments. BMJ: 324(7340): 780 pmid: 11924662.
20. Chang DC, Knight V, Ziegfeld S, Haider A, Warfield D, et al. (2004) The tip of the iceberg for child abuse: the critical roles of the pediatric trauma service and its registry. J Trauma. 57(6): 1189–1198, discussion 1198.
21. Louwers EC, Korfage IJ, Affourtit MJ, Scheewe DJ, van de Merwe MH, et al. (2011) Detection of child abuse in emergency departments: a multi-centre study. Arch Dis Child. 96(5): 422–425.
22. The Agency for Healthcare Research and Quality (AHRQ) (2013) NEDS is a component database of the Healthcare Cost and Utilization Project (HCUP). Available: http://www.hcup-us.ahrq.gov/nedsoverview.jsp. Accessed 2013 October 5.
23. Schnitzer PG, Slusher PL, Kruse RL, Tarleton MM (2011) Identification of ICD codes suggestive of child maltreatment. Child Abuse Negl. Jan; 35(1): 3–17.
24. Hooft A, Ronda J, Schaeffer P, Asnes AG, Leventhal JM (2013) Identification of physical abuse cases in hospitalized children: accuracy of International Classification of Diseases codes. J Pediatr. Jan; 162(1): 80–5.
25. Scott D, Tonmyr L, Fraser J, Walker S, McKenzie K (2009) The utility and challenges of using ICD codes in child maltreatment research: A review of existing literature. Child Abuse Negl. Nov; 33(11): 791–808.
26. McKenzie K, Enraght-Moony EL, Walker SM, McClure RJ, Harrison JE (2009) Accuracy of external cause-of-injury coding in hospital records. Inj Prev. Feb; 15(1): 60–4.
27. Panel on Research on Child Abuse and Neglect, Commission on Behavioral and Social Sciences and Education National Research Council (1993) Understanding Child Abuse and Neglect. Washington, DC: National Academy Press: 208.
28. Kolko DJ (1992) Characteristics of child victims of physical violence: research findings and clinical implications. J Interpers Violence.7: 244–276.
29. Perez CM, Widom CS (1994) Childhood victimization and long-term intellectual and academic outcomes. Child Abuse Negl.18: 617–633.
30. Feldman KW, Bethel R, Shugeman RP, Grossman DC, Grady MS (2001) The cause of infant and toddler subdural hemorrhage: a prospective study. Pediatrics.108: 636–646.
31. Reece RM, Sege R (2000) Childhood head injuries: accidental or inflicted. Arch Pediatr Adolesc Med.154: 11–15.
32. Canty TG Sr, Canty TG Jr, Brown C (1999) Injuries of the gastrointestinal tract from blunt trauma in children: a 12-year experience at a designated pediatric trauma center. J Trauma: 46: 234–240.
33. Alexander RC, Levitt CJ, Smith W (2001) Abusive head trauma. In: Reece RM, Ludwig S, eds. Child Abuse: Medical Management and Diagnosis. 2nd ed. Philadelphia, PA: Lippincott, Williams & Wilkins: 47–80.
34. Finkelhor D, Ormrod R, Turner H, Hamby SL (2005) The victimization of children and youth: a comprehensive, national survey [published correction appears in Child Maltreat: 10: 207]. Child Maltreat; 10: 5–25.
35. US Department of Health and Human Services, Administration on Children, Youth, and Families (2004) Child Maltreatment. Washington, DC: US Government Printing Office; 2006.
36. National Center on Child Abuse and Neglect. Study Findings (1998) Study of National Incidence and Prevalence of Child Abuse and Neglect. Washington, DC: US Department of Health and Human Services, Administration on Children, Youth, and Families.
37. Schnitzer PG, Ewigman BG (2005) Child deaths resulting from inflicted injuries: household risk factors and perpetrator characteristics. Pediatrics.116(5).
38. Norman RE, Byambaa M, De R, Butchart A, Scott J, et al. (2012) The Long-Term Health Consequences of Child Physical Abuse, Emotional Abuse, and Neglect: A Systematic Review and Meta-Analysis. PLoS Med 9(11): e1001349. doi:10.1371/journal.pmed.1001349.
39. Shein SL, Bell MJ, Kochanek PM, Tyler-Kabara EC, Wisniewski SR, et al. (2012) Risk Factors for Mortality in Children with Abusive Head Trauma. The Journal of Pediatrics: 161(4), October, Pages 716–722. e1.
40. Kellogg N and the Committee on Child Abuse and Neglect (2005) The Evaluation of Sexual Abuse in Children Pediatrics: 116: 2506–512.

# 12

# Early Hospital Mortality among Adult Trauma Patients Significantly Declined between 1998-2011

**Martin Gerdin[1]\*, Nobhojit Roy[1,2,3], Satish Dharap[4], Vineet Kumar[4], Monty Khajanchi[5], Göran Tomson[1,6], Li Felländer Tsai[7], Max Petzold[8], Johan von Schreeb[1]**

1 Health Systems and Policy, Department of Public Health Sciences, Karolinska Institutet, Stockholm, Sweden, 2 Department of Surgery, Bhabha Atomic Research Centre Hospital, Mumbai, India, 3 School of Habitat, Tata Institute of Social Sciences, Mumbai, India, 4 Department of Surgery, Lokmanya Tilak Municipal Medical College and General Hospital, Mumbai, India, 5 Department of Surgery, Seth G. S. Medical College & King Edward Memorial Hospital, Mumbai, India, 6 Medical Management Centre, Department of Learning, Informatics, Management and Ethics, Karolinska Institutet, Stockholm, Sweden, 7 Division of Orthopedics and Biotechnology, Department of Clinical Science Intervention and Technology, Karolinska Institutet, Stockholm, Sweden, 8 Centre for Applied Biostatistics, Occupational and Environmental Medicine, Sahlgrenska Academy at University of Gothenburg, Gothenburg, Sweden

## Abstract

*Background:* Traumatic injury causes more than five million deaths each year of which about 90% occur in low- and middle-income countries (LMIC). Hospital trauma mortality has been significantly reduced in high-income countries, but to what extent similar results have been achieved in LMIC has not been studied in detail. Here, we assessed if early hospital mortality in patients with trauma has changed over time in an urban lower middle-income setting.

*Methods:* We conducted a retrospective study of patients admitted due to trauma in 1998, 2002, and 2011 to a large public hospital in Mumbai, India. Our outcome measure was early hospital mortality, defined as death between admission and 24-hours. We used multivariate logistic regression to assess the association between time and early hospital mortality, adjusting for patient case-mix. Injury severity was quantified using International Classification of Diseases-derived Injury Severity Score (ICISS). Major trauma was defined as ICISS $< 0.90$.

*Results:* We analysed data on 4189 patients out of which 86.5% were males. A majority of patients were between 15 and 55 years old and 36.5% had major trauma. Overall early hospital mortality was 8.9% in 1998, 6.0% in 2002, and 8.1% in 2011. Among major trauma patients, early hospital mortality was 13.4%, in 1998, 11.3% in 2002, and 10.9% in 2011. Compared to trauma patients admitted in 1998, those admitted in 2011 had lower odds for early hospital mortality (OR = 0.56, 95% CI = 0.41–0.76) including those with major trauma (OR = 0.57, 95% CI = 0.41–0.78).

*Conclusions:* We observed a significant reduction in early hospital mortality among patients with major trauma between 1998 and 2011. Improved survival was evident only after we adjusted for patient case-mix. This finding highlights the importance of risk-adjustment when studying longitudinal mortality trends.

**Editor:** Yu-Kang Tu, National Taiwan University, Taiwan

**Funding:** This research was funded through grants from the Second Assist and the Swedish National Board of Health and Welfare. The funders had no role in study design, data collection and analysis, decision to publish, or preparation of the manuscript.

**Competing Interests:** The authors have declared that no competing interests exist.

\* E-mail: martin.gerdin@ki.se

## Background

Traumatic injury is a major threat to global public health [1,2]. More people die annually from traumatic injuries than from HIV/AIDS, tuberculosis, malaria, and obstetric conditions combined [1]. Over 90% of the five million annual deaths from traumatic injuries occur in low- and middle-income countries (LMIC) [3,4]. A recent study estimated that almost two million lives could be saved each year, if hospital care for the injured, i.e. trauma care in LMIC can be improved and reach the same level as in high-income countries (HIC) [5]. However, it is currently unclear how such reduction can be achieved.

Although a large part of trauma mortality occurs at the injury-site and during pre-hospital transportation, around 30-50% of trauma mortality occurs in hospital [6,7]. In HIC, hospital trauma mortality has been significantly reduced in recent years [8,9]. Among the most important explanations for this reduction are implementation of trauma care systems and improved medical and surgical treatment [10,11], including management of traumatic brain injury [12], haemorrhage control [13], and musculoskeletal injuries [14,15]. These improvements in clinical care have been driven, in large part, by research progress, from the basic sciences to the systems and policy level.

Hospital trauma registers have played a key role in the advancement of patient-based research and trauma care in HIC [16,17]. Trauma registers offer a unique opportunity to document patient characteristics and audit outcomes [18], thereby creating a platform for innovative clinical research. Moreover, trauma registers in HIC have been used to study longitudinal trends in hospital mortality [9]. Such studies are important as they form the basis for further research on factors underlying changes in hospital mortality. In contrast, few trauma registers exist in LMIC [19,20], which limit the potential for studies of longitudinal trends in hospital mortality in these countries.

Studies from HIC have stressed the importance of risk-adjustment when comparing trauma hospital mortality rates between hospitals or over time [21,22]. Risk-adjustment is commonly done by incorporating measures of patient case-mix including injury severity or mortality risk in the analysis [23]. Several different methods for assigning mortality risk exist but the evidence for which one to use is inconclusive [24]. Recent research from HIC has used the data-driven score International Classification of Disease (ICD) based Injury Severity Score (ICISS) to adjust for mortality risk [25], but there is no consensus regarding the appropriate approach in studies from LMIC. We adopted an explorative approach to risk-adjustment using ICISS, with the aim to assess if early hospital mortality in patients with trauma has changed over time in an urban lower middle-income setting.

## Methods

### Study design

We conducted a retrospective study of patients presenting to Lokmanya Tilak Municipal General Hospital (LTMGH), Mumbai, India (Figure 1).

### Ethics statement

The institutional ethics committee of LTMGH approved the collation of the 2011 database, reference number IEC/22/10, and approved new analyses of all three dataset in an amendment to IEC/22/10. The ethics committee granted a waiver of consent.

### Setting

India is the world's second most populous country, classified as a lower middle-income country by the World Bank [26]. In 2011, it was estimated that more than 500,000 people died from traumatic injuries in India [27]. In 2015, around 200,000 Indians are expected to die from road traffic injuries (RTI) [28]. Furthermore, in India, more than 50% of mortality from RTI occur in hospitals [29]. Mumbai is the most populous city in India, with more than18 million inhabitants [30]. Lokmanya Tilak Municipal General Hospital (Figure 2) is one of the four biggest public hospitals in Mumbai.

### Data

We retrospectively analysed three datasets of patient cohorts admitted to LTMGH trauma ward during 1998, 2002, and 2011 (Table 1). All three datasets were collated for previous research. At least one of the authors (NR, VK, or SD) of this study supervised collection of all three datasets. The three datasets were merged and duplicate entries were detected and removed using the automated approach suggested in STATA's FAQ [31].

### Eligibility criteria

All non-duplicate observations were considered eligible. Observations falling outside of accepted value ranges were set to missing.

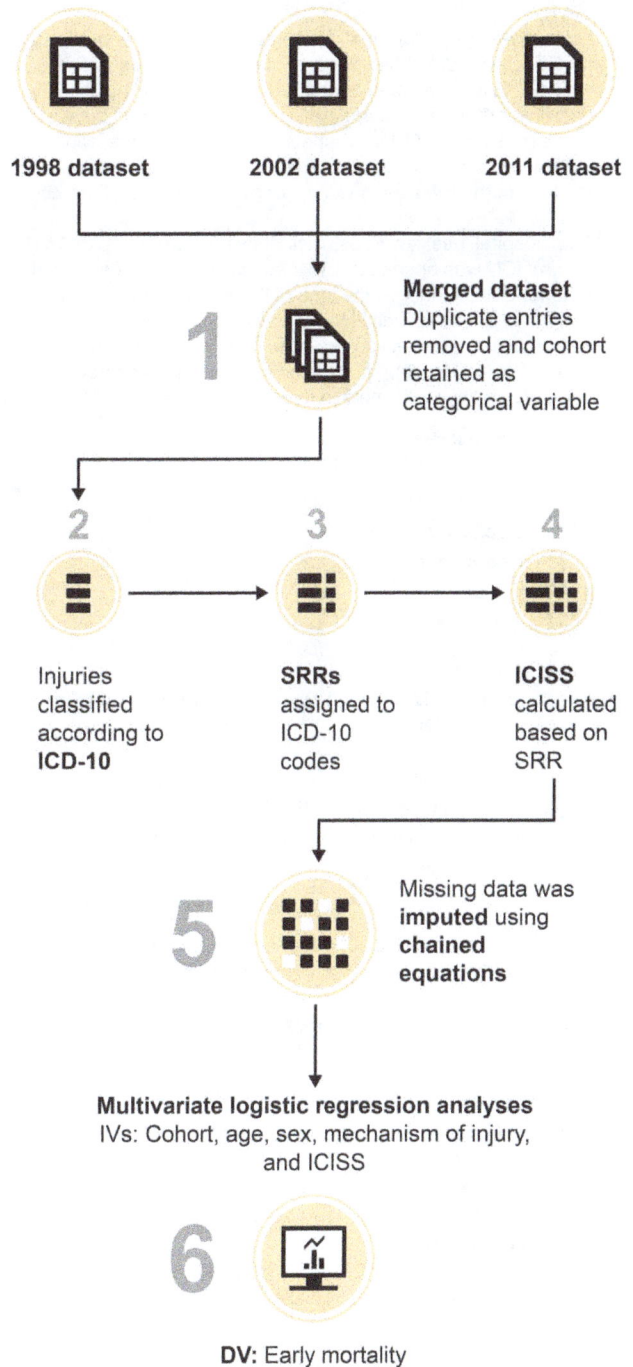

**1998 dataset        2002 dataset        2011 dataset**

**Merged dataset**
Duplicate entries removed and cohort retained as categorical variable

**2**
Injuries classified according to **ICD-10**

**3**
SRRs assigned to ICD-10 codes

**4**
ICISS calculated based on SRR

**5**
Missing data was **imputed** using **chained equations**

**Multivariate logistic regression analyses**
IVs: Cohort, age, sex, mechanism of injury, and ICISS

**6**

**DV:** Early mortality

**Figure 1. Flowchart providing a simplified outline of the study process.** Abbreviations: DV Dependent Variable, ICD International Classification of Disease, ICISS ICD-derived Injury Severity Score, IV Independent Variables, SRR Survival Risk Ratio.

### Variables

Our outcome of interest was early hospital mortality, defined as death between admission and 24 hours. According to Haider et al. [23], risk adjusted outcome studies should account for sex, age, mechanism of injury, and physiological- and anatomical injury severity. We were able to include all except physiological injury severity as covariates. Age was defined as a categorical variable, with the conventionally used cut-offs <15, 15–55, and >55 years.

Lokmanya Tilak Municipal General Hospital is public and provides subsidized health care, catering to a population of which 70% lives in some of Asia's biggest slums. The socially sensitive areas Dharavi and Koliwada are located on the west and east side of LTMGH, respectively. Being the first tertiary care hospital on the highway leading into the city, it receives the bulk of the road crash victims from the outskirts of the city.

The hospital has ten ICUs, including the trauma ICU. The trauma ICU was opened in 1974, as one of the first dedicated trauma ICUs in India. At the time of this study, the trauma ICU had 14 beds and six ventilators. At all times, the trauma ICU is staffed by two general surgeons, one orthopedic surgeon, two anesthesiologists, four nurses, two nursing assistants, four servants and two sweepers in three shifts each.

### Basic hospital data
- 1416 beds
- 257 medical students per year.
- 291 hospital faculty members
- 506 resident doctors
- 881 nurses
- 31 departments

**Figure 2. Characteristics of Lokmanya Tilak Municipal General Hospital.** Abbreviations: ICU Intensive Care Unit.

Mechanism of injury was defined as a nominal variable, categorised as fall, railway injury (RI), road traffic injury (RTI), assault, other, and unknown.

## Anatomical injury severity

We used ICISS to quantify anatomical injury severity [32]. Our rationale was that ICISS has been shown to perform well compared to the more conventional Injury Severity Score (ISS) and other established injury severity measures such as Trauma and Injury Severity Score (TRISS) [33,34], while also being easily computed using ICD-codes. To calculate ICISS, each ICD-code is assigned a survival risk ratio (SRR). Each SRR is equal to the proportion of patients who survived with a specific ICD-code in a reference population. In studies with large samples, the study sample is often used as the reference population [35,36]. Smaller studies may use published SRRs from a larger, similar, reference population [37]. In literature searches, we found no published SRRs from a LMIC trauma population and therefore we decided to use our own sample as the reference population. Because our sample was small, this analysis should be considered explorative and we are well aware of the same-sample bias that potentially is introduced using this approach.

MG coded all patients' injuries using ICD-10: 2010 edition, down to the fourth level. We calculated SRRs by dividing the number of survivors with a specific ICD-code with the total number of patients with the same ICD-code. This was done separately for each cohort to account for potential differences in factors such as transport time and care that might have influenced outcomes in the three time periods. We used the ICISS1 version of ICISS, which means that for overall scoring of patients' injury severity we counted only the worst injury (lowest SRR). We chose ICISS1 because this version has been showed to have a higher predictive value compared to versions that take into account all of a patient's injuries [38]. We defined major trauma as ICISS<0.9 [39].

**Table 1.** Characteristics of the 1998, 2002, and 2011 datasets.

| | 1998 dataset | 2002 dataset | 2011 dataset |
|---|---|---|---|
| **Purpose** | Research | Research | Research |
| **Time period (days)** | 1 Jan 1998 - 31 Dec 1998 (365) | 1 Aug 2001 - 31 May 2002 (304) | 15 Oct 2010 - 31 Dec 2011 (443) |
| **Inclusion criteria** | Admitted to LTMGH trauma ICU | Admitted to LTMGH trauma ICU | Admitted to LTMGH trauma ICU with life or limb threatening injury[1] |
| **Number of patients included (after duplicates removed)** | 2009 (2009) | 1075 (1063) | 1130 (1117) |
| **Data collection methods** | The surgical registrar of each unit collected data on patients admitted during his or her unit's duty. | The surgical registrar of each unit collected data on patients admitted during his or her unit's duty. | One dedicated data collector performed all data collection. Her timings in the trauma ward were randomized, covering eight hours each day, five days a week. She retrieved data from patients admitted during her off shift periods from intake forms. |
| **Categories of variables collected** | Demographics, mechanism of injury, level of consciousness, injuries, and early hospital mortality | Demographics, mechanism of injury, physiologic status, injuries, and early hospital mortality. | Demographics, mechanism of injury, physiologic status, length of stay in ICU and hospital, procedures and investigations performed, injuries, mortality, and time to death |
| **Sources for injury diagnoses** | Patient chart, x-rays, CT-scan findings, intraoperative findings and procedures | Patient chart, x-rays, CT-scan findings, intraoperative findings and procedures | Patient chart, x-rays, CT-scan findings, intraoperative findings and procedures |
| **Mode of injury recording** | Free text, categorized under head injury, orthopedic injury, chest injury, abdominal injury, and faciomaxillar inury | Free text, categorized under CT-findings, abdominal injury, pelvic injury, amputations, degloving injury, other orthopedic injury, and faciomaxillar injury | Free text |
| **Length of follow up** | 24 hours | 24 hours | Discharge or death |

[1]A list of injury mechanisms in combination with certain physiological signs (such as hypotension) was used to define life or limb threatening injury. Abbreviations: CT Computer Tomography, ICU Intensive Care Unit, ICU Intensive Care Unit, LTMGH Lokmanya Tilak Municipal General Hospital.

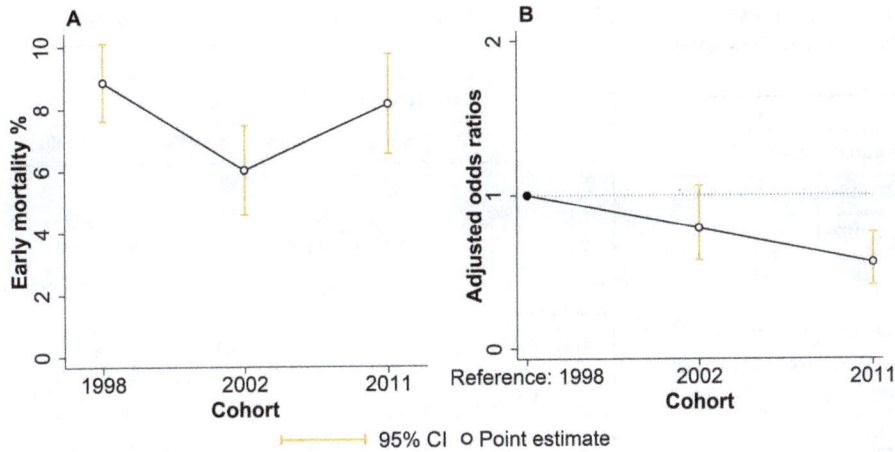

Figure 3. Unadjusted and adjusted comparison of early hospital mortality across cohorts. A. Unadjusted early hospital mortality rates across cohorts. B. Odds ratios for the 2002 and 2011 cohorts when treated as indicator variables in a multivariate logistic regression analysis with early hospital mortality as the dependent variable. The model was adjusted for sex, age, mechanism of injury and ICISS. Abbreviations: ICD International Classification of Disease, ICISS ICD-derived Injury Severity Score.

## Statistical methods

We used STATA (STATA 12, StataCorp, Texas) for statistical analyses. Where applicable, a significance level of 5% and a confidence level of 95% were used. Sample characteristics are reported for each cohort. Continuous variables are reported using their median, inter-quartile range, and range because they were found to be non-normally distributed. Categorical variables are reported as proportions.

We assessed the univariate associations between covariates and early hospital mortality using logistic regression and report their unadjusted odd-ratios (OR). We used multivariate logistic regression to evaluate the association between time and early hospital mortality. Dummy variables were created for the three

cohorts and the 2002 and 2011 cohorts were included in the logistic regression model and compared early hospital mortality with the early hospital mortality in 1998. Age, sex, mechanism of injury, and ICISS were included as covariates [23]. We conducted 13 subgroup analyses and assessed early hospital mortality trends separately in patients with and without major trauma, males, females, each age category, and in patients with history of fall, railway injury, and road traffic injury.

We used multiple imputation using chained equations to handle missing data. For each variable with missing data, we assessed the association between the probability of missing data and early hospital mortality using logistic regression. We found no significant associations, i.e. P-value>0.05 in all analyses, and hence deemed

**Table 2.** Patient characteristics*.

|  | 1998 | 2002 | 2011 | All cohorts |
|---|---|---|---|---|
| **Number of patients** | 2009 | 1063 | 1117 | 4189 |
| **Males %$^\alpha$** | 87.3 | 83.9 | 87.7 | 86.5 |
| **Age in years %$^\beta$** |  |  |  |  |
| <15 | 9.8 | 13.1 | 13.0 | 11.4 |
| 15–55 | 84.9 | 78.1 | 78.1 | 81.5 |
| >55 | 5.3 | 8.8 | 8.9 | 7.1 |
| **Mechanism of injury %$^\gamma$** |  |  |  |  |
| Fall | 24.0 | 26.5 | 24.4 | 24.8 |
| Railway injury | 27.5 | 22.6 | 26.9 | 26.1 |
| Road traffic injury | 37.7 | 38.7 | 31.5 | 36.3 |
| Assault | 9.0 | 8.3 | 13.4 | 10.0 |
| Other | 0.7 | 2.8 | 2.7 | 1.1 |
| Unknown | 1.0 | 1.1 | 3.9 | 1.8 |
| **Median ICISS (IQR:range)** | 0.96 (0.87–0.99:0.00–1.00) | 0.97 (0.93–0.98:0.00–1.00) | 0.89 (0.86–0.93:0.00–1.00) | 0.93 (0.88–0.98:0.00–1.00) |
| **Major trauma %** | 37.6 | 15.8 | 54.2 | 36.5 |
| **Early hospital mortality %** | 8.9 | 6.0 | 8.1 | 7.9 |

*Values are expressed as medians (IQR:range) or proportions (%) where appropriate. $^\alpha$0.1% missing data. $^\beta$5.4% missing data. $^\gamma$<0.1% missing data. Abbreviations: ICD International Classification of Disease, ICISS ICD-derived Injury Severity Score, IQR Inter Quartile Range.

**Table 3.** Results from univariate logistic regression assessing associations between patient characteristics and early hospital mortality.

| | Complete case analysis | | Imputed values | |
|---|---|---|---|---|
| | OR (95% CI) | P-value | OR (95% CI) | P-value |
| **Male** | 1.13 (0.79–1.60) | 0.510 | 1.15 (0.82–1.62) | 0.417 |
| **Age in years** | | | | |
| Reference: <15 | 1.00 | . | 1.00 | . |
| 15–55 | 1.17 (0.79–1.73) | 0.439 | 1.17 (0.80–1.72) | 0.420 |
| >55 | 1.81 (1.07–3.05) | 0.026 | 1.82 (1.09–3.05) | 0.022 |
| **Mechanism of injury** | | | | |
| Reference: Fall | 1.00 | . | 1.00 | . |
| Railway injury | 3.21 (2.26–4.57) | <0.001 | 3.18 (2.27–4.45) | <0.001 |
| Road traffic injury | 1.78 (1.24–2.55) | 0.002 | 1.74 (1.23–2.45) | 0.002 |
| Assault | 0.48 (0.23–1.00) | 0.050 | 0.45 (0.22–0.93) | 0.032 |
| Other | 1.22 (0.28–5.22) | 0.792 | 0.96 (0.23–4.07) | 0.954 |
| Unknown | 3.04 (1.42–6.51) | 0.004 | 3.12 (1.51–6.45) | 0.002 |
| **ICISS per 0.01 increase** | 0.95 (0.94–0.96) | <0.001 | 0.95 (0.94–0.96) | <0.001 |
| **Major trauma** | 2.44 (1.93–3.09) | <0.001 | 2.37 (1.89–2.97) | <0.001 |

Abbreviations: CI Confidence Interval, ICD International Classification of Disease, ICISS ICD-derived Injury Severity Score, OR Odds Ratio.

**Table 4.** Multivariate logistic regression model parameters.

| | Complete case analysis | | Imputed values | |
|---|---|---|---|---|
| | OR (95% CI) | P-value | OR (95% CI) | P-value |
| **Cohort** | | | | |
| Reference: 1998 | 1.00 | . | 1.00 | . |
| 2002 | 0.64 (0.45–0.92) | 0.015 | 0.78 (0.58–1.06) | 0.118 |
| 2011 | 0.56 (0.42–0.76) | <0.001 | 0.56 (0.41–0.75) | <0.001 |
| **Age in years** | | | | |
| Reference: <15 | 1.00 | . | 1.00 | . |
| 15–55 | 0.71 (0.46–1.09) | 0.116 | 0.71 (0.46–1.08) | 0.111 |
| >55 | 1.38 (0.79–2.39) | 0.254 | 1.32 (0.76–2.29) | 0.322 |
| **Male** | 1.15 (0.78–1.70) | 0.472 | 1.17 (0.80–1.70) | 0.416 |
| **Mechanism of injury** | | | | |
| Reference: Fall | 1.00 | . | 1.00 | . |
| Railway injury | 2.78 (1.90–4.05) | <0.001 | 2.85 (1.98–4.10) | <0.001 |
| Road traffic injury | 1.52 (1.05–2.22) | 0.028 | 1.54 (1.07–2.21) | 0.021 |
| Assault | 0.46 (0.21–1.00) | 0.050 | 0.44 (0.21–0.95) | 0.038 |
| Other | 1.36 (0.31–5.96) | 0.683 | 0.99 (0.23–4.30) | 0.994 |
| Unknown | 2.62 (1.14–6.01) | 0.023 | 2.86 (1.30–6.28) | 0.009 |
| **ICISS per 0.01 increase** | 0.95 (0.94–0.96) | <0.001 | 0.95 (0.94–0.96) | <0.001 |

Abbreviations: CI Confidence Interval, ICD International Classification of Disease, ICISS ICD-derived Injury Severity Score, OR Odds Ratio.

multiple imputation as appropriate. Each cohort was imputed separately. We specified our imputation model to impute sex using logistic regression, and age and mechanism of injury using multinominal logistic regression. We performed 20 imputations to achieve stable estimates.

## Results

We analysed data on 4189 patients (Table 2), out of which 86.5% were male. Road traffic injury was the most common mechanism of injury across cohorts, followed by railway injury and falls. Out of all patients, 81.5% were between 15 and 55 years old. Early hospital mortality among all patients was 7.9% (Figure 3A), the median ICISS was 0.93, and 36.5% had major trauma (ICISS<0.9). The early hospital mortality rate among major trauma patients was 12.2% overall and 13.4%, 11.3%, and 10.9% in 1998, 2002, and 2011 respectively.

### Univariate analysis

Our univariate logistic regression analyses (Table 3) showed that patients over 55 years of age had significantly higher odds of early hospital mortality compared to patients younger than 15 years of age (OR = 1.81, P-value = 0.026, 95% CI = 1.07–3.05). Patients with railway injury (OR = 3.21, P-value<0.001, 95% CI = 2.26–4.57), road traffic injury (OR = 1.78, P-value = 0.002, 95% CI = 1.24–2.55), or an unknown mechanism of injury (OR = 3.04, P-value = 0.004, 95% CI = 1.42–6.51) had significantly higher odds of early hospital mortality compared to patients with fall. Every 0.01 unit increase in ICISS was significantly associated with lower odds of early hospital mortality (OR = 0.95, P-value<0.001, 95% CI = 0.94–0.96), and having major trauma was significantly associated with higher odds of early hospital mortality (OR = 2.44, P-value<0.001, 95% CI = 1.93–3.09).

### Multivariate analysis

Compared to 1998, the multivariate logistic regression model showed lower adjusted odds of early hospital mortality in 2002 (OR = 0.78, P-value = 0.118, 95% CI = 0.58–1.06) and significantly lower odds in 2011 (OR = 0.56, P-value<0.001, 95% CI = 0.41–0.75), (Table 4, Figure 3B). Males did not have significantly higher odds of early hospital mortality compared to females. There was no significant difference in odds of early hospital mortality difference between either older (>55 years) or younger (15–55 years) compared to the youngest (<15 years) patients. Railway injury (OR = 2.85, P-value<0.001, 95% CI = 1.98–4.10) and road traffic injury (OR = 1.54, P-value = 0.021, 95% CI = 1.07–2.21) retained largely the same effect sizes and remained significantly associated with early hospital mortality in multivariate analysis. Assault was significantly associated with lower odds of early mortality (OR = 0.46, P-value = 0.038, 95% CI = 0.21–0.95). Also, every 0.01 unit increase in ICISS remained significantly associated with lower odds of early hospital mortality (OR = 0.95, P-value<0.001, 95% CI = 0.94–0.96). Model estimates for each cohort analysed separately are available as Table S1-S3.

### Subgroup analysis

Among patients with major trauma, the odds of early hospital mortality were significantly lower in 2011 (OR = 0.44, P-value<0.001, 95% CI = 0.30–0.66) compared to 1998 (Figure 4A). Males had significantly lower odds of early hospital mortality in 2011 (OR = 0.57, P-value<0.001, 95% CI = 0.41–0.78) compared to 1998 (Figure 4B). In patients between 15 and 55 years of age the odds of early hospital mortality were significantly lower in 2011 (OR = 0.52, P-value<0.001, 95% CI = 0.37–0.74) compared to 1998 (Figure 4C). For patients with

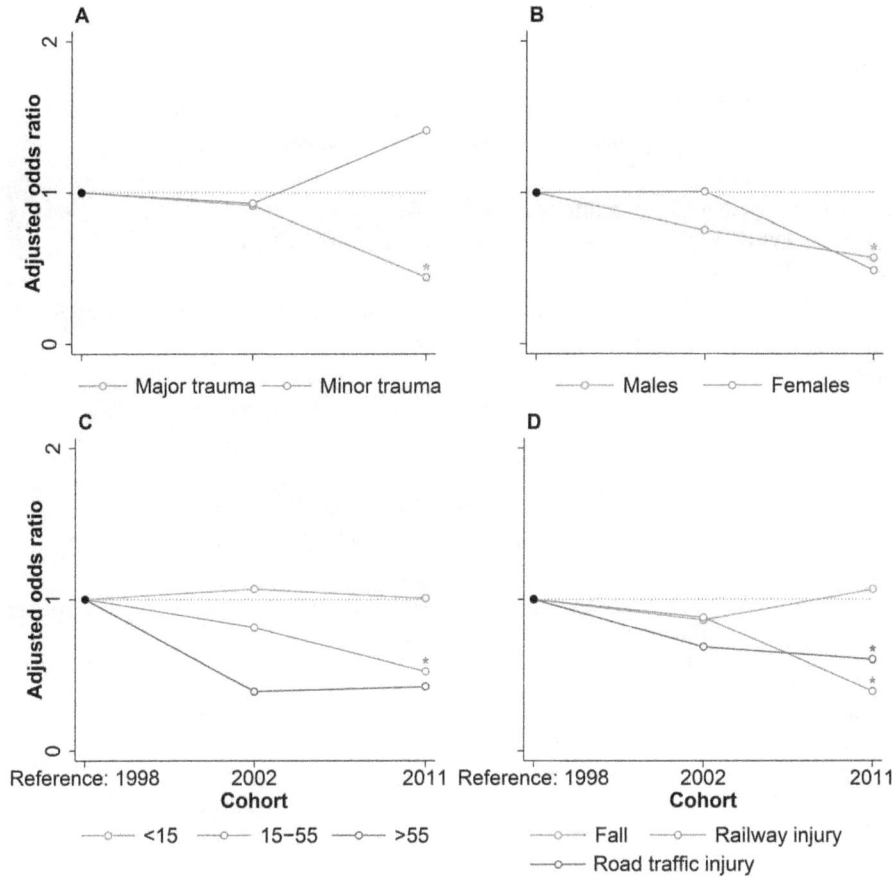

**Figure 4. Comparison of early hospital mortality odds ratios in subgroup analyses.** Odds ratios are early hospital mortality odds ratios. **A.** Major trauma was defined as ICISS<0.9. The model was adjusted for sex, age, mechanism of injury, and ICISS. **B.** The model was adjusted for age, mechanism of injury, and ICISS. **C.** The model was adjusted for sex, mechanism of injury, and ICISS. **D.** The model was adjusted for sex, age, and ICISS. Abbreviations: ICD International Classification of Disease, ICISS ICD-derived Injury Severity Score. *P-value<0.05, compared to the reference category.

railway injury the odds were significantly lower in 2011 (OR = 0.39, P-value<0.001, 95% CI = 0.24–0.64) compared to 1998 (Figure 4D). Patients with road traffic injury had significantly lower odds in 2011 (OR = 0.60, P-value = 0.047, 95% CI = 0.36–1.00) compared to 1998. Full model estimates for all subgroups, including non-significant results, are available as Table S4-13.

## Discussion

Our study showed that early hospital mortality in trauma patients decreased over a 13-year period in an urban lower middle-income setting. This trend was not observed in unadjusted analysis and our study therefore highlights the importance of risk-adjustment when comparing mortality rates over time. However, we used an explorative approach to compute ICISS as a measure of anatomical injury severity and this should be kept in mind when interpreting our results. The observed reduction in early hospital mortality was most pronounced in patients with major trauma, while no significant changes could be detected in patients with minor trauma. Similar trends as the one shown here have been observed for other major conditions in the same geographical area. For example, the infant mortality rate and under-five mortality rate in Maharashtra dropped by 25% and 34% respectively between 1992 and 2006 [40]. Similarly, Maharashtra's maternal mortality rate dropped by 23% between 1998 and

2009 [41,42]. It is important to note that these figures are not risk-adjusted.

The implementation of trauma systems has been widely claimed as a major reason for reduced trauma mortality over time in HIC [11,22,43,44]. The trauma system concept originates from the designation of dedicated trauma centres in the US some 40 years ago [45]. Today such systems ideally include streamlined preventive, prehospital, hospital, and rehabilitative measures [8]. Interestingly, the reduction in early hospital mortality observed in our study has occurred in the absence of a comprehensive trauma system. On the hospital level, LTMGH does employ a trauma team model, and one hypothetical explanation for the observed trend might be a maturation of trauma care efforts at institutional level, with improved equipment and enforced education of residents according to advanced trauma life support principles.

A functioning prehospital system is generally considered a vital component of a modern trauma system and improvements in prehospital triage and care may influence overall mortality rates. A recent systematic review found that the implementation of prehospital systems in LMIC has led to reduced overall mortality rates [46]. However, there is no organised prehospital system in Mumbai and most trauma patients arrive to hospital in taxis or are brought by the police [47]. Ambulances are used almost exclusively for inter-hospital transfers and are largely used as transport vehicles without any resuscitation equipment [47]. Therefore, the reduced odds of early hospital mortality can most likely not be attributed to improvements in prehospital care, but rather improved hospital trauma care.

A high proportion of the patients in this study were males. This finding is consistent with other research from LMIC [48–50]. Interestingly, the proportion of females seems to be higher in HIC trauma than in our study population [9,51]. This discrepancy might be partly due to more women involved in work outside of the home in HIC compared to LMIC. Lastly, we found that RTI, falls, and RI were the most common mechanisms of injury. Although RTI and falls are major causes of trauma around the world, RI appears to be rather unique for Mumbai, and thus interesting to explore further as a subset of the Mumbai trauma population.

## Methodological considerations and limitations

First, the difference in inclusion criteria between the three cohorts is a major limitation. To adjust for this limitation and to minimize bias, we adjusted our analyses for case-mix and also conducted several subgroup analyses. Second, we used ICISS to adjust for anatomical injury severity and used our own data to calculate SRRs and generate finals scores. As we highlighted in the methodology section this approach might have introduced a same-sample bias that in part can explain the good fit of ICISS. Our approach should therefore be considered explorative in nature. However, we argue that this was a more sensible approach compared to using SRRs derived from a completely different trauma population. Third, we analysed available datasets and were therefore not able to choose our time-points. Unfortunately, retrospective inquires into patient files spanning more than ten years back constitute a more or less impossible undertaking as files are paper based and stored under variable conditions over time. Finally, the data did not allow us to explore outcome measures beyond mortality between admission and 24 hours. We do acknowledge that later mortality and functional outcomes are important and should be the focus of prospective studies in the same setting.

## Conclusions

In our study, we observed a significant reduction in early trauma mortality among patients with major trauma between 1998 and 2011. Improved survival was evident after adjusting for patient case-mix and this finding therefore highlights the importance of risk-adjustment in studies of mortality over time. Furthermore, as one of few studies from an urban lower-middle income setting spanning more than ten years, we show that survival has improved despite the absence of a trauma system and functioning prehospital organisation.

## Supporting Information

**Table S1** Multivariate logistic regression model parameters, 1998 cohort analysed separately.

**Table S2** Multivariate logistic regression model parameters, 2002 cohort analysed separately.

**Table S3** Multivariate logistic regression model parameters, 2011 cohort analysed separately.

**Table S4** Multivariate logistic regression model parameters, patients with major trauma analysed separately.

**Table S5** Multivariate logistic regression model parameters, patients with minor trauma analysed separately.

**Table S6** Multivariate logistic regression model parameters, males analysed separately.

**Table S7** Multivariate logistic regression model parameters, females analysed separately.

**Table S8** Multivariate logistic regression model parameters, age<15 years analysed separately.

**Table S9** Multivariate logistic regression model parameters, age 15–55 years analysed separately.

**Table S10** Multivariate logistic regression model parameters, age>55 years analysed separately.

**Table S11** Multivariate logistic regression model parameters, patients with fall analysed separately.

**Table S12** Multivariate logistic regression model parameters, patients with railway injury analysed separately.

**Table S13** Multivariate logistic regression model parameters, patients with road traffic injury analysed separately.

## Acknowledgments

We would like to acknowledge the support by the Dean and Staff and Research Society of LTMGH. We would also like to thank scientific editor Angelika Hofmann for professional proofreading, Siddarth Daniels David, and our reviewers for insightful and helpful comments.

## Author Contributions

Conceived and designed the experiments: MG NR JvS. Performed the experiments: NR SD VK. Analyzed the data: MG MP. Contributed reagents/materials/analysis tools: NR SD VK MK. Wrote the paper: MG NR GT JvS. Substantial contribution to interpretation of data: NR SD VK MK GT MP LFT JvS. Revised the article critically for important intellectual content: MG NR SD VK MK GT MP LFT JvS. Gave final approval of the version to be published: MG NR SD VK MK GT MP LFT JvS.

## References

1. Lozano R, Naghavi M, Foreman K, Lim S, Shibuya K, et al. (2013) Global and regional mortality from 235 causes of death for 20 age groups in 1990 and 2010: a systematic analysis for the Global Burden of Disease Study 2010. Lancet 380: 2095–2128.
2. World Health Organization (2004) World report on road traffic injury prevention. Geneva: World Health Organization.
3. Mathers C, Boerma T, Ma Fat D (2008) The global burden of disease: 2004 update. Geneva: World Health Organization.
4. World Health Organization (2010) Injuries and violence: the facts. Geneva: World Health Organization.
5. Mock C, Joshipura M, Arreola-Risa C, Quansah R (2012) An estimate of the number of lives that could be saved through improvements in trauma care globally. World J Surg 36: 959–963.
6. Pfeifer R, Tarkin IS, Rocos B, Pape HC (2009) Patterns of mortality and causes of death in polytrauma patients—has anything changed? Injury 40: 907–911.

7. Ker K, Kiriya J, Perel P, Edwards P, Shakur H, et al. (2012) Avoidable mortality from giving tranexamic acid to bleeding trauma patients: an estimation based on WHO mortality data, a systematic literature review and data from the CRASH-2 trial. BMC Emerg Med 12: 3.

8. Gruen RL, Gabbe BJ, Stelfox HT, Cameron PA (2012) Indicators of the quality of trauma care and the performance of trauma systems. Br J Surg 99 Suppl 1: 97–104.

9. Glance LG, Osler TM, Mukamel DB, Dick AW (2012) Outcomes of adult trauma patients admitted to trauma centers in Pennsylvania, 2000-2009. Arch Surg 147: 732–737.

10. Nathens AB, Jurkovich GJ, Cummings P, Rivara FP, Maier RV (2000) The effect of organized systems of trauma care on motor vehicle crash mortality. JAMA 283: 1990–1994.

11. Celso B, Tepas J, Langland-Orban B, Pracht E, Papa L, et al. (2006) A systematic review and meta-analysis comparing outcome of severely injured patients treated in trauma centers following the establishment of trauma systems. J Trauma 60: 371–378; discussion 378.

12. Rosenfeld JV, Maas AI, Bragge P, Morganti-Kossmann MC, Manley GT, et al. (2012) Early management of severe traumatic brain injury. The Lancet 380: 1088–1098.

13. Gruen RL, Brohi K, Schreiber M, Balogh ZJ, Pitt V, et al. (2012) Haemorrhage control in severely injured patients. The Lancet 380: 1099–1108.

14. Balogh ZJ, Reumann MK, Gruen RL, Mayer-Kuckuk P, Schuetz MA, et al. (2012) Advances and future directions for management of trauma patients with musculoskeletal injuries. The Lancet 380: 1109–1119.

15. Gruen RL, Fitzgerald MC (2012) Towards a maturation of trauma research. The Lancet 380: 1033–1034.

16. Cameron PA, Gabbe BJ, Cooper DJ, Walker T, Judson R, et al. (2008) A statewide system of trauma care in Victoria: effect on patient survival. Med J Aust 189: 546–550.

17. Rutledge R (1995) The goals, development, and use of trauma registries and trauma data sources in decision making in injury. Surg Clin North Am 75: 305–326.

18. Gliklich RE, Dreyer NA (2007) Registries for Evaluating Patient Outcomes: A User's Guide. Rockville, MD: Agency for Healthcare Research and Quality.

19. O'Reilly GM, Cameron PA, Joshipura M (2012) Global trauma registry mapping: a scoping review. Injury 43: 1148–1153.

20. O'Reilly GM, Joshipura M, Cameron PA, Gruen R (2013) Trauma registries in developing countries: A review of the published experience. Injury.

21. Christensen MC, Parr M, Tortella BJ, Malmgren J, Morris S, et al. (2010) Global differences in causes, management, and survival after severe trauma: the recombinant activated factor VII phase 3 trauma trial. J Trauma 69: 344–352.

22. Moore L, Hanley JA, Turgeon AF, Lavoie A (2010) Evaluation of the long-term trend in mortality from injury in a mature inclusive trauma system. World J Surg 34: 2069–2075.

23. Haider AH, Saleem T, Leow JJ, Villegas CV, Kisat M, et al. (2012) Influence of the National Trauma Data Bank on the study of trauma outcomes: is it time to set research best practices to further enhance its impact? J Am Coll Surg 214: 756–768.

24. Tohira H, Jacobs I, Mountain D, Gibson N, Yeo A (2012) Systematic review of predictive performance of injury severity scoring tools. Scand J Trauma Resusc Emerg Med 20: 63.

25. Ciesla DJ, Tepas JJ, 3rd, Pracht EE, Langland-Orban B, Cha JY, et al. (2013) Fifteen-year trauma system performance analysis demonstrates optimal coverage for most severely injured patients and identifies a vulnerable population. J Am Coll Surg 216: 687–695; discussion 695–688.

26. The World Bank (2013) Country and Lending Groups. Geneva: The World Bank.

27. National Crime Records Bureau (2011) Accidental deaths and suicides in India. New Delhi: Ministry of Home Affairs, Government of India.

28. Gururaj G (2008) Road traffic deaths, injuries and disabilities in India: current scenario. Natl Med J India 21: 14–20.

29. Gururaj G (2005) Injuries in India: A national perspective. Background Papers: Burden of Disease in India Equitable Development - Healthy Future. New Delhi: National Commission on Macroeconomics and Health, Ministry of Health & Family Welfare, Government of India. pp. 325–347.

30. Press Information Bureau (2011) INDIA STATS : Million plus cities in India as per Census 2011. Government of India.

31. Gould W (1999) How do I identify duplicate observations in my data? Texas: StataCopr LP.

32. Osler T, Rutledge R, Deis J, Bedrick E (1996) ICISS: an international classification of disease-9 based injury severity score. J Trauma 41: 380–386; discussion 386–388.

33. Rutledge R, Osler T, Emery S, Kromhout-Schiro S (1998) The end of the Injury Severity Score (ISS) and the Trauma and Injury Severity Score (TRISS): ICISS, an International Classification of Diseases, ninth revision-based prediction tool, outperforms both ISS and TRISS as predictors of trauma patient survival, hospital charges, and hospital length of stay. J Trauma 44: 41–49.

34. Meredith JW, Evans G, Kilgo PD, MacKenzie E, Osler T, et al. (2002) A comparison of the abilities of nine scoring algorithms in predicting mortality. J Trauma 53: 621–628; discussion 628–629.

35. Blomberg H, Svennblad B, Michaelsson K, Byberg L, Johansson J, et al. (2013) Prehospital trauma life support training of ambulance caregivers and the outcomes of traffic-injury victims in sweden. J Am Coll Surg 217: 1010–1019 e1012.

36. Gedeborg R, Thiblin I, Byberg L, Melhus H, Lindback J, et al. (2010) Population density and mortality among individuals in motor vehicle crashes. Inj Prev 16: 302–308.

37. Wong SS, Leung GK (2008) Injury Severity Score (ISS) vs. ICD-derived Injury Severity Score (ICISS) in a patient population treated in a designated Hong Kong trauma centre. Mcgill J Med 11: 9–13.

38. Kilgo PD, Osler TM, Meredith W (2003) The worst injury predicts mortality outcome the best: rethinking the role of multiple injuries in trauma outcome scoring. J Trauma 55: 599–606; discussion 606–597.

39. Diggs BS, Mullins RJ, Hedges JR, Arthur M, Newgard CD (2008) Proportion of seriously injured patients admitted to hospitals in the US with a high annual injured patient volume: a metric of regionalized trauma care. J Am Coll Surg 206: 212–219.

40. International Institute for Population Sciences and Macro International (2008) National Family Health Survey (NFHS-3), India, 2005-06: Maharashtra. Mumbai: International Institute for Population Sciences.

41. Sample Registration System (2011) Special Bulletin on Maternal Mortality in India 2007-2009. New Delhi: Office of Registrar General, India.

42. Sample Registration System (2000) SRS Bulletin. Volume 33. Issue 1. New Delhi: Office of Registrar General, India.

43. Gabbe BJ, Simpson PM, Sutherland AM, Wolfe R, Fitzgerald MC, et al. (2012) Improved functional outcomes for major trauma patients in a regionalized, inclusive trauma system. Ann Surg 255: 1009–1015.

44. Shackford SR, Hollingworth-Fridlund P, Cooper GF, Eastman AB (1986) The effect of regionalization upon the quality of trauma care as assessed by concurrent audit before and after institution of a trauma system: a preliminary report. J Trauma 26: 812–820.

45. West JG, Trunkey DD, Lim RC (1979) Systems of trauma care. A study of two counties. Arch Surg 114: 455–460.

46. Henry JA, Reingold AL (2012) Prehospital trauma systems reduce mortality in developing countries: a systematic review and meta-analysis. J Trauma Acute Care Surg 73: 261–268.

47. Roy N, Murlidhar V, Chowdhury R, Patil SB, Supe PA, et al. (2010) Where there are no emergency medical services-prehospital care for the injured in Mumbai, India. Prehosp Disaster Med 25: 145–151.

48. Marson AC, Thomson JC (2001) The influence of prehospital trauma care on motor vehicle crash mortality. J Trauma 50: 917–920; discussion 920–911.

49. Demyttenaere SV, Nansamba C, Nganwa A, Mutto M, Lett R, et al. (2009) Injury in Kampala, Uganda: 6 years later. Can J Surg 52: E146–150.

50. Ichikawa M, Chadbunchachai W, Marui E (2003) Effect of the helmet act for motorcyclists in Thailand. Accid Anal Prev 35: 183–189.

51. Brennan PW, Everest ER, Griggs WM, Slater A, Carter L, et al. (2002) Risk of death among cases attending South Australian major trauma services after severe trauma: the first 4 years of operation of a state trauma system. J Trauma 53: 333–339.

# 13

# Risk of Maltreatment-Related Injury: A Cross-Sectional Study of Children under Five Years Old Admitted to Hospital with a Head or Neck Injury or Fracture

Joseph Jonathan Lee, Arturo Gonzalez-Izquierdo, Ruth Gilbert*

Institute of Child Health, University College London, London, United Kingdom

## Abstract

***Objectives:*** To determine the predictive value and sensitivity of demographic features and injuries (indicators) for maltreatment-related codes in hospital discharge records of children admitted with a head or neck injury or fracture.

***Methods:*** Study design: Population-based, cross sectional study. Setting: NHS hospitals in England. Subjects: Children under five years old admitted acutely to hospital with head or neck injury or fracture. Data source: Hospital Episodes Statistics, 1997 to 2009. Main outcome measure: Maltreatment-related injury admissions, defined by ICD10 codes, were used to calculate for each indicator (demographic feature and/or type of injury): i) the predictive value (proportion of injury admissions that were maltreatment-related); ii) sensitivity (proportion of all maltreatment-related injury admissions with the indicator).

***Results:*** Of 260,294 childhood admissions for fracture or head or neck injury, 3.2% (8,337) were maltreatment-related. With increasing age of the child, the predictive value for maltreatment-related injury declined but sensitivity increased. Half of the maltreatment-related admissions occurred in children older than one year, and 63% occurred in children with head injuries without fractures or intracranial injury.

***Conclusions:*** Highly predictive injuries accounted for very few maltreatment-related admissions. Protocols that focus on high-risk injuries may miss the majority of maltreated children.

**Editor:** Lisa Hartling, Alberta Research Centre for Health Evidence, University of Alberta, Canada

**Funding:** The funders had no role in study design, data collection and analysis, decision to publish, or preparation of the manuscript. AGI was supported by funding from the Department of Health (http://www.dh.gov.uk/en/index.htm) Clinical Strategies and Clinical Audit Division) and the Policy Research Programme through funding to the Policy Research Unit in the Health of Children, Young People and Families. This is an independent report commissioned and funded by the Department of Health. The views expressed are not necessarily those of the Department. There was no other external funding of this project.

**Competing Interests:** The authors have declared that no competing interests exist.

* E-mail: r.gilbert@ucl.ac.uk

## Introduction

Clinicians must have a low threshold for considering physical abuse or neglect in injured children as prompt intervention may reduce the risk of further harm. [1] Detection requires clinical experience, but most injured children presenting to hospital are seen by relatively inexperienced 'frontline' trainee paediatricians or emergency department staff. Their first-hand experience of maltreatment is limited because abuse or neglect account for less than one in every 100 emergency department attendances for injury. [2] The literature frequently cites certain features of injury, such as intracranial injury or fracture in a young child, as indicative of a high risk of maltreatment. Some hospitals use guidelines that recommend these features should trigger further investigation of possible child maltreatment; for example, by asking a paediatrician who is experienced in child protection to assess the child. [1,3,4] An advantage of such guidance is that it focuses the scarce resources of experienced staff on children at high risk of child maltreatment. A disadvantage is that clinicians may give less attention to children with injury characteristics that indicate a relatively low risk of child maltreatment. If most maltreated children present with low risk characteristics such guidance could result in more cases of child maltreatment being missed than if the recommendations were not followed.

Balancing the need for indicators (patient characteristics such as age or type of injury) to have high predictive value (i.e. a high proportion of injury admissions with the indicator are maltreatment-related), with high sensitivity (the indicator picks up a high proportion of truly maltreated children), is well recognised in the evaluation of screening tests. In this report, we use national data for injured children admitted to hospital in England to quantify the predictive value and sensitivity for child maltreatment of indicators based on age and type of injury.

## Methods

### Overview

We firstly took the perspective of a clinician faced with an injured child, and determined the predictive value of age and type of injury for maltreatment-related admission, which was defined by ICD10 codes taken from electronic discharge records. We also used a multivariable model take into account age, sex, and socio-economic status. Second, we took a broader view (such as when writing a clinical guideline), and determined the sensitivity of each of the indicators. This was done by determining the proportion of all maltreatment-related injury admissions detected by the indicator. Third, we considered a public health perspective and calculated the incidence of maltreatment-related injures for each type of injury indicator at each age, using Poisson regression. In order to take account of developmental differences, we stratified all analyses by developmental age bands.

## Population

We conducted a cross-sectional study of all acute hospital admissions to the NHS in England of children aged one week to five years using hospital administrative data for 1997 to 2009 (known as Hospital Episode Statistics (HES) http://www.hesonline.nhs.uk/). The study population was restricted to children with head or neck injury or fracture because these injuries are readily recognisable and therefore unlikely to be affected by miscoding. They also reflect the most frequent and serious injury presentations in young children and are associated with an increased risk of maltreatment. [4–8] Estimates of the denominator population of children resident in England at each year of age and calendar year, were extrapolated from census data provided by the Office of National Statistics. [9]

## Outcome

The primary outcome measure, maltreatment-related injury admission, was defined as the presence of any code from two exclusive clusters of ICD-10 codes recorded as a diagnostic code in the child's electronic discharge record (Table S1). [10,11] The most specific cluster contained codes for maltreatment syndrome or assault. The second cluster contained codes that reflected investigation for undetermined intent or concerns about the child's adverse social circumstances. Both clusters of codes were used together to define the main outcome measure, maltreatment-related codes.

These maltreatment-related ICD-10 codes were selected to be consistent with 'alert' features listed in UK national guidance from NICE (National Institute of Clinical Excellence) that should prompt the clinician to 'consider' or 'suspect' child maltreatment and take further action. [1] These codes therefore reflect clinical concern about possible maltreatment but do not reflect a definitive diagnosis of abuse. They identify children who should be investigated further, and who require further assessment and information sharing. This classification reflects clinical reality where the cause of injury may not be known for certain until sometime after admission, if at all. To exclude these children from the analysis would bias estimates of predictive values, increasing estimates in the most suspicious injuries and decreasing them in less clear cut cases. To assess the robustness of our findings, we repeated analyses using the more specific set of codes for maltreatment syndrome or assault (Table S1, results in figures S1 and S2).

In a separate validation study in one hospital, both clusters of maltreatment-related codes were compared with clinician-entered text in electronic records. The codes were highly specific (90%, 20/22; personal communication, Gilbert), similar to findings from validation studies in the US and Australia. [12–14] Comparisons of rates and risk factors for these maltreatment-related codes in different countries have shown consistent results. [10,11]

## Age and type of injury indicators

Previous studies have shown that an injured child's risk of maltreatment declines with age and is strongly related to development. [6,8,15] Types of injury also vary with developmental age. [1,6] We therefore performed analyses separately for children admitted before six months of age (pre-mobile), between six to 12 months (mobility increasing), and between one to four years of age (mobile). Within these strata, we included indicators for age (one week to one month, one to three months and quarterly till 12 months, then each year of age).

We included indicators for types of injury that have been associated with a high risk of maltreatment in systematic reviews, for example, intracranial injury (ICI), skull fracture, long bone fracture, and thoracic or rib fractures. [4–8] Smaller groupings were avoided to prevent spurious findings due to multiple testing and small cell sizes. Because we restricted analyses to children with head or neck injury or fracture, the baseline category for comparison was children without other indicators: i.e. children with head injury without ICI or fracture. Such children could have any other form of head injury including bruising, laceration, incision and soft tissue injuries.

## Statistical analyses

All analyses were based on data for the entire 12-year period. The incidence of maltreatment-related injury admission and the injury grouping were stable over this time. [10] Each analysis was performed separately for the three age strata.

The crude predictive value was calculated as the proportion of all acute admissions with each type of injury that had maltreatment-related codes (Table 1). Adjusted estimates of the predictive value were calculated using logistic regression models with age, sex and quintile of multiple deprivation as *a priori* confounders for each age stratum. These models were used to assess the association between each type of injury and maltreatment-related codes by computing adjusted odds ratios (table 2). They were also used to predict the median probability (with $5^{th}$ to $95^{th}$ centiles) of maltreatment-related injury for each age and injury indicator (figures 1, 2, and 3).

The sensitivity of each injury or age indicator was calculated as the proportion of all maltreatment-related admissions with the indicator. To reflect the public health burden of maltreatment-related injury, we estimated incidence rates of admission for each age-injury indicator, using Poisson regression offset by population estimates. The variance and mean were approximately equal and there was no evidence of over-dispersion. Admissions were not clustered by child as multiple admissions were rare.

Analyses were conducted in Stata 11 and R 2.13.0.

## Results

The 260,294 admissions with head or neck injury or fracture comprised 52.8% of all acute hospital admissions for injury in children aged one week to four completed years. Overall, 8,337 admissions (3.2%) had maltreatment-related codes, of which 45% were coded for maltreatment syndrome or assault. 94% of admissions were the first admission for injury and 2.4% of admissions had no code for the cause of injury.

## Predictive value

Table 1 shows that the predictive value for maltreatment-related injury admission given any type of head or neck injury or fracture declined with age from 9.9% in children less than six months old to 1.2% in children aged four years old. Results were similar for boys and girls. Predictive values for maltreatment-

**Table 1.** Characteristics of children admitted to hospital with head or neck injury or fracture in England 1997–2009.

| Characteristic | | Number (%) with characteristic | Predictive Value (% MR)* |
|---|---|---|---|
| **Age 1 week–6 months: All** | | **27,128 (100)** | **9.9** |
| **Age** | 1 w to <1 m | 3,781 (13.9) | 7.0 |
| | 1 m to <3 m | 11,947 (44.0) | 10.7 |
| | 3 m to <6 m | 11,400 (42.0) | 10.1 |
| **Sex** | Female | 12,524 (46.2) | 9.3 |
| | Male | 14,604 (53.8) | 10.5 |
| **Deprivation quintile** | Most deprived 1 | 9,260 (34.1) | 12.8 |
| | 2 | 5,918 (21.8) | 10.9 |
| | 3 | 4,474 (16.5) | 9.3 |
| | 4 | 3,847 (14.2) | 6.3 |
| | Least deprived 5 | 3,629 (13.4) | 5.8 |
| **All admissions aged 6–12 m:** | | **27,198 (100)** | **5.4** |
| **Age** | 6 m to <9 m | 12,710 (46.7) | 6.5 |
| | 9 m to <12 m | 14,488 (53.3) | 4.6 |
| **Sex** | Female | 12,362 (45.5) | 5.3 |
| | Male | 14,836 (54.5) | 5.6 |
| **Deprivation quintile** | Most deprived 1 | 9,295 (34.2) | 7.5 |
| | 2 | 5,912 (21.7) | 5.4 |
| | 3 | 4,517 (16.6) | 4.2 |
| | 4 | 3,694 (13.6) | 3.6 |
| | Least deprived 5 | 3,780 (13.9) | 3.8 |
| **All admissions aged 1–5 yrs:** | | **205,968 (100)** | **2.0** |
| **Age** | 1 to <2 yrs | 57,297 (27.8) | 3.1 |
| | 2 to <3 yrs | 51,922 (25.2) | 2.0 |
| | 3 to <4 yrs | 47,189 (22.9) | 1.6 |
| | 4 to <5 yrs | 49,560 (24.1) | 1.2 |
| **Sex** | Female | 85,275 (41.4) | 1.9 |
| | Male | 120,693 (58.6) | 2.1 |
| **Deprivation quintile** | Most deprived 1 | 64,547 (31.3) | 3.1 |
| | 2 | 42,148 (20.5) | 2.2 |
| | 3 | 34,277 (16.6) | 1.6 |
| | 4 | 31,460 (15.3) | 1.2 |
| | Least deprived 5 | 33,536 (16.3) | 1.0 |

*%MR: The percentage of admissions maltreatment-related.

related admission increased steeply according to quintile of deprivation.

The types of injury indicator with the highest predictive value for maltreatment-related codes (table 2) were intracranial injury (30.7% in children under six months old) and thoracic fractures (rib, sternum or thoracic spine) in children aged less than one year (59.3% in children less than six months old, 49.3% in children six months to one year old). No injury indicators in children over six months old had a predictive value above 10% apart from thoracic injury. Head or neck injury without fracture or intracranial injury (ICI) had a low predictive value for maltreatment-related admission, even in children less than six months old (6.4%) (table 2). Table S2 shows the predictive value for each type of injury indicator for narrow age bands as plotted in figures 1, 2, and 3. The predictive values for all injuries peaked in children aged one to three months old and declined thereafter.

Among children under one year, adjusted odds ratios revealed that ICI was associated with a two- to five-fold increased risk of maltreatment-related injury admission compared with head or neck injury without ICI injury or fracture (table 2). However, there was no evidence of an association with ICI in children aged one to five years old. Thoracic fractures were associated with a six- to seventeen-fold increased risk of maltreatment-related admission, depending on age group (Table 2). Long bone fracture was associated with a four-fold increased risk of maltreatment-related admission in children under 12 months old, but in children aged one to five years was associated with a decreased risk, compared with head or neck injury without ICI or fracture. Skull fractures were not associated with maltreatment-related codes in children less than six months of age, but were weakly associated in children aged six months to one year.

**Table 2.** Association between type of injury and maltreatment-related (MR) codes.

| Type of injury by age group | Number (%) | Predictive Value (%)# | MR incidence per 100,000 child years (95% CI)^ | Sensitivity (% of all MR)~ | Adjusted odds ratio$ (95% CI) |
|---|---|---|---|---|---|
| **1 week to 6 months** | | | | | |
| **All injuries and fractures** | 27128 (100) | 9.9 | 76.2 (64.0–88.5) | 32.3 | |
| All head and neck injuries | 24771 (91.3) | 8.4 | 59.5 (51.6–68.9) | 25 | |
| Any fracture | 6869 (25.3) | 17.1 | 33.3 (27.8–40.1) | 14.1 | |
| **High risk injuries** | | | | | |
| Head or neck without ICI or fracture | 19125 (70.5) | 6.4 | 36.4 (32.3–41.0) | 14.8 | Baseline |
| ICI | 1800 (6.6) | 30.7 | 15.6 (13.1–18.8) | 6.6 | 5.42 (4.81–6.10)** |
| Skull fracture | 3337 (12.3) | 9.2 | 8.7 (7.1–10.6) | 3.7 | 0.93 (0.81–1.06) |
| Long bone | 2217 (8.2) | 28.8 | 18.1 (15.4–21.3) | 7.7 | 4.75 (4.25–5.31)** |
| Thoracic | 484 (1.8) | 59.3 | 8.1 (6.6–10.1) | 3.4 | 11.24 (9.15–13.81)** |
| **6 to 12 months** | | | | | |
| **All injuries and fractures** | 27198 (100) | 5.4 | 41.1 (32.1–50.1) | 17.8 | |
| All head and neck injuries | 23430 (86.1) | 5.1 | 31.8 (26.9–37.9) | 14.3 | |
| Any fracture | 6910 (25.4) | 7.8 | 14.3 (11.7–17.9) | 6.4 | |
| **High risk injuries** | | | | | |
| Head or neck without ICI or fracture | 19459 (71.5) | 4.5 | 24.3 (21.0–28.2) | 10.5 | Baseline |
| ICI | 1134 (4.2) | 9.7 | 3.0 (2.3–4.1)) | 1.3 | 2.15 (1.74–2.65)** |
| Skull fracture | 2220 (8.2) | 6.9 | 4.2 (3.2–5.4) | 1.8 | 1.34 (1.12–1.60)* |
| Long bone | 3672 (13.5) | 8.7 | 8.7 (7.1–10.7) | 3.8 | 1.99 (1.74–2.27)** |
| Thoracic | 75 (0.3) | 49.3 | 1.0 (0.7–1.5) | 0.4 | 17.25 (10.72–27.77)** |
| **1 to 5 years** | | | | | |
| **All injuries and fractures** | 205968 (100) | 2 | 14.6 (9.3–20.0) | 49.9 | |
| All head and neck injuries | 138427 (67.2) | 2.6 | 11.4 (10.3–12.7) | 42.7 | |
| Any fracture | 75606 (36.7) | 1.2 | 2.9 (2.5–3.5) | 10.6 | |
| **High risk injuries** | | | | | |
| Head or neck without ICI or fracture | 126320 (61.3) | 2.5 | 10.6 (9.6–11.6) | 37.8 | Baseline |
| ICI | 5344 (2.6) | 2.2 | 0.4 (0.3–0.5) | 1.4 | 0.85 (0.71–1.03) |
| Skull fracture | 3662 (1.8) | 3.2 | 0.4 (0.3–0.5) | 1.4 | 1.22 (1.01–1.47)* |
| Long bone | 63886 (31) | 1 | 2.1 (1.8–2.4) | 7.5 | 0.45 (0.42–0.50)** |
| Thoracic | 149 (0.1) | 12.8 | 0.06 (0.03–0.13) | 0.2 | 6.58 (4.02–10.78)** |

MR: Maltreatment-Related admissions, with codes for maltreatment, assault or adverse social circumstances.
#The percentage of admissions with each injury classified as maltreatment-related in each age group.
^Incidence of maltreatment-related admissions in children of each age group in England, by injury type.
~The contribution to the total of all 8,337 maltreatment-related admissions of children aged 1 w–5 y made by children in each age group with each injury, expressed as a percentage: the sensitivity of the injury.
$Adjusted for injuries shown, socioeconomic status (deprivation quintiles), age and sex.
*p<0.05,
**p<0.001.

## Sensitivity

Children aged from one to five years accounted for 49.9% of maltreatment-related admissions, while the highest risk age group (one week to six months) accounted for 32.3% (table 2). This was partly driven by the larger number of admissions in the age category one to five years compared with less than six months or six to twelve months.

Head injury without ICI or fracture was the most sensitive indicator in all three age strata: when added together it accounted for 63.1% of maltreatment-related injury admissions in children under five years old. Although thoracic fractures were associated with the highest predictive value, they accounted for only four percent of maltreatment-related injury admissions

(table 2). Predictive value and sensitivity are contrasted in figures 4 and 5. The age and injury indicators that were associated with a low predictive value for maltreatment-related codes accounted for the large majority of maltreatment-related injury admissions. This pattern was similar in the analyses restricted to the diagnostic codes for maltreatment syndrome or assault (figures S1 and S2).

## Incidence

The incidence of maltreatment-related admission head or neck injury or fracture was 58 per 100,000 children per year in children under one year of age, peaking at 104 per 100,000 between one and three months and then declining in older children (table S2,

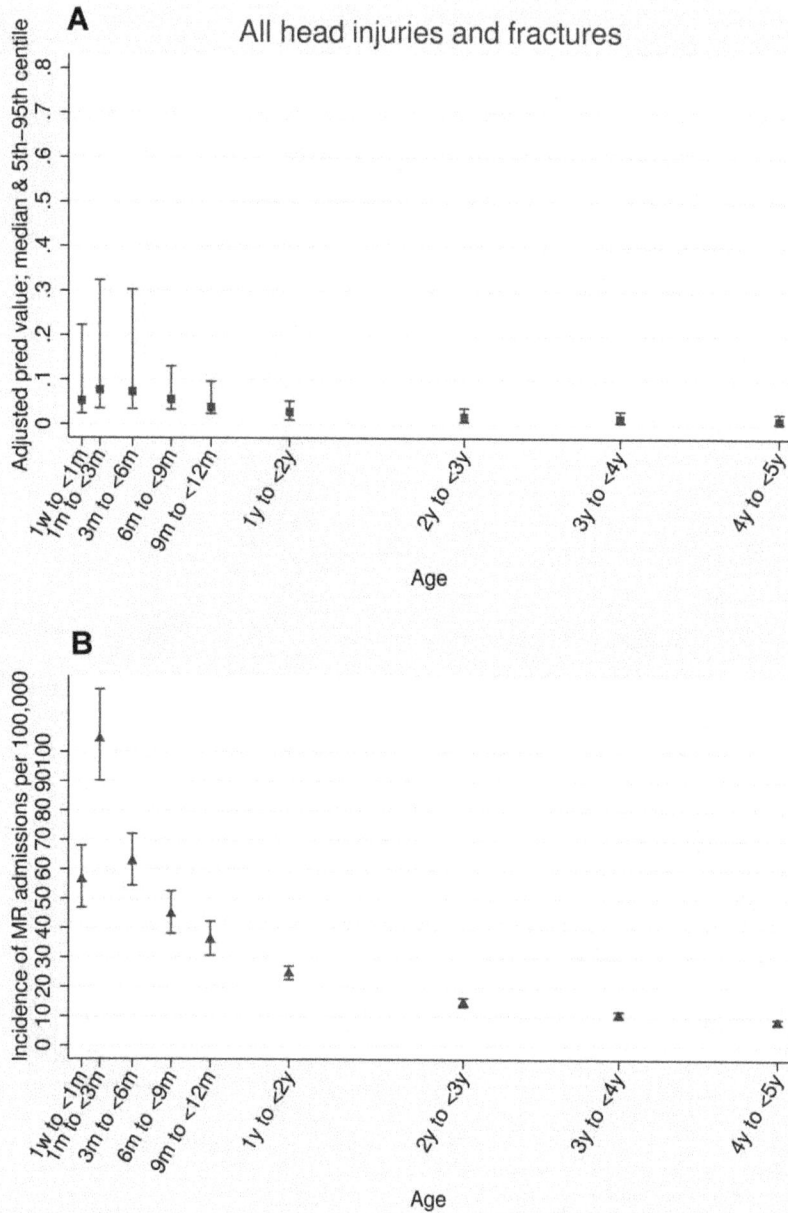

**Figure 1. All injuries.** Estimated predictive value and incidence of maltreatment-related admission by age (adjusted for sex, deprivation, and type of injury): all admissions for head or neck injury or fracture.

figures 1, 2, and 3). Children with head or neck injuries without ICI or fractures had the highest incidence of a single maltreatment-related injury, peaking at 49 per 100,000 (95% CI 43.7–54.9) in children aged one to three months. These injuries had a low predictive value for maltreatment, less than seven per cent at any age. In contrast, injuries with a high predictive value for maltreatment-related admission had low incidence rates. 61.6% of children with thoracic fractures in children aged one to three months had maltreatment-related admissions but the incidence was low (only 14 per 100,000 children) (table 2, figure 2, and table S2).

## Discussion

Half of the maltreatment-related admissions occurred in children aged one to five years old, particularly in children with types of injury that had a low predictive value for maltreatment. Few indicators for type of injury had a predictive value of more than 10%, rendering them of limited diagnostic use for clinicians deciding on the need for further assessment.

## Limitations

It is likely that maltreatment-related codes are under-recorded in hospital administrative data. Under-recording is also likely to vary with age and type of injury. [10,13,14,16] The predictive

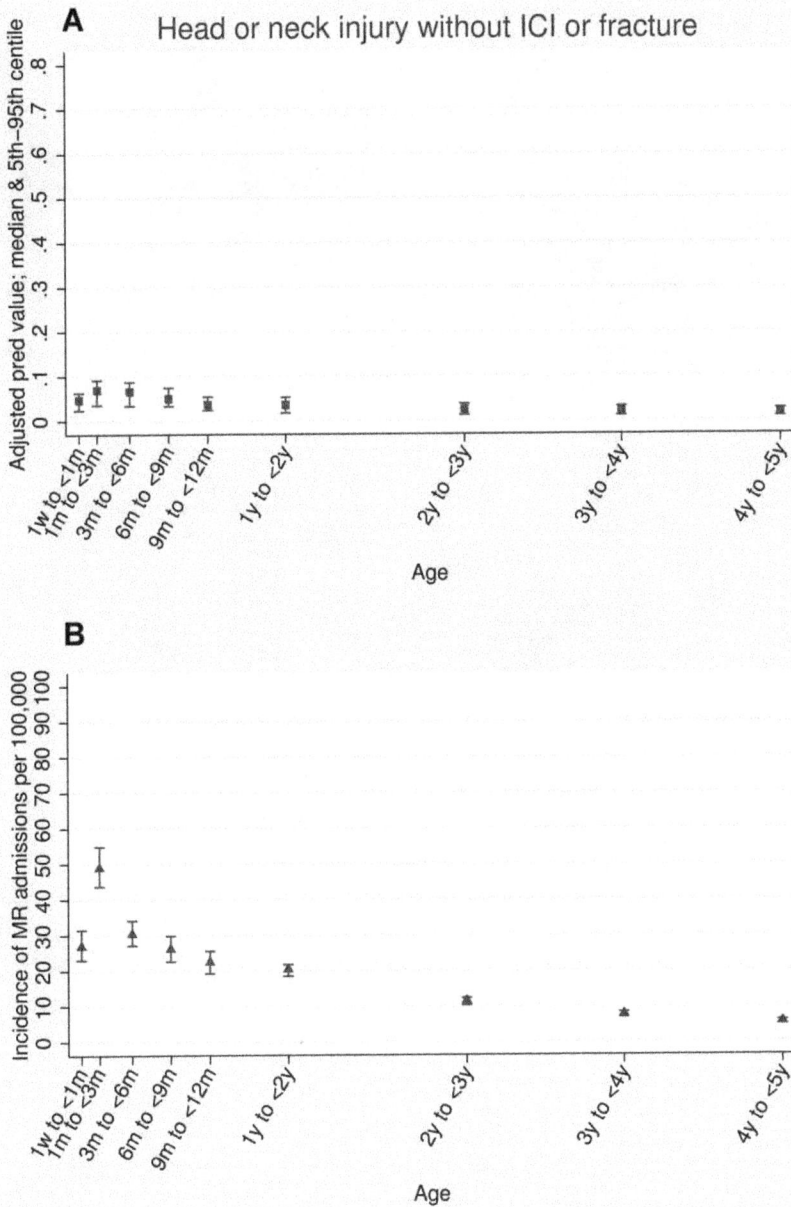

**Figure 2. Head and neck injuries.** Estimated predictive value and incidence of maltreatment-related admission by age (adjusted for sex, deprivation, and type of injury): all admissions for head or neck injury without intracranial injury or fracture.

values in our analyses should therefore be regarded as minimum estimates. Recording of maltreatment is likely to be best in the youngest children with high-risk injuries, as these groups are given most attention in guidelines. Our estimates of predictive value and incidence are therefore low-end estimates, particularly so for older children and those with injuries considered to be low risk.

Variation in under-recording with age differentially biases estimates of sensitivity. For example, our estimate that half of all maltreatment-related injuries occur in older children is likely to be an underestimate, as clinicians are less likely to recognise or record maltreatment in older age groups than in infants. A further source of error is that older children may be less likely than infants to be admitted when maltreatment is considered. Older children with recognised maltreatment-related injury are more likely than

younger children to be discharged from the emergency department, with safeguarding follow-up in the community. [17,18] These children could not be analysed in our database as emergency department attendances are not collated or coded in the same way as hospital admissions.

Detection bias increases estimates of predictive value because children not suspected of abuse are subject to different investigations than those who are under suspicion. For instance, only children suspected of maltreatment are subject to skeletal surveys. This phenomenon is most problematic for injuries that are unlikely to be apparent clinically, particularly rib fractures, and has been previously recognised by other studies. [5]

The inverse relationship between predictive value and sensitivity persisted when analyses were confined to the more specific cluster

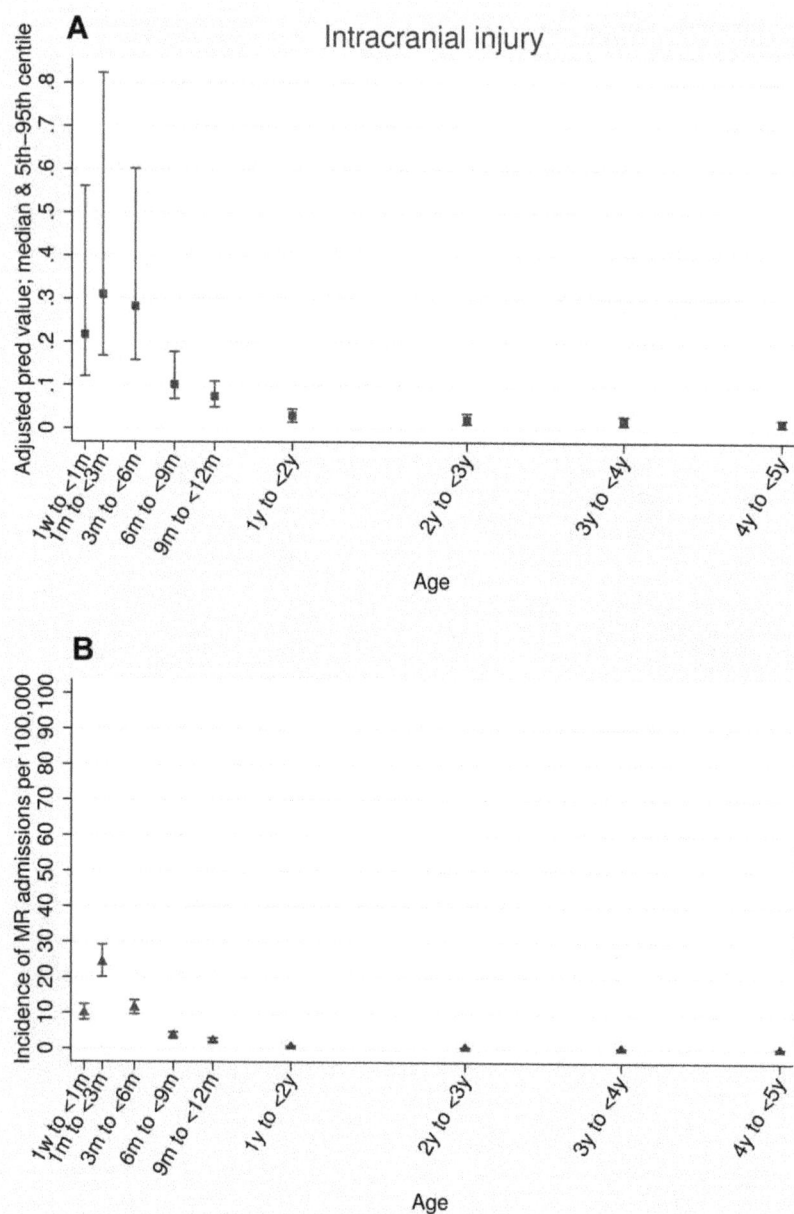

**Figure 3. Intracranial injuries.** Estimated predictive value and incidence of maltreatment-related admission by age (adjusted for sex, deprivation, and type of injury): all admissions for intracranial injury.

of ICD10 codes for maltreatment syndrome or assault (table S1, figures S1 and S2). We favoured the broader category of maltreatment-related injury admissions as we have previously shown evidence suggestive of diagnostic transfer between the specific cluster and the broader cluster of codes for undetermined intent or adverse social circumstances. These changes may have been due to a requirement for coders to record only definite or probable diagnoses from 2002 onwards. [10]

Our estimates of predictive value are lower than those seen in case series, but consistent with those from population-based studies. In a similar population-based study of inpatients in the USA, Leventhal *et al* found 24.8% of children aged less than three years with traumatic brain injuries or fractures were abused, and

revealed the importance of fine age categories for the predictive value of maltreatment. [6] Case series report predictive values for maltreatment ranging from 30% to 67% for long bone fractures and 19% for head injuries. [3–5]

We found that predictive value, incidence and odds ratios were all highest in younger children, with a striking peak at one to three months of age (Figures 1, 2, and 3, table S2). We note that our findings are similar to those of Barr *et al*, who found that the peak incidence of maltreatment follows shortly after the peak of inconsolable crying in infants. [19] Additionally, a study of babies aged one to six months by Reijneveld *et al* found evidence for excessive crying as a trigger for potentially harmful carer behaviours such as smothering, slapping or shaking. [20]

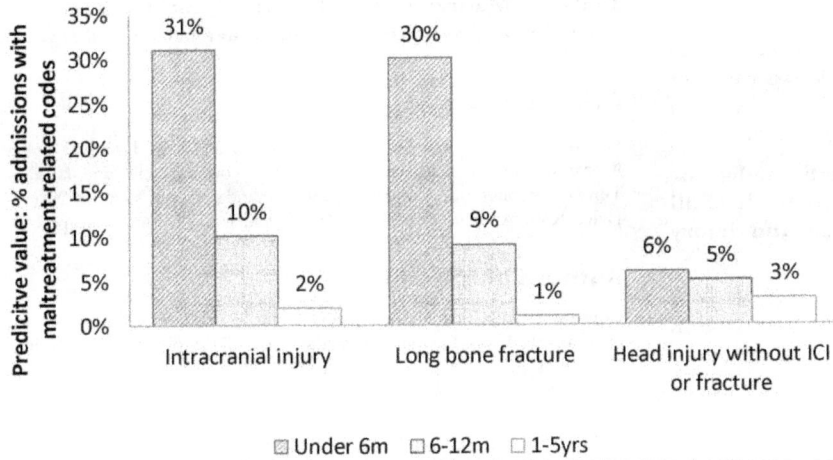

**Figure 4. Predictive value of type of injury by age group.**

## Implications

Our findings illustrate the potential harms of protocols that focus consideration of child maltreatment on the youngest children or children with high-risk injuries, as most maltreated children do not have these characteristics. To focus on incidence rates rather than predictive values does not solve this problem unless the size of the population at risk is also taken into account. Instead, all children presenting with injury should be assessed by clinicians with sufficient expertise to fully assess the child and their interaction with their parent for indicators of neglect, emotional abuse and physical maltreatment.

Our estimates of the predictive value of indicators for maltreatment-related injury are lower than reported in systematic reviews. The discrepancy is explained partly by under-recording of maltreatment in hospital administrative data

reducing our estimates, and partly by selection biases in the case series and high-risk cohorts included in the reviews. Case series and high-risk cohorts are unlikely to include all accidental injuries, leading to artificially small denominators and overestimates of predictive value. [2,10,21] When used for judicial evidence, professionals should be aware that true predictive values are likely to lie between estimates from population-based administrative data and estimates reported in case series and high-risk cohorts.

## Conclusions

Guidance that focusses clinician attention on children at highest risk of maltreatment-related injury may falsely reassure clinicians and divert their attention from children with low-risk types of injury who make up the majority of maltreatment-related admissions.

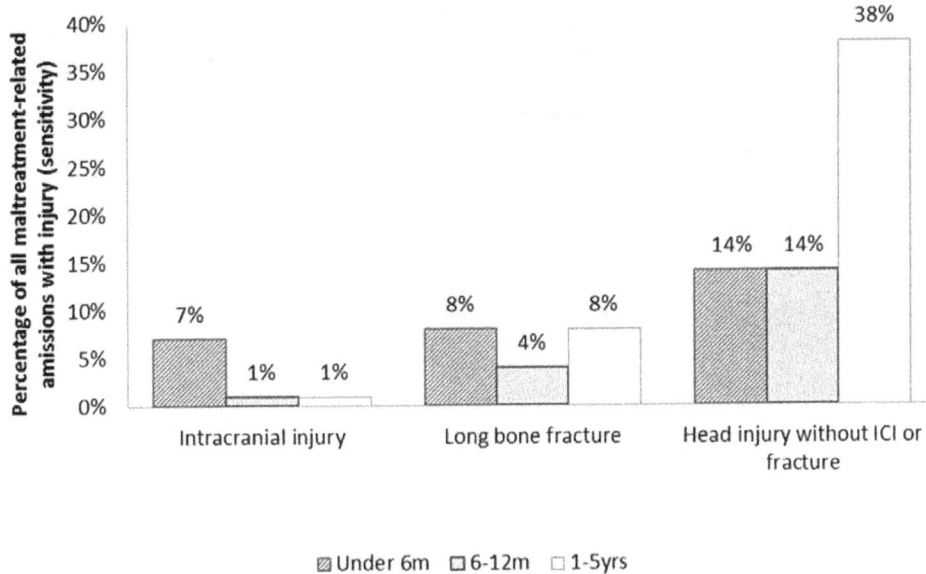

**Figure 5. Sensitivity (% of all MR admissions represented by each age and injury group).**

## Supporting Information

**Figure S1 Repeated analysis using specific codes for maltreatment syndrome or assault: predictive value of type of injury by age group.**

**Figure S2 Repeated analysis using specific codes for maltreatment syndrome or assault: sensitivity (% of all MR admissions represented by each age and injury group).**

**Table S1 Hierarchy of ICD 10 diagnostic codes\* used to classify cause of injury related to child victimization.**

**Table S2 Maltreatment-related (MR) incidence, predictive value and sensitivity by finest age group and injury.**

## Acknowledgments

We would like to thank members of University College London's Policy Research Unit for the health of children, young people and families: Terence Stephenson, Catherine Law, Amanda Edwards, Steve Morris, Helen Roberts, Catherine Shaw, Russell Viner and Miranda Wolpert.

## Author Contributions

Conceived and designed the experiments: JL AGI RG. Performed the experiments: JL AGI. Analyzed the data: JL AGI. Wrote the paper: JL RG. Guarantor: RG.

## References

1. Saperia J, Lakhanpaul M, Kemp A, Glaser D (2009) When to suspect child maltreatment: summary of NICE guidance. BMJ (Clinical research ed) 339: b2689. Available: http://www.pubmedcentral.nih.gov/articlerender. fcgi?artid = 2754329&tool = pmcentrez&rendertype = abstract.

2. Woodman J, Pitt M, Wentz R, Taylor B, Hodes D, et al. (2008) Performance of screening tests for child physical abuse in accident and emergency departments. Health technology assessment (Winchester, England) 12: iii, xi–xiii 1–95. Available: http://www.ncbi.nlm.nih.gov/pubmed/18992184.

3. Coffey C, Haley K, Hayes J, Groner JI (2005) The risk of child abuse in infants and toddlers with lower extremity injuries. Journal of pediatric surgery 40: 120–123. Available: http://www.ncbi.nlm.nih.gov/pubmed/15868570. Accessed: 18 July 2011.

4. Reece RM, Sege R (2000) Childhood head injuries: accidental or inflicted? Archives of pediatrics & adolescent medicine 154: 11–15. Available: http://www.ncbi.nlm.nih.gov/pubmed/10632244.

5. Kemp AM, Dunstan F, Harrison S, Morris S, Mann M, et al. (2008) Patterns of skeletal fractures in child abuse: systematic review. BMJ (Clinical research ed) 337: a1518. Available: http://www.pubmedcentral.nih.gov/articlerender. fcgi?artid = 2563260&tool = pmcentrez&rendertype = abstract. Accessed: 12 August 2011.

6. Leventhal JM, Martin KD, Asnes AG (2010) Fractures and traumatic brain injuries: abuse versus accidents in a US database of hospitalized children. Pediatrics 126: e104–15. Available: http://www.ncbi.nlm.nih.gov/pubmed/20530077. Accessed: 18 July 2011.

7. Minns R a, Jones P a, Mok JY-Q (2008) Incidence and demography of non-accidental head injury in southeast Scotland from a national database. American journal of preventive medicine 34: S126–33. Available: http://www.ncbi.nlm. nih.gov/pubmed/18374262. Accessed: 15 July 2011.

8. Strait T, Siegel M, Shapiro A (1995) Humeral Fractures Without Obvious Etiologies in Children Less Than 3 Years of Age : When Is It Abuse? Pediatrics 96: 667–671.

9. Office of National Statistics (n.d.). Available: http://www.statistics.gov.uk/. Accessed: 10 Oct 2012.

10. González-Izquierdo A, Woodman J, Copley L, van der Meulen J, Brandon M, et al. (2010) Variation in recording of child maltreatment in administrative records of hospital admissions for injury in England, 1997–2009. Archives of disease in childhood 95: 918–925. Available: http://www.ncbi.nlm.nih.gov/pubmed/20647257. Accessed: 18 July 2011.

11. Gilbert R, Fluke J, O'Donnell M, Gonzalez-Izquierdo A, Brownell M, et al. (2012) Child maltreatment: variation in trends and policies in six developed countries. Lancet 379: 758–772. Available: http://www.ncbi.nlm.nih.gov/ pubmed/22169108. Accessed: 31 July 2012.

12. McKenzie K, Scott D a, Waller GS, Campbell M (2011) Reliability of routinely collected hospital data for child maltreatment surveillance. BMC public health 11: 8. Available: http://www.pubmedcentral.nih.gov/articlerender. fcgi?artid = 3022700&tool = pmcentrez&rendertype = abstract. Accessed: 30 July 2012.

13. Hooft B, Ronda J, Schaeffer M, Asnes A IJ (2012) Identification of physical abuse cases in hospitalized children: accuracy of ICD codes. Pediatrics In press.

14. Schnitzer PG, Slusher PL, Kruse RL, Tarleton MM (2011) Identification of ICD codes suggestive of child maltreatment. Child abuse & neglect 35: 3–17. Available: http://www.ncbi.nlm.nih.gov/pubmed/21316104. Accessed: 11 September 2012.

15. Jayawant S, Rawlinson a, Gibbon F, Price J, Schulte J, et al. (1998) Subdural haemorrhages in infants: population based study. BMJ (Clinical research ed) 317: 1558–1561. Available: http://www.pubmedcentral.nih.gov/articlerender. fcgi?artid = 28734&tool = pmcentrez&rendertype = abstract.

16. Scott D, Tonmyr L, Fraser J, Walker S, McKenzie K (2009) The utility and challenges of using ICD codes in child maltreatment research: A review of existing literature. Child abuse & neglect 33: 791–808. Available: http://www. ncbi.nlm.nih.gov/pubmed/19853915. Accessed: 18 July 2011.

17. Gilbert R, Kemp A, Thoburn J, Sidebotham P, Radford L, et al. (2009) Recognising and responding to child maltreatment. Lancet 373: 167–180. Available: http://www.ncbi.nlm.nih.gov/pubmed/19056119. Accessed: 27 June 2011.

18. Louwers ECFM, Korfage IJ, Affourtit MJ, Scheewe DJH, van de Merwe MH, et al. (2011) Detection of child abuse in emergency departments: a multi-centre study. Archives of disease in childhood 96: 422–425. Available: http://www. pubmedcentral.nih.gov/articlerender.fcgi?artid = 3075563&tool = pmcentrez& rendertype = abstract. Accessed: 31 July 2012.

19. Barr RG, Trent RB, Cross J (2006) Age-related incidence curve of hospitalized Shaken Baby Syndrome cases: convergent evidence for crying as a trigger to shaking. Child abuse & neglect 30: 7–16. Available: http://www.ncbi.nlm.nih. gov/pubmed/16406023. Accessed: 5 June 2012.

20. Reijneveld SA, Wal MFVD, Brugman E, Sing RAH, Verloove-vanhorick SP (2004) Infant crying and abuse. Lancet 364: 1340–1342.

21. Maguire SA, Kemp AM, Lumb RC, Farewell DM (2011) Estimating the probability of abusive head trauma: a pooled analysis. Pediatrics 128: e550–64. Available: http://www.ncbi.nlm.nih.gov/pubmed/21844052. Accessed: 30 July 2012.

# 14

# HGF-Transgenic MSCs can Improve the Effects of Tissue Self-Repair in a Rabbit Model of Traumatic Osteonecrosis of the Femoral Head

**Qian Wen[1], Dan Jin[2], Chao-Ying Zhou[1], Ming-Qian Zhou[1], Wei Luo[1], Li Ma[1]***

**1** Institute of Molecular Immunology, Southern Medical University, Guangzhou, People's Republic of China, **2** Department of Orthopaedics and Traumatology, Nanfang Hospital, Southern Medical University, Guangzhou, People's Republic of China

## Abstract

*Background:* Osteonecrosis of the femoral head (ONFH) is generally characterized as an irreversible disease and tends to cause permanent disability. Therefore, understanding the pathogenesis and molecular mechanisms of ONFH and developing effective therapeutic methods is critical for slowing the progress of the disease.

*Methodology/Principal Findings:* In this study, an experimental rabbit model of early stage traumatic ONFH was established, validated, and used for an evaluation of therapy. Computed tomography (CT) and magnetic resonance (MR) imaging confirmed that this model represents clinical Association Research Circulation Osseous (ARCO) phase I or II ONFH, which was also confirmed by the presence of significant tissue damage in osseous tissue and vasculature. Pathological examination detected obvious self-repair of bone tissue up to 2 weeks after trauma, as indicated by revascularization (marked by CD105) and expression of collagen type I (Col I), osteocalcin, and proliferating cell nuclear antigen. Transplantation of hepatocyte growth factor (HGF)-transgenic mesenchymal stem cells (MSCs) 1 week after trauma promoted recovery from ONFH, as evidenced by a reversed pattern of Col I expression compared with animals receiving no therapeutic treatment, as well as increased expression of vascular endothelial growth factor.

*Conclusions/Significance:* These results indicate that the transplantation of HGF-transgenic MSCs is a promising method for the treatment for ONFH and suggest that appropriate interference therapy during the tissue self-repair stage contributes to the positive outcomes. This study also provides a model for the further study of the ONFH etiology and therapeutic interventions.

**Editor:** Bart O. Williams, Van Andel Institute, United States of America

**Funding:** This work was supported by the Cooperation Project in Industry, Education and Research of Guangdong province and Ministry of Education of People's Republic of China (2011B090400013), Science and Technology Project of Guangzhou (2009Z1-E441) and State 863 Projects (2007AA02Z458). The funders had no role in study design, data collection and analysis, decision to publish, or preparation of the manuscript.

**Competing Interests:** The authors have declared that no competing interests exist.

* E-mail: maryhmz@126.com

## Introduction

Traumatic osteonecrosis of the femoral head (ONFH) is a progressive pathological process primarily caused by interrupted blood circulation in the femoral head that leads to apoptosis of endothelial cells [1] and hemopoietic/osseous tissue necrosis [2]. The pathology then progresses through several stages [2]. First, there is a repair stage, which generally begins shortly after cell death and is accompanied by the proliferation of undifferentiated mesenchymal cells as well as capillary buds containing endothelial cells around the fracture. Next, there is a remodeling stage, which is established by the concomitant appearance of osteoclasts (OCs), mesenchymal cells, and capillaries; this stage involves repeated trabecular microfractures due to the action of mechanical factors on the femoral head, which is comprised of various materials of diverse elasticities. Finally, there is a joint impairment stage, during which impairment originates from the fracture at the junction between dead and live bone due to their differing elastic moduli and compliance; this impairment usually occurs after a substantial delay, approximately 2 years after the femoral neck fracture. Without timely, effective treatment, the patient may be left with a permanent disability. Clinical signs typically include hip pain, followed by progressive lameness that results in the partial or complete inability to bear weight on the affected limb.

Many challenges remain in the treatment of ONFH. Firstly, effective therapeutic methods are lacking. This lack may be due to insufficient understanding of the pathogenesis of osteonecrosis (e.g. the posttraumatic molecular events). Secondly, regarding treatment selection, it is unclear whether surgery is the best therapy for ONFH. Other treatment options, such as an auxiliary means of activating the patient's healing systems, may be better. Furthermore, because there is usually no need to change the articulus of patients with artificial one during the early stage of traumatic ONFH, it is difficult to acquire tissue samples for diagnosis. Molecular level events at the lesion site have not been well addressed and there is insufficient information available to improve the timing and efficacy of treatment. An animal model of early ONFH that truly simulates the clinical situation would provide a platform for the study of the pathogenesis and molecular mechanisms of the disease, and would contribute to the development of an optimal treatment regimen.

To establish a traumatic ONFH model, several methods for blocking the blood supply to the femoral head have been reported; these involve tightening the femoral blood vessels, circulation of liquid nitrogen around the femoral head, and dislocation of the hip and detachment of the soft tissue [3,4,5,6,7,8,9]. Nishino *et al.* compared several methods for establishing a traumatic ONFH model using hematoxylin and eosin (H&E) staining; they found that a combination of dislocation and ligation of femoral vessels, but not either one alone, led to empty lacunae, significant necrosis, and vigorous appositional bone formation in 80% of animals after 2 weeks [10]. Their results suggested that none of the methods ensured that all animals would exhibit the typical symptoms of ONFH, and that a relatively severe method is needed. In the present study, the femoral neck was broken completely, including the round ligament, severely disrupting blood circulation in the femoral head. This method is relatively more acute than other methods, has a higher success rate in a shorter time, and is convenient for further studies. In addition, the model can be treated through fixation with a small splint to assess the efficacy of therapeutic regimens.

Clinically, the lack of effective therapy for ONFH has become an issue that needs to be overcome. Several methods for the treatment of early stage traumatic ONFH have been attempted, including drug therapy, surgical core decompression, vascularized bone grafting, and osteotomy. However, none of these has been effective in preventing the disease. Femoral heads usually collapse in the late stage of ONFH and the only feasible treatment is arthroplasty. However, the failure rate after 5 years is 10%–50%, and the best artificial femoral heads only last for 10–15 years. Thus, patients often need two or three replacements, entailing pain and a further economic burden. Thus finding early treatment that could save the femoral head would represent an important advance.

Mesenchymal stem cells (MSCs) are pluripotent and can differentiate into several lineages of cells, including osteocytic, chondrocytic, and adipocytic cells. They are present in the adult bone marrow and have shown potency in the treatment of ischemic diseases, such as myocardial infarction [11,12] and ONFH [13,14]. In our previous work, we treated early stage hormone-induced ONFH with the transplantation of MSCs infected with replication-deficiency adenoviral vectors carrying the hepatocyte growth factor (HGF) gene, with relatively satisfactory therapeutic efficacy [15]. In that study, after MSC transplantation, changes in HGF protein levels in the region of the disease correlated with the sequential activation or inhibition of the p-ERK1/2 or p-Akt pathways. These sequential changes contribute greatly to the function of MSCs in the recovery of injured tissue [16].

In the present study, a rabbit model was established to study molecular events during the pathogenesis of traumatic ONFH and to assess the efficacy of transplantation of HGF-transgenic MSCs. The model was validated by radiological and histopathological examinations, which suggested the occurrence of tissue self-repair. Coordinated with self-repair, we found HGF-transgenic MSC transplantation to be efficacious in the treatment of the traumatic ONFH model.

## Materials and Methods

### Animals

Healthy, male New Zealand rabbits aged 3 months and weighing between 2.8–3.3 kg were provided by the Experimental Animal Centre of Nanfang Hospital, Southern Medical University

(Guangzhou, China), and were maintained under specific pathogen-free conditions. All animals received humane care in compliance with the Guide for the Care and Use of Laboratory Animals, published by the US National Institutes of Health (Publication No. 85-23, revised 1996). The experiment protocol was approved by the Animal Ethics Committee at Southern Medical University.

### Operation performance

Five rabbits were set aside as intact controls, while 40 rabbits underwent traumatic surgery and were evaluated using radiological and histopathological examinations at different time-points up to 3 weeks as indicated in Table 1. Animals were anaesthetized with an intravenous injection of 30 mg·kg$^{-1}$ body weight 30% pentobarbitone sodium (Sigma, MO, USA). A posterolateral incision was made in the left hip under aseptic conditions, and a 3 cm incision was made in the joint capsule to expose the femoral head. All soft tissue attachments, including the annular ligament, were detached, and the femoral neck was severed at the base. An unabsorbable suture was used to secure the separated femoral head into the acetabulum, and the wound was copiously irrigated with penicillin before being closed in layers. Animals received $2 \times 10^5$ U of penicillin intramuscularly as prophylaxis. During the post-operative period, all animals were free to move, and recovery from anaesthesia without post-operative infection was observed. However, difficulty in jumping was observed.

### CT examinations

Radiographs were obtained at various intervals post-operatively using a Lightspeed 16 spiral CT scanner (GE Company, New York, USA). After injection of 1.5 mL veterinary Sumianxin II, a compound anesthetic preparation consisting of haloperidol, Baoding Ning, dihydrocodeine Eto'o, etc., into the gluteal muscle for anesthesia, animals were fixed in the supine position, with hip joints positioned as symmetrically and laterally as possible. Transect scanning of the entire hip joint was performed at 100 kV and 220 mA. The screw pitch was 0.625:1, the combination detector was 16×0.625 mm, the bed speed was 5.62 mm·r-1, the reconstruction layer was 1.25 mm thick, and the diameter of the field-of-view (FOV) was 9.6 cm.

### MRI examinations

A Magnetom Vision PLUS 1.5 T superconducting MRI machine (Siemens, Germany) was used. After being anaesthetized in the same session for the CT, animals were placed supine on a bed and the centre of an orthogonal head coil was located on the hip joint. Sequences included T1-weighted spin-echo (TR = 440.0, TE = 6.9), fat suppressed T2-weighted fast spin-echo (TR = 4000.0, TE = 87.0). Images were collected twice in the coronal position. The layer thickness was 3 mm and the FOV was 100×100 mm. Due to truncation of the femoral neck, no contrast agent could be administered into the femoral head to perform post-contrast MR imaging.

### Histopathological examinations

Femoral head specimens were fixed in 4% buffered paraformaldehyde, decalcified in buffered 10% ethylenediamine tetraacetic acid disodium salt (Na$_2$-EDTA) for more than 20 d. After being dehydrated stepwise and turned transparent by dimethylbenzene, the samples were embedded in wax and sectioned into coronal planes (4 μm). Sections were stained with H&E to observe histological changes after injury. Image-Pro Plus 6.0 software (IPP 6.0, Media Cybernetics, MD, USA) was used to

**Table 1.** Animal observation groups.

| Observation group | Total number of hips (animals) per group | Number of hips (animals) in analysis groups | |
| --- | --- | --- | --- |
| | | Radiology | Histology (H&E/IHC) |
| Normal | 10(5) | 4(2) | 6(3) |
| 3 days post operation | 10(10) | 4(4) | 6(6) |
| 1 week post operation | 10(10) | 4(4) | 6(6) |
| 2 week post operation | 10(10) | 4(4) | 6(6) |
| 3 week post operation | 10(10) | 4(4) | 6(6) |

quantify the number of empty lacunae and haematopoietic cell nuclei observed at 100× magnification in ten randomly selected fields per section. The width and area of trabeculae and the area of grey scale in the trabeculae mainly under cartilage were also calculated.

Immunohistochemistry (IHC) was performed using antibodies specific for: collagen type I (Col I) (I-8H5; Calbiochem, Darmstadt, Germany), osteocalcin (OCN) (OCG4; Abcam plc., Cambridge, UK), von willebrand factor (vWF) (F8/86), phosphorylated-ERK1/2 (p-ERK1/2) (E-4) (Santa Cruz Biotechnology, CA, USA), CD105 (SN6h), proliferating cell nuclear antigen (PCNA) (PC10) (Invitrogen co. Ltd., CA, USA), HGF, Vascular endothelial growth factor (VEGF) (BOSTER Bioengineering Co. Ltd., Wuhan, China) and phosphorylated-Akt (p-Akt) (D9E; Cell Signaling Technology, MA, USA). Briefly, sections were incubated with primary antibodies at 4°C overnight, washed 3 times, then incubated with biotinylated secondary IgGs (Maxim Bio., Fujian, China). Sections were washed again, then developed with 3,3'-diaminobenzidine (DAB) (Zhongshan Goldenbridge Biotechnology, Beijing, China). Sections incubated without primary antibodies were used as a negative control. All specimens were consistently maintained in liquid to prevent edge effects. Each section was imaged at 200× magnification, and IPP 6.0 was used for quantitation using a single blind method. In bone marrow cavities of ten randomly selected fields, staining was quantitated based on integrated optical density (IOD). The corresponding cavity area was also measured, and the expression ratio was calculated by dividing IOD by the cavity area. For Col I, the expression ratio for both bone marrow and trabeculae were calculated.

## Isolation and culture of MSCs and Differentiation assays

Allogeneic MSCs were achieved and adenoviral vectors (Ad-vectors) carrying or not HGF gene (Ad-HGF) were prepared as described before with some modification [15]. Briefly, bone marrow was aspirated from the bilateral posterior superior iliac spine of rabbits and washed with Dulbecco's modified Eagle's medium-low glucose (Hyclone Ltd, Logan, UT, USA) containing 10% fetal bovine serum (FBS; Hyclone) and 100 U/ml penicillin, 100 mg/ml streptomycin and 2 mM L-glutamine (Invitrogen). The adherent cells were cultured for two generations and then infected with Ad-vectors or Ad-HGF at a multiplicity of infection (MOI) of 300 before transplantation. For identifying the pluripotency of MSCs, cells were induced to differentiate into osteoblasts, chondroblasts and adipocytes respectively according to the methods described before [16].

## Treatment of traumatic ONFH with transplantation of allogeneic MSCs

For treatment, traumatic ONFH was induced in 48 rabbits. One week later, $10^6$ cells in 100 μL culture medium without FBS were transplanted into the necrotic femoral head exposed and closed in the same way as model establishment. Three animals were left untreated as model controls (ONFH). Fifteen animals were transplanted with HGF-transgenic MSCs (ONFH+MSC+HGF). Another 15 rabbits received adenoviral vector-infected MSCs as vector controls (ONFH+MSC+vector). The remaining 15 animals were transplanted with uninfected MSCs as treatment controls (ONFH+MSC). Then the leg was fixed with a small splint and the animals were carefully fed. Four weeks later, the treatment efficacy was assessed through pathological examination. During the experiment, no animal unintentionally died. At 2 d, 2 weeks, and 4 weeks after transplantation, euthanization were performed by air injection through ear vein to obtain the femoral head samples. Paraffin samples and sections were sequentially prepared for H&E staining and IHC assays.

## Statistical analysis

SPSS statistical software (version 16.0; SPSS, Chicago, IL, USA) was used. Data are expressed as the mean ± standard deviation of the mean. One-way ANOVA was applied to determine statistical significance. Least-significant differences, or Dunnett's T3 tests, were performed for post-hoc multiple comparisons. A $P$-value less than 0.05 was considered statistically significant.

## Results

### Radiological inspection of traumatic ONFH model

To verify whether the model represents the typical clinical Association Research Circulation Osseous (ARCO) phase I or II of ONFH, we conducted CT and MR imaging.

CT examinations of normal rabbits showed symmetrical femoral heads, clear and distinct joint surface and epiphyseal line, and a smooth and intact cortex. In contrast, femoral heads that had undergone a severance of the annular ligament and the femoral neck to severely damage blood circulation, exhibited an increasingly heterogeneous density of cancellous bone, a gradual loss of symmetry, thinning of the bone cortex, and the epiphyseal line was blurred (Figure 1, left column).

MR imaging features of the normal femur include uniformly high signal intensities compared with muscle. Pathological changes are characterized by inhomogeneous intermediate to high signal intensity on MR FS T2-weighted images in which the subcortical high intensity fat signal is suppressed and is reversed on T1-weighted images within the femur compared with muscle. On T2-

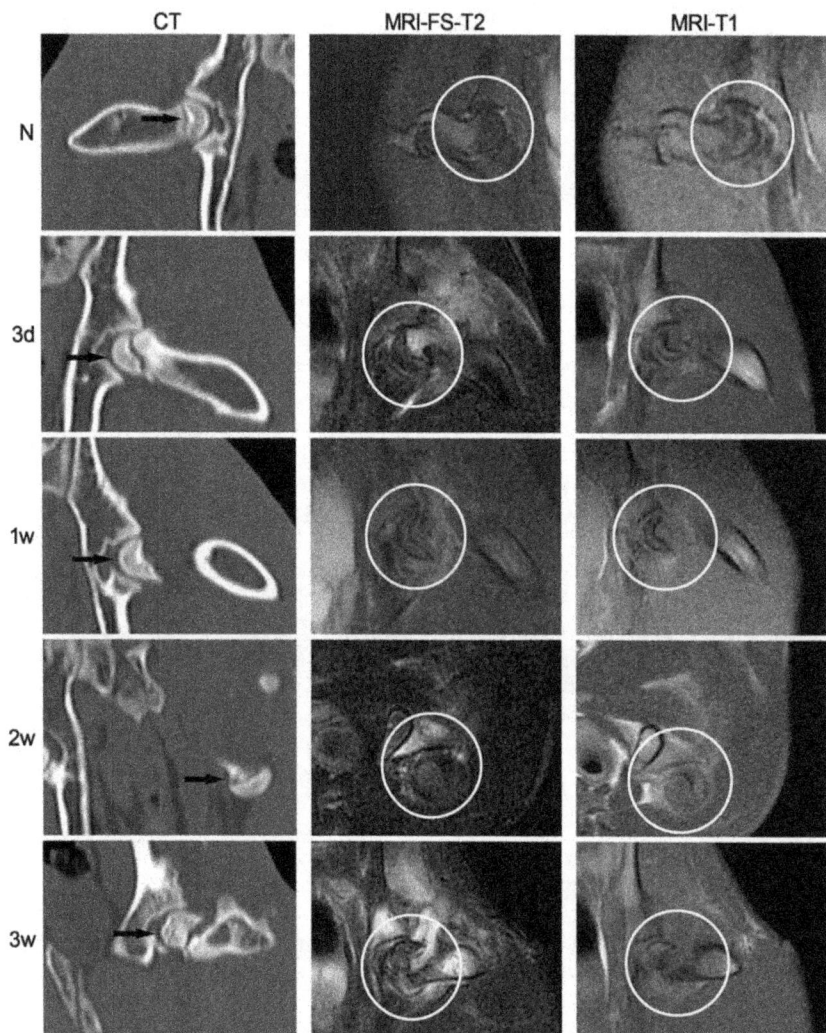

**Figure 1. Conventional CT and MR examination of the traumatic ONFH rabbit model established in this study.** Left column: Conventional CT examination (coronal reconstruction). With progression of the disease, the density of cancellous bone became more heterogeneous and eventually lost its symmetry. Arrows indicate the femoral head. Middle column: MR-FS T2-weighted imaging (coronal plane) detected a signal that became increasingly uneven for up to 2 weeks after trauma. A signal with high intensity was observed at the fracture line, suggesting edema was present in the bone marrow. Right column: MR T1-weighted imaging (coronal plane) detected a loss of normal signal within the femoral head. Circles indicate the femoral head. N: normal group; 3 d, 1 w, 2 w, 3 w: 3 days, 1 week, 2 weeks, 3 weeks post-trauma, respectively.

weighted images, originally uniform signal intensity within the operative coxofemoral joint began to increase unevenly 2 weeks after trauma, especially within the fracture line, suggesting the presence of marrow edema (Figure 1, middle column). Similarly, on T1-weighted images, the injured femoral head had a smooth surface that became inhomogeneous 2 weeks after trauma, except for a band-like area of low signal intensity in the distal stump marrow of the femoral neck, which was seen as early as 3 days after trauma (Figure 1, right column). Similar changes were observed at up to 3 weeks on both sequences in all traumatized rabbits, more than two-thirds of which also lacked signal intensity locally in the subchondral bone. In comparison, the unaffected femurs of these rabbits maintained a uniform signal. Overall, prominent changes in signals associated with cancellous bone were detected by week 3, consistent with the report of Nishino *et al* [10] and the imaging features of ONFH in ARCO phase I and II [17,18,19].

## Pathological examination validated the ONFH model

H&E staining confirmed the presence of osteonecrosis in all sections of traumatized femoral heads; obvious pathological changes were observed as early as 3 days after trauma. For example, the operative medulla on both sides of the epiphyseal plate was found to be loose and greatly diminished, and was worse 1 week after trauma, accompanied by a change of shape or fusion of most medullary cells (Figure 2A, B-a). Hemorrhage was evident and increased for 2 weeks, after which it became limited. Simultaneously, immature fibrous tissue was observed in the medulla under the cartilage. To further examine alterations in the vasculature, microvessels (MVs) were labeled with vWF stain [20], a marker of endothelial cells, and observed by immunohistochemistry (IHC) (Figure 2C, D). MVs were abundant in normal tissues, but decreased rapidly after trauma. Loss of cell nuclei marked by hematoxylin staining, along with non-regular spacing of vascular endothelial cells (VECs), was observed at the end of the study. The three-layer structure of arteries was observed only up to 3 days after trauma, and gradually broke down thereafter. Until 3 weeks after trauma, the MVs marked by CD105, a specific marker of new blood vessels, could still be observed but were limited in number in the injured femoral head (Figure 2E, F).

In injured tissue, concomitant increases in OCs inferred by morphological features and empty lacunae up to week 2 after trauma were observed (Figure 2A, B-b), accompanied by the gradually increased thinning of the trabeculae (Figure 2B-c) and enlargement of the medullary cavities from 1 week after trauma. These findings were consistent with the lack of focal signal intensity at the subchondral bone on radiological examination and may be associated with loss of heavy-loading capacity. Beginning 3 days after trauma, small regions within the trabeculae near the cartilage exhibiting a grey color similar to cartilage appeared, and increased markedly 2 weeks after trauma (Figure 2B-d). Some of these regions stained with eosin, indicating new bone formation. Appositional bone formation was also observed in the metaphysis, but had decreased greatly by week 3 post-trauma. Spindle-shaped osteoblasts (OBs) were readily observed in an orderly arrangement near the epiphyseal plate, although they were reduced in number up to 1 week after trauma and became distant to the trabeculae over time (Figure 2). An obvious and noteworthy concomitant increase in OBs was observed 2 weeks after trauma, especially under the cartilage where OBs were originally sparse.

Both radiological and pathological examination confirmed that a model of early stage traumatic ONFH had been established. Several pathological observations suggested the occurrence of self-tissue repair, including the appearance of revascularization and the increases in immature fibrous tissue in the medulla, grey regions in the trabeculae and OBs under the cartilage.

## Tissue self-repair in the local region after trauma

As tissue self-repair is important for the choice of timing and method of treatment in ONFH, it is worth clarifying its temporal and spatial features. For this purpose, markers of OB regeneration were determined by IHC, including the cell proliferation marker proliferating cell nuclear antigen (PCNA) and the bone formation markers, collagen type I (Col I) and osteocalcin (OCN).

High levels of PCNA were detected in normal hematopoietic tissue, but not in osteocytes or OBs. Following trauma, PCNA levels decreased significantly ($P<0.01$) then were maintained at a relatively stable and low level, especially in hematopoietic tissues. In OBs, PCNA expression began to be detected 2 weeks after trauma and was maintained throughout the remaining observation period, although the number of OBs had decreased by the end of observation (Figure 3A, B).

As the most abundant protein in the extracellular matrix of bone and skin, the large diameter fibrils of Col I are responsible for tissue stabilization and regeneration. Col I levels were low in normal medullary cavities, but increased immediately after trauma and then decreased over the remaining observation period. Col I levels, which were low in the OCs of normal tissues, increased markedly as early as 3 days post-trauma and continued to increase for up to 2 weeks, which indicated an increase in OC activity [21] and the presence of bone remodeling [2]. In contrast, Col I was barely detectable in OBs in normal tissue. After trauma, the Col I level was initially low, but it had increased markedly by 2 weeks post-trauma; this increase was concomitant with PCNA expression and suggested the presence of new OBs in the early stage of OB differentiation. Compared with marrow cells, Col I expression in the trabeculae was elevated following trauma, and remained significantly higher than in normal femoral heads during the third week ($P<0.01$), suggesting decreased OB activity and a failure to degrade Col I for matrix mineralization by the end of the

observation period. In VECs, it was notable that, instead of the varied expression of Col I seen in normal tissues, there were uniformly high levels of Col I following trauma (Figure 3C, D).

The level of Col I represents a measure of bone tissue status. Similarly, OCN is a specific marker of bone formation during bone turnover [22], and characterizes the initial osteogenic differentiation of MSCs [23]. In normal femoral head sections, expression of OCN was mainly in perivascular vessels and in a subset of osteocytes. However, 3 days after trauma, OCN levels decreased significantly ($P<0.05$), and this was concomitant with the decrease in the number of OBs. Subsequently, OCN levels returned to normal, and then increased to a higher level again 2 weeks after trauma, although they had decreased significantly overall by the end of week 3. In general, the highest levels of OCN expression were consistently observed in perivascular vessels and in fibrous medulla, regions associated with localization of MSCs [24]. In addition, the re-elevation of OCN expression was coordinated with the increase in the number of OBs (Figure 3E, F), suggesting that osteogenic differentiation of MSCs remained active in the injured tissue.

## Efficacy of transplantation of HGF-transgenic MSCs

The above IHC results, including increased PCNA and Col I in OBs and the repeated increase of OCN, suggest that there was a relatively strong tissue self-repair for up to 2 weeks after trauma. Thus, we treated ONFH model animals with transplantation of transgenic MSCs 1 week after trauma with the aim of improving self-repair.

Before transplantation, the pluripotency of the MSCs was verified by inducing their differentiation into osteoblasts, chondroblasts, or adipocytes (Figure 4). H&E-stained specimens collected 4 weeks after transplantation showed virtually no hematopoietic tissue, no live osteocytes, and misarranged, thinning trabeculae in the ONFH group that did not receive any treatment. In contrast, in all treated groups, there was an increase in OBs with an orderly arrangement near the trabeculae, and partial recovery of hematopoietic tissue; in addition, the thinning of the trabeculae was attenuated. However, only in the ONFH+MSC+HGF group did the number of empty lacunae decrease and hematopoietic tissue recover significantly compared with the ONFH group ($P<0.05$). Moreover, normal bone marrow including tri-lineage hematopoietic elements was observed locally, which may have resulted, at least in part, from the sequentially transient increase in HGF-mediated p-ERK/Akt signaling described below. Meanwhile, the trabeculae exhibited a more organized arrangement and more new capillaries were observed in animals treated with HGF-transgenic MSCs compared with the other two treatment groups (Figure 5A, B-a, B-b). The expression of CD105 also increased after MSC transplantation, which suggested the occurrence of new MVs. Although angiogenesis did not recover to normal levels, the amounts of MVs marked by CD105 in the ONFH+MSC+HGF group were significantly stronger than the other two treatment groups in addition to the untreated ONFH group (Figure 5C, D).

VEGF is a specific mitogen that acts on endothelial cells. It has multiple functions, including inducing endothelial cell growth, angiogenesis, and vasculogenesis, promoting cell migration and inhibiting apoptosis. VEGF plays important roles in vasculogenesis during the healing of and recovery from bone fracture. It also promotes OB migration through an interaction with the flt-1 receptor, which is highly expressed on the surface of OBs. Thus, elevated VEGF expression after trauma will contribute to healing. In the ONFH model, expression of VEGF after trauma greatly decreased compared with the normal group. However, VEGF

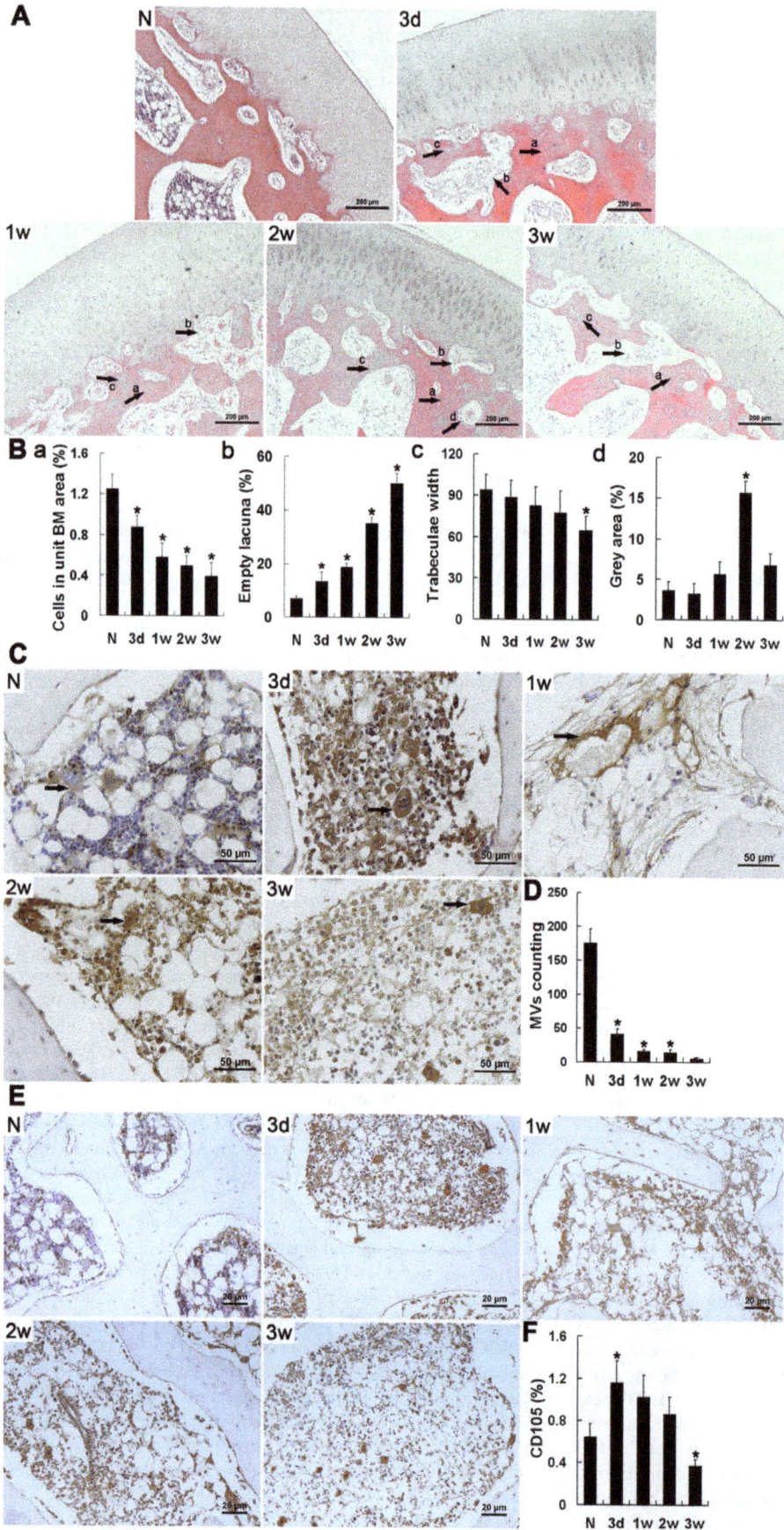

**Figure 2. Histopathological images of the traumatic ONFH rabbit model, and immunohistochemical staining and semi-quantitative analysis of vWF and CD105.** (A) Representative images of a section of femoral head including cartilage stained with H&E. Scale bar = 200 μm. In the injured femoral head, the number of empty lacunae increased and hematopoietic tissue diminished significantly, but cartilage did not exhibit any obvious pathological changes. Immature fibrotic tissue and appositional bone formation were observed under the cartilage from 3 days after trauma, followed by an increase in the number of OBs 2 weeks later. a. empty lacuna; b. immature fibrotic tissue; c. appositional bone formation; d. OBs. (B) Bar graphs represent the ratio of bone marrow cells to the area of bone marrow (a), the ratio of empty lacunae to the area of trabeculae (b), thinning trabeculae (c) and grey scale (d), respectively. (C) Immunohistochemical assays of vWF expression. Scale bar = 50 μm. (D) Blood vessels were counted according to positive staining of vWF in combination with appropriate vessel structure. Following trauma, the structure of the blood vessels became increasingly compromised and the number of blood vessels decreased. Arrows = microvessels or arteries. (E) Immunohistochemical assays of vWF expression. Scale bar = 20 μm. (F) Bar graphs represent the expression density of CD105 as unit area of bone marrow or unit area of bone trabeculae. The expression of CD105 until 3 weeks after trauma suggested the presence of revascularization in the injured femoral head. N: normal group; 3 d, 1 w, 2 w, 3 w: 3 days, 1 week, 2 weeks, 3 weeks post-trauma, respectively. Quantification was based on at least 10 fields per section. *$P < 0.05$ vs. normal group.

levels were markedly increased after MSC transplantation. The greatest levels of expression were observed in animals treated with HGF-transgenic MSCs, which also exhibited the greatest promotion of vasculogenesis (Figure 6A, B).

Col I in medullary cavities also increased gradually after treatment for 2 weeks and was higher in animals in the ONFH+MSC+HGF group than in the other two treatment groups ($P < 0.05$) (Figure 6C, D-a). In the trabeculae, treatment by transplantation of HGF-transgenic MSCs decreased, but did not completely inhibit, accumulation of Col I. The most significant decrease of Col I in trabeculae was detected in the ONFH+MSC+HGF group, in which the Col I level increased slightly but was not significantly higher than that in the normal group (Figure 6 C, D-b). These results suggest that animals in the ONFH+MSC+HGF group had the strongest activity of OBs, which promote new bone formation.

## HGF-induced sequential activation of ERK1/2 and Akt contributed to the efficacy of HGF-transgenic MSC transplantation

Our previous work showed that HGF levels in the femoral head region in hormone-induced ONFH changed after transplantation with HGF-transgenic MSCs which promotes the function of MSCs in tissue repair. At the beginning of treatment, high levels of HGF enhance MSC proliferation by strongly activating ERK1/2 signaling; a gradually decreasing HGF level then promotes MSC osteogenic differentiation through preferential activation of the Akt pathway [16].

To investigate whether a similar mechanism exists in the traumatic ONFH model, we explored the mechanism by which HGF-transgenic MSC transplantation achieves its therapeutic effect. Firstly, we measured HGF expression levels in all treated tissues. Unexpectedly, HGF protein expression increased slightly in the traumatic ONFH model group before eventually declining, distinguishing the present model from hormone-induced ONFH. Significant increases in HGF expression were observed in all of the treated animals as early as 2 days after transplantation and decreased approximately 2 weeks later (Figure 7A). The greatest levels of HGF were observed in animals treated with HGF-transgenic MSCs. Unlike HGF, which increased after trauma, p-ERK1/2 levels, which were high in the normal group, were greatly decreased in the ONFH group. Transplantation of MSCs greatly increased activation of the ERK1/2 pathway; the highest p-ERK1/2 levels were still seen in the animals treated with HGF-transgenic MSCs, concomitant with a significant elevation of HGF expression (Figure 7B). Although lower than in the normal group, Akt pathway activation was still extensive in the ONFH group, and was elevated after MSC transplantation. However, a significant increase in Akt pathway activation was observed only in the ONFH+MSCs+HGF group after 2 weeks (Figure 7C),

accompanied by a decline in HGF expression in the local region. These observations demonstrate that the transplantation of HGF-transgenic MSCs contributed to recovery from traumatic ONFH through a mechanism similar to that seen with treatment of hormone-induced ONFH [16].

## Discussion

In this study, a model of early stage traumatic ONFH representing clinical ARCO phase I or II ONFH was established in rabbits and confirmed by CT and MR imaging and pathological examination. Based on the differing distributions of necrotic lesions on the two flanks of the epiphyseal plate in this model and the preserved cartilage, which are consistent with human ONFH, this model can be regarded as a mimic of early stage clinical ONFH. Based on the apparent occurrence of self-repair after trauma, we selected the best time for treatment of the model with the transplantation of HGF-transgenic MSCs. Local inspection of the treated tissues confirmed the efficacy of this therapeutic method and the feasibility of assessing its efficacy in this traumatic ONFH model.

Complicated cellular interactions in the injured femoral head contribute to the development of ONFH. According to the histological definition of osteonecrosis, including empty lacunae in the osseous matrix and necrosis of marrow elements [25,26], osteonecrosis occurred within 3 days after trauma. During the progression of traumatic ONFH, there was obvious evidence of tissue self-repair. For example, pathological inspection with H&E staining showed the presence of local bone formation as well as the reoccurrence of OBs, which was especially obvious under the cartilage. Furthermore, expression of CD105, a specific marker of new blood vessels [27,28,29], increased around the MVs until 3 weeks after trauma, which suggested the emergence of revascularization. In addition, although PCNA levels decreased following traumatic surgery, the increase in OBs from the second week indicated their proliferation during the early stage of OB differentiation. At the same time, as a marker of initiation of osteogenic differentiation, which is elevated in the early stage of bone synthesis after trauma [23], expression of OCN also reached its highest level 2 weeks after trauma. All of these observations indicate that there was ongoing tissue self-repair in the injured femoral head until for 2 weeks after trauma. Our assessment of tissue self-repair was based mainly on the expression of marker molecules. Nonetheless, as the trauma operation did not injure the medullary cavity, the residual MSCs, the intact cartilage, the epiphyseal plate, and the connective tissue around or infiltrating into the femoral head, may also play roles in this process. However, a continual decrease in the MVs marked by vWF indicated that there was an increased rate of apoptosis of endothelial cells after trauma. Additionally, the continued increase in OCs and empty lacunae as well as thinning of the trabeculae

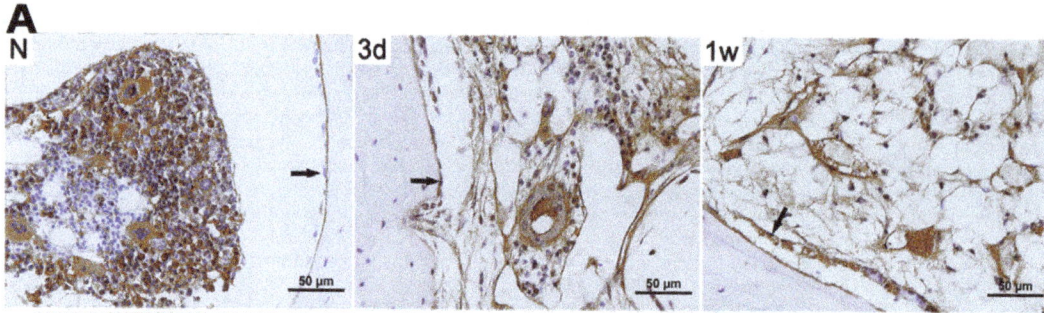

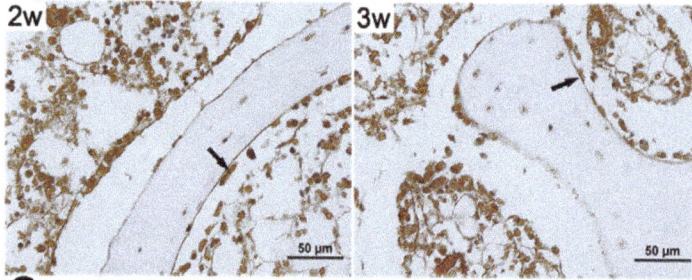

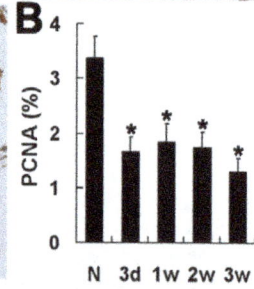

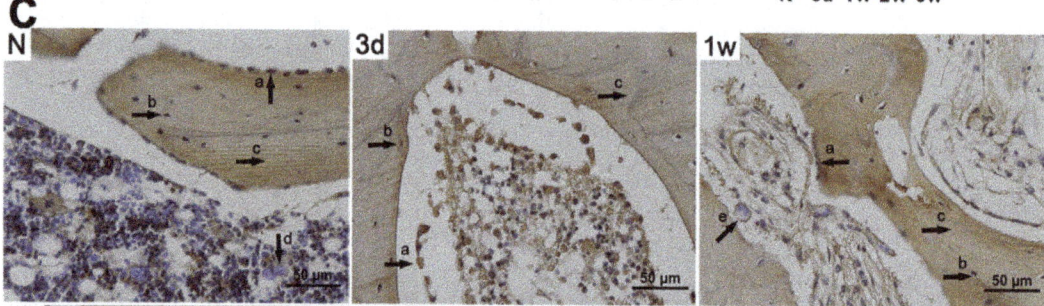

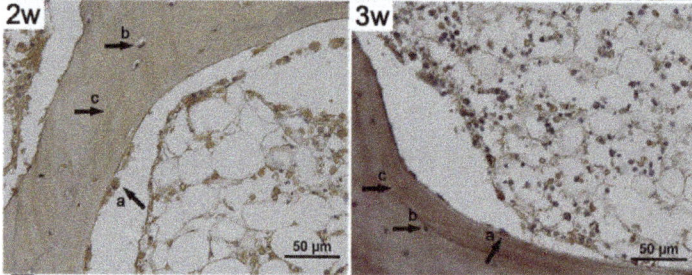

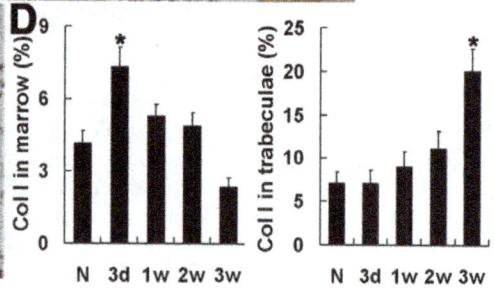

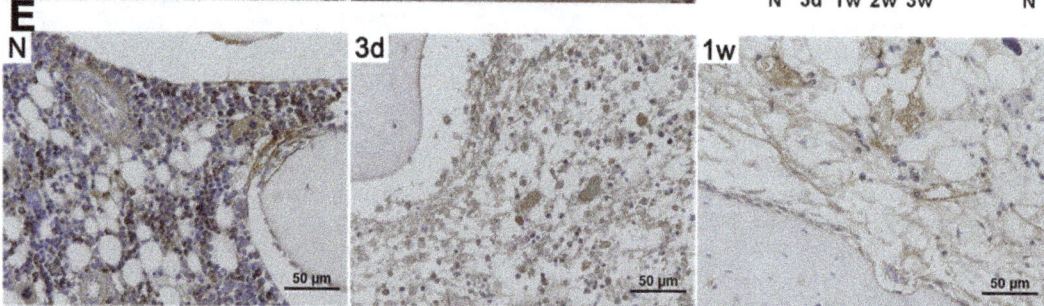

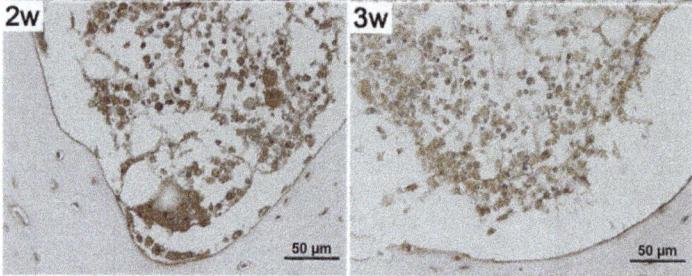

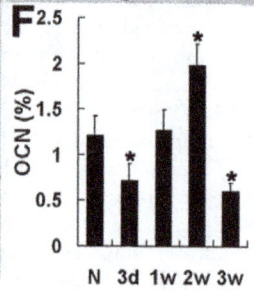

**Figure 3. Tissue self-repair after trauma indicated by immunohistochemical staining and semi-quantitative analysis of PCNA, Col I and OCN.** (A, C, E) Immunohistochemical assays of the expression of PCNA (A), Col I (C) and OCN (E). (B, D, F) Bar graphs represent their expression density in unit area of bone marrow or unit area of bone trabeculae. (A) OBs; (C) a. OBs, b. osteocytes, c. trabeculae, d. VECs, e. OCs. The expression of PCNA decreased after trauma, and began to be detected in OBs 2 weeks after trauma and was maintained during the following time. Col I increased in the bone marrow for less than 1 week after trauma, and was significantly accumulated in the trabeculae by the end of the study. Both OBs and OCs also expressed increased levels of Col I following trauma. A significant decrease in OCN was detected 3 days after trauma, but it increased significantly 2 weeks later. High levels of OCN were consistently associated with peri-VECs and the fibrous medulla. N: normal group; 3 d, 1 w, 2 w, 3 w: 3 days, 1 week, 1 weeks, 3 weeks post-trauma, respectively. Quantification was based on at least 10 fields per section. *$P < 0.05$ vs. normal group.

suggest that there was an imbalance between osteogenesis and osteoclastic absorption, which may account for the bone loss. Due to the complete disruption of vascularization, self-repair could not keep pace with the ongoing tissue necrosis and became abortive, resulting in irreversible progression of the disease.

It is proposed that a treatment that promotes revascularization and bone tissue repair before the peak level of self-repair at approximately 2 weeks after trauma would improve the efficacy of tissue self-repair, impede the progression of the disease, and potentially rescue a necrotic femoral head. The course of self-tissue repair provided an excellent time point to intervene in the development of the disease and suggested that pluripotent MSCs could play important roles in this process. Accordingly, we treated the traumatic ONFH model animals with transplanted MSCs transfected with HGF early after trauma before the reparative phase was histologically observed. One week after trauma, the injured tissue had recovered more with transplantation of HGF-transgenic MSCs than with uninfected or Ad-vector-infected MSCs. Changes in HGF expression were also observed; HGF levels increased immediately after transplantation and declined approximately 2 weeks later. This pattern of HGF expression was the same as that seen *in vitro* with Ad-HGF-transfected MSCs and *in vivo* treatment of hormone-induced ONFH [16]. Our previous work demonstrated that the elevation of HGF promotes MSC proliferation to meet the cell's requirement for tissue reconstruction through the activation of the ERK1/2 signaling pathway. The subsequent decrease in HGF promotes MSC differentiation by activating the Akt signaling pathway in the osteogenic microenvironment, favoring re-establishment of bone tissue, as demonstrated by increased numbers of OBs. These results suggest that changes in HGF concentration enhance the ability of MSCs to contribute to femoral head tissue repair in ONFH. Similar

phenomena were also observed in the untreated animals up to 2 weeks after trauma, but they were much less extensive, suggesting that coordination between the therapy and self-repair promoted recovery in the treated animals. The activation of the ERK1/2 and Akt pathways during the treatment of traumatic ONFH was also similar to that observed in the treatment of hormone-induced ONFH with the transplantation of HGF-transgenic MSCs [16]; that is, ERK1/2 activation increased simultaneously with increased HGF expression after transplantation, but decreased about 2 weeks later. In contrast, there was less activation of the Akt pathway after MSC transplantation than 2 weeks later, and these changes in Akt activations were accompanied by changes in HGF levels. These observations suggest that, in traumatic ONFH, HGF affects the activity of MSCs through a mechanism similar to that seen in hormone-induced ONFH. That is, high concentrations of HGF enhance activation of the ERK1/2 signaling pathway and inhibit that of Akt, which promotes MSC proliferation but suppresses osteogenic differentiation. However, low concentrations of HGF can activate Akt and promote osteogenic differentiation [16]. It should be noted that the changes in Akt activation observed in traumatic ONFH were not as significant as in hormone-induced ONFH. The reason may be the presence of tissue self-repair. It was observed that, although declining, expression of Akt was still higher in our animals than in hormone-induced ONFH [16]. For this reason, the increase of Akt activation resulting from transgenic HGF was limited.

The self-repair observed in the traumatic ONFH model suggested that significant MSC activity was present in the injured tissue. Strong signals persisted around VECs until the end of the observation period, consistent with the presence of MSCs [24]. Such phenomena were not observed in hormone-induced ONFH, suggesting that MSCs may have been inactivated after hormone

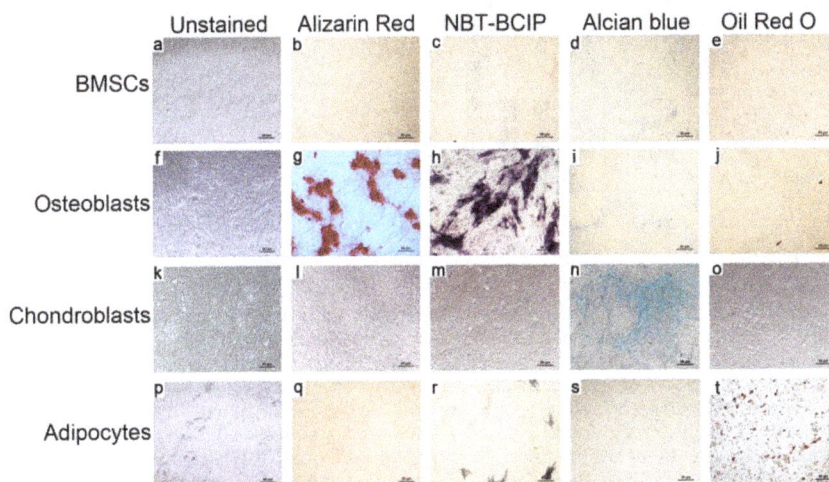

**Figure 4. Identification of MSC pluripotent potential.** Undifferentiated MSCs (a–e), osteoblasts (f–j), chondroblasts (k–o), and adipocytes (p–t) were left unstained (a, f, k, & p), or stained with Alizarin Red at day 21 (b, g, l, & q), NBT-BCIP at day 14 (c, h, m, & r), Alcian blue at day 27 (d, i, n, & s), or Oil Red O at day 27 (e, j, o, & t). Scale bar = 50 μm.

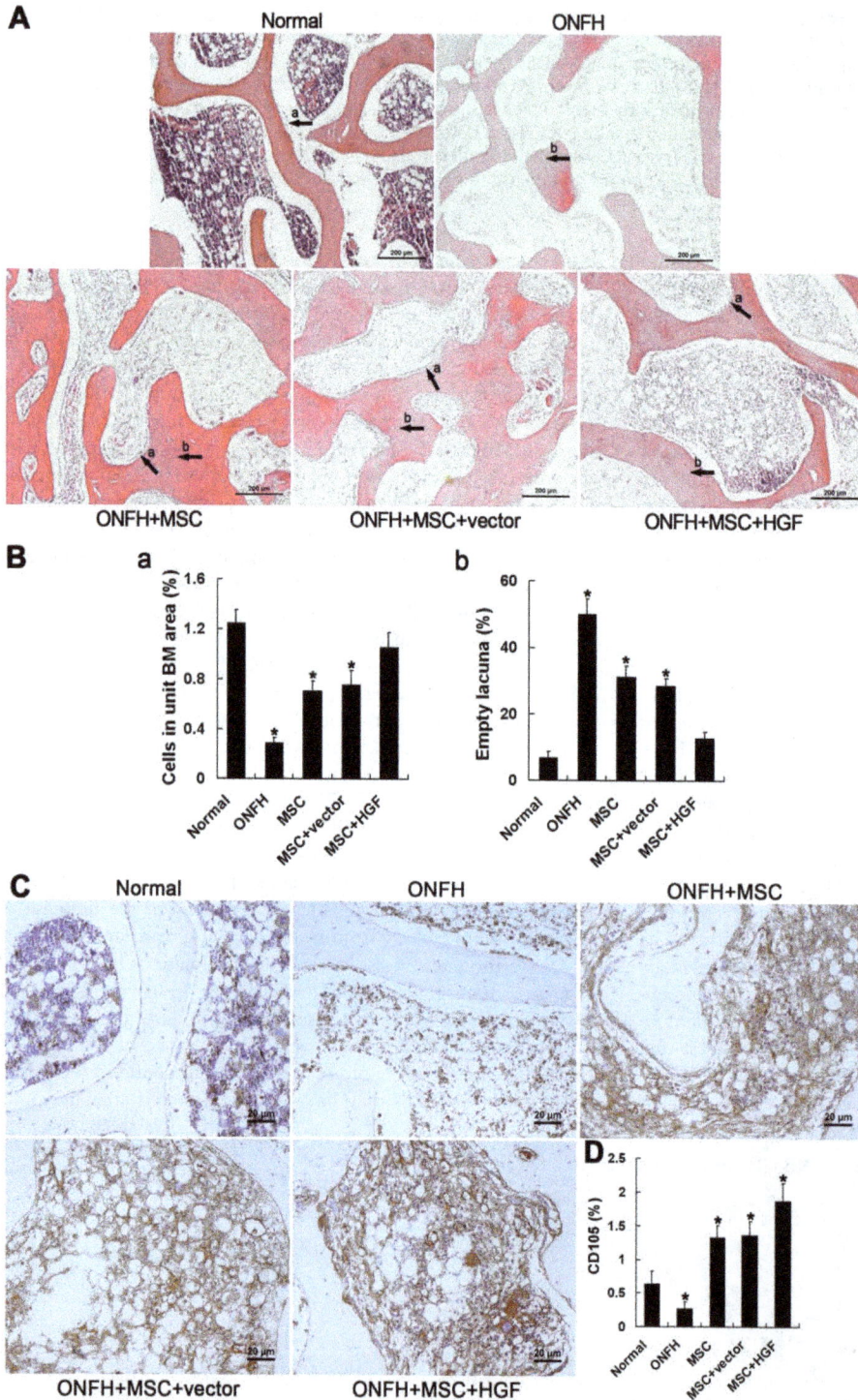

**Figure 5. Histopathological examination of treatment efficacy in traumatic ONFH by H&E staining, and immunohistochemical staining and semi-quantitative analysis of CD105.** (A) Representative image of a section of femoral head stained with H&E. Scale bar = 200 μm. In the treated femoral head, the number of empty lacunae decreased and hematopoietic tissue partially recovered, accompanied by an increase in the number of OBs, which was most significant in animals that received HGF-transgenic MSCs. a. empty lacuna; b. OBs. (B) Bar graph (left panel) represents the ratio of bone marrow cells to the area of bone marrow. A second bar graph (right panel) represents the ratio of empty lacunae to the area of trabeculae. (C) Immunohistochemical assays of CD105 expression. Scale bar = 20 μm. (D) Bar graphs represent the expression density of CD105 as unit area of bone marrow or unit area of bone trabeculae. After MSC transplantation, the expression of CD105 increased compared with that of untreated ONFH group, indicating the occurrence of revascularization. Quantification was based on at least 10 fields per section. *$P < 0.05$.

treatment. This possibility is consistent with the report of Weinstein *et al.* [30], and such findings suggest that MSC activity is important for recovery from ONFH. In traumatic ONFH, the

use of MSC transplantation to coordinate tissue self-repair could improve the effects of the latter, and the pro-osteogenic function on MSCs of HGF could further increase the efficacy of the

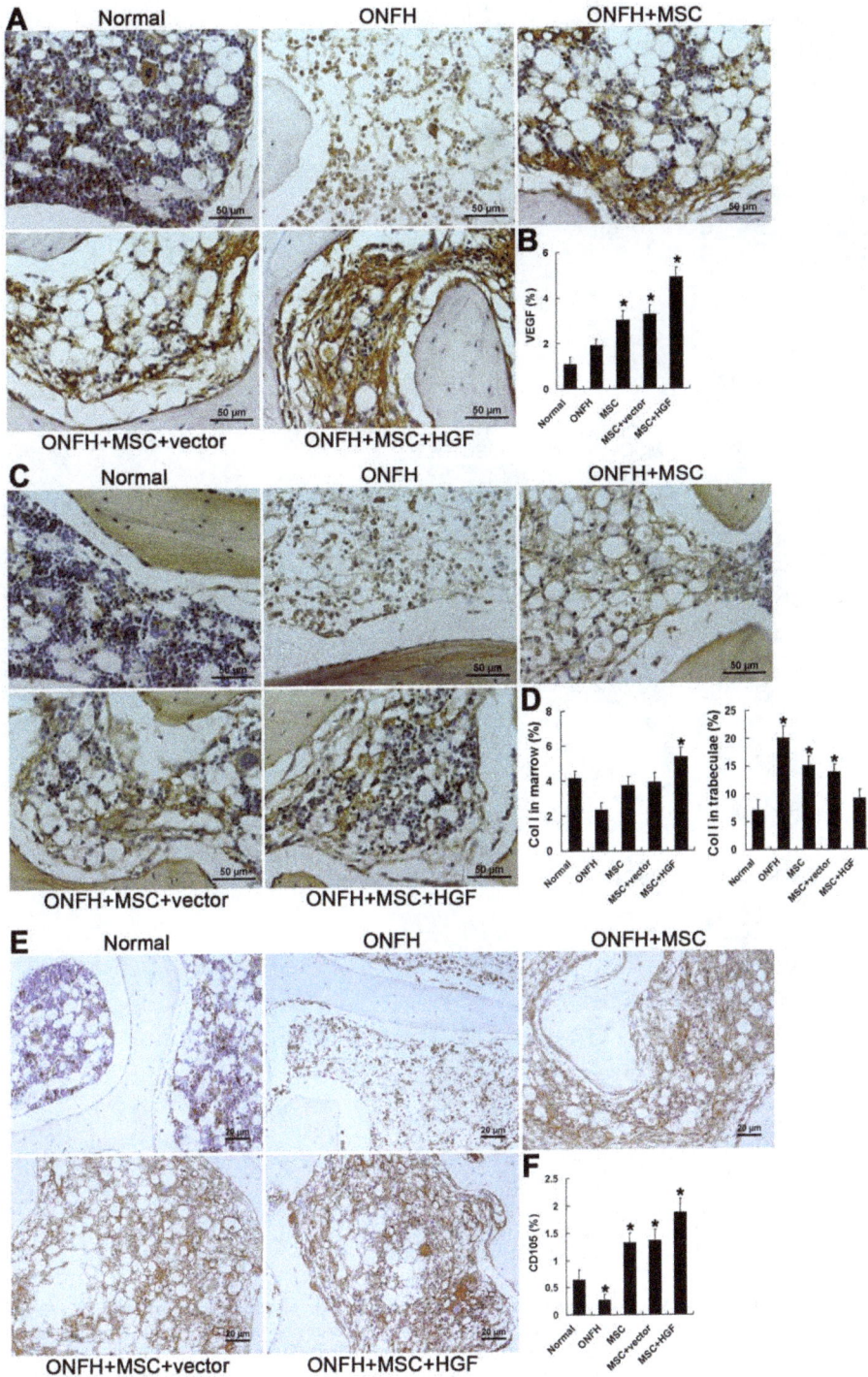

**Figure 6. Immunohistochemical staining and semi-quantitative analysis of VEGF and Col I.** (A, C) Immunohistochemical assays of the expression of VEGF (A) and Col I (C). (B, D) Bar graphs represent the expression density of VEGF and Col I as unit area of bone marrow or unit area of bone trabeculae. Transplantation of MSCs reversed the decline of VEGF and Col I expression in the marrow, but decreased the accumulation of Col I in the trabeculae. The most significant recovery was seen in the ONFH+MSC+HGF group. Quantification was based on at least 10 fields per section. *$P < 0.05$ vs. normal group.

treatment. Besides the effects on MSCs, previous studies have reported that HGF can induce secretion of VEGF through activation of its receptor c-Met, which is followed by the activation of both the ERK1/2 and Akt signaling pathways [31,32,33,34]. In bone marrow, c-Met is extensively expressed on MSCs and endothelial cells as well as other cell types. The transplantation of HGF-transgenic MSCs is therefore a promising potential therapy for traumatic ONFH. In the future, further investigations of the etiology of ONFH and the effects of the therapeutic transplantation of HGF-transgenic MSCs will provide a deeper understand-

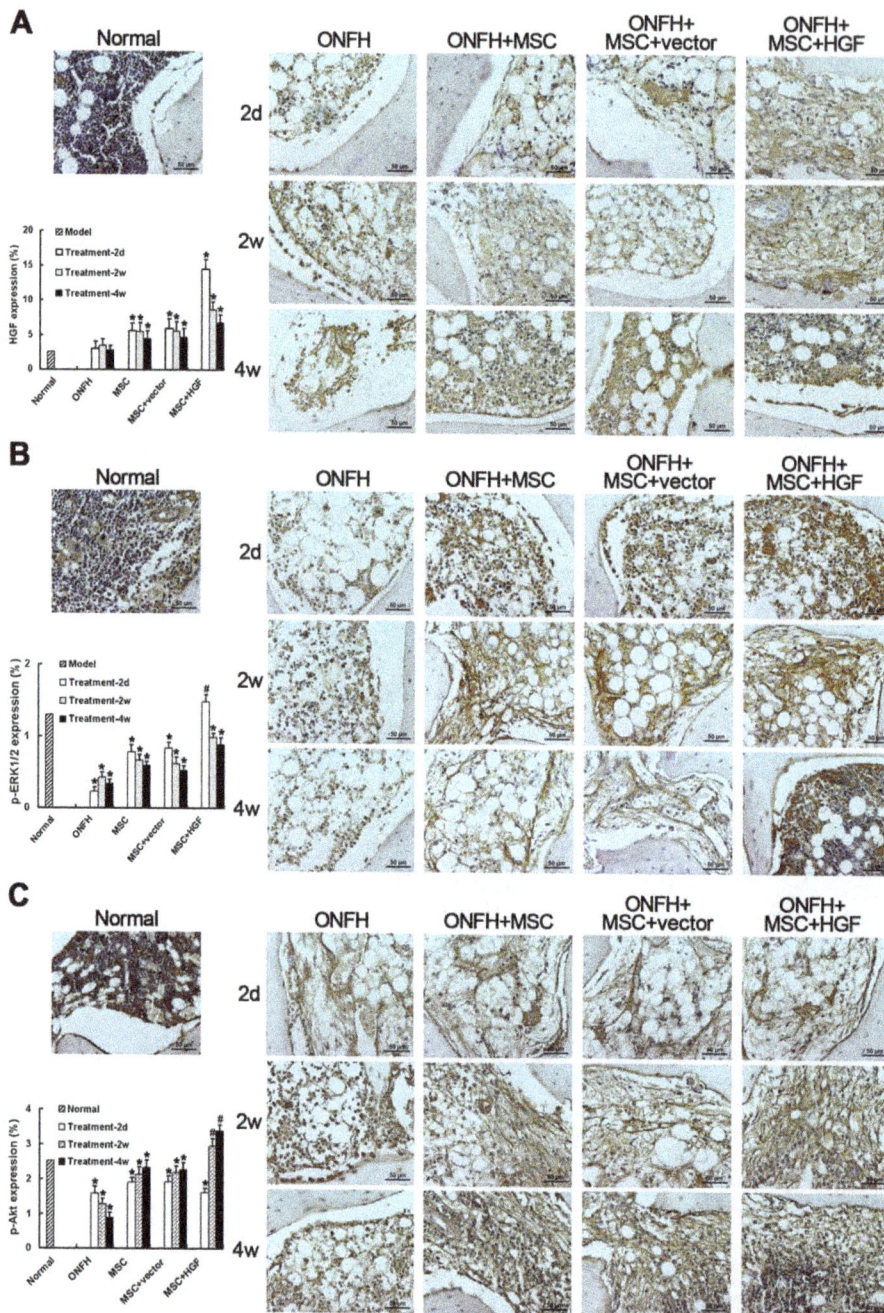

**Figure 7. Immunohistochemical detection and semi-quantitative analysis of HGF expression (A), phosphorylation of ERK1/2 (p-ERK1/2) (B) and Akt (p-Akt) (C).** There was a little increase in HGF after trauma. After the transplantation of MSCs, the HGF level increased significantly at as early as 2 days, which was concomitant with increased p-ERK1/2. The HGF level decreased gradually for 2 weeks after transplantation, followed by a significant increase in Akt activation. The effects were most marked in the animals treated with HGF-transgenic MSCs. *$P<0.05$, compared with the normal group. #$P<0.05$, compared with the non-infected MSC-treated group. Scale bar = 50 μm.

ing of the progression of ONFH after treatment and will be of assistance in designing more effective therapeutic regimens.

## Conclusions

In this study, a rabbit model of early stage traumatic ONFH was established. Based on radiological inspection and the distribution and features of necrotic lesions, this model can be considered to represent clinical ARCO phase I or II ONFH and to be suitable for pathophysiological studies and the assessment of therapeutic regimens. Histological findings and the expression profiles of specific molecules indicate that self-repair was initiated in the femoral head as early as 3 days after trauma and peaked at 2 weeks. The use of this therapeutic window will be critical for designing therapeutic regimens. Transplantation of HGF-transgenic MSCs was performed 1 week after trauma and contributed greatly to the recovery of the injured femoral head. These results provide valuable insights into the development of effective treatment strategies for ONFH.

## Acknowledgments

We are grateful to the Department of Orthopaedics and Traumatology staff of the Nanfang Hospital, Southern Medical University, for assistance with animal studies.

## References

1. Kerachian M, Harvey E, Cournoyer D, Chow T, Séguin C (2006) Avascular necrosis of the femoral head: vascular hypotheses. Endothelium 13: 237–244.
2. Bachiller F, Caballer A, Portal L (2002) Avascular necrosis of the femoral head after femoral neck fracture. Clin Orthop Relat Res 399: 87–109.
3. Nakamura T, Matsumoto T, Nishino M, Tomita K, Kadoya M (1997) Early magnetic resonance imaging and histologic findings in a model of femoral head necrosis. Clin Orthop Relat Res 334: 68–72.
4. Nadel S, Debatin J, Richardson W, Hedlund L, Senft C, et al. (1992) Detection of acute avascular necrosis of the femoral head in dogs: dynamic contrast-enhanced MR imaging vs spin-echo and STIR sequences. AJR Am J Roentgenol 159: 1255–1261.
5. Malizos K, Quarles L, Seaber A, Rizk W, Urbaniak J (1993) An experimental canine model of osteonecrosis: characterization of the repair process. J Orthop Res 11: 350–357.
6. Freeman M, England J (1969) Experimental infarction of the immature canine femoral head. Proc R Soc Med 62: 431–433.
7. Dahners L, Hillsgrove D (1989) The effects of drilling on revascularization and new bone formation in canine femoral heads with avascular necrosis: an initial study. J Orthop Trauma 3: 309–312.
8. Mont M, Jones L, Elias J, Inoue N, Yoon T, et al. (2001) Strut-autografting with and without osteogenic protein-1: a preliminary study of a canine femoral head defect model. J Bone Joint Surg Am 83: 1013–1022.
9. Huffman K, Bowers J, Dailiana Z, Huebner J, Urbaniak J, et al. (2007) Synovial fluid metabolites in osteonecrosis. Rheumatology (Oxford) 46: 523–528.
10. Nishino M, Matsumoto T, Nakamura T, Tomita K (1997) Pathological and hemodynamic study in a new model of femoral head necrosis following traumatic dislocation. Arch Orthop Trauma Surg 116: 259–262.
11. Stamm C, Westphal B, Kleine H, Petzsch M, Kittner C, et al. (2003) Autologous bone-marrow stem-cell transplantation for myocardial regeneration. Lancet 361: 45–46.
12. Sch chinger V, Erbs S, Els sser A, Haberbosch W, Hambrecht R, et al. (2006) Intracoronary bone marrow-derived progenitor cells in acute myocardial infarction. N Engl J Med 355: 1210–1221.
13. Gangji V, Hauzeur J, Matos C, De Maertelaer V, Toungouz M, et al. (2004) Treatment of osteonecrosis of the femoral head with implantation of autologous bone-marrow cells. A pilot study. J Bone Joint Surg Am 86: 1153–1160.
14. Daltro G, Fortuna V, Araújo M, Lessa P, Borojevic R (2008) Femoral head necrosis treatment with autologous stem cells in sickle cell disease. Acta Ortop Bras 16: 23–27.
15. Wen Q, Ma L, Chen Y, Yang L, Luo W, et al. (2008) Treatment of avascular necrosis of the femoral head by hepatocyte growth factor-transgenic bone marrow stromal stem cells. Gene Ther 15: 1523–1535.
16. Wen Q, Zhou L, Zhou C, Zhou M, Luo W, et al. (2011) Change in hepatocyte growth factor concentration promote mesenchymal stem cell-mediated osteogenic regeneration. J Cell Mol Med doi: 10.1111/j.1582-4934.2011.01407.x. Epub ahead of print.
17. Gardeniers J (1991) ARCO committee on terminology and staging (report from the Nijmegen meeting). ARCO News Letter 3: 153–159.
18. Gardeniers J (1992) A new international classification of osteonecrosis of the ARCO-committee on terminology and classification. ARCO News 4: 41–46.
19. Gardeniers J (1993) Report of the Committee of Staging and Nomenclature. ARCO News Letter 5: 79–82.
20. Barkalow F, Goodman M, Mayadas T (1996) Rapid Communication Cultured Murine Cerebral Microvascular Endothelial Cells Contain von Willebrand Factor-Positive Weibel-Palade Bodies and Support Rapid Cytokine-Induced Neutrophil Adhesion. Microcirculation 3: 19–28.
21. Arabmotlagh M, Sabljic R, Rittmeister M (2006) Changes of the biochemical markers of bone turnover and periprosthetic bone remodeling after cemented hip arthroplasty. J Arthroplasty 21: 129–134.
22. Kusumi T, Kusumi A (2004) Osteocalcin/bone Gla protein (BGP). Nihon Rinsho 62 Suppl 2: 136–140.
23. Yin L, Li Y, Wang Y (2006) Dexamethasone-induced adipogenesis in primary marrow stromal cell cultures: mechanism of steroid-induced osteonecrosis. Chin Med J (Engl) 119: 581–588.
24. Ehninger A, Trumpp A (2011) The bone marrow stem cell niche grows up: mesenchymal stem cells and macrophages move in. J Exp Med 208: 421–428.
25. Glimcher M, Kenzora J (1979) The biology of osteonecrosis of the human femoral head and its clinical implications: II. The pathological changes in the femoral head as an organ and in the hip joint. Clin Orthop Relat Res 139: 283–312.
26. Inoue A, Ono K (1979) A histological study of idiopathic avascular necrosis of the head of the femur. J Bone Joint Surg Br 61-B: 138–143.
27. Barbara N, Wrana J, Letarte M (1999) Endoglin is an accessory protein that interacts with the signaling receptor complex of multiple members of the transforming growth factor-beta superfamily. J Biol Chem 274: 584–594.
28. Li C, Guo B, Wilson P, Stewart A, Byrne G, et al. (2000) Plasma levels of soluble CD105 correlate with metastasis in patients with breast cancer. Int J Cancer 89: 122–126.
29. Minhajat R, Mori D, Yamasaki F, Sugita Y, Satoh T, et al. (2006) Organ-specific endoglin (CD105) expression in the angiogenesis of human cancers. Pathol Int 56: 717–723.
30. Weinstein R, Jilka R, Parfitt A, Manolagas S (1998) Inhibition of osteoblasto-genesis and promotion of apoptosis of osteoblasts and osteocytes by glucocorticoids. Potential mechanisms of their deleterious effects on bone. J Clin Invest 102: 274–282.
31. Van Belle E, Witzenbichler B, Chen D, Silver M, Chang L, et al. (1998) Potentiated angiogenic effect of scatter factor/hepatocyte growth factor via induction of vascular endothelial growth factor: the case for paracrine amplification of angiogenesis. Circulation 97: 381–390.
32. Wojta J, Kaun C, Breuss J, Koshelnick Y, Beckmann R, et al. (1999) Hepatocyte growth factor increases expression of vascular endothelial growth factor and plasminogen activator inhibitor-1 in human keratinocytes and the vascular endothelial growth factor receptor flk-1 in human endothelial cells. Lab Invest 79: 427–438.
33. Dong G, Chen Z, Li Z, Yeh N, Bancroft C, et al. (2001) Hepatocyte growth factor/scatter factor-induced activation of MEK and PI3K signal pathways contributes to expression of proangiogenic cytokines interleukin-8 and vascular endothelial growth factor in head and neck squamous cell carcinoma. Cancer Res 61: 5911–5918.
34. Sengupta S, Sellers L, Li R, Gherardi E, Zhao G, et al. (2003) Targeting of mitogen-activated protein kinases and phosphatidylinositol 3 kinase inhibits hepatocyte growth factor/scatter factor-induced angiogenesis. Circulation 107: 2955–2961.

## Author Contributions

Conceived and designed the experiments: QW LM. Performed the experiments: QW DJ MZ. Analyzed the data: QW CZ WL. Contributed reagents/materials/analysis tools: QW LM. Wrote the paper: QW LM.

# 15

# Comparison of Road Traffic Injury Characteristics between Local versus Floating Migrant Patients in a Tertiary Hospital between 2007 and 2010

**Chungui Xu, Yanhua Wang, Na Han, Yuhui Kou, Xiaofeng Yin, Peixun Zhang, Tianbing Wang\*, Dianying Zhang, Baoguo Jiang\***

Department of Trauma and Orthopaedics, Peking University People's Hospital, Beijing, China

## Abstract

*Background:* The aim of this study is to give a description of the road traffic injuries (RTIs) characteristics of floating migrant population by comparing with those of local residents in a harbor city of China.

*Methods:* A population-based descriptive study was carried out between 2007 and 2010 with RTI patient records from the Fifth Center Hospital of Tianjin. Inpatient diagnoses of RTI patients were defined using the International Classification of Diseases, Tenth Revision (ICD-10) codes. We analyzed the demographics and general characteristics of RTI patients that were in the hospital during the four years. In order to compare the group differences between local resident patients and floating migrant patients, the distribution of their ages, diagnoses, severity of injuries, duration of inpatient stays, hospitalization cost were analyzed.

*Results:* People between the ages of 16 and 55 were the most likely to suffer RTIs. The floating migrant patients between the ages of 16 and 45 had a higher incidence of accidents, while local resident patients between 46 and 55 had a higher incidence of accidents. Compared to local resident patients, floating migrant patients were more vulnerable to open injuries and severe traffic injuries. With the severity of injuries ranked from mild to severe, floating migrant patients had lower duration of inpatient stay, but higher hospitalization costs compared to local resident patients.

*Conclusions:* Floating migrant patients had a different age distribution, severity of injuries, diseases, inpatient duration and hospitalization cost compared with local resident patients. Compared to local resident patients, floating migrants had a higher risk to RTIs and were more vulnerable to severer traffic accidents at lower ages.

**Editor:** Robert K. Hills, Cardiff University, United Kingdom

**Funding:** This research project was funded by the Specific Research Project of Health Pro Bono Sectors, Ministry of Health, China (No. 201002014), the National Natural Science Fund of China (31171150, 31271284, 81171146, 30971526, 31100860, 31040043, 30801169) and the Chinese Education Ministry New Century Excellent Talent Support Project (BMU20110270), the Chinese National Natural Science Fund for Outstanding Young (30625036), the Beijing City Science & Technology New Star Classification A-2008-10 and the Chinese 973 Project Planning (2005CB522604). The funders had no role in study design, data collection and analysis, decision to publish, or preparation of the manuscript.

**Competing Interests:** The authors have declared that no competing interests exist.

\* E-mail: jiangbaoguo@vip.sina.com (BJ); wangtianbing@medmail.com.cn (TW)

## Introduction

Over nearly the last three decades, a new demographic phenomenon in China has attracted increasing attention [1]. The 'floating population' (or *liudong renkou* in Chinese) refers to the large and increasing number of migrants without local household registration status (namely *hukou*). According to the report of China National Bureau of Statistics, China had 230 million people in its floating population in 2011, representing 19% of the total population [2]. As a result of the gap between rural and urban incomes, the 'floating' migrant population came from the countryside to the cities in pursuit of a better life [3]. This rural-urban migration poses significant challenges, especially for China's welfare system concerning both local and migrant residents. Without local household registration, the floating migrants are not entitled to some of the benefits that local people enjoy. They face

daunting problems, particularly with access to healthcare, adequate housing, employment opportunities, pension plans and school enrollment for their children. Recently, the National People's Congress of China has highlighted the plight of the 'floating population' and outlined policies for education and basic health services.

Some epidemiological investigation has been done on the health problems of floating population in China, such as some infected diseases [4,5], unintentional injuries under six years old children [6] and so on. However, the characteristics of road traffic injuries (RTIs) among floating population have never been reported. There may be two reasons. First, such a massive migration of people from undeveloped regions to developed regions was scarcely seen in the other countries of the world except China. Second, most studies about the floating population health were focused on the infected diseases, because the migration of people is closely related to the spread of infected diseases, and the impact of infected diseases is obviously seen. An example is the SARS in 2003 of China [7,8]. However RTIs could happen on any people independent of the household registration, so research regarding the differences in RTIs, between local resident patients and floating migrant patients, has been scarce. But the floating population of China had a fast increase from 7 million in 1982 to 22 million in 1990 to 79 million in 2000 and 230 million in 2011 [1]. Due to the high mobility characteristics of these people, the fast expansion of floating population could be a factor contributing to the high frequency of road traffic accidents. In China, there were 3.9 million traffic accidents reported in 2010, in which 65 thousand people died and 2.5 million peoples were injured with a direct property loss of around 143 million dollars [9]. A sampling survey of injury deaths in Chinese people also found that, from 1991 to 2005, the proportion of all injury deaths due to traffic accident increased from 15.00% to 33.79% clearly showing a rising trend [10]. So it will make sense to have an investigation on the RTIs characteristics of the floating population that was unclear before.

In this study, we collected the hospital records of RTI patients from the emergency department of the Fifth Center Hospital of Tianjin, and analyzed the RTIs characteristics of floating population in comparison with those of local residents. This hospital is located in the Binhai New District of Tianjin city. It is largest tertiary hospital in this district. More than one-third of the RTI patients in this district were treated in this hospital. Other RTI patients were scattered among the hospitals near the accident spots. As an important harbor in north China, masses of freight were transported from neighboring regions to this district, which lead RTIs here having particular characteristics. This area provides a good sample for research comparing RTIs between local residents and floating population in this district.

## Materials and Methods

### Ethics statement

The study was approved by the Research Ethics Committee at PKUPH and met international biomedical ethics guidelines. Both the Hospital and the Biostatistics Department of Peking University Health Science Center supervised the acquisition of data. The written consent was given by the patients and the next of kin for their information to be stored in the hospital database and used for research.

### Data source

This descriptive study was performed based on the hospital records of RTI patients who suffered from motor vehicle accidents between the beginning of 2007 and the end of 2010. The RTI patients were transferred to the Fifth Center Hospital of Tianjin, by ambulance or by themselves. When patients arrived at the hospital, their personal information and general condition of the road traffic accidents was recorded on an emergency card by the patients themselves or by the accident witnesses. After the initial treatment in the emergency ward, patients were transferred to other departments of this hospital for follow-up treatment. All the emergency patients were treated at best regardless of their household registration. There were no differences for dealing with local resident patients or floating migrant patients. Patient condition was classified as one of the following severity levels according to the examination results: mild, moderate, severe and dead. Traffic accidents sufferers who died before arriving at the hospital were not included, because the persons dead at the scene were not transferred to hospital.

The RTI patients' data were extracted from the medical records database of this hospital. Medical records of all RTI patients were reviewed and diagnosis codes were assigned by trained coders using the International Classification of Diseases 10th Revision (ICD-10). The following database information was provided to the research team: medical record number, date of birth, gender, date of admission, household status, severity of injury, injured parts of the body, admission diagnosis, inpatient diagnoses, ICD-10 diagnoses codes, inpatient duration, hospitalization cost and outcomes at discharge.

### Statistical methods

We used the Excel software to collect the hospital records data and perform the basic statistical analysis. Descriptive statistics included means, median, 25% percentile, 75% percentile, standard deviations, and table and chart design. The parameters observed were age, gender, household status, severity of injury, injured parts of the body, diagnosis, inpatient duration, and hospitalization cost.

## Results

### Demographics and general characteristics

Between 2007 and 2010, there were a total of 2,224 RTI patients transferred to the emergency department of this hospital. The maximum and the minimum number of patients per year were 598 and 507 in 2007 and 2010, respectively. No increasing or decreasing trend in the number of patients per year was found. Patients examined over the four years, included 1,550 male and 674 female patients. The number of male and female patients over the four years is shown in Figure 1. The proportion of female patients of local residents ranged yearly between 30.6% and 37.7%, while that of female patients of floating migrants ranged yearly between 17.4% and 28.6%. There were 1,295 local resident patients and 929 floating migrant patients seen over the four years. The proportion of floating migrant patients was 42.8%, 42.1%, 44.1% and 37.5% for each year of the study. According to the *Tianjin Statistical Yearbooks* [11–14], there were 507 thousand, 517 thousand, 529 thousand and 494 thousand people with local household registration in each year from 2007 to 2010. In contrast, the amounts of floating migrants in these four years were 107 thousand, 245 thousand, 272 thousand and 300 thousand people respectively. So the average risks of RTI over the four years for local residents and floating migrants were 0.632 and 1.005 per thousand people.

### Age distribution of RTIs patients

The age distribution of local and floating migrant RTI patients over the four years was calculated and is shown in Figure 2. The age range of RTI patients was between 0 and 84 years. Patients under the age of 16 were divided into two groups according to age: preschool age, which was defined as 0 to 6 years old and school age, which was defined as 7 to 15 years old. This is because most children in China go to school at the age of 7 and receive nine years of compulsory education. From 16 to the eldest age, patients were divided into seven groups with each group comprising approximately 10 years. The results showed that, before the age of 16, the preschool age population had a higher distribution of RTIs compared to the school age population. The age distributions of local resident patients and floating migrant patients were also calculated. These distributions were compared and patients were divided into three groups according to age: younger than age 16, age 16 to 45, and age 46 to 84. There were a greater number of local resident patients in the first and the last age groups than

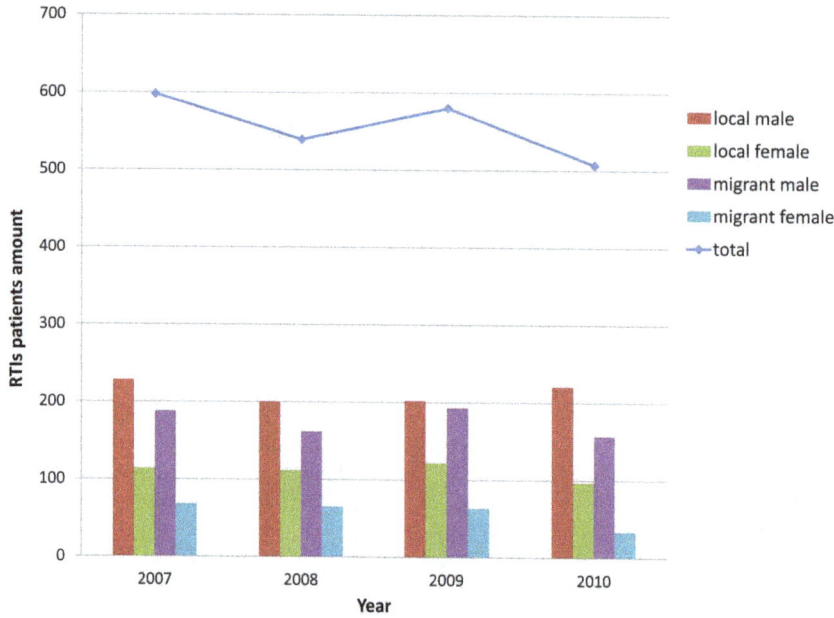

**Figure 1. Distribution of male and female RIT patients between 2007 and 2010.**

floating migrant patients. The number of floating migrant patients was no fewer than that of local resident patients in the 16 to 45 age groups. The peak number of local patients emerged between the ages of 46 and 55, while that of floating migrant patients occurred between the ages of 16 and 45.

## Monthly distribution of RTIs patients

Over the 4 years, the number of patients each month was counted and the sum over 12 months was calculated. The results are shown in Figure 3. The 3 months that had the most patients were October (218), March (217) and June (216). In contrast, the 2 months that had the least patients were February (107) and January (146). The proportion of floating migrant patients was also calculated for each month during the 4 years. In January and February, the proportions of floating migrant patients were just 27.4% and 33.6%, which were less than those of other months.

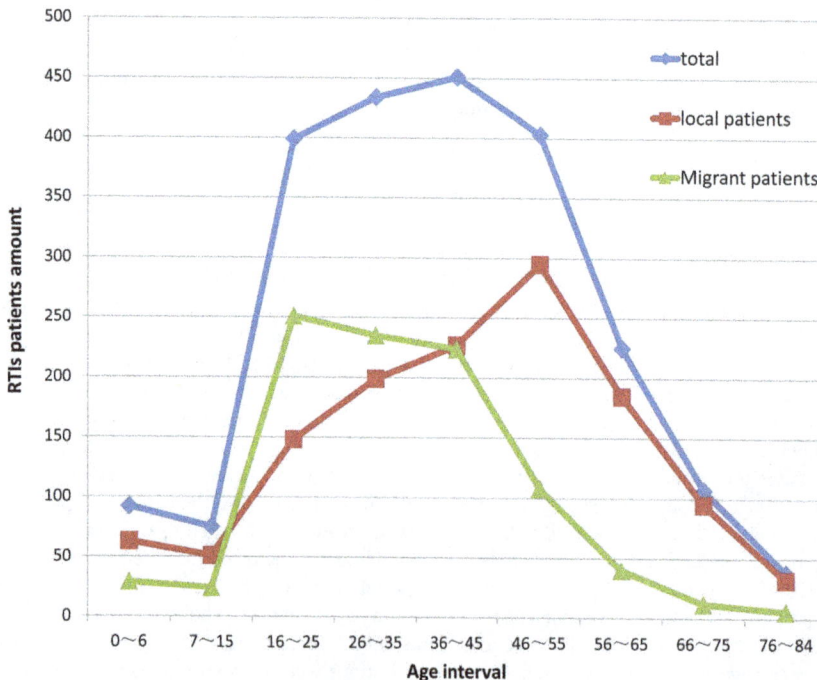

**Figure 2. Age distribution of local and floating migrant RTI patients from 2007 to 2010.**

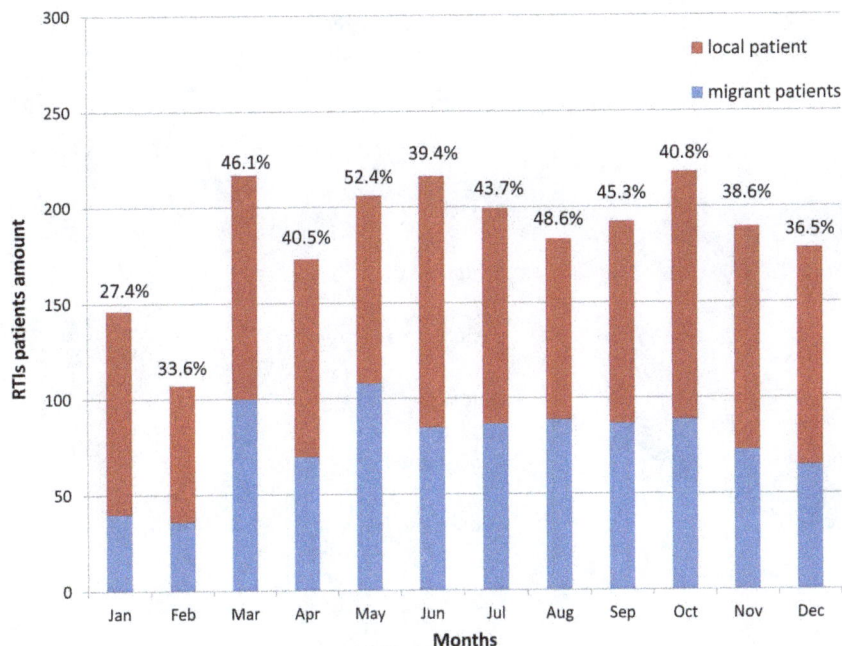

**Figure 3. Monthly distribution of RTI patients in the four years from 2007 to 2010 (the data above the columns were proportions of floating migrant population of the 12 months).**

## Distribution of injured regions of the body in traffic accidents

Information regarding injured regions of the body was registered for all of the patients who were in traffic accidents. Patients were divided into 11 groups according to the injured regions: head, neck, thorax, abdomen, lower back, lumbar spine and pelvis, shoulder and upper arm, elbow and forearm, wrist and hand, hip and thigh, knee and lower leg, ankle and foot, and multiple regions of the body. The proportion of injured regions in RTIs is shown in Figure 4. Most RTI patients had injuries to the head or had injuries to multiple regions of the body. These two groups of patients accounted for 37% and 34.6% of all the patients, respectively. The injury severity and residence of these two groups of patients were analyzed and are shown in Table 1. Except for one patient that died as a result of traumatic rupture of the liver and another patient that died from a sudden cardiac event, patient deaths were caused by head injuries or multiple body region injuries. In the head injury group, the proportions of floating migrant patients classified as mild, moderate and severe were 40.1%, 48.4% and 50% respectively. In the multiple body regions injury group, these proportions were 39.3%, 42.1% and 46.3%, respectively.

## Injury characteristics among RTI patients

The hospital diagnoses of all RTI patients were analyzed. In total, 561 types of injuries were diagnosed. Frequently diagnosed injuries were classified as those that occurred no less than 20 times. There were 100 types of injuries that met this criteria. A total of 10 diagnosed injuries involved the head or thorax (e.g. scalp hematoma and rib fracture). These injuries are listed in Table S1 and ranked according to the proportion of floating migrant patients with each injury. The average, median, 25% percentile, 75% percentile and standard deviation of the age of the patients, that had each injury, were also calculated. For some injuries, there were apparent age differences between local and floating migrant

patients. For example, the average age of local patients suffered from fracture of pelvis was $47.2\pm18.1$ years old, while that of floating migrant patients was just $33.9\pm7.6$ years old.

Open injuries need more care in the emergency ward because an open wound provides easy access for bacterial infections. The total number of open injuries, among all injuries, was calculated. The result showed that there were 326 local resident patients and 406 floating migrant patients that had open injuries. Table 2 lists the open injuries that occurred in at least 10 cases. The amounts of floating migrant patients were more than those of local resident patients in each of the open injuries except open wound of thigh and elbow, indicating that floating migrant patients were more vulnerable to open injuries.

Fractures that appeared in at least 20 cases were sifted out. These fractures are listed in Table S1 (Lines with yellow background). There were 30 kinds of fractures left after the selection. The ribs and clavicle are the most vulnerable parts of body to fracture and accounted for 11.4% and 5.1% of all traffic injuries, respectively.

## Inpatient duration and hospitalization cost distribution of traffic injury patients

Inpatient duration and hospitalization cost were analyzed for all RTI patients. These patients were grouped according to the severity of injuries and their household status. The average, median, 25% percentile, 75% percentile and standard deviation of inpatient duration and total cost distribution of mild, moderate, severe and deceased groups were calculated and are listed in Table S2. From the mild to severe group, the average, median, 25% percentile, 75% percentile and standard deviation of inpatient duration and total cost increased with the enhancement of severity. In these three groups, the difference in these parameters, between local and floating migrant patients, was more apparent.

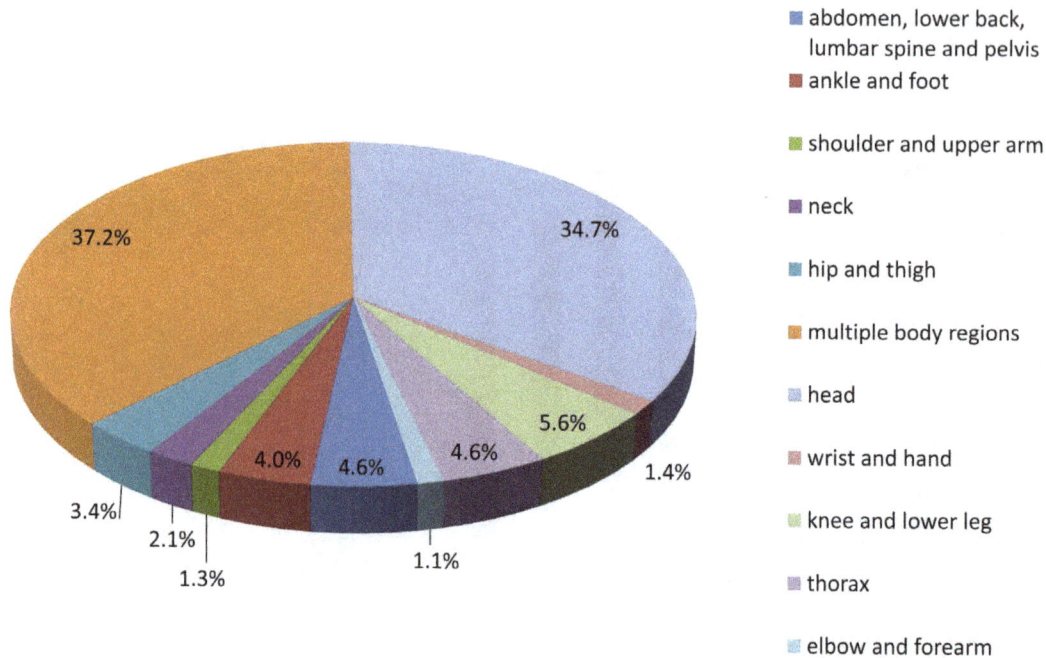

**Figure 4. Area of the body injured, as a proportion of total RTIs, from 2007 to 2010.**

## Discussion

Motor vehicle accident is a common cause of road traffic injuries and deaths throughout the world. According to a WHO report, traffic accidents cause 1.27 million deaths and 20 to 50 million injuries around the world annually [15]. In China, with the recent economic boom, vehicle volume and the number of traffic accident fatalities have become the highest in the world. Wang el al. [16]estimated that deaths from vehicle collisions increased 97-fold from 1951 to 1999 in China; and RTIs had become a leading cause of death, accounting for 3.25 percent of all deaths and one third of all injury-related deaths between 2002 and 2006. With such a severe situation in China's road traffic safety, there is an urgent need to study the RTIs characteristics and risk factors that determine traffic violations and traffic accident severity.

A lot of factors contribute to the fast increase of road traffic accidents and injuries in recent China. With the development of the social economy and increased living standard, the ownership of motor vehicles has quickly risen among the middle class population, which has resulted in more road traffic congestion and accidents [17,18]. Besides, increases in travel between the city and outside is one factor contributing to the high frequency of accidents [19]. In big Chinese cities, such as Beijing and Shanghai, the floating migrants make up a large section of the entire population of the city. Due to the high mobility characteristics of these people, the fast expansion of floating population could be a factor contributing to the high frequency of road traffic accidents. On the other hand, most of the floating migrants were from rural area. They were less educated and involved in low-level physical labor such as freight transportation [1]. A study about the risk factors of traffic accident severity in China showed that driver's gender, education level, household status and occupation were associated with traffic violations and injury severity [20]. So migrant workers exhibited a high risk for severe accidents.

In our study, the RTIs characteristics of floating migrant population were analyzed through comparison with those of local residents. From 2007 to 2010, there were between 500 and 600 RTI patients seen by this hospital annually. Floating migrant patients accounted for 41.6% of RTIs during the four years. This proportion reflected that a great deal of exchange was occurring between this harbor city and outside. The average risks of RTIs over the four years for local residents and floating migrants were different (0.632 versus 1.005 per thousand people). This result indicated that floating population exhibited a higher risk of RTIs compared to local residents. In view of the gender distribution of RTIs patients, the proportion of male patients in these four years ranged between 2/3 and 3/4. Male patients made up the majority of traffic accident sufferers, likely because men are generally the

**Table 1.** Severity distribution of the head injury group and multiple body regions injury group from 2007 to 2010.

| severity | Head and face injuries | | | | Multiple sites injuries | | | |
|---|---|---|---|---|---|---|---|---|
| | mild | moderate | severe | dead | mild | moderate | severe | dead |
| Local resident patients | 251 | 132 | 35 | 13 | 105 | 297 | 65 | 10 |
| Floating migrant patients | 168 | 124 | 35 | 11 | 68 | 216 | 56 | 6 |
| Proportion of floating migrant patients(%) | 40.1 | 48.4 | 50.0 | 45.8 | 39.3 | 42.1 | 46.3 | 37.5 |

**Table 2.** Open injuries that occurred at least 10 times from 2007 to 2010.

| RTIs | T | Local patients | | | Migrant patients | | | |
| | | N | A* | STD* | N | A* | STD* | Prop. |
| --- | --- | --- | --- | --- | --- | --- | --- | --- |
| Open wound of ankle | 17 | 4 | 46.5 | 27 | 13 | 27.6 | 7.9 | 0.76 |
| Open wound of auricle Pinna | 10 | 3 | 33 | 19.1 | 7 | 31.3 | 12.5 | 0.70 |
| Open wound of lower leg | 45 | 15 | 47.5 | 15.9 | 30 | 32.4 | 10.3 | 0.67 |
| Open wound of finger(s) | 10 | 4 | 51.8 | 19.4 | 6 | 29.8 | 10.7 | 0.60 |
| Open fracture of tibia | 10 | 4 | 31.5 | 20.4 | 6 | 32.7 | 9.4 | 0.60 |
| Open wound of head | 137 | 57 | 43.6 | 14.2 | 80 | 33.3 | 13 | 0.58 |
| Open fracture of tibial and fibula | 36 | 15 | 49.7 | 15.9 | 21 | 37.4 | 12.5 | 0.58 |
| Open wound of foot | 63 | 27 | 42.1 | 22.2 | 36 | 28.3 | 11.8 | 0.57 |
| Open wound of nose | 46 | 20 | 31.2 | 13 | 26 | 30 | 10.9 | 0.57 |
| Open intracranial injuries | 18 | 8 | 46.4 | 19 | 10 | 30.1 | 11.7 | 0.56 |
| Open wound of ear | 39 | 18 | 38.3 | 13.7 | 21 | 36.2 | 10.7 | 0.54 |
| Open wound of upper arm | 13 | 6 | 36.8 | 18.5 | 7 | 33.4 | 16.5 | 0.54 |
| Open wound of forearm | 17 | 8 | 40.4 | 25 | 9 | 30.3 | 6.5 | 0.53 |
| Open wound of knee | 31 | 15 | 37.3 | 11.8 | 16 | 31.1 | 16 | 0.52 |
| Open wound of lip | 106 | 52 | 35.7 | 17 | 54 | 31.6 | 11.7 | 0.51 |
| Open wound of thigh | 21 | 11 | 39.6 | 15.4 | 10 | 28.3 | 4.6 | 0.48 |
| Open wound of elbow | 19 | 11 | 39.5 | 17.1 | 8 | 32.5 | 12.5 | 0.42 |

(T = total amount, N = number of local or floating migrant patients, A = average, STD = standard deviation, Prop. = proportion of floating migrant patients with each injury).
*The unit of A and STD is years old.

main laborers in society. This phenomenon was more obvious in the floating migrant patients, because female RTIs patients with local household were less than those of floating migrants in each of the four years.

Patients between 16 and 55 years of age constituted the majority of RTI patients likely because people in this age range are the main labor force in society. This was also demonstrated in a recent study examining RTIs in Shanghai [21]. Pre-school children had a higher accident incidence compared to school-children under the age of 16. The probable reason is that compulsory education in China starts in primary school. Before that age, pre-school children are not all taken to the nursery and some children stay at home with parents or grandparents. The age distribution of local and floating migrant patients was also different. Floating migrant patients had a higher accident incidence between ages 16 and 45, while local resident patients had a higher accident incidence between ages 46 and 55. The reason for this difference is likely that the majority of floating migrants in this city are mostly young people who came to the city for business. The detailed age distributions of locals and floating migrant population in this district were not available in any public dataset or yearbook. But according to the report of China National Bureau of Statistics in 2001, among 121 million floating population over the country in 2000, 83% were of working age(from 15 to 64 years). So we believed that the difference spread by age was partly due to different population demographics between local and floating migrant patients. For the local residents, increased age was related to the likelihood of injury from a traffic accident [22].

March, June and October were found to be the months with the most RTI patients with 217, 216 and 218 patients for each month, respectively. February and January were the months that had fewer RTI patients with 107 and 146 patients, respectively. The proportions of floating migrant patients were just 27.4% and

33.6% in these two months, which were less than those of other months too. This is because January and February are usually the months in which the lunar calendar Spring Festival of China occurs. Most floating migrants go back home, thus there are fewer RTIs during these two months. This monthly distribution result is also in accordance with that found in Beijing from 2004 to 2008 [23], which is near Tianjin.

In a traffic accident, any part of body may be injured. The data in this paper showed that most patients had head or multiple body region injuries. These two groups accounted for 34.6% and 37% of all patients. The numbers of local resident patients and floating migrant patients in these two groups were counted and classified according to the severity of injuries: mild, moderate, severe and deceased. The proportion of floating migrant patients increased as the severity of injury increased from mild to severe. We supposed that this was due to the fact that floating migrant patients likely traverse, not only the city district, but also between the city and outside. On the highways, the speed limit is over that of city roads and there is no traffic regulation. Accidents that happen on the highway usually cause severe injuries or death [24]. Meanwhile, many floating migrants have lower level of education. They lack the knowledge and consciousness of safe-driving. This is also a risk factor for traffic violation and accident severity. Therefore, floating migrants are more vulnerable to severe RTIs compared with local residents.

Statistical analysis of RTIs means a lot to emergency clinics. Injuries that had occurred at least 20 times were reviewed. For each of these injuries, we calculated the floating migrant patient proportion with each injury, and the mean, median, 25% percentile and 75% percentile ages in both the local resident patient and floating migrant patient groups. The results showed that the top injuries with higher proportion of floating migrant patients were mostly associated with high energy accidents, for example traumatic spleen rupture, fracture of acetabulum, contusion of kidney or fracture of the shaft of the femur. In contrast, the injuries with smaller proportions were generally upper extremity or neck injuries, or injuries or diseases associated with aging, for example fracture of humerus, superficial injury of neck, hypertension and type 2 diabetes. Among these injuries, the open injuries, except open wound of thigh and open wound of elbow, had the proportions more than 0.5, which indicated that floating migrant patients were more vulnerable to open injuries. For fractures, those with larger proportions were usually associated with high-energy crashes. However, fractures with smaller proportions were usually associated with low-energy crashes or with aging, such as fracture of lumbar vertebra and intertrochanteric fracture of the femur. To sum up, statistical analysis results of RTIs supports that local resident patients are usually associated with low-energy accidents while floating migrant patients are usually associated with high-energy accidents, and that ages have an impact on the RTI distribution among local resident patients.

Due to the reasons mentioned above, inpatient duration and hospitalization costs were different for local versus floating migrant patients. Hospitalization costs for floating migrant patients increased with the severity of injury (mild to severe) from below to a great deal above that of local residents. For the inpatient duration, there was an increase in both the local residents and floating migrants with injury, but that it increased more slowly among floating migrants.

## Conclusion

In the current paper the hospital records of RTI patients seen in a tertiary hospital in a harbor city of China between the year of 2007 and 2010, were analyzed. The results showed that floating migrant patients had different characteristics than local resident patients in terms of age, the type and severity of injuries, inpatient

duration, hospitalization cost. We attribute this to the fact that most floating migrants are young businessmen from out of the city and they spend more time on the road, especially on the highway. In contrast, the population of local residents consists of different ages and elder people who are more vulnerable to injuries resulting from traffic accidents compared to younger people. In light of this study, further research should be done and more consideration given to the health of floating migrants.

## Supporting Information

**Table S1 Age distribution of diagnosed injuries that occurred at least 20 times among all patients.** (T = total number of patients in each disease, N = the number of local or migrant patients in each disease, A = average, M = median, Q = 25% percentile, 3Q = 75% percentile, S = standard deviation) * The unit of A, M, Q, 3Q and S is years old.

**Table S2 Inpatient duration and total cost distribution for mild, moderate, severe injury and deceased groups for both local and floating migrant patients.** * The unit of duration is day. ** The unit of expense is USD.

## Acknowledgments

Mrs. Haiyan Zhang and Mr. Feng Su at the fifth center hospital of Tianjin are acknowledged for their assistance with data preparation.

## Author Contributions

Conceived and designed the experiments: BJ DZ TW. Performed the experiments: CX. Analyzed the data: YW NH YK. Contributed reagents/materials/analysis tools: XY PZ. Wrote the paper: CX.

## References

1. Liang Z, Ma ZD (2004) China's floating population: new evidence from the 2000 census. Population and Development Review, 30, 467–488.
2. Report on China's Migrant Population Development 2012 (2012) China Population Publishing House. [In Chinese]
3. Wang JW, Cui ZT, Cui HW, Wei CN, Harada K, et al. (2010) Quality of life associated with perceived stigma and discrimination among the floating population in Shanghai, China: a qualitative study. Health Promot Int, 25(4):394–402
4. Li X, Zhang H, Jiang S, Wang J, Liu X, et al. (2010) Active pulmonary tuberculosis case detection and treatment among floating population in China: an effective pilot. J Immigr Minor Health, 12(6):811–5.
5. Anderson AF, Qingsi Z, Hua X, Jianfeng B (2003) China's floating population and the potential for HIV transmission: a social-behavioural perspective. AIDS Care, 15(2):177–85.
6. Xu T, Gong L, Wang H, Zhang R, Wang X, et al. (2013) Epidemiology of Unintentional Injuries Among Children Under Six Years Old in Floating and Residential Population in Four Communities in Beijing: A Comparative Study. Matern Child Health J, 22.
7. Fang LQ, de Vlas SJ, Feng D, Liang S, Xu YF, et al. (2009) Geographical spread of SARS in mainland China. Trop Med Int Health, 14 Suppl 1:14–20.
8. Zhong NS, Zheng BJ, Li YM, Poon, Xie ZH, et al. (2003) Epidemiology and cause of severe acute respiratory syndrome (SARS) in Guangdong, People's Republic of China, in February, 2003. Lancet, 362(9393):1353–8.
9. Annuals of Road Traffic Accidents of the People's Republic of China, 2010 (2011) Traffic Management Bureau, the Ministry of Public Security of the People's Republic of China.
10. Wang LJ, Hu N, Wan X, Zhou MG, Wang J (2010) Status and trend of injury deaths among Chinese population, 1991–2005. Zhonghua Yu Fang Yi Xue Za Zhi 44(4): 309–313. [In Chinese]
11. Tianjin Statistical Yearbook 2008 (2008) Tianjin Municipal Bureau of Statistics & Survey Office of National Bureau of Statistics in Tianjin.
12. Tianjin Statistical Yearbook 2009 (2009) Tianjin Municipal Bureau of Statistics & Survey Office of National Bureau of Statistics in Tianjin.

13. Tianjin Statistical Yearbook 2010 (2010) Tianjin Municipal Bureau of Statistics & Survey Office of National Bureau of Statistics in Tianjin.
14. Tianjin Binhai New Area Statistical Yearbook 2011 (2011) Tianjin Binhai New Area Bureau of Statistics.
15. World Report on Road Traffic Injury Prevention (2004) World Health Organization, Geneva. Available: http://www.who.int/world-health-day/2004/infomaterials/world_report/.
16. Wang SY, Li YH, Chi GB, Xiao SY, Ozanne-Smith J, et al. (2008) Injury-related fatalities in China: an under-recognized public-health problem. Lancet 372:1765–1773.
17. Jiang BG (2011) Status of road traffic injury rescue and current work in China. Chin Med J (Engl) 124(23): 3850–3851.
18. Wang C, Chi GB, Wang SY, Dong XM (2011) The relationship between secular trend of road traffic injuries and gross domestic product per capita in China. Zhonghua Yu Fang Yi Xue Za Zhi 45(4): 350–353. [In Chinese]
19. Global status report on road safety: time for action (2013) World Health Organization, Geneva. Available: http://www.who.int/violence_injury_prevention/road_safety_status/2013.
20. Zhang G, Yau KK, Chen G (2013) Risk factors associated with traffic violations and accident severity in China. Accid Anal Prev, 59:18–25.
21. Li YH, Rahim Yousif, Lu W, Song GX, Yu Y, et al. (2006) Pattern of traffic injuries in Shanghai: implications for control. Int J Inj Contr Saf Promot 13(4): 217–225.
22. Nagata T, Takamori T, Berg H-Y, Hasselberg M (2012) Comparing the impact of socio-demographic factors associated with traffic injury among older road users and the general population in Japan. BMC Public Health 12: 887.
23. Peng JP, Wang YH, Zhang ZJ, Wang J, Zhang PX, et al. (2011) Time distribution characteristics of traffic injury in different age groups in Beijing from 2004 to 2008. Beijing Da Xue Xue Bao 43(5): 739–742.
24. Zhao J, Deng W (2012) Traffic accidents on expressways: new threat to China. Traffic Inj Prev 13(3): 230–238.

# 16

# Prevalence and Predictors of Sub-Acute Phase Disability after Injury among Hospitalised and Non-Hospitalised Groups

**Sarah Derrett**[1]*, **Ari Samaranayaka**[1], **Suzanne Wilson**[1], **John Langley**[1], **Shanthi Ameratunga**[2], **Ian D. Cameron**[3], **Rebbecca Lilley**[1], **Emma Wyeth**[4], **Gabrielle Davie**[1]

1 Injury Prevention Research Unit, Department of Preventive and Social Medicine, Dunedin School of Medicine, University of Otago, Dunedin, New Zealand, 2 School of Population Health, Faculty of Medical and Health Sciences, University of Auckland, Auckland, New Zealand, 3 Rehabilitation Studies Unit, Sydney Medical School, University of Sydney, Sydney, Australia, 4 Te Roopū Rangahau Hauora Māori a Ngāi Tahu (Ngāi Tahu Māori Health Research Unit), Department of Preventive and Social Medicine, Dunedin School of Medicine, University of Otago, Dunedin, New Zealand

## Abstract

*Introduction:* To reduce the burden on injury survivors and their supporters, factors associated with poor outcomes need to be identified so that timely post-injury interventions can be implemented. To date, few studies have investigated outcomes for both those who were hospitalised and those who were not.

*Aim:* To describe the prevalence and to identify pre-injury and injury-related predictors of disability among hospitalised and non-hospitalised people, three months after injury.

*Methods:* Participants in the Prospective Outcomes of Injury Study were aged 18–64 years and on an injury entitlement claims register with New Zealand's no-fault injury compensation insurer, following referral by healthcare professionals. A wide range of pre-injury demographic, health and injury-related characteristics were collected at interview. Participants were categorised as 'hospitalised' if they were placed on New Zealand's National Minimum Data Set within seven days of the injury event. Injury severity scores (NISS) and 12 injury categories were derived from ICD-10 codes. WHODAS assessed disability. Multivariable analyses examined relationships between explanatory variables and disability.

*Results:* Of 2856 participants, 2752 (96%) had WHODAS scores available for multivariable analysis; 673 were hospitalised; 2079 were not. Disability was highly prevalent among hospitalised (53.6%) and non-hospitalised (39.4%) participants, three-months after injury. In both groups, pre-injury disability, obesity and higher injury severity were associated with increased odds of post-injury disability. A range of other factors were associated with disability in only one group: e.g. female, ≥2 chronic conditions and leg fracture among hospitalised; aged 35–54 years, trouble accessing healthcare, spine or lower extremity sprains/dislocations and assault among non-hospitalised.

*Significance:* Disability was highly prevalent among both groups yet, with a few exceptions, factors associated with disability were not common to both groups. Where possible, including a range of injured people in studies, hospitalised and not, will increase understanding of the burden of disability in the sub-acute phase.

**Editor:** Jerson Laks, Federal University of Rio de Janeiro, Brazil

**Funding:** This study is funded by the Health Research Council of New Zealand (2007-2013), and was co-funded by the Accident Compensation Corporation, New Zealand (2007–2010). The views and conclusions expressed herein are the authors' and may not reflect those of the funders. EW was supported by a Health Research Council of New Zealand Eru Pomare Research Fellowship, RL by an ACC Early Research Career Post-Doctoral Fellowship and IDC by an Australian National Health and Medical Research Council Practitioner Fellowship. The Accident Compensation Corporation sent out invitations to eligible potential participants on the research team's behalf, and also provided, following participants' consent, information from the electronic record about participants' injuries. The funders had no role in study design, analysis, decision to publish, or preparation of the manuscript.

**Competing Interests:** The authors have declared that no competing interests exist.

* E-mail: sarah.derrett@otago.ac.nz

## Introduction

For most countries, injury is the leading cause of mortality among younger people [1]. Injuries are also known to have important consequences for survivors of injury; particularly for those whose injury does not heal promptly and precludes return to pre-injury function, activity and participation in life [2,3]. More needs to be known about the factors associated with poor outcomes at a population level [4–6]. In addition, to reduce burden among injury survivors and their families/supporters, characteristics associated with poor outcomes need to be identified so that timely and effective post-injury interventions can be implemented.

Despite the acknowledged gap in understanding the burden associated with poor outcomes following injury, few studies have investigated outcomes for people with 'all types of injury' [7,8].

Furthermore, research considering 'all injury' has tended to focus on general health, functional or employment outcomes rather than disability [7,9–12].

In studies of injury outcome, few have investigated outcomes for non-hospitalised people; perhaps because of an assumption that injured people who are not hospitalised are likely to have short recovery periods [13]. In the Netherlands, researchers found that people followed up after an emergency department (ED) visit for an injury had recovered, on a global measure of functional status, to a level equivalent to the general population, whereas people admitted to hospital for their injury had not [14]. However, a meta-analysis of data from studies of functioning after injury in a number of countries, found poor outcomes associated with injuries not commonly involving hospitalisation, such as sprains and strains [8]. A study of outcomes for survivors of car crashes found that among those with 'minor' injuries (Abbreviated Injury Scale; AIS = 1), as many as 10% had a permanent medical impairment [15]. The prospective UK Burden of Injury Study recruited injured participants from hospital in-patient admissions and emergency-department (ED) attendees [6]. This study found that disability was greater among in-patients yet, at the level of the population, considerable disability burden was estimated for those attending ED without a hospital admission [6].

To date, we do not know about the risk of adverse disability outcomes for those who are not hospitalised following injury. The Prospective Outcomes of Injury Study (POIS) provides an ideal opportunity to investigate factors associated with disability for both hospitalised and non-hospitalised injured people.

POIS is a longitudinal cohort study in New Zealand with the primary objective of identifying factors associated with disability following injury. The aims of this paper are threefold: 1) To determine whether there are differences in pre-injury and injury-related characteristics between hospitalised and non-hospitalised sub-groups of POIS participants; 2) To describe the prevalence of disability in the sub-acute phase, three months after injury, for both hospitalised and non-hospitalised groups; and 3) To identify

pre-injury and injury-related predictors of disability among hospitalised and non-hospitalised sub-groups.

## Methods

### Study Participants

The study was undertaken following approval from the New Zealand Health and Disability Multi-Region Ethics Committee (MEC/07/07/093). Following feedback from participants in the pilot study and to be inclusive of all people (including those with poor vision or limited literacy), and with the approval of the Ethics Committee, all participants granted oral consent to participate after receiving comprehensive information about the study. Oral consent was documented by interviewers, and all participants received copies of the consent form. POIS design, recruitment and participants' characteristics have been described previously [16,17]. Briefly, potential participants were aged 18–64 years and lived in one of five regions in New Zealand. Following referral by an accredited primary or secondary healthcare professional, participants had all been placed onto an injury (entitlement claims) register at the Accident Compensation Corporation (ACC), the organisation responsible for New Zealand's no-fault compensation scheme. All injured people in New Zealand are eligible for accident compensation by law; approximately 1.75 million injury claims are lodged with ACC annually; 'entitlement claimants' comprise approximately 7% of injuries referred to ACC [18,19]. These people have injuries serious enough to potentially require 'on-going support', such as income compensation (if in paid employment), medical treatment costs and social and vocational services [19]. People were not eligible for the study if they had been placed on the sensitive claims register (e.g. people who have been sexually assaulted) or if their injury was the result of self-harm [17].

Between December 2007 and August 2009, 7875 entitlement claimants were sent letters about the study by ACC, of whom 4881 people were able to be contacted by the research team; 2856 (59%)

**Table 1.** Pre-injury socio-demographic characteristics of participants according to hospitalisation status (n = 2752).

| Explanatory variables | | Hospitalised | | Non-hospitalised | | P value** |
|---|---|---|---|---|---|---|
| | | n | %* | n | %* | |
| Age | 18–34 years | 266 | 27.9 | 689 | 72.1 | 0.007 |
| | 35–54 years | 284 | 22.1 | 1002 | 77.9 | |
| | 55–64 years | 123 | 24.1 | 388 | 75.9 | |
| Gender | Male | 458 | 27.1 | 1231 | 72.9 | <0.001 |
| | Female | 215 | 20.2 | 848 | 79.8 | |
| Education | None | 106 | 25.4 | 311 | 74.6 | 0.909 |
| | Secondary school | 159 | 23.7 | 512 | 76.3 | |
| | Other | 397 | 24.5 | 1226 | 75.5 | |
| Living arrangements | Alone | 74 | 28.2 | 188 | 71.8 | 0.483 |
| | With non-family | 60 | 24.1 | 189 | 75.9 | |
| | With family | 537 | 24.1 | 1693 | 75.9 | |
| Paid employment | Yes | 610 | 24.1 | 1922 | 75.9 | 0.258 |
| | No | 63 | 28.8 | 156 | 71.2 | |
| Financial status | Sufficient | 604 | 24.5 | 1866 | 75.5 | 0.026 |
| | Insufficient | 57 | 22.3 | 199 | 77.7 | |

*Row percentage.
**P value from Chi2 test to compare hospitalised and non-hospitalised groups between variable categories.

**Table 2.** Pre-injury health and psychosocial characteristics of participants according to hospitalisation status (n = 2752).

| Explanatory variables | | Hospitalised | | Non-hospitalised | | P value** |
|---|---|---|---|---|---|---|
| | | n | %* | n | %* | |
| General health | Excellent/ Very good/ Good | 642 | 24.7 | 1960 | 75.3 | 0.540 |
| | Fair/ Poor | 30 | 20.7 | 115 | 79.3 | |
| Chronic conditions | 0 | 361 | 26.0 | 1025 | 74.0 | 0.046 |
| | 1 | 184 | 25.0 | 551 | 75.0 | |
| | ≥2 | 111 | 20.4 | 433 | 79.6 | |
| Depressive-type episode | No | 537 | 24.4 | 1663 | 75.6 | 0.895 |
| | Yes | 135 | 24.7 | 411 | 75.3 | |
| Optimism | Yes | 598 | 25.0 | 1798 | 75.0 | 0.192 |
| | No | 69 | 21.8 | 248 | 78.2 | |
| Self-efficacy | Not poor | 619 | 25.0 | 1853 | 75.0 | 0.085 |
| | Poor | 50 | 19.8 | 202 | 80.2 | |
| Comfort in faith or spiritual beliefs | Very much/ Quite a bit | 214 | 23.0 | 718 | 77.0 | 0.323 |
| | Somewhat/ A little bit/ Not at all | 435 | 25.4 | 1277 | 74.6 | |
| | Missing | 24 | 22.2 | 84 | 77.8 | |
| Family involvement | Very large/ Large | 586 | 24.2 | 1836 | 75.8 | 0.632 |
| | Small/ Very small | 83 | 26.6 | 229 | 73.4 | |
| Social relationships | Satisfied | 630 | 24.5 | 1945 | 75.5 | 0.852 |
| | Not satisfied | 39 | 23.8 | 125 | 76.2 | |
| Sense of community | Strong | 189 | 22.8 | 639 | 77.2 | 0.627 |
| | In-between | 282 | 25.2 | 839 | 74.8 | |
| | Very little | 169 | 25.3 | 499 | 74.7 | |
| | Missing | 33 | 24.4 | 102 | 75.6 | |
| Physical activity | ≥5 days | 378 | 25.4 | 1109 | 74.6 | 0.440 |
| | <5 days | 282 | 23.3 | 926 | 76.7 | |
| Sleep | ≥5 nights | 512 | 24.9 | 1543 | 75.1 | 0.557 |
| | <5 nights | 148 | 22.9 | 498 | 77.1 | |
| BMI | Underweight/ Normal/ Overweight | 477 | 24.2 | 1497 | 75.8 | 0.552 |
| | Obese | 162 | 24.6 | 497 | 75.4 | |
| | Missing | 34 | 28.6 | 85 | 71.4 | |
| Smoking | No | 465 | 24.2 | 1458 | 75.8 | 0.858 |
| | Yes | 206 | 25.1 | 616 | 74.9 | |
| Alcohol use | Low | 287 | 22.5 | 987 | 77.5 | 0.007 |
| | Moderate | 216 | 23.7 | 695 | 76.3 | |
| | High | 163 | 30.0 | 381 | 70.0 | |
| Recreational drug use | No | 524 | 23.6 | 1697 | 76.4 | 0.099 |
| | Yes | 147 | 28.1 | 377 | 71.9 | |

*Row percentage.
**P value from Chi2 test to compare hospitalised and non-hospitalised groups between variable categories.

participated in the first interview three months (on average) after injury [17].

## Outcome

The measure of disability was the brief World Health Organization Disability Assessment Schedule II 12-item instrument (WHODAS) [20]. This assesses activity limitations and participation restrictions over the past 30 days along six dimensions (understanding and communication, self-care, mobility, interpersonal relationships, work and household roles, and community roles), with 12 questions (concerning standing, household responsibilities, learning, community activities, emotionally affected by health problems, concentrating, walking a long distance, washing whole body, getting dressed, dealing with unknown people, friendships, day to day work). Each of the twelve questions has five difficulty-level response options: 'None = 0, Mild = 1, Moderate = 2, Severe = 3 or Extreme/Cannot do = 4'. The 12 response scores were summed using the simple-summed approach to provide a total score with a possible range from 0 (no disability) to 48 (maximum disability) [21]. Participants missing a response to one of the 12 items had their average score, from the 11 completed responses, imputed for the missing response; if more

**Table 3.** Injury-related characteristics of participants according to hospitalisation status (n = 2752).

| Explanatory variables | | Hospitalised | | Non-hospitalised | | P value** |
|---|---|---|---|---|---|---|
| | | n | %* | n | %* | |
| Injury cause | Accidental | 620 | 23.6 | 2010 | 76.4 | <0.001 |
| | Assault | 51 | 46.4 | 59 | 53.6 | |
| Threat to life | No | 506 | 21.2 | 1881 | 78.8 | <0.001 |
| | Yes/ Maybe | 144 | 44.7 | 178 | 55.3 | |
| Threat of severe longer-term disability | No | 312 | 19.8 | 1267 | 80.2 | <0.001 |
| | Yes/ Maybe | 339 | 30.2 | 784 | 69.8 | |
| Access to healthcare services | No trouble | 586 | 23.9 | 1863 | 76.1 | 0.184 |
| | Trouble/Mixed | 80 | 28.9 | 197 | 71.1 | |
| Injury severity | NISS 1–3 | 174 | 15.7 | 936 | 84.3 | <0.001 |
| | NISS 4–6 | 321 | 27.6 | 842 | 72.4 | |
| | NISS >6 | 162 | 41.9 | 225 | 58.1 | |
| *Injury categories#* | | | | | | |
| Intracranial | No | 624 | 23.5 | 2030 | 76.5 | <0.001 |
| | Yes | 49 | 50.0 | 49 | 50.0 | |
| Head/neck superficial | No | 624 | 23.5 | 2030 | 76.5 | <0.001 |
| | Yes | 49 | 50.0 | 49 | 50.0 | |
| Spine sprain/ strain or dislocation | No | 623 | 26.9 | 1691 | 73.1 | <0.001 |
| | Yes | 50 | 11.4 | 388 | 88.6 | |
| Upper extremity fracture | No | 499 | 22.0 | 1771 | 78.0 | <0.001 |
| | Yes | 174 | 36.1 | 308 | 63.9 | |
| Upper extremity sprain/ strain or dislocation | No | 602 | 25.5 | 1756 | 74.5 | 0.001 |
| | Yes | 71 | 18.0 | 323 | 82.0 | |
| Upper extremity open wound | No | 597 | 23.1 | 1992 | 76.9 | <0.001 |
| | Yes | 76 | 46.6 | 87 | 53.4 | |
| Upper extremity superficial | No | 642 | 24.5 | 1978 | 75.5 | 0.790 |
| | Yes | 31 | 23.5 | 101 | 76.5 | |
| Lower extremity fracture | No | 474 | 20.8 | 1810 | 79.2 | <0.001 |
| | Yes | 199 | 42.5 | 269 | 57.5 | |
| Lower extremity sprain/ strain or dislocation | No | 583 | 28.2 | 1486 | 71.8 | <0.001 |
| | Yes | 90 | 13.2 | 593 | 86.8 | |
| Lower extremity open wound | No | 624 | 23.6 | 2018 | 76.4 | <0.001 |
| | Yes | 49 | 44.5 | 61 | 55.5 | |
| Lower extremity superficial | No | 638 | 24.8 | 1932 | 75.2 | 0.090 |
| | Yes | 35 | 19.2 | 147 | 80.8 | |
| Other | No | 472 | 20.7 | 1803 | 79.3 | <0.001 |
| | Yes | 201 | 42.1 | 276 | 57.9 | |

*Row percentage.
**P value from Chi2 test to compare hospitalised and non-hospitalised groups between variable categories.
# Multiple injury categories possible.

than one response was missing, the participant's scores were not summed for analysis [21]. Participants were asked to report WHODAS status in the 30 days pre-injury and in the 30 days before the interview (three months after injury). For multivariable analysis, participants were dichotomised into 'disability' or 'no disability' groups based on whether their WHODAS score was greater than, or equal to, 10 [21].

## Hospital

Participants in this study were categorised as 'hospitalised' if they appeared in New Zealand's National Minimum Data Set (NMDS) which: "For the purposes of the national collections, healthcare users who receive assessment and/or treatment for three hours or more, or who have a general anaesthetic, are to be admitted. This also applies to healthcare users of Emergency Departments" [22]. To identify those admitted in proximal response to the injury, a threshold of admission within seven days from the date of the injury event was used [23]. POIS data were

**Table 4.** Prevalence (and 95%CI) of participants with WHODAS disability scores ≥10 according to pre-injury socio-demographic characteristics and hospitalisation status (n = 2752).

| Explanatory variables | | Hospitalised | | | Non-hospitalised | | |
|---|---|---|---|---|---|---|---|
| | | % | 95% CI | | % | 95% CI | |
| Age | 18–34 years | 52.6 | 46.6 | 58.4 | 34.7 | 31.1 | 38.2 |
| | 35–54 years | 53.2 | 47.4 | 59.0 | 43.4 | 40.3 | 46.5 |
| | 55–64 years | 56.9 | 48.1 | 65.7 | 37.1 | 32.3 | 41.9 |
| Gender | Male | 49.6 | 45.0 | 54.1 | 36.4 | 33.7 | 39.1 |
| | Female | 62.3 | 55.8 | 68.8 | 43.6 | 40.2 | 47.0 |
| Education | None | 53.8 | 44.2 | 63.3 | 45.7 | 40.1 | 51.2 |
| | Secondary school | 49.7 | 41.9 | 57.5 | 36.3 | 32.2 | 40.5 |
| | Other | 55.4 | 50.5 | 60.3 | 39.1 | 36.3 | 41.8 |
| Living arrangements | Alone | 48.7 | 37.2 | 60.1 | 37.2 | 30.3 | 44.2 |
| | With non-family | 60.0 | 47.5 | 72.5 | 36.5 | 29.6 | 43.4 |
| | With family | 53.5 | 49.2 | 57.7 | 39.9 | 37.6 | 42.3 |
| Paid employment | Yes | 52.8 | 48.8 | 56.8 | 39.0 | 36.8 | 41.2 |
| | No | 61.9 | 49.8 | 74.0 | 43.0 | 35.2 | 50.7 |
| Financial status | Sufficient | 53.8 | 49.8 | 57.8 | 38.3 | 36.1 | 40.5 |
| | Insufficient | 54.4 | 41.3 | 67.4 | 48.7 | 41.8 | 55.7 |

probabilistically linked to NMDS data to identify hospitalised participants.

## Explanatory variables

Explanatory variables were grouped according to pre-injury socio-demographic, pre-injury health and psychosocial and injury-related characteristics.

**Pre-injury socio-demographic characteristics.** Participants self-reported their socio-demographic characteristics including age at time of interview, gender, education and living arrangements, based on questions from the New Zealand Census [24]. Education was grouped as 'none', 'secondary school' (i.e. high school) level or 'other' qualifications (if these took three months or more to obtain). 'Living arrangements' were grouped as 'alone', with 'non-family' or with 'family' (including partner or spouse). People working full-time (≥30 hours per week) or part-time (<30 hours per week) were classified as being in 'paid employment'; the remaining as 'not in paid employment' [25]. 'Financial status' was classified as 'sufficient' if participants reported they had 'just enough, enough or more than enough' total household income to meet their every day needs; and 'insufficient' if they reported 'not enough' pre-injury [25].

**Pre-injury health and psychosocial characteristics.** Participants rated their pre-injury 'general health' on a five-point scale ('excellent', 'very good', 'good', 'fair' or 'poor') [26]. Pre-injury 'chronic conditions' was assessed using questions modified from the New Zealand Health Survey 2006/ 2007 [27]. Participants reported whether they had been told by a doctor that they had one or more of a list of 22 chronic illnesses or diseases (e.g. asthma, cancer, diabetes, depression or anxiety) that had lasted, or was expected to last, for more than six months.

Participants were classified as having a 'depressive-type episode' if they responded affirmatively to at least one of two screening questions asking whether nearly every day, for a period of two weeks or more in the year before injury, they had felt 'sad, blue or depressed', and/or 'loss of interest in things like work or hobbies or

things they usually like to do for fun' [28]. Pre-injury 'optimism' was measured by asking a single question from the Life Orientation Test [29]. Participants who 'strongly agreed' or 'agreed' with the statement that "Overall, I expect more good things to happen to me than bad" were compared with the rest. 'Self-efficacy' was based on the General Self-Efficacy Scale, a scale that assesses problem-solving capabilities in relation to a variety of difficult demands in ten aspects of life [30]. The responses 'strongly disagree', 'disagree', 'neutral/mixed', 'agree', and 'strongly agree' were scored from 0 to 4 respectively and summed to provide a total score. Poor self-efficacy was defined as a score ≤25, out of a possible score of 40. Participants were asked if they found "comfort in faith and spiritual beliefs", using a single question from the FACIT-Sp (permission granted by www.facit.org), which had five options ranging from 'not at all' to 'very much' [31].

'Family involvement' was assessed by asking whether family played a 'very large', 'large', 'small' or 'very small' part in participants' lives pre-injury [25]. Participants rated their overall satisfaction with 'social relationships' (including contact with relatives and friends, quality of relationships with your partner and/or family and frequency of social contact). Those stating they were 'completely' or 'mostly' satisfied were classified as 'satisfied'; those stating they were 'neither satisfied nor dissatisfied', 'mostly' or 'completely' dissatisfied were classified as 'not satisfied'. People stated whether they felt their neighbourhood's 'sense of community' was 'strong', 'very little' or 'something in-between' [32].

Participants reported pre-injury 'physical activity' according to the number of days in the seven-day period prior to injury that they had engaged in either 30 minutes of moderate activity (including brisk walking) or 15 minutes of vigorous activity [33]. Pre-injury 'sleep' was assessed by asking participants to report the number of nights per week that they (usually) had seven or more hours sleep. Participants reported pre-injury height and weight; derived Body Mass Index ('BMI') categories were underweight (BMI<18.5), normal (18.5–24.9), overweight (25–29.9) and obese (≥30), with the first three combined for analyses [34]. Pre-injury

**Table 5.** Prevalence (and 95%CI) of participants with WHODAS disability scores ≥10 according to pre-injury health and psychosocial characteristics and hospitalisation status (n = 2752).

| Explanatory variables | | Hospitalised | | | Non-hospitalised | | |
|---|---|---|---|---|---|---|---|
| | | % | 95% CI | | % | 95% CI | |
| General health | Excellent/ Very good/ Good | 53.6 | 49.6 | 57.5 | 38.9 | 36.7 | 41.1 |
| | Fair/ Poor | 53.3 | 34.3 | 71.7 | 46.1 | 36.7 | 55.6 |
| Chronic conditions | 0 | 49.9 | 45.0 | 55.0 | 35.8 | 32.9 | 38.7 |
| | 1 | 52.2 | 44.9 | 59.4 | 38.8 | 34.8 | 42.9 |
| | ≥2 | 68.5 | 59.8 | 77.2 | 48.7 | 44.0 | 53.4 |
| Depressive-type episode | No | 51.8 | 47.5 | 56.0 | 38.0 | 35.7 | 40.3 |
| | Yes | 60.7 | 52.5 | 69.0 | 45.3 | 40.4 | 50.1 |
| Optimism | Yes | 53.3 | 49.3 | 57.3 | 38.9 | 36.7 | 41.2 |
| | No | 58.0 | 46.2 | 69.7 | 44.4 | 38.2 | 50.6 |
| Self-efficacy | Not poor | 52.8 | 48.9 | 56.8 | 38.8 | 36.6 | 41.0 |
| | Poor | 66.0 | 52.7 | 79.3 | 45.5 | 38.6 | 52.4 |
| Comfort in faith or spiritual beliefs | Very much/ Quite a bit | 62.6 | 55.8 | 69.1 | 43.7 | 40.1 | 47.4 |
| | Somewhat/ A little bit/ Not at all | 49.9 | 45.1 | 54.6 | 37.5 | 34.8 | 40.2 |
| | Missing | 41.7 | 22.1 | 63.4 | 29.8 | 20.2 | 40.7 |
| Family involvement | Very large/ Large | 54.1 | 50.1 | 58.1 | 38.8 | 36.5 | 41.0 |
| | Small/ Very small | 50.6 | 39.8 | 61.4 | 43.2 | 36.8 | 49.7 |
| Social relationships | Satisfied | 52.9 | 49.0 | 56.8 | 38.9 | 36.7 | 41.0 |
| | Not satisfied | 61.5 | 46.1 | 77.0 | 46.4 | 37.6 | 55.2 |
| Sense of community | Strong | 53.4 | 46.3 | 60.6 | 39.3 | 35.5 | 43.1 |
| | In-between | 51.4 | 45.6 | 57.3 | 38.3 | 35.0 | 41.6 |
| | Very little | 57.4 | 49.9 | 64.9 | 40.3 | 36.0 | 44.6 |
| | Missing | 54.6 | 37.3 | 71.8 | 44.1 | 34.4 | 53.8 |
| Physical activity | ≥5 days | 55.6 | 50.5 | 60.6 | 40.5 | 37.6 | 43.4 |
| | <5 days | 50.7 | 44.9 | 56.6 | 38.1 | 35.0 | 41.3 |
| Sleep | ≥5 nights | 52.9 | 48.6 | 57.3 | 40.4 | 38.0 | 42.9 |
| | <5 nights | 56.8 | 48.7 | 64.8 | 35.9 | 31.7 | 40.2 |
| BMI | Underweight/ Normal/ Overweight | 50.1 | 45.6 | 54.6 | 36.3 | 33.9 | 38.8 |
| | Obese | 63.6 | 56.1 | 71.0 | 47.9 | 43.5 | 52.3 |
| | Missing | 55.9 | 38.9 | 72.8 | 42.4 | 31.8 | 52.9 |
| Smoking | No | 56.3 | 51.8 | 60.9 | 37.9 | 35.4 | 40.4 |
| | Yes | 48.1 | 41.2 | 54.9 | 43.0 | 39.1 | 46.9 |
| Alcohol use | Low | 56.5 | 50.7 | 62.2 | 40.5 | 37.4 | 43.6 |
| | Moderate | 53.2 | 46.6 | 59.9 | 38.1 | 34.5 | 41.7 |
| | High | 50.3 | 42.6 | 58.0 | 38.3 | 33.4 | 43.2 |
| Recreational drug use | No | 54.2 | 49.8 | 58.5 | 40.2 | 37.4 | 42.6 |
| | Yes | 52.4 | 44.0 | 60.7 | 35.5 | 30.7 | 40.6 |

'smoking' was determined by asking whether or not people smoke cigarettes regularly [35]. The brief Alcohol Use Disorders Identification Test (AUDIT-C) was used to categorise participants into three 'alcohol use' groups according to their drinking patterns in the year before injury: low (males AUDIT-C score 0–4; females 0–3), moderate (males 5–7; females 4–6) or high (males 8–12; females 7–12) [36]. Participants were asked about the frequency of 'recreational drug use', i.e. marijuana/cannabis and other recreational drugs such as methamphetamine, speed, ecstasy, LSD or cocaine, with responses being: 'never', 'monthly or less', '2–4 times a month', '2–3 times a week', '4 or more times a week'.

Those who responded they never used substances in the year before injury were classified as 'no'.

**Injury characteristics.** At interview, participants were asked to report if the 'injury cause' was accidental or a physical assault; whether, at the time of injury, they felt the injury was a 'threat to their life'; and whether they felt the injury was a 'threat of severe longer-term disability'. For each of these questions those responding 'yes' or 'maybe/possibly' were grouped together and compared with those responding 'no'. Information about 'access to healthcare services' was obtained by asking people if they had

**Table 6.** Prevalence (and 95%CI) of participants with WHODAS disability scores ≥10 according to injury-related characteristics and hospitalisation status (n = 2752).

| Explanatory variables | | Hospitalised | | | Non-hospitalised | | |
|---|---|---|---|---|---|---|---|
| | | % | 95% CI | | % | 95% CI | |
| Injury cause | Accidental | 53.6 | 49.6 | 57.5 | 38.8 | 36.7 | 40.9 |
| | Assault | 52.9 | 39.1 | 66.8 | 55.9 | 43.1 | 68.7 |
| Threat to life | No | 50.4 | 46.0 | 54.8 | 38.0 | 35.8 | 40.2 |
| | Yes/ Maybe | 59.0 | 51.0 | 67.1 | 52.8 | 45.5 | 60.2 |
| Threat of severe longer-term disability | No | 45.5 | 40.0 | 51.0 | 35.8 | 33.2 | 38.5 |
| | Yes/ Maybe | 59.0 | 53.8 | 64.2 | 44.1 | 40.7 | 47.6 |
| Access to healthcare services | No trouble | 53.4 | 49.4 | 57.5 | 37.8 | 35.6 | 40.0 |
| | Trouble/ Mixed | 55.0 | 44.0 | 66.0 | 52.3 | 45.3 | 59.3 |
| Injury severity | NISS 1–3 | 35.6 | 28.5 | 42.8 | 34.8 | 31.8 | 37.9 |
| | NISS 4–6 | 57.0 | 51.6 | 62.4 | 40.4 | 37.1 | 43.7 |
| | NISS >6 | 65.4 | 58.1 | 72.8 | 52.9 | 46.3 | 59.4 |
| *Injury categories#* | | | | | | | |
| Intracranial | No | 53.2 | 49.3 | 57.1 | 39.2 | 37.0 | 41.3 |
| | Yes | 59.2 | 45.3 | 73.1 | 46.9 | 32.8 | 61.1 |
| Head/neck superficial | No | 53.0 | 49.1 | 57.0 | 39.4 | 37.3 | 41.5 |
| | Yes | 61.2 | 47.4 | 75.0 | 36.7 | 23.1 | 50.4 |
| Spine sprain/ strain or dislocation | No | 52.5 | 48.6 | 56.4 | 36.7 | 34.4 | 38.9 |
| | Yes | 68.0 | 54.9 | 81.1 | 51.0 | 46.0 | 56.0 |
| Upper extremity fracture | No | 56.9 | 52.6 | 61.3 | 40.4 | 38.1 | 42.7 |
| | Yes | 44.3 | 36.8 | 51.7 | 33.1 | 27.9 | 38.4 |
| Upper extremity sprain/ strain or dislocation | No | 55.3 | 51.3 | 59.3 | 39.9 | 37.6 | 42.2 |
| | Yes | 39.4 | 28.0 | 51.0 | 36.5 | 31.3 | 41.8 |
| Upper extremity open wound | No | 55.4 | 51.4 | 59.4 | 40.0 | 37.8 | 42.1 |
| | Yes | 39.5 | 28.4 | 50.5 | 25.3 | 16.1 | 34.5 |
| Upper extremity superficial | No | 52.5 | 48.6 | 56.4 | 39.5 | 37.4 | 41.7 |
| | Yes | 77.4 | 62.5 | 92.4 | 35.6 | 26.3 | 45.0 |
| Lower extremity fracture | No | 44.9 | 40.5 | 49.4 | 39.6 | 37.4 | 41.9 |
| | Yes | 74.4 | 68.3 | 80.5 | 37.6 | 31.7 | 43.3 |
| Lower extremity sprain/ strain or dislocation | No | 51.6 | 47.6 | 55.7 | 37.4 | 34.9 | 39.8 |
| | Yes | 66.7 | 56.9 | 76.5 | 44.4 | 40.3 | 48.4 |
| Lower extremity open wound | No | 54.2 | 50.3 | 58.1 | 39.6 | 37.5 | 41.8 |
| | Yes | 46.9 | 32.8 | 61.1 | 29.5 | 18.0 | 41.0 |
| Lower extremity superficial | No | 53.6 | 49.7 | 57.5 | 39.2 | 37.0 | 41.4 |
| | Yes | 54.3 | 37.5 | 71.0 | 41.5 | 33.5 | 49.5 |
| Other | No | 52.3 | 47.8 | 56.8 | 39.5 | 37.2 | 41.7 |
| | Yes | 56.7 | 49.8 | 63.6 | 38.4 | 32.7 | 44.2 |

# Multiple injury categories possible.

trouble getting to or contacting health services; 'yes' or 'mixed' were grouped together and compared with those who said 'no'.

All injury diagnosis information for each participant was collected from ACC in the form of Read, International Classification of Diseases ICD-9 or ICD-10 codes allocated by healthcare professionals [37]. To ensure all codes were in the same format, Read codes were mapped to ICD-10 (3-character level) using a mapping file provided by ACC; ICD-9 codes were mapped to ICD-10 using publicly-available mapping files from New Zealand's Ministry of Health. Of the 4794 ICD-10 codes thus obtained, 405 were either not within, or did not map to, S or T

injury codes. Typically, these were injury sequelae (e.g. a diagnosis of cellulitis secondary to the injury) or medical procedures. These diagnoses were recoded to the index injury identified from the text accompanying the ACC diagnosis or from participants' own descriptions of their injury. Injuries without an S or T code were manually recoded (e.g. hernia was recoded to 'other injury of abdomen') to fit within the 'diagnosis and body part' matrix described below. There were 112 S and T codes which did not specify either the injury or the part of the body (e.g. unspecified injury of lower leg, fracture of unspecified body region); these were also recoded to fit the matrix based on participants' own

**Table 7.** Multivariable analyses of pre-injury and injury-related characteristics associated with disability three months after the injury event for each sub-group, hospitalised (n = 590) and non-hospitalised (n = 1838).

| Explanatory variables | | Hospitalised | | | Non-hospitalised | | |
|---|---|---|---|---|---|---|---|
| | | OR | 95% CI | | OR | 95% CI | |
| Pre-injury WHODAS disability score | | 1.13 | 1.04 | 1.23 | 1.17 | 1.13 | 1.22 |
| Age | 18–34 years | 1.00 | reference | | | | |
| | 35–54 years | 0.87 | 0.57 | 1.34 | 1.40 | 1.11 | 1.78 |
| | 55–64 years | 0.94 | 0.52 | 1.69 | 1.04 | 0.76 | 1.43 |
| Gender | Male | 1.00 | reference | | | | |
| | Female | 1.78 | 1.14 | 2.80 | 1.23 | 0.99 | 1.52 |
| Financial status | Sufficient | 1.00 | reference | | | | |
| | Insufficient | 1.14 | 0.55 | 2.34 | 1.51 | 1.06 | 2.14 |
| General health | Excellent/ Very good/ Good | 1.00 | reference | | | | |
| | Fair/Poor | 0.39 | 0.15 | 1.02 | 0.61 | 0.36 | 1.01 |
| Chronic conditions | 0 | 1.00 | reference | | | | |
| | 1 | 1.14 | 0.72 | 1.79 | 1.02 | 0.79 | 1.30 |
| | ≥2 | 1.92 | 1.06 | 3.46 | 1.17 | 0.88 | 1.56 |
| Comfort in faith or spiritual beliefs | Very much/ Quite a bit | 1.00 | reference | | | | |
| | Somewhat/ A little bit/ Not at all | 0.53 | 0.34 | 0.83 | 0.75 | 0.60 | 0.93 |
| | Missing | 1.15 | 0.29 | 4.63 | 0.84 | 0.45 | 1.57 |
| Physical activity | ≥5 days | 1.00 | reference | | | | |
| | <5 days | 0.79 | 0.54 | 1.18 | 0.79 | 0.64 | 0.97 |
| Sleep | ≥5 nights | 1.00 | reference | | | | |
| | <5 nights | 0.95 | 0.59 | 1.53 | 0.70 | 0.55 | 0.90 |
| BMI | Underweight/ Normal/ Overweight | 1.00 | reference | | | | |
| | Obese | 1.93 | 1.19 | 3.13 | 1.49 | 1.17 | 1.89 |
| | Missing | 0.92 | 0.34 | 2.48 | 0.66 | 0.35 | 1.25 |
| Injury cause | Accidental | 1.00 | reference | | | | |
| | Assault | 1.49 | 0.71 | 3.12 | 3.04 | 1.54 | 6.01 |
| Threat to life | No | 1.00 | reference | | | | |
| | Yes/ Maybe | 0.92 | 0.55 | 1.53 | 1.52 | 1.02 | 2.26 |
| Threat of severe longer-term disability | No | 1.00 | reference | | | | |
| | Yes/ Maybe | 1.61 | 1.07 | 2.41 | 1.20 | 0.96 | 1.49 |
| Access to healthcare services | No trouble | 1.00 | reference | | | | |
| | Trouble/ Mixed | 0.72 | 0.39 | 1.33 | 1.92 | 1.37 | 2.69 |
| Injury severity | NISS 1–3 | 1.00 | reference | | | | |
| | NISS 4–6 | 2.17 | 1.23 | 3.82 | 1.65 | 1.23 | 2.20 |
| | NISS >6 | 2.69 | 1.30 | 5.56 | 2.01 | 1.40 | 2.88 |
| *Injury categories#* | | | | | | | |
| Intracranial | | 0.57 | 0.22 | 1.50 | 0.89 | 0.41 | 1.92 |
| Head/neck superficial | | 1.96 | 0.85 | 4.49 | 0.65 | 0.27 | 1.57 |
| Spine sprain/ strain or dislocation | | 1.94 | 0.89 | 4.22 | 2.21 | 1.57 | 3.11 |
| Upper extremity fracture | | 0.57 | 0.32 | 1.01 | 0.78 | 0.53 | 1.15 |
| Upper extremity sprain/ strain or dislocation | | 0.64 | 0.33 | 1.25 | 1.14 | 0.82 | 1.59 |
| Upper extremity open wound | | 0.96 | 0.49 | 1.87 | 0.62 | 0.34 | 1.14 |
| Upper extremity superficial | | 2.23 | 0.77 | 6.46 | 1.11 | 0.67 | 1.83 |
| Lower extremity fracture | | 3.50 | 1.91 | 6.42 | 1.09 | 0.74 | 1.60 |
| Lower extremity sprain/ strain or dislocation | | 1.75 | 0.91 | 3.37 | 1.64 | 1.19 | 2.28 |
| Lower extremity open wound | | 0.70 | 0.32 | 1.51 | 0.70 | 0.35 | 1.41 |
| Lower extremity superficial | | 0.88 | 0.36 | 2.14 | 1.25 | 0.83 | 1.88 |

**Table 7.** Cont.

| Explanatory variables | Hospitalised | | | Non-hospitalised | | |
|---|---|---|---|---|---|---|
| | OR | 95% CI | | OR | 95% CI | |
| Other | 1.47 | 0.88 | 2.46 | 1.00 | 0.69 | 1.45 |

# Each of the injury category odds ratios are with reference to those not having an injury of that category.

descriptions of their injury. If the specific index injury was coded elsewhere in the diagnosis list, the sequelae, procedure or non-specific codes were not used.

As all diagnoses were collected, participants could have more than one injury type (e.g. both a fracture and a sprain) or more than one part of their body injured (e.g. both an arm and a leg). Twelve injury categories were developed using the ICD-10 codes to describe both the injured body region and nature of injury, based on the ICD-10 injury mortality diagnosis matrix and the Barell injury diagnosis matrix [38,39]. The 12 injury categories were: intracranial, head/neck superficial, spine sprain/strain or dislocation, upper extremity fracture, upper extremity sprain/ strain or dislocation, upper extremity open wound, upper extremity superficial, lower extremity fracture, lower extremity sprain/strain or dislocation, lower extremity open wound, lower extremity superficial, and other anatomical region/nature. 'Upper extremity' includes the shoulder; 'lower extremity' the hip. The first 11 injury categories comprise all those containing more than 100 cases; all remaining injuries (e.g. crush, amputation, burn) were collapsed into the heterogeneous 'other' category. For analysis, all participants were classified according to whether or not they had sustained an injury in any of the 12 categories following the same approach used by Holtslag et al [40].

A New Injury Severity Score (NISS) was also derived for each participant [41]. ICD-10 codes were converted to AIS scores using a computer program [42]. Codes which did not map to an AIS score using the program were reviewed using the AIS manual [43]. Where an AIS score could not be derived for all ICD-10 codes of a participant, that person was considered missing for the purposes of calculating NISS. Potential AIS scores range from 1 (minor) to 6 (maximum (currently untreatable)) [44]. NISS was calculated as the sum of the squares of an individual's three highest AIS scores (or all their AIS scores if they have fewer than four diagnoses) [41], and grouped for analysis into three severity categories: 1–3 (least severe; AIS = 1 injuries only), 4–6 (middle severity; one AIS = 2 injury plus none, one or two AIS = 1 injuries) and >6 (most severe; at least two AIS = 2 injuries or one AIS≥3 injury) [41].

## Analysis

Bivariate analyses (chi-squared tests) were completed to compare the proportions of participants hospitalised and non-hospitalised according to each of the explanatory variables. Proportions reporting WHODAS disability three months after injury are presented with 95% confidence intervals (95%CI). Discussion of bivariate results is focused on results with p-values of less than 0.01 or discrete (non-overlapping) 95%CI.

For multivariable analyses exploring relationships between explanatory variables and WHODAS disability for the hospitalised and non-hospitalised groups, a two-step process was used. First, two separate multivariable logistic regression models were built for each of the hospitalised and non-hospitalised groups using a stepwise backward selection procedure with a threshold p-value of ≤0.1. All explanatory variables listed in Tables 1, 2, 3 were

considered for inclusion in each of these two independent models. When more than 100 responses were missing for any explanatory variable (e.g. sense of community), a separate category was presented and labelled 'missing' to allow participants missing such variables to be included in the model. If ≤100 responses were missing for any variable, participants with missing data for that variable were not included in this initial model-building (results not presented).

Second, all variables retained in either the hospitalised and non-hospitalised groups' independent models were entered into two further 'consistent variable' models. This allows us to present the odds ratio (OR), and 95%CI, of WHODAS disability after injury consistently for both groups. These two models include all cases with non-missing responses in retained variables (subjected to the above ≤100 criterion). In all four models, 'time between the injury event and interview' was adjusted for, as this was known to vary between participants and also to be associated with disability. Age, gender, NISS and the 12 injury categories were also retained in all models. Stata 11.1 was used for analysis [45].

## Results

Of 2856 POIS participants, 104 were missing either a pre-injury or three-month post-injury WHODAS score, leaving data from 2752 (96%) available for analysis.

### Bivariate analyses

Tables 1, 2, 3 present the proportions of the hospitalised (n = 673; 24.5%) and non-hospitalised (n = 2079; 75.5%) groups according to each of the listed variables. Of the pre-injury socio-demographic characteristics (Table 1), a greater proportion of people in the youngest age group (18–34 years) and males were treated in hospital as a consequence of their injury; conversely, people in the middle age group (35–54 years) were less likely to be hospitalised. Considering pre-injury health and psychosocial characteristics (Table 2), a greater proportion of those with high alcohol use were hospitalised. Among injury-related variables (Table 3), a greater proportion of those reporting their injury resulted from assault and was a threat to their life or of disability, and those with NISS of four or more, were hospitalised; NISS in this study ranged from 1 to 22. For the 12 injury categories a greater proportion of those with intracranial injury, head or neck superficial injuries, extremity fractures, open wounds, and 'other' injuries were hospitalised. Conversely, a smaller proportion of those with sprains, strains or dislocations were hospitalised. No differences in proportions were apparent for either upper or lower extremity superficial injury.

Before injury, the prevalence of disability (WHODAS summed score ≥10) was 4.5% for the hospitalised group and 5.3% for the non-hospitalised group. Tables 4, 5, 6 present the prevalence of disability three months after the injury event, according to each explanatory variable. Overall, sub-acute phase disability was more prevalent among injured participants treated at hospital (53.6%)

than those not. However, among the non-hospitalised group disability was experienced by more than one-third (39.4%) three months after the injury event.

## Multivariable analyses

Table 7 presents the multivariable models for the hospitalised and non-hospitalised groups. After applying the '≤100 missing' restriction described above, data were missing for at least one of the independent variables (presented in Tables 1, 2, 3) for 324 participants; including 92 who were missing a NISS score, one of the variables deliberately retained in each model. Consequently, data from 590 hospitalised and 1838 non-hospitalised participants were available for multivariable analysis. P-values for Hosmer-Lemeshow goodness-of-fit for the hospitalised and non-hospitalised models are acceptable; $p = 0.17$ and $0.64$ respectively. The area under the curve for each model indicates reasonable disability discrimination: 80.0% and 72.5% respectively.

**Pre-injury disability.** In both the hospitalised and non-hospitalised groups, pre-injury disability was associated with increased odds of post-injury disability. For every point increase in pre-injury WHODAS score, there was a 13% increase in odds of disability among the hospitalised and a 17% increase among the non-hospitalised.

**Pre-injury socio-demographic characteristics.** Among the hospitalised group, age did not appear to be associated with the odds of disability. However, among the non-hospitalised group being in the middle age group (35–54 years) was associated with increased disability (OR = 1.40). In the hospitalised model, but not the non-hospitalised, being female increases the odds of disability after injury (OR = 1.78). Having insufficient finances pre-injury was associated with increased disability among the non-hospitalised group only (OR = 1.51). Other socio-demographic characteristics (education, living arrangements and paid employment) were not retained in either model.

**Pre-injury health and psychosocial characteristics.** Having two or more chronic conditions resulted in nearly twice the odds of disability for the hospitalised group only (compared to those with no chronic conditions; OR = 1.92). Reporting less comfort in faith or spiritual beliefs was associated with lower odds of disability among both groups (compared to those with quite a bit or very much comfort; OR = 0.53 for hospitalised and 0.75 for non-hospitalised). In the non-hospitalised group only, compared to the relevant reference categories, not engaging in regular physical activity and not having enough sleep pre-injury reduced the odds of disability (OR = 0.79 and 0.70 respectively). Being obese was associated with disability among both the hospitalised and non-hospitalised groups (compared to non-obese; OR = 1.93 for hospitalised; OR = 1.49 for non-hospitalised).

A number of pre-injury health and psychosocial variables were not retained in the models; namely pre-injury general health, depressive-type episodes in the year before injury, optimism, self-efficacy, family involvement, social relationship satisfaction, sense of community, smoking, alcohol use and recreational drug use.

**Injury-related characteristics.** A three-fold increased odds of disability was experienced by non-hospitalised participants reporting their injury to be the result of an assault (OR = 3.04) compared to those reporting an unintentional injury. The non-hospitalised group were also at increased odds when they perceived a threat to their life (OR = 1.52) and the hospitalised group when they perceived a threat of longer-term disability (OR = 1.61). Trouble accessing health services among the non-hospitalised group was associated with nearly twice the odds of disability (OR = 1.92).

In both the hospitalised and non-hospitalised groups having a NISS score of either 4–6 or >6 (compared to those with scores of 1–3; OR = 2.17 and 2.69 respectively for hospitalised, and 1.65 and 2.01 for non-hospitalised) is independently associated with disability after injury. However, among the 12 injury categories, only three were independently associated with disability. A 3.5-fold increased odds of disability is experienced by hospitalised people with a lower extremity fracture (OR = 3.50) compared to those without such an injury. Having a spine or lower extremity sprain/strain or dislocation (OR = 2.21 and 1.64 respectively) was associated with increased odds of disability in the non-hospitalised group.

## Discussion

We compared a wide range of pre-injury and injury-related characteristics among people with injuries, including both those who were hospitalised as a consequence of their injury (n = 673) and those who were not (n = 2079). Bivariate analyses revealed few differences between the hospitalised and non-hospitalised groups in pre-injury socio-demographic, health and psychosocial characteristics; more variation was apparent among the injury-related characteristics (Tables 1, 2, 3). Disability was experienced by 53.6% of the hospitalised group three months, on average, after injury. It is noteworthy that more than one-third of the people not hospitalised (39.4%) were also experiencing disability at this time.

Pre-existing disability is a strong and independent predictor of disability in the sub-acute post-injury period for both those treated at hospital and those not (Table 7). Analysis of data from the large National Health Interview Survey in the United States found that adults with pre-existing disability had poorer access to health care, and calls were made for removal of barriers to access for people with disability [46]. In our study all participants had to have had at least some contact with health professionals to become registered with ACC and thereby eligible for possible recruitment to POIS. Assessment of pre-injury disability could be useful in effectively targeting people at risk of poor outcome for a more comprehensive and/or tailored package of treatment and rehabilitation services.

Aside from pre-injury disability, a number of other characteristics were independently associated with disability three months after injury for the hospitalised group (Table 7). These included being female, having two or more pre-existing chronic conditions, obesity, perceiving a threat of disability, a NISS score >3 and a lower extremity fracture. We, and others, have previously found being female places people at increased risk of other types of poor outcome [9,47,48]. However, a smaller Norwegian study of longer-term disability outcomes among people with NISS>15, did not find an association between WHODAS (36-item version) and gender [49]. Worse outcomes may be associated with poorer care being provided to women [48,50].

For the non-hospitalised group, in contrast to the hospitalised group, being female, having pre-existing chronic conditions or a perceived threat of disability were not independently associated with disability. Further research is required to understand why these independent relationships were not observed among our non-hospitalised participants while accounting for a wide range of other characteristics including age, NISS and injury category. Associations with increased odds of disability in the sub-acute phase are only similar between the hospitalised and non-hospitalised groups for pre-injury disability, obesity and NISS.

More associations were apparent in the model for the non-hospitalised group than the hospitalised group, although the smaller size of the hospitalised group may have led to insufficient power to detect associations that do, in fact, exist. Among the non-hospitalised, people aged 35–54 years were at increased odds of disability, as were those with insufficient finances, injury due to assault, perceived threat to their life, trouble accessing healthcare services and those with spine or lower extremity sprains/strains or dislocations. Of particular note were people reporting assault as the cause of their injury. This group were at three-fold increased odds of disability compared to those not reporting assault, after accounting for other factors including injury severity. To our knowledge, this is the first study to examine the relationship between assault and disability in a non-hospitalised injured population. Further research needs to be undertaken to understand the reason for the increased odds of disability. For example, it is plausible that such poor odds among the non-hospitalised may arise as a consequence of appropriate support being less available to the non-hospitalised assaulted group than to those who were assaulted but treated at hospital.

Certain characteristics were associated with lower odds of disability. Among both the hospitalised and non-hospitalised groups, having little comfort in faith or spiritual beliefs reduced the odds of disability. Faith and spirituality are complex concepts [51]. While acknowledging that 'religion' is not the same concept as 'faith', certain religious practices may have a positive relationship with health or provide a sense of meaning when adverse health events occur (consolation model) [51]. Conversely, for some people adverse health events may be interpreted as a punishment by God (punishment model) [51,52]. In their study investigating relationships between the FACIT-Sp-12 and health outcomes reported by cancer survivors, Edmondson et al found the two components of the FACIT, religious and existential well-being, were conceptually distinct with different effects on cancer survivors' health [53]. Existential well-being was more strongly associated with health outcomes than was religious well-being [53]. The single question used in our study is from the religious well-being component, which may explain our result. We encourage others to include a wider range of spirituality questions in studies of outcome following injury to confirm, or otherwise, the association between injury and disability outcome.

Counter-intuitively, not engaging in regular pre-injury physical activity or having adequate sleep were also associated with lower odds of disability among the non-hospitalised group only. Previously, we have found similar (protective) associations between low levels of pre-injury physical activity and functional and work outcomes [48,54]. We wonder if such an association indicates that those who were not exercising or sleeping well pre-injury are not suffering as much from their loss post-injury; in contrast to those who were exercising and sleeping well before injury. These findings may also have arisen by chance. Future analyses will examine whether or not these associations continue into the longer-term.

In summary, we found a wide range of pre-injury demographic, health and injury-related characteristics associated with increased odds of disability in the sub-acute phase. It is interesting to observe that of the 12 injury categories only three (lower extremity fracture for hospitalised; spine or lower extremity sprain/strains/dislocations for the non-hospitalised) are independently associated with increased odds of disability outcomes; whereas overall injury severity (NISS) is a consistent predictor of outcome among both the hospitalised and non-hospitalised groups. With a few exceptions, the characteristics associated with increased odds of disability are not consistent between the hospitalised and non-hospitalised groups. This indicates that caution should be used in generalising results from studies of hospitalised patients to people with injuries not resulting in hospital treatment.

## Strengths and limitations

A strength of our study is the inclusion of both people who were hospitalised and people who were not. Further, many injury outcome studies have focused on very specific injury types (e.g. traumatic brain injury or hip fracture) or causes (e.g., falls, road crashes), rather than 'all injury' types as we have done. Another strength of our study is that we were able to include injury severity, and a comprehensive range of pre-injury and injury-related factors.

Our study has some limitations. First, the fact that participants were asked to recall pre-injury characteristics three months after injury introduced the possibility of recall bias. Although most pre-injury factors (e.g. level of education, living arrangements) did not rely on 'subjective' ratings, the measure of pre-injury disability did. In a study considering other health status outcomes, researchers have found peoples' recalled pre-injury health status was (re-)attained when they also reported having recovered, suggesting reasonable recall of pre-injury states [55]. However, their study was investigating recall using a different measure to the WHODAS and we cannot discount some bias in relation to recall of pre-injury disability. Despite this limitation, it is a strength that we have used the WHODAS, an instrument specifically developed to assess disability, as an outcome measure [56,57]. Few injury studies have considered disability as an outcome; and fewer still have used validated measures of disability [49,58,59]. The WHODAS was developed by the World Health Organization in conjunction with advisors, including groups of people experiencing disability [21,60].

Our classification of hospitalisation excludes cases who sought treatment or assessment at hospital, but whose visit lasted less than three hours, because these are not required to be reported to NMDS. People with injuries that typically require treatment in the acute phase only, without the need for more than a week off work, or on-going treatment, were also excluded from our study [13]. Another limitation is that few people in our cohort had injuries with very high severity scores (highest NISS being 22). Consequently, although a strength of our study is that we have been able to include people with (all) injuries whether or not they resulted in hospitalisation, it also means caution should be used when interpreting our odds of disability for those with NISS >6. A study in Denmark found no association between higher injury severity (ISS) categories and health-related quality of life outcomes among injured participants with ISS≥9 [61]. Similar research is required to understand relationships between higher NISS and disability. Furthermore, although the inclusion of a wide range of pre-injury characteristics was a strength of our study, this also led to a limitation. To minimise burden to participants it was not possible to include lengthy sets of questions about every characteristic included. We did not find associations between pre-injury psychological variables and disability outcomes, or between a number of other characteristics, such as smoking and alcohol use, and disability using the measures employed in the POIS study. Future analyses of data collected at subsequent POIS follow-up points (12- and 24-months) will ascertain whether relationships exist between psychosocial characteristics present three months after injury and longer-term poor outcomes, as others have found [59,62].

## Conclusions

Our study is one of a small, but growing, number to report disability outcomes following all-injury using a measure developed specifically for disability, the WHODAS. Our study suggests that it would be unwise to generalise results from the hospitalised population to the non-hospitalised population. The UK Burden of Injury Study estimated considerable collective burden following injury for people seen at ED but not hospitalised, in part because of the greater numbers with injuries not resulting in hospitalisation [6]. Our study suggests that a considerable proportion of non-hospitalised individuals carry a significant disability burden following injury. It would be desirable for other studies, where possible, to investigate outcomes following injury for those who are not hospitalised. Elsewhere, others have called for longer-term assessment of outcome following injury [63]. Our research group is now analysing disability (and other outcomes) to 12-month and 24-month follow-up points, and will also examine trajectories of recovery (or not) over time, as undertaken in a smaller New Zealand study examining health status following car crashes [64].

## References

1. World Health Organization (2008) The global burden of disease: 2004 update. Geneva: World Health Organization.
2. MacKenzie E (2000) Epidemiology of injuries: Current trends and future challenges. Epidemiologic Reviews 22: 112–119.
3. Krug EG, Sharma GK, Lozano R (2000) The global burden of injuries. American Journal of Public Health 90: 523–526.
4. Cripps R, Harrison J (2008) Injury as a chronic health issue in Australia. Cat. no. INJCAT 118. Canberra: AIHW.
5. World Health Organization, The World Bank (2011) World Report on Disability 2011.
6. Lyons R, Kendrick D, Towner E, Christie N, Macey S, et al. (2011) Measuring the Population Burden of Injuries–Implications for Global and National Estimates: A Multicentre Prospective UK Longitudinal Study. PLoS Med 8: e1001140.
7. Polinder S, Haagsma J, Belt E, Lyons R, Erasmus V, et al. (2010) A systematic review of studies measuring health-related quality of life of general injury populations. BMC Public Health 10: 783.
8. Black J, Herbison G, Lyons R, Polinder S, Derrett S (2011) Recovery after Injury: An individual patient data meta-analysis of general health status using the EQ-5D. Journal of Trauma 71: 1003–1010.
9. Vles W, Steyerberg E, Essink-Bot M-L, van Beeck E, Meeuwis J, et al. (2005) Prevalence and determinants of disabilities and return to work after major trauma. Journal of Trauma 58: 126–135.
10. Meerding WJ, Mulder S, van Beeck EF (2006) Incidence and costs of injuries in The Netherlands. The European Journal of Public Health 16: 271–277.
11. MacKenzie E, Morris J, Jurkovich G, Yasui Y, Cushing B, et al. (1998) Return to work following injury: the role of economic, social, and job-related factors. American Journal of Public Health 88: 1630–1637.
12. Holbrook T, Anderson J, Sieber W, Browner D, Hoyt D (1999) Outcome after major trauma: 12-month and 18-month follow-up results from the Trauma Recovery Project. Journal of Trauma 46: 765–773.
13. Langley J, Cryer C (2012) A consideration of severity is sufficient to focus our prevention efforts. Injury Prevention 18: 73–74.
14. Polinder S, van Beeck E, Essink-Bot M, Toet H, Looman C, et al. (2007) Functional outcome at 2.5, 5, 9, and 24 months after injury in the Netherlands. Journal of Trauma 62: 133–141.
15. Malm S, Krafft M, Kullgren A, Ydenius A, Tingvall C (2008) Risk of permanent medical impairment (RPMI) in road traffic accidents. Annals of Advances in Automotive Medicine 52: 93–100.
16. Derrett S, Langley J, Hokowhitu B, Ameratunga S, Hansen P, et al. (2009) Prospective Outcomes of Injury Study. Injury Prevention 15: 351.
17. Derrett S, Davie G, Ameratunga S, Wyeth E, Colhoun S, et al. (2011) Prospective Outcomes of Injury Study: recruitment, and participant characteristics, health and disability status. Injury Prevention 17: 415–418.
18. Accident Compensation Corporation (2009) Annual Report 2009 Wellington.
19. Accident Compensation Corporation (2010) Annual Report 2010. Wellington: Accident Compensation Corporation.
20. Üstün T, Kostanjsek N, Chatterji S, Rehm J, editors (2010) Measuring Health and Disability: Manual for WHO Disability Assessment Schedule (WHODAS 2.0). Malta: WHO Press.
21. Andrews G, Kemp A, Sunderland M, Von Korff M, Üstün T (2009) Normative data for the 12 item WHO Disability Assessment Schedule 2.0. PLoS One 4: e8343.
22. Ministry of Health (2011) National Collections Glossary: Appendix B Glossary Wellington: Ministry of Health.
23. Meerding WJ, Looman CWN, Essink-Bot M-L, Toet H, Mulder S, et al. (2004) Distribution and determinants of health and work status in a comprehensive population of injury patients. Journal of Trauma 56: 150–161.
24. Statistics New Zealand (2006) 2006 Census of Population and Dwellings. Wellington. http://www.stats.govt.nz/census.aspx.

25. Ministry of Social Development (2000) Direct Measurement Of Living Standards: The New Zealand ELSI Scale – Survey of Working Age People in 2000. Wellington: Ministry of Social Development.
26. Ware J, Kosinski M, Gandek B (2000) SF-36® Health Survey: Manual and Interpretation Guide. Lincoln, RI: QualityMetric Incorporated.
27. Ministry of Health (2008) A Portrait of Health. Key Results from the 2006/07 New Zealand Health Survey. Wellington.
28. American Psychiatric Association Committee of Nomenclature and Statistics (1980) Diagnostic and statistical manual of mental disorder-3rd edition (DSM-3). Washington DC: American Psychiatric Association.
29. Scheier M, Carver C, Bridges M (1994) Distinguishing optimism from neuroticism (and trait anxiety, self-mastery, and self-esteem): A reevaluation of the Life Orientation Test. Journal of Personality and Social Psychology 67: 1063–1078.
30. Schwarzer R, M J (1995) Generalized Self-Efficacy Scale. In: Weinman J, Johnston M, editors. Measures in health psychology: A user's portfolio Causal and control beliefs. Windsor, England: NFER-NELSON. 35–37.
31. Peterman A, Fitchett G, Brady M, Hernandez L, Cella D (2002) Measuring spiritual well-being in people with cancer: the functional assessment of chronic illness therapy – Spiritual Well-being Scale (FACIT-Sp). Annals of Behavioral Medicine 24: 49–58.
32. Portney K, Berry J (1997) Mobilizing minority communities. The American Behavioral Scientist 40: 632–644.
33. Sport and Recreation New Zealand (2004) The New Zealand Physical Activity Questionnaires. Wellington: SPARC.
34. World Health Organization (2011) BMI Classification World Health Organization,.
35. Statistics New Zealand (2006) 2006 Census questionnaires. Statistics New Zealand,.
36. Bradley KA, DeBenedetti AF, Volk RJ, Williams EC, Frank D, et al. (2007) AUDIT-C as a Brief Screen for Alcohol Misuse in Primary Care. Alcoholism: Clinical and Experimental Research 31: 1208–1217.
37. Robinson D, Schulz E, Brown P, Price C (1997) Updating the Read Codes: User-interactive Maintenance of a Dynamic Clinical Vocabulary. Journal of the American Medical Informatics Association 4: 465–472.
38. Fingerhut L, Warner M (2006) The ICD-10 injury mortality diagnosis matrix. Injury Prevention 12: 24–29.
39. Barell V, Aharonson-Daniel L, Fingerhut LA, Mackenzie EJ, Ziv A, et al. (2002) An introduction to the Barell body region by nature of injury diagnosis matrix. Injury Prevention 8: 91–96.
40. Holtslag H, van Beeck E, Lindeman E, Leenen L (2007) Determinants of Long-Term Functional Consequences After Major Trauma. Journal of Trauma 62: 919–927.
41. Stevenson M, Segui-Gomez M, Lescohier I, Di Scala C, McDonald-Smith G (2001) An overview of the injury severity score and the new injury severity score. Injury Prevention 7: 10–13.
42. European Center for Injury Prevention (2011) ICD Map. Pampolona: Universidad de Navarra.
43. Association for the Advancement of Automotive Medicine (1990) The Abbreviated Injury Scale 1990 Revision. Des Plaines, Illinois, USA: Association for the Advancement of Automotive Medicine.
44. Gennarelli T, Wodzin E (2008) The Abbreviated Injury Scale 2005. Update 2008. Des Plaines: Association for the Advancement of Automotive Medicine.
45. StataCorp (2009) Stata: Release 11 Statistical Software. College Station: StataCorp.
46. Smith D (2008) Disparities in health care access for women with disabilities in the United States from the 2006 National Health Interview Survey. Disability and Health Journal 1 (2008) 79e88 1.
47. Holbrook TL, Hoyt DB (2004) The impact of major trauma: quality-of-life outcomes are worse in women than in men, independent of mechanism and injury severity. Journal of Trauma 56: 284–290.

## Acknowledgments

We are most grateful to the study participants for sharing their information with us, and to the study interviewers for their role in data collection. We thank Paul Hansen, Helen Harcombe and Hank Weiss for their comments on an earlier draft of this paper.

## Author Contributions

Conceived and designed the experiments: SD JL SA RL EW GD. Performed the experiments: SD JL SA RL EW GD. Analyzed the data: AS SD SW JL SA IDC RL EW GD. Wrote the paper: SD. Contributed to the writing of the manuscript: SD AS SW JL SA IDC RL EW GD. ICMJE criteria for authorship read and met: SD AS SW JL SA IDC RL EW GD. Agree with manuscript results and conclusions: SD AS SW JL SA IDC RL EW GD.

48. Langley J, Derrett S, Davie G, Ameratunga S, Wyeth E (2011) A cohort study of short-term functional outcomes following injury: the role of pre-injury socio-demographic and health characteristics, injury and injury-related healthcare. Health and Quality of Life Outcomes 9.

49. Soberg H, Bautz-Holter E, Roise O, Finset A (2007) Long-term multidimensional functional consequences of severe multiple injuries two years after trauma: a prospective longitudinal cohort study. Journal of Trauma 62: 461–470.

50. Pukk K, Lundberg J, Penaloza-Pesantes RV, Brommels M, Gaffney FA (2003) Do women simply complain more? National patient injury claims data show gender and age differences. Quality Management in Health Care 12: 225–231.

51. Fitchett G, Rybarczyk B, DeMarco G, Nicholas J (1999) The role of religion in medical rehabilitation outcomes: a longitudinal study. Rehabilitation Psychology 44: 333–353.

52. Pargament KI, Tarakeshwar N, Ellison CG, Wulff KM (2001) Religious coping among the religious: The relationships between religious coping and well-being in a National Sample of Prebyterian clergy, elders and members. Journal for the Scientific Study of Religion 40: 497–513.

53. Edmondson D, Park CL, Blank TO, Fenster JR, Mills MA (2008) Deconstructing spiritual well-being: existential well-being and HRQOL in cancer survivors. Psycho-Oncology 17: 161–169.

54. Lilley R, Davie G, Ameratunga S, Derrett S (2012) Factors predicting work status three months after injury: Results from the Prospective Outcome of Injury Study. BMJ Open 2.

55. Watson WL, Ozanne-Smith J, Richardson J (2007) Retrospective baseline measurement of self-reported health status and health-related quality of life versus population norms in the evaluation of post-injury losses. Injury Prevention 13: 45–50.

56. Krahn GL, Fujiura G, Drum CE, Cardinal BJ, Nosek MA (2009) The dilemma of measuring perceived health status in the context of disability. Disability and Health Journal 2: 49–56.

57. Federici S, Meloni F (2010) A note on the theoretical framework of World Health Organization Disability Assessment Schedule II. Disability and Rehabilitation 32: 687–691.

58. Gofin R, Adler B (1997) A seven item scale for the assessment of disabilities after child and adolescent injuries. Injury Prevention 3: 120–123.

59. O'Donnell ML, Creamer M, Elliott P, Atkin C, Kossman T (2005) Determinants of quality of life and role-related disability after injury: Impact of acute psychological responses. The Journal of Trauma 59: 1328–1335.

60. World Health Organisation (2001) ICF: International Classification of Functioning, Disability and Health. Geneva: World Health Organisation.

61. Overgaard M, Hoyer C, Christensen E (2011) Long-Term Survival and Health-Related Quality of Life 6 to 9 Years After Trauma. Journal of Trauma 71: 435–441.

62. Michaels A, Michaels C, Smith J, Moon C, Peterson C, et al. (2000) Outcome from Injury: General Health, Work Status, and Satisfaction 12 Months after Trauma. Journal of Trauma 48: 841–850.

63. Pape H-C, Probst C, Lohse R, Zelle B, Panzica M, et al. (2010) Predictors of Late Clinical Outcome Following Orthopedic Injuries After Multiple Trauma. Journal of Trauma 69: 1243–1251.

64. Ameratunga S, Norton R, Connor J, Robinson E, Civil I, et al. (2006) A population-based cohort study of longer-term changes in health of car drivers involved in serious crashes. Annals of Emergency Medicine 48 729–736.

# 17

# Persistent, Long-term Cerebral White Matter Changes after Sports-Related Repetitive Head Impacts

**Jeffrey J. Bazarian**[1]*, **Tong Zhu**[2], **Jianhui Zhong**[3], **Damir Janigro**[4], **Eric Rozen**[5], **Andrew Roberts**[6], **Hannah Javien**[7], **Kian Merchant-Borna**[1], **Beau Abar**[1], **Eric G Blackman**[8]

1 Emergency Medicine, University of Rochester School of Medicine and Dentistry, Rochester, New York, United States of America, 2 Imaging Sciences, University of Rochester School of Medicine and Dentistry, Rochester, New York, United States of America, 3 Imaging Sciences, Biomedical Engineering, and Physics, University of Rochester, Rochester, New York, United States of America, 4 Cleveland Clinic Lerner Research Institute, Cleveland, Ohio, United States of America, 5 Athletics and Recreation, University of Rochester, Rochester, New York, United States of America, 6 University of Rochester, Rochester, New York, United States of America, 7 Hamilton College, Clinton, New York, United States of America, 8 Physics and Astronomy, University of Rochester, Rochester, New York, United States of America

## Abstract

*Introduction:* Repetitive head impacts (RHI) sustained in contact sports are thought to be necessary for the long-term development of chronic traumatic encephalopathy (CTE). Our objectives were to: 1) characterize the magnitude and persistence of RHI-induced white matter (WM) changes; 2) determine their relationship to kinematic measures of RHI; and 3) explore their clinical relevance.

*Methods:* Prospective, observational study of 10 Division III college football players and 5 non-athlete controls during the 2011-12 season. All subjects underwent diffusion tensor imaging (DTI), physiologic, cognitive, and balance testing at pre-season (Time 1), post-season (Time 2), and after 6-months of no-contact rest (Time 3). Head impact measures were recorded using helmet-mounted accelerometers. The percentage of whole-brain WM voxels with significant changes in fractional anisotropy (FA) and mean diffusivity (MD) from Time 1 to 2, and Time 1 to 3 was determined for each subject and correlated to head impacts and clinical measures.

*Results:* Total head impacts for the season ranged from 431–1,850. No athlete suffered a clinically evident concussion. Compared to controls, athletes experienced greater changes in FA and MD from Time 1 to 2 as well as Time 1 to 3; most differences at Time 2 persisted to Time 3. Among athletes, the percentage of voxels with decreased FA from Time 1 to 2 was positively correlated with several helmet impact measures. The persistence of WM changes from Time 1 to 3 was also associated with changes in serum ApoA1 and S100B autoantibodies. WM changes were not consistently associated with cognition or balance.

*Conclusions:* A single football season of RHIs without clinically-evident concussion resulted in WM changes that correlated with multiple helmet impact measures and persisted following 6 months of no-contact rest. This lack of WM recovery could potentially contribute to cumulative WM changes with subsequent RHI exposures.

**Editor:** Hugo Theoret, University of Montreal, Canada

**Funding:** This study was supported by funds from the National Football League Charities https://www.nflcharities.org/. The funders had no role in study design, data collection and analysis, decision to publish, or preparation of the manuscript.

**Competing Interests:** The following author(s) have conflicts of interest related to the subject matter presented in the study: Bazarian - Patent Pending, "Method of Diagnosing Mild Traumatic Brain Injury", US serial number 61/467,224. This patent involves the use the peripheral protein Apolipoprotein A1 to aid in the diagnosis of concussion.

* E-mail: jeff_bazarian@urmc.rochester.edu

## Introduction

Although concussions are a frequent occurrence among athletes involved in contact sports such as American football, ice hockey, soccer, and lacrosse (1.6–3.8 million/year [1]), repetitive head impacts (RHI) that do not result in concussion are even more common. Using helmet-based accelerometers, estimates of the average number of RHIs in a single football season range from 244 to 1,444 per collegiate athlete [2,3], and from 175 to 1,410 per high school athlete [2,4]. In comparison, football-related concussion rates range from 64 to 76.8 per 100,000 athlete-exposures [5,6], translating to approximately 0.05 concussions per athlete per season. Thus football players incur roughly 3,500–28,000 RHIs for every one concussion.

Several studies suggest that RHIs may be harmful to the brain in the short term. Head hits incurred during a boxing match without concussion have been associated with cognitive dysfunction [7] and acute brain injury [8]. Among high school athletes who did not experience concussion, RHIs during a single season of football were associated with abnormal regional cortical activation patterns on functional MRI [9,10]. The magnitude of this activation correlated with the number of RHIs sustained during the season, and resembled that previously reported in subjects with frank concussion [11]. In a separate cohort, new learning on the

California Verbal Learning Test declined over a single season of RHIs among collegiate football players who did not experience concussion [12]. Using helmet mounted accelerometers, poorer post-season reaction time and scores on the Trail Making test of visual attention and task switching were found to be associated with greater head impact exposures [12].

Evidence linking RHIs to longer-term brain problems such as chronic traumatic encephalopathy (CTE) is more tenuous. When traumatic neurodegeneration was first described among boxers in 1928 it was presumed that RHIs were responsible [13]. More recent autopsy series have detected CTE in other sports (American football, hockey, and wrestling [14,15]), and also among individuals engaged in other activities such as repetitive head-banging [14]. In common to all of these cases was exposure to RHIs. Although frank concussions can occur with these activities, a pre-mortem history of concussion was absent in some of these cases [16,17], raising the possibility that RHIs played a role in CTE [16], independent of concussion. Further, early-onset dementia has not been reported among athletes involved in sports such as rugby and Australian-rules football, where concussions are common but RHIs are not. (CTE has been reported in two rugby players but both also played American football [17]). Recognizing that RHIs play a key role in the development of CTE, but that not all athletes exposed to them develop CTE [17,18], researchers at The Center for the Study of CTE at Boston University have concluded that repetitive brain trauma is "necessary but not sufficient," for the development of CTE [19].

The mechanism by which RHIs might impair neurologic outcomes is not known. White matter (WM) changes detected on diffusion tensor imaging (DTI) after RHIs suggest a parallel to frank concussion. Reductions in fractional anisotropy (FA) [20], increases in mean diffusivity (MD) [20–23], and both [24] have been reported after RHIs in humans. These changes are thought to reflect traumatically-induced structural alterations in the neuronal axon and microenvironment [25]. However, the relationship of head impact forces and physiologic factors to these WM changes is not clear. Additionally it is unclear if these WM changes are transient or resolve with time.

To address these gaps, we performed DTI on a group of collegiate football players outfitted with helmet impact sensors prior to and after a single season of football, and then again after 6 months of no-contact rest. Our objectives were to: 1) quantify and characterize RHI-related WM changes at the end of the football season, and determine the persistence of these changes after a period of prolonged rest; 2) determine the relationship between kinematic measures of RHI and these WM changes; and 3) explore the clinical relevance of the observed WM changes in terms of cognitive function, balance, and select physiologic factors.

## Methods

We conducted a prospective study of 10 college football players and 5 non-athlete controls at the University of Rochester during the 2011 football season (August to December) and a subsequent 6-month no-contact rest period (December to May). Helmet impact measure data were collected from all athletes throughout the season using helmet-mounted accelerometers. WM changes and clinical correlates were assessed on each subject at the beginning of the football season (Time 1), at the end of the football season (Time 2), and after 6 months of rest from contact sports (Time 3). The University of Rochester Institutional Review Board approved this study and the process of informed consent; written informed consent was obtained from all participants.

## Subjects

Male athletes were recruited from the University of Rochester (UR) football team, which competes in National Collegiate Athletic Association Division III. Male controls were recruited from the UR general student body. Available resources and the novel nature of this investigation limited the maximum enrollment in this study to 15 subjects. Twice as many athletes as controls were chosen to maximize the power to detect significant correlations between helmet impact measures and WM changes. Ten active UR varsity football players were asked to participate and all agreed. These athletes were chosen for the variety of positions and anticipated head impacts they would experience during the season, which was informed by prior studies [3,26]. Controls were selected based on response to a campus-wide call for research volunteers. Of the 10 student who responded, 5 were not eligible (4 had contraindications to MRI scanning, 1 played club rugby) and the remaining 5 were enrolled. Subjects, including controls, who were <18 years old or sustained a clinically diagnosed traumatic brain injury (TBI) of any severity within 2 weeks prior to the 2011 football season were excluded. History of prior TBI was determined by self-report using a previously validated survey tool [27].

## Primary Outcome: Changes in White Matter

Change in WM structure was the primary outcome and DTI was employed to measure these changes. This imaging modality is uniquely suited to detect the stretch-induced axonal damage thought to underlie all forms of TBI [28,29]. This process results in the destruction of neurofilaments and microtubules spanning the length of the axon and leads to axonal swelling, followed by axonal disconnection and retraction. The linear arrangement of the axonal cytoskeleton is disrupted, as is the flow of water molecules down the axon [30]. These events are not detectable with computed tomography (CT) or conventional magnetic resonance imaging (MRI) [31]. DTI measures water movement in six or more non-collinear directions, allowing the determination of three mutually perpendicular eigenvalues, which coincide with the main water movement direction in white matter. Combinations of these three eigenvalues allow the derivations of two principle diffusion indices: fractional anisotropy (FA, represented by values ranging from 0 [random, multi-directional movement] to 1.0 [movement in one particular direction]), and mean diffusivity (MD, represented by a numerical value ranging from 0 [no movement] to $1.5 \times 10^{-2}$ mm$^2$/sec [totally unrestricted movement]).

For this study, DTI was acquired with a 3T Siemens Trio scanner using a single-shot pulsed-gradient SE-EPI sequence to measure FA and MD changes in WM. From the DTI images, voxel-wise comparisons of FA and MD were analyzed on a subject-specific basis. DTI data were analyzed using the wild bootstrapping permutation test, in which statistical significance of subject-specific voxel-wise changes in FA and MD were determined (described in detail elsewhere [24]). From this output, we calculated the percentage of all WM voxels with a statistically significant change (increase and/or decrease) in FA or MD from Time 1 to Time 2 and from Time 1 to Time 3 within each subject.

## Helmet Impact Measures

Each athlete was outfitted with a Riddell Revolution IQ helmet (Riddell Corporation; Elyria, OH) equipped with the Head Impact Telemetry System (HITS) encoders (Simbex LLC; Lebanon, NH) for the duration of the season, including all practices and games. These accelerometers record 40 milliseconds of data (8 milliseconds pre-trigger and 32 milliseconds post-trigger) at 1000 Hz for each head impact. Only impacts in which the calculated translational acceleration at the center of gravity of the player's head exceeded 10 g-forces (g) were recorded for analysis. Linear and rotational acceleration, the Gadd Severity Index (GSI), the Head Injury Criterion (HIC), and the Head Impact Technology suspect profile (HITsp) [2], were computed from the accelerometer data. The peak linear and peak rotational accelerations are the maximum magnitude of linear and rotational accelerations measured during an impact. The GSI and the HIC both measure a time integral of the linear acceleration to the 2.5 power but differ in the choice of time interval of integration [32]. The GSI is calculated by integrating over the full time of the impact, whereas the HIC is calculated by integrating only over the 15 milliseconds spanning the peak acceleration (and is thus commonly referred to as HIC15). The HIC is less likely than GSI to overestimate brain injury severity after low-intensity, long-duration impacts. Finally, the HITsp is a single metric computed from a principal component analysis and represents a weighted combination of peak linear acceleration, peak rotational acceleration, GSI, and HIC, along with information about impact location. This metric is an empirical metric that was shown to correlate with concussion in a previous study of football impacts [2].

## Clinical Measures

Subjects were also evaluated on the following clinical measures at all three study time points:

**Cognitive performance.** Cognitive performance was measured using the Immediate Post-Concussion Assessment and Cognitive Testing (ImPACT) test, a proprietary software program consisting of a concussion symptom inventory and six test modules measuring attention, memory and reaction time [33]. These modules are collectively used to generate three composite scores ranging from 0–100% (verbal memory, visual memory, visual motor speed), mean reaction time in seconds, and an impulse control score based on the sum of errors committed on two test modules (X's and 0's, color match). The cognitive efficiency index measures the interaction between accuracy and speed on one of the test modules (symbol match), with values ranging from zero to approximately 0.70. Finally, the concussion symptom inventory (CSI) is used to generate a post-concussive symptom score based on the frequency and severity of symptoms with total scores ranging from 0–132. These seven cognitive performance metrics were evaluated in each subject.

**Balance.** Postural stability was measured using the Balance Error Scoring System (BESS) and the Wii Balance Board (WBB). The BESS requires the subject to stand in three different stances (double leg, single leg, and in tandem) for 20 seconds with eyes closed and hands on hips [34]. Each stance was performed once on a firm surface and once on a 10-cm thick piece of medium-density foam. The BESS score is calculated by adding 1 error point for each performance error to a maximum of 60. The BESS has excellent intra-tester (0.88) and inter-tester (0.83) reliability [35]. The WBB was interfaced with a computer using custom-written software (Labview 8.5 National Instruments; Austin, TX, U.S.A.) while subjects performed 4 standing balance tasks: 1) single leg standing, eyes closed, 2) single leg standing, eyes open, 3) double leg standing, eyes closed and 4) double leg standing, eyes open. Data were collected for 10 seconds during single leg trials and for 30 seconds during double leg trials. The primary metric was center of pressure path length (cm) totaled for the 4 stances [36]. Longer path lengths indicate worse postural stability.

**Physiologic Factors.** Four milliliters of venous blood were drawn into sterile Vacutainer serum separator tubes and immediately placed on 0°C ice. Within 60 minutes, the blood was centrifuged (3000 rpm, 10 minutes), and the serum separated

and stored at –80°C until sample analysis. Serum S100B concentrations were determined by ELISA manufactured by Diasorin (Stillwater, MN). 96 well plates were used and the analyte was sandwiched between two monoclonal antibodies directed against the beta-chain of the S100 dimer. Anti-human ELISA kits from Diasorin were read using a multi-plate fluorescent reader (at 450 nm). Fluorescent signals were converted into ng/mL as per standard curve concentrations. The detection limit of this ELISA is 0.01 ng/ml. The intra-assay coefficient of variance of this test is around 6%. S100B autoantibody and apoA-I concentrations were also measured in serum samples by ELISA. Maxisorp ELISA 96 wells plates were coated with a PBS solution containing S100B protein (human brain, catalog number-559291, EMD Chemicals), and serum apoA-I concentrations were measured in duplicate by ELISA (Mabtech; Cincinnati, OH). Apoε genotype was performed on DNA extracted from intra-oral cheek cells using the Hixson and Vernier method [37].

## Analysis

For each subject, the percentage of whole brain WM voxels with statistically significant changes from Time 1 to Time 2 and Time 1 to Time 3 were calculated for each of the of the following metrics: ↑ FA, ↓ FA, ↑ MD, and ↓ MD. Median percent changes were compared in athletes and controls using the Wilcoxon Rank Sum test. The percentage of WM voxels with significant interval changes in FA and MD was correlated to: 1) helmet impact metrics; and 2) clinical outcomes (including balance, cognitive performance, S100B, auto-S100B antibodies, and ApoA1 concentrations) using Spearman's correlation coefficient. Cognition and balance were correlated only to contemporaneous DTI changes, while physiologic variables were correlated to DTI changes occurring at all study time points. We posited that changes in clinical performance would be a result of WM changes and never preceded them. However, we anticipated that the physiologic milieu could not only be a result of WM changes (occurring contemporaneously or after) but could also influence the degree of WM changes (occurring before them).

Analyses were performed using SAS Software Version 9.3 (SAS Institute Inc.; Cary, NC, USA) and GraphPad Prism Version 5.02 for Windows (GraphPad Software; La Jolla, CA, USA). Statistical significance was defined as p<0.05, with p<0.10 also substantively important and interpreted as marginally significant given the small sample size. With a sample size of 10 athletes and 5 controls (assuming α = 0.05), we estimated approximately 90% power to detect a difference in the mean percentage of WM voxels with significant changes in FA between athletes and controls ranging from 0.6 to 0.8, and a difference in the mean percentage of WM voxels with significant changes in MD ranging from 0.80 to 1.0. Although wild bootstrapping includes an adjustment for multiple comparisons in brain voxels when calculating percentages of increased and decreased FA and MD, the correlation analysis linking DTI changes to head hits, serum biomarkers, and cognitive impairments was not adjusted for multiple comparisons. Rather, these correlations were presented graphically in a heat map table denoting tertile and direction of statistically significant r-values so that patterns could be more clearly discerned.

## Results

Baseline comparison to controls revealed that athletes had significantly higher body mass index and lower auto-S100B antibody titers, and lower impulse control (**Table 1**); athletes and controls were otherwise similar in the measured physiologic variables and clinical components. Two athletes and two controls

**Table 1.** Baseline comparison of athlete (n = 10) and control (n = 5) subjects.

| Parameter | Athletes | | Controls | | |
| --- | --- | --- | --- | --- | --- |
| | Mean | (SD) | Mean | (SD) | p-value |
| Age (years) | 20.4 | (1.08) | 20.6 | (1.14) | 0.81 |
| Body Mass Index (kg/m$^2$) | 30.74 | (1.58) | 24.22 | (2.02) | 0.03 |
| **Clinical Correlates** | | | | | |
| *Physiologic Measures* | | | | | |
| ApoE4 Positive, n (%) | 2 | (20.00) | 2 | (40.00) | 0.56 |
| ApoA1 (mg/dL) | 122.5 | (8.01) | 149.2 | (10.42) | 0.07 |
| S100B (ug/L) | 0.107 | (0.03) | 0.059 | (0.01) | 0.34 |
| S100B AutoAb Titer (Abs) | 1.11 | (0.27) | 2.52 | (0.06) | 0.01 |
| *Balance* | | | | | |
| Balance Error Scoring System | 17.1 | (4.70) | 13.4 | (5.30) | 0.19 |
| Center of Pressure Total Path Length (cm) | 288.6 | (33.00) | 342.2 | (132.00) | 0.23 |
| *Cognitive Performance* | | | | | |
| Visual Memory Score | 74.3 | (15.10) | 70.2 | (14.60) | 0.63 |
| Verbal Memory Score | 90.4 | (6.20) | 85.6 | (9.70) | 0.26 |
| Visual Motor Speed Score | 47.2 | (6.10) | 43.8 | (6.20) | 0.33 |
| Reaction Time (sec) | 0.49 | (0.05) | 0.52 | (0.04) | 0.17 |
| Impulse Control | 3.0 | (4.10) | 6.6 | (2.10) | 0.04 |
| Symptom | 0.20 | (0.63) | 3.20 | (5.20) | 0.09 |
| Cognitive Efficiency Score | 0.45 | (0.12) | 0.39 | (0.11) | 0.40 |

were heterozygous for the ApoE4 allele. Only one athlete had a history of concussion (>2 weeks prior to study).

## WM Changes

Compared to controls, athletes experienced greater WM changes in FA and MD from baseline (Time 1) to the end of the season (Time 2), as seen in **Figure 1, A and C**. These group differences were statistically significant for percentage of voxels with ↓FA (p = 0.024), ↓MD (p = 0.017), and ↑MD (p = 0.003), as shown in **Figure 2**. ↓FA and ↑MD co-localized to the same brain voxels, especially in the corpus callosum (**Figure 3**).

Athletes also had greater voxel changes in FA and MD from baseline (Time 1) to the end of the 6-month no-contact rest period (Time 3), as seen in **Figure 1, panels B and D**. These group differences were statistically significant for ↓FA (p = 0.043), ↓MD (p = 0.017), and ↑MD (p = 0.003) (**Figure 2**). The difference in percentage of voxels with ↑FA was marginally significant (p = 0.076). Viewing the longitudinal trajectory in DTI changes in **Figure 2**, the significant differences observed at the end of the season (Time 2) in ↑MD, ↓MD and ↓FA persisted after 6 months of no-contact rest (Time 3).

## Helmet Impact Measures and Correlation with WM Change

Total head hits for the season ranged from 431 to 1,850. Summary helmet impact measures accrued during the 2011 football season for each athlete are shown in **Table 2**. Notably, none of the athletes suffered a clinically evident concussion during the study period.

Among athletes, changes in FA and MD from Time 1 to Time 2 were associated with several helmet impact measures during the football season (**Figure 4**). Most of these significant correlations

were related to the amount of FA decrease from Time 1 to Time 2. The impact measures with the most robust correlations were number of head hits with a peak rotational acceleration exceeding 4500 rad/sec$^2$ (r = 0.91, p<0.001) and the number of head hits with a peak rotational acceleration exceeding 6000 rad/sec$^2$ (r = 0.81, p<0.001). The direction of these correlations indicates that greater helmet impact measures were associated with greater percentage of voxels with *FA decrease*. The percentage of WM with decreased FA exceeded that of controls when the number of helmet impacts resulting in a peak rotational acceleration >4500 rads/sec$^2$ exceeded 30–40 for the season, and when the number of helmet impacts resulting in a peak rotational acceleration >6000 rads/sec$^2$ exceeded 10-15 for the season. A smaller number of helmet impact measures were significantly correlated to *MD decrease*. The direction of these correlations indicates that greater helmet impact measures were associated with a smaller percentage of voxels with ↓MD. DTI changes between Times 1 and 3 were not consistently associated with helmet impact measures.

## Clinical Correlates and WM Change

Several clinical correlates were also associated with Time 1 to Time 3 WM changes (**Figure 5**). Greater ↓FA was associated with an increase in serum ApoA1 from Time 1 to Time 2 (r = 0.661, p = 0.038) as well as from Time 1 to Time 3 (r = 0.648, p = 0.043). Greater ↑FA was associated with changes in ApoA1 in the opposite direction, that is, with a decrease from Time 1 to Time 2 (r = −0.612, p = 0.060), as well as from Time 1 to Time 3 (r = −0.612, p = 0.060). Greater ↑FA was also associated with lower S100B autoantibody titers at Time 2 (r = −0.624, p = 0.054). Greater ↓MD was associated lower S100B autoantibody titers at Time 1 (r = −0.673, p = 0.033). Greater ↑MD was

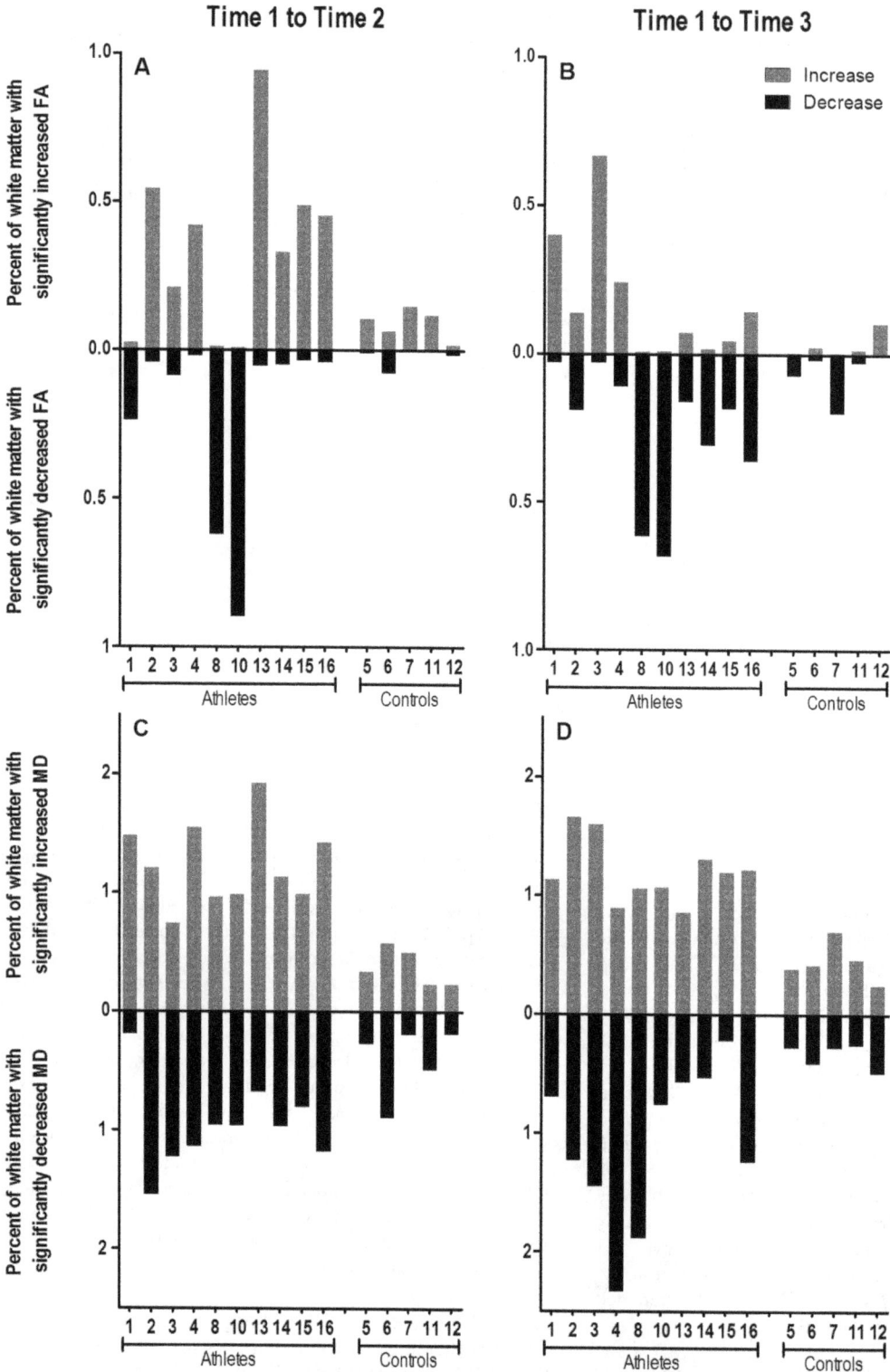

**Figure 1. Subject-Specific DTI Changes.** Subject-specific changes in FA (A and B) and MD (C and D) from Time 1 to Time 2 (A and C) and from Time 1 to Time 3 (B and D). Bars in each graph represent the percentage of white matter voxels in each individual subject with significantly decreased (black) and increased (grey) FA and MD over the specified time interval.

associated with increased levels of serum ApoA1 at Time 1 (r = 0.612, p = 0.060) and Time 3 (r = 0.600, p = 0.067).

WM changes were not systematically associated with balance and cognitive performance measures among athletes at Time 2 or

Time 3, but several patterns did emerge (**Figure 5**). DTI changes between Time 1 and Time 2 were not significantly correlated with most clinical outcome measures examined. However, DTI changes between Time 1 and Time 3 were correlated with both

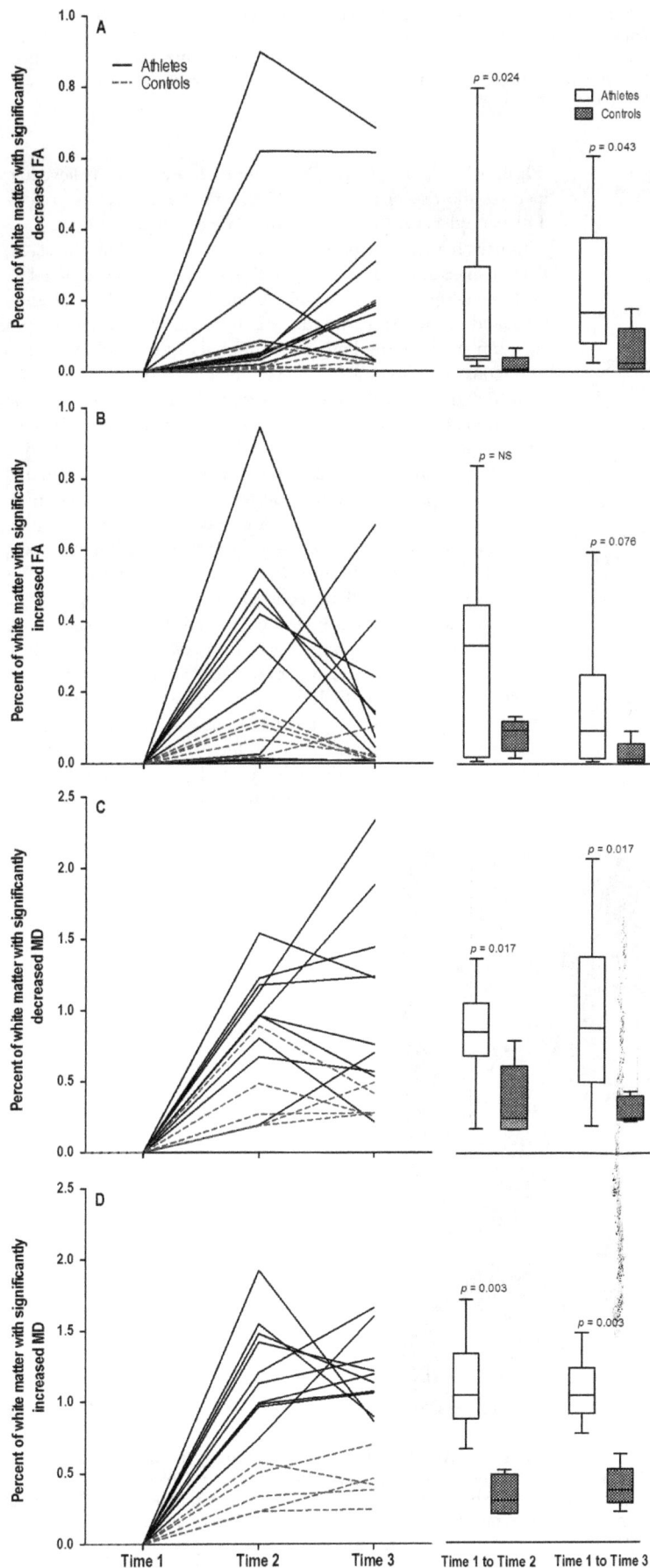

**Figure 2. Trajectory of Subject-specific DTI Changes and Comparison by Subject Group.** Line graphs show the percentage of WM voxels in each athlete (solid lines) and each control (hatched line) with significantly decreased (A and C) and increased (B and D) FA (A and B) and MD (C and D) from Time 1 to Time 2, and from Time 1 to Time 3. Box-and-whisker plots show the maximum and minimum (whiskers), inter quartile range (box) and median (line within box) values for the percentage of WM voxels in athletes (clear) and controls (black) with significantly decreased (A and C) and increased (B and D) FA (A and B) and MD (C and D) from baseline (Time 1) to 6 months of rest (Time 3).

improved ( ↑ FA, ↑ MD) and worsened ( ↓ FA) clinical outcomes as measured by cognitive performance.

## Discussion

In the current study we demonstrate that a single football season of RHIs resulted in significant changes in the structure of WM that persisted despite 6 months of no-contact rest. Post-season WM changes correlated with multiple head impact measures implying a potential causal relationship between helmet impact forces during a season of collegiate football and WM injury, despite no clinically evident concussion.

That these late, persistent changes in WM structure did not correlate with most clinical outcome measures suggests that they are for the most part clinically silent. This makes it difficult to establish with certainty whether these DTI changes are detrimental (i.e. represent damage or potential neuropathology) or in some way adaptive (i.e. represent neural plasticity). However, there were a few significant clinical correlations suggesting that some DTI changes may be detrimental while others are perhaps adaptive. For example, greater ↑ FA between Time 1 and Time 3 was associated with improvements in verbal memory score and impulse control, while greater ↓ FA was associated with worsening impulse control (**Figure 5**). Reciprocal changes in physiologic variables also support this concept. Greater ↑ FA was associated with decreases in serum ApoA1 between Time 1 and Time 3 while greater ↓ FA was associated with increases in serum ApoA1

(**Figure 5**). Although low serum ApoA1 levels are believed to increase the risk of dementia [38,39], their relationship to post-TBI neurodegeneration has yet to be determined.

Others have also reported similar, sometimes clinically silent, DTI changes after non-concussive RHIs. Zhang et al compared 49 professional boxers to 19 healthy controls and found significantly increased mean MD and decreased mean FA in the corpus callosum and posterior limb of the internal capsule [20]. All boxers were considered free of neurologic disease although the methods used to make this determination were not described. Koerte et al compared pre- and postseason DTI scans among 17 male professional ice hockey players, three of whom experienced a clinically diagnosed concussion during the season [22]. Compared to preseason, postseason scans revealed significantly elevated trace, radial diffusion, and axial diffusion in the right precentral region, right corona radiata, and the anterior and posterior limbs of the internal capsule. Results were not given separately for the 14 players who did not suffer a concussion nor was their neurologic status. Additionally, Koerte et al compared the DTI scans of 12 male elite-level club soccer players to 8 male competitive swimmers, none of whom reported a history of concussion [21]. Soccer players had multiple brain regions with increased mean radial and axial diffusivity but none with significant changes in MD or FA. The neurologic status of the players was not reported. Our research group compared pre- and postseason DTI scans among nine high school football and hockey players (one of whom

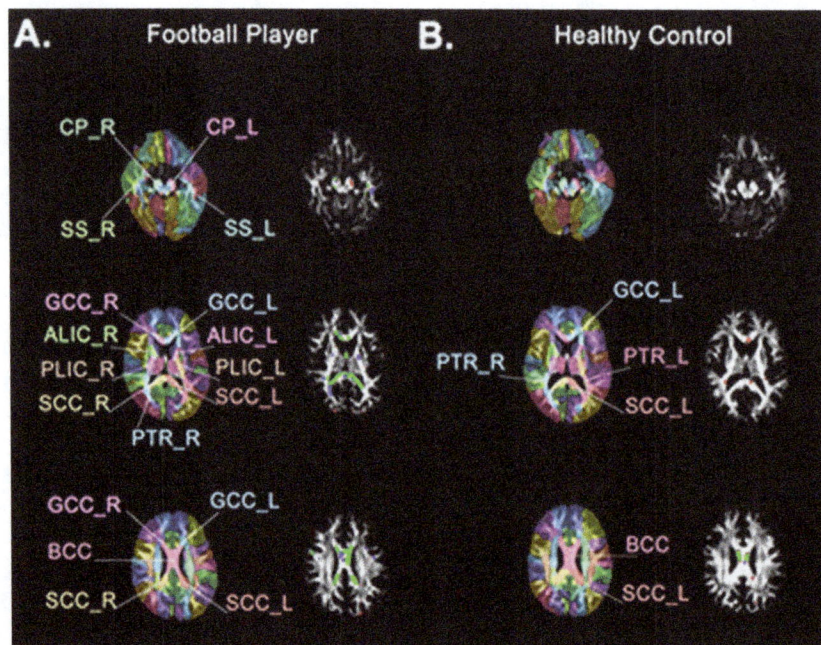

**Figure 3. Spatial Distribution of WM Voxels with Decreased FA and Increased MD.** WM structures (left), and significant DTI changes from Time 1 to Time 2 (right) in a football player (A) and a control subject (B). Columns 2 and 4 depict voxels with significant ↓ FA (blue), significant ↑ MD (red) and both ↓ FA and ↑ MD (green). ALIC: anterior limb of internal capsule; BCC: body of corpus callosum; CP: cerebral peduncle; GCC: genu of corpus callosum; PLIC: posterior limb of internal capsule; PTR: posterior thalamic radiation; SCC: splenium of corpus callosum; SS: sagittal stratum (includes inferior longitudinal fasciculus and inferior fronto-occipital fasciculus).

**Table 2.** Helmet impact measures among athlete subjects (n = 10).

| Position | Total Head Hits | Mean (SD) Linear Acceleration/Hit (g) | Mean (SD) Rotational Acceleration/Hit (rad/sec²) | Total Linear Acceleration (g) | Total Rotational Acceleration (rad/sec²) |
|---|---|---|---|---|---|
| Running Back | 431 | 29.78 (20) | 1880.53 (1513) | 12,836.0 | 810,511 |
| Tight End | 572 | 31.41 (20) | 1815.66 (1279) | 18,033.0 | 1,042,191 |
| Linebacker | 612 | 37.53 (25) | 1973.65 (1438) | 22,969.3 | 1,207,879 |
| Defensive Line | 617 | 27.09 (14) | 1704.77 (1034) | 16,742.4 | 1,053,554 |
| Defensive Line | 649 | 28.23 (17) | 1691.95 (1216) | 18,325.1 | 1,098,081 |
| Full Back | 1,042 | 31.84 (22) | 1877.13 (1572) | 33,250.3 | 1,959,725 |
| Linebacker | 1,142 | 35.24 (24) | 2071.71 (1578) | 40,245.5 | 2,365,894 |
| Defensive Line | 1,423 | 34.36 (20) | 2021.55 (1188) | 48,903.4 | 2,876,675 |
| Offensive Tackle | 1,431 | 26.91 (14) | 1726.87 (1026) | 38,516.7 | 2,471,157 |
| Center | 1,850 | 31.88 (18) | 1837.52 (1076) | 58,994.1 | 3,399,421 |

suffered a concussion during the season) and five healthy controls [24]. Among the eight athletes who did not suffer concussion, increases and decreases in both FA and MD were observed, but without significant changes in post-concussive symptoms or cognitive performance. Total changes in FA and MD among these athletes were over three times that of controls and also correlated to self-reported head hits during the season. Thus, while several studies have examined DTI in the setting of RHIs, few have related these changes to clinical outcomes.

Even fewer studies have linked DTI changes to head impact measures after RHI. However, McAllister et al compared DTI scans before and after a sport season in 80 non-concussed collegiate football and ice hockey players to 79 noncontact sport athletes. There was a significant athlete-group increase in MD in the corpus callosum. Postseason FA and MD in brain regions of interest were correlated with several helmet impact measures including total hits for the season, number of hits during the 14 days prior to scanning, seasonal 95th percentile rotational acceleration, HITsp, and linear acceleration [23].

If RHIs are related to neurodegeneration many years later, a long clinically silent period between the onset of neuronal injury and overt symptoms of dementia would not be unexpected. During this clinically silent period however, indicators of dysfunction on a cellular level are typically demonstrable. For example alterations in CSF levels of tau, phosphorylated tau, amyloid $\beta_{42}$ and calbindin precede the development of overt symptoms of Alzheimer's disease [40,41]. Our finding of altered ApoA1 and S100B autoantibodies in the serum may thus be analogous to these pre-AD changes in the CSF, potentially heralding the early stages of CTE. Pending confirmation in a long-term longitudinal study tracking athletes prospectively for years to decades looking for manifestations of early cognitive dysfunction and dementia, we believe our results suggest that these persistent DTI changes are likely detrimental.

If borne out in future research, the long-term persistence of these WM changes would mean that athletes returning to play the following season would be at risk for expanded RHI-related WM changes, undetectable by conventional assessments. Could the lack of WM recovery we observed result in cumulative WM damage with subsequent football seasons of RHI exposures? If so, could this cumulative WM damage be related to the long-term development of CTE? While we await confirmation for the long-term adverse effects of these WM changes, efforts to limit the development of RHI-related WM changes by monitoring helmet impact measures would seem prudent, and has already been suggested by The Sports Legacy Institute [42]. However rather than monitor total head hits, as has been suggested, it may be more effective to monitor those hits that are most likely to produce WM changes in excess of that seen among controls. In our relatively small sample, the percentage of WM with ↓ FA exceeded that of controls when the number of helmet impacts resulting in a peak rotational acceleration >4500 rads/sec² exceeded 30–40 for the season, and when the number of helmet impacts resulting in a peak rotational acceleration >6000 rads/sec² exceeded 10–15 for the season.

There are several possible explanations for the long-term persistence of WM changes after a football season of RHIs. As a group, athletes did not show significant reduction in Time 1 to Time 2 WM changes during the six-month no-contact rest period. However, individually, some athletes demonstrated a return to baseline levels. Thus for some athletes, six months of rest may be sufficient for recovery, but for others more time may be necessary for postseason changes to return to baseline. In addition, our results suggest that changes in immunity may impact WM

|  | Pre-Season to Post- | | | | Pre-Season to 6 Months | | | |
|---|---|---|---|---|---|---|---|---|
| Helmet Impact Measure | FA↓ | FA↑ | MD↓ | MD↑ | FA↓ | FA↑ | MD↓ | MD↑ |
|  | r | r | r | r | r | r | r | r |
| **Total Hits** | | | | | | | | |
| **Linear Acceleration (g)** | | | | | | | | |
| Total | | | | | | | | |
| Mean Per Hit | | | | | | | | |
| Peak | | | | | | | | |
| Number of Hits > 50 | | | | | | | | |
| Number of Hits > 100 | | | | | | | | |
| Number of Hits > 150 | | | | | | | | |
| Number of Hits > 200 | | | | | | | | |
| **Rotational Acceleration (rad/sec²)** | | | | | | | | |
| Total | | | | | | | | |
| Mean Per Hit | | | | | | | | |
| Peak | | | | | | | | |
| Number of Hits > 1500 | | | | | | | | |
| Number of Hits > 3000 | | | | | | | | |
| Number of Hits > 4500 | | | | | | | | |
| Number of Hits > 6000 | | | | | | | | |
| **Head Injury Criterion** | | | | | | | | |
| Total | | | | | | | | |
| Mean Per Hit | | | | | | | | |
| Number of Hits > 150 | | | | | | | | |
| Number of Hits > 300 | | | | | | | | |
| Number of Hits > 450 | | | | | | | | |
| Number of Hits > 600 | | | | | | | | |
| **Gadd Severity Index** | | | | | | | | |
| Total | | | | | | | | |
| Mean Per Hit | | | | | | | | |
| Number of Hits > 150 | | | | | | | | |
| Number of Hits > 300 | | | | | | | | |
| Number of Hits > 450 | | | | | | | | |
| Number of Hits > 600 | | | | | | | | |
| **Head Impact Technology severity profile** | | | | | | | | |
| Total | | | | | | | | |
| Mean Per Hit | | | | | | | | |
| Number of Hits > 50 | | | | | | | | |
| Number of Hits > 100 | | | | | | | | |
| Number of Hits > 150 | | | | | | | | |
| Number of Hits > 200 | | | | | | | | |

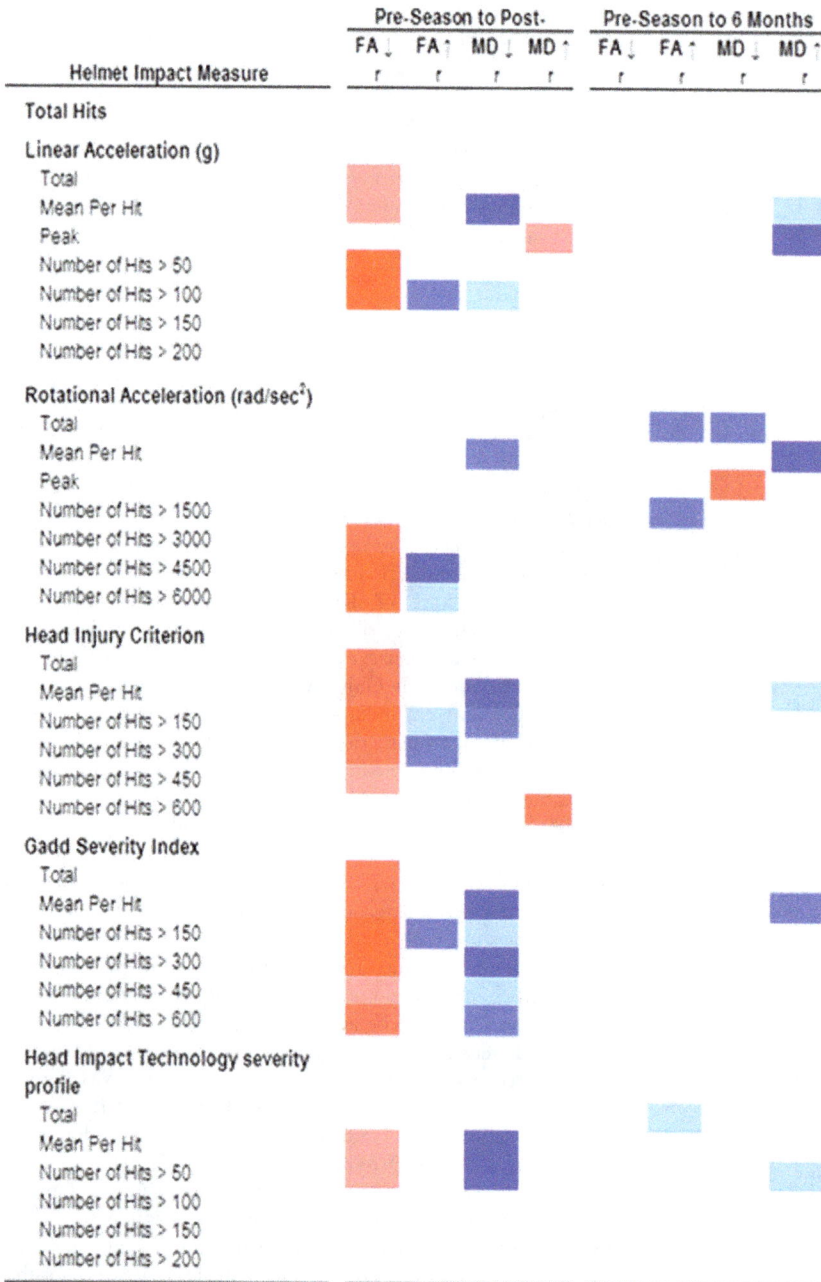

* Correlations with p-values > 0.10 are not reported

* All DTI metrics refer to the proportion of white matter with the FA or MD change indicated

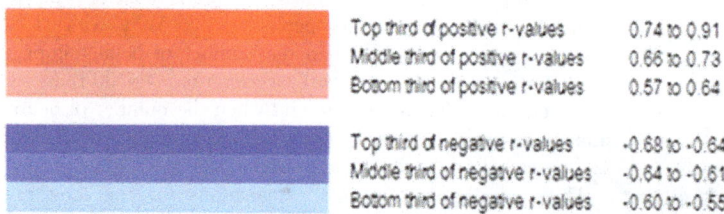

| | |
|---|---|
| Top third of positive r-values | 0.74 to 0.91 |
| Middle third of positive r-values | 0.66 to 0.73 |
| Bottom third of positive r-values | 0.57 to 0.64 |
| Top third of negative r-values | -0.68 to -0.64 |
| Middle third of negative r-values | -0.64 to -0.61 |
| Bottom third of negative r-values | -0.60 to -0.55 |

**Figure 4. Heat map display of correlations between helmet impact measures and DTI changes between pre- and post-season (T1 to T2), and pre- and 6 months post-season (T1 to T3).** Color and shading reflect direction and strength of correlation, as indicated by the figure key. Correlations with p-values>0.10 are not reported. All DTI metrics refer to the proportion of white matter with the FA or MD change indicated.

|  | (T1 to T2)* | | | | Season (T1 to T3)* | | | |
|---|---|---|---|---|---|---|---|---|
| Physiologic Covariate | FA↓ r | FA↑ r | MD↓ r | MD↑ r | FA↓ r | FA↑ r | MD↓ r | MD↑ r |
| Age | | | | | | | | |
| BMI | | | | | | | | |
| ApoE4 | | | | | | | | |
| **S-100B** | | | | | | | | |
| S-100B Pre-Season | | | | | | | | |
| S-100B Post-Season | | | | | | | | |
| S-100B Change (Pre- to Post- Season) | | | | | | | | |
| **S-100B Auto-Antibody** | | | | | | | | |
| S-100B Auto-Ab Pre-Season | | | | | | | | |
| S-100B Auto-Ab Post-Season | | | | | | | | |
| S-100B Auto-Ab Change (Pre- to Post- Season) | | | | | | | | |
| **ApoA1** | | | | | | | | |
| ApoA1 Pre-Season | | | | | | | | |
| ApoA1 Post-Season | | | | | | | | |
| ApoA1 6 Months Post-Season | | | | | | | | |
| ApoA1 Change (Pre- to Post- Season) | | | | | | | | |
| ApoA1 Change (Pre- to 6 Months Post- Season) | | | | | | | | |
| **Clinical Outcome at Post-Season (T2)** | | | | | | | | |
| BESS Total | | | | | | | | |
| Wii Total | | | | | | | | |
| Verbal Memory Score | | | | | | | | |
| Visual Memory Score | | | | | | | | |
| Visual Memory Speed Score | | | | | | | | |
| Reaction Time | | | | | Not Analyzed | | | |
| Impulse Control Score | | | | | | | | |
| Total Symptom Score | | | | | | | | |
| Cognitive Efficiency Index | | | | | | | | |
| **Clinical Outcome at Post-Season (T3)** | | | | | | | | |
| BESS Total | | | | | | | | |
| Wii Total | | | | | | | | |
| Verbal Memory Score | | Not Analyzed | | | | | | |
| Visual Memory Score | | | | | | | | |
| Visual Memory Speed Score | | | | | | | | |
| Reaction Time | | | | | | | | |
| Impulse Control Score | | | | | | | | |
| Total Symptom Score | | | | | | | | |
| Cognitive Efficiency Index | | | | | | | | |

* Correlations with p-values > 0.10 are not shown
† All DTI metrics refer to the percentage of white matter with the FA or MD change indicated

Top third of positive r-values — 0.66 to 0.71
Middle third of positive r-values — 0.61 to 0.65
Bottom third of positive r-values — 0.57 to 0.60

Top third of negative r-values — -0.67 to -0.80
Middle third of negative r-values — -0.62 to -0.67
Bottom third of negative r-values — -0.60 to -0.62

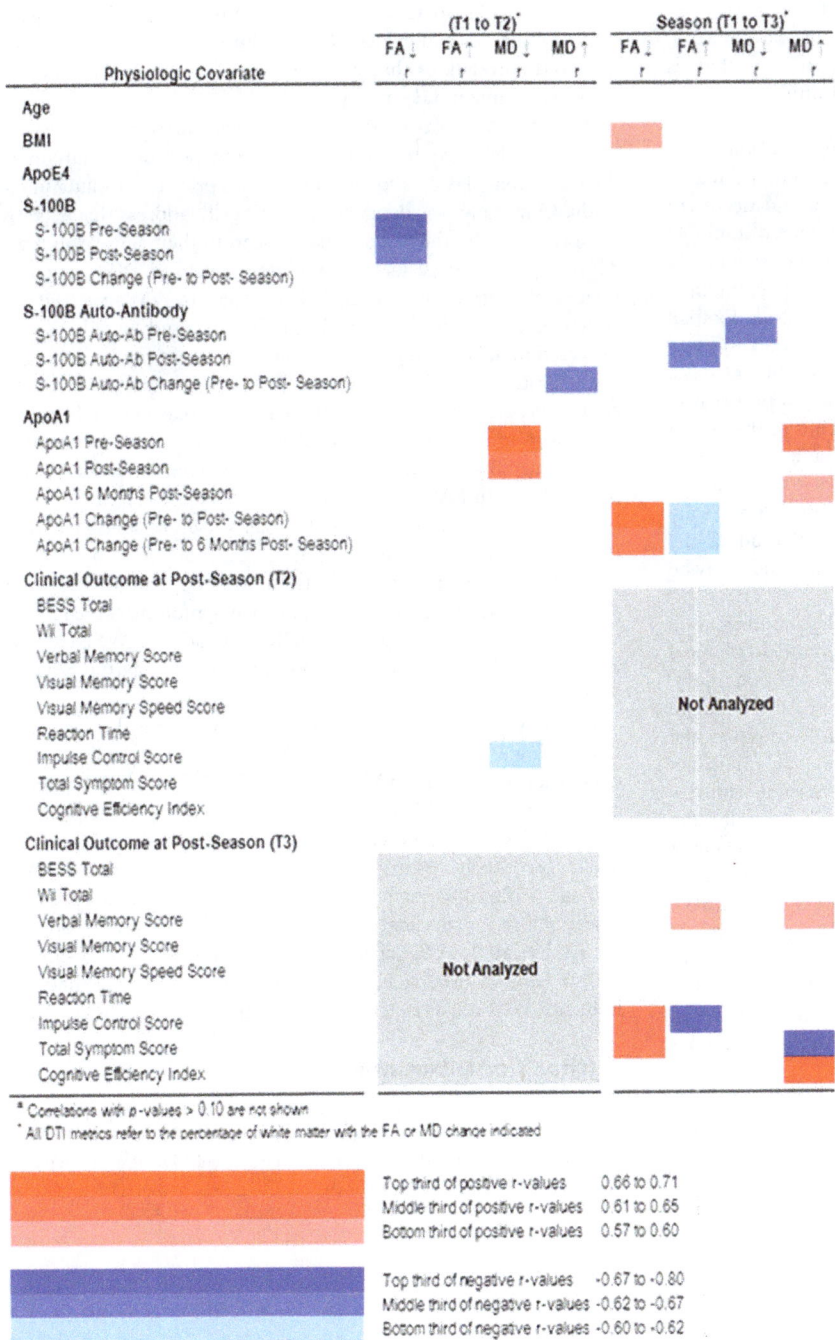

**Figure 5. Physiologic and clinical correlations of DTI changes among athletes.** Color and shading reflect direction and strength of correlation, as indicated by the figure key. Correlations with p-values>0.10 are not reported. All DTI metrics refer to the proportion of white matter with the FA or MD change indicated.

recovery. The significant correlations between S100B autoanti-bodies and WM changes suggest RHIs influence the immune response to repetitive antigen exposure. We have previously demonstrated that RHIs can result in intermittent low-level S100B release in football players [43]. Increased levels of serum S100B following in-season injury appears to lead to the elicitation of anti-S100B autoantibodies, and it is likely these athletes have encountered RHIs during prior seasons. As an innate and adaptive immune response, significant induction of regulatory T cells and other endogenous mechanisms that counteract autoimmunity and promote CNS repair during the off-season likely suppress the humoral response to this antigen, resulting in the lower autoantibody titers we observed among athletes as compared to controls at baseline (Time 1). Low Time 2 S100B autoantibody titers were associated with greater ↑ FA between Time 1 and Time 3, while declines in S100B autoantibody titers between Time 1 and Time 2 were associated with greater ↑ MD during that same time interval. Because the observed DTI changes were mostly clinically silent, the clinical implications of these associations are not clear. If the immune responses induced by

RHIs contribute to the long-term neurodegeneration observed in those with CTE, as has been hypothesized [43], the mechanism(s) by which this adaptive response transitions to one that is maladaptive needs to be identified, and is a fruitful avenue for future research.

In the current study, we speculate that observed whole-brain DTI changes represent a mixture of cellular events. The seemingly paradoxical subject-specific concomitant increases and decreases in both FA and MD are likely due to the occurrence of multiple axonal injuries separated spatially in the brain and temporally across the 3 month football season. For any single athlete, multiple head impacts accrued over the course of the 3 month football season have the potential to injure more than one spatially-distinct area of brain. If injurious head impacts occur on different days, which they likely do, the time interval from injury to post-season scanning will vary for each injured brain area. Thus at the end of the football season each injured brain area will be in unique and possibly different stages in the evolution of traumatic axonal injury and/or repair. Thus the DTI scan of the whole brain done at the end of the football season likely reflects a combination of the cellular events occurring in the injured brain regions which may be at different axonal injury stages.

A limitation of our study is the use of non-athlete controls. The WM changes observed in athletes could have been due to physical exertion associated with college football in addition to brain injury. The clear separation observed between controls and athletes in the percentage of WM with ↑ MD may be more likely to reflect the effect of physical, sports-related exertion on brain water diffusion rather than brain injury, as this DTI metric correlated with few helmet impact measures. Other DTI metrics, especially the percentage of WM with ↓ FA, were more closely linked to helmet impact measures and thus may be less sensitive to the effects of exertion. Indeed, Gons et al reported significant changes in MD, but not FA, among 440 older adults reporting the highest levels of physical exercise [44]. Others have proposed the use of non-contact athletes as controls [21], but to our knowledge there has been no published reports demonstrating a significant difference in subject-specific DTI metrics between age-matched healthy non-athletes and non-contact athletes.

Additionally, although wild bootstrapping includes an adjustment for multiple voxel-wise comparisons, the analysis correlating DTI changes to head hits, antibodies, and cognitive impairments was not adjusted for multiple comparisons due to limited power afforded by the small sample size and the nascent state of the

literature in this area. Regardless, many of the correlations were quite robust, with p-values <0.001. Furthermore, many of the observed correlations that were non-significant displayed moderate-to-large magnitude (r's> |0.50|).

Although one player admitted to having a prior concussion, there is no definitive method to exclude the possibility that any of the remaining players also had concussions prior to enrolling in the study. Our study was designed to specifically address this issue by comparing each athlete's postseason scan to their preseason scan. Thus, rather than evaluating absolute changes in WM structure, relative changes were examined. The effects on WM structure of a concussion occurring prior to beginning the study would not be expected to affect changes in WM structure from the beginning of the season to later time points. Finally, our ability to detect cognitive changes associated with a football season of RHIs may have been improved by the use of more sophisticated pencil-and-paper cognitive testing, rather than the computerized format afforded by ImPACT. For example, McAllister et al detected cognitive changes after a single football season of RHIs by using the California verbal learning test[12]. It may also have been improved by following subjects beyond 6 months for the development of delayed post concussive symptoms or cognitive deficits. The relationship between RHI-associated WM changes and more subtle cognitive changes is yet another fertile area for future research.

Collectively, in this preliminary study, we have demonstrated that a single football season of RHIs without clinically evident concussion resulted in WM changes on DTI. These DTI changes correlated with multiple helmet impact measures and persisted despite 6 months of no-contact rest. This lack of WM recovery could potentially contribute to progressive, cumulative WM damage with subsequent RHI exposures. If this relationship is confirmed in longitudinal studies, efforts to limit the development of RHI-related WM changes by monitoring helmet impact measures, and further elucidation of modifiable factors that may influence WM recovery, could mitigate the long-term risk of CTE.

## Author Contributions

Conceived and designed the experiments: JJB. Performed the experiments: TZ ER AR HJ KMB DJ. Analyzed the data: JJB TZ JZ BA HJ KMB EGB. Contributed reagents/materials/analysis tools: DJ. Wrote the paper: JJB AR JZ EGB BA KMB ER DJ.

## References

1.  Langlois JA, Rutland-Brown W, Wald MM (2006) The epidemiology and impact of traumatic brain injury: a brief overview. Journal of Head Trauma Rehabilitation 21: 375–378.
2.  Greenwald RM, Gwin JT, Chu JJ, Crisco JJ, Greenwald RM, et al. (2008) Head impact severity measures for evaluating mild traumatic brain injury risk exposure. Neurosurgery 62: 789–798; discussion 798.
3.  Crisco JJ, Fiore R, Beckwith JG, Chu JJ, Brolinson PG, et al. (2010) Frequency and location of head impact exposures in individual collegiate football players. Journal of Athletic Training 45: 549–559.
4.  Broglio SP, Schnebel B, Sosnoff JJ, Shin S, Fend X, et al. (2010) Biomechanical properties of concussions in high school football. Medicine & Science in Sports & Exercise 42: 2064–2071.
5.  Marar M, McIlvain N, Fields S, Comstock D (2012) Epidemiology of Concussions Among United States High School Athletes in 20 Sports. The American Journal of Sports Medicine 40: 747–755.
6.  Meehan WP, 3rd, d'Hemecourt P, Collins CL, Comstock RD (2011) Assessment and management of sport-related concussions in United States high schools. Am J Sports Med 39: 2304–2310.
7.  McCrory P, Zazryn T, Cameron P, McCrory P, Zazryn T, et al. (2007) The evidence for chronic traumatic encephalopathy in boxing. Sports Medicine 37: 467–476.
8.  Zetterberg H, Hietala MA, Jonsson M, Andreasen N, Styrud E, et al. (2006)

Neurochemical aftermath of amateur boxing. Archives of Neurology 63: 1277–1280.
9.  Talavage TM, Nauman EA, Breedlove EL, Yoruk U, Dye AE, et al. (2010) Functionally-Detected Cognitive Impairment in High School Football Players Without Clinically-Diagnosed Concussion. Journal of Neurotrauma doi: 10.1089/neu.2010.1512.
10. Breedlove EL, Robinson M, Talavage TM, Morigaki KE, Yoruk U, et al. (2012) Biomechanical correlates of symptomatic and asymptomatic neurophysiological impairment in high school football. Journal of Biomechanics 45: 1265–1272.
11. Jantzen KJ (2010) Functional magnetic resonance imaging of mild traumatic brain injury. Journal of Head Trauma Rehabilitation 25: 256–266.
12. McAllister TW, Flashman LA, Maerlender A, Greenwald RM, Beckwith JG, et al. (2012) Cognitive effects of one season of head impacts in a cohort of collegiate contact sport athletes. Neurology 78: 1777–1784.
13. Martland HS (1928) Punch Drunk. JAMA 91: 1103–1107.
14. McKee AC, Cantu RC, Nowinski CJ, Hedley-Whyte ET, Gavett BE, et al. (2009) Chronic traumatic encephalopathy in athletes: progressive tauopathy after repetitive head injury. Journal of Neuropathology & Experimental Neurology 68: 709–735.
15. Omalu B, Bailes J, Hamilton RL, Kamboh MI, Hammers J, et al. (2011) Emerging histomorphologic phenotypes of chronic traumatic encephalopathy in American athletes. Neurosurgery 69: 173–183; discussion 183.

16. Baugh CM, Stamm JM, Riley DO, Gavett BE, Shenton ME, et al. (2012) Chronic traumatic encephalopathy: neurodegeneration following repetitive concussive and subconcussive brain trauma. Brain Imaging & Behavior 6: 244–254.

17. McKee AC, Stein TD, Nowinski CJ, Stern RA, Daneshvar DH, et al. (2012) The spectrum of disease in chronic traumatic encephalopathy. Brain 136: 43–64.

18. Hazrati L-N TM, Diamandis P, Davis KD, Green RE, Wennberg R WJ, Ezerins L, Tator CH. (2013) Absence of chronic traumatic encephalopathy in retired football players with multiple concussions and neurological symptomatology. Frontiers in Human Neuoscience 2: 1–9.

19. Stern RA, Riley DO, Daneshvar DH, Nowinski CJ, Cantu RC, et al. (2011) Long-term consequences of repetitive brain trauma: chronic traumatic encephalopathy. Pm & R 3: S460–467.

20. Zhang L, Heier LA, Zimmerman RD, Jordan B, Ulug AM (2006) Diffusion anisotropy changes in the brains of professional boxers. Ajnr: American Journal of Neuroradiology 27: 2000–2004.

21. Koerte IK, Ertl-Wagner B, Reiser M, Zafonte R, Shenton ME (2012) White matter integrity in the brains of professional soccer players without a symptomatic concussion. JAMA 308: 1859–1861.

22. Koerte IK KD, Hartl E, Bouix S, Pasternak O, Kubicki M, Rauscher A, Li D, Dadachanji SB, Taunton JA, Forwell LA, Johnson AM, Echlin PS, Shenton ME. (2012) A prospective study of physician-observed concussion during a varsity university hockey season: white matter integrity in ice hockey players. Part 3 of 4. Neurosugical Focus 33: E3.

23. McAllister TW FJ, Flashman LA, Maerlender A, Greenwald RM, Beckwith JG, Bolander RP, Tosteson TD, Turcl JH, Raman R, Jain S. (2013) Effect of head impacts on diffusivity measures in a cohort of collegiate contact sport athletes. Neurology DOI 10.1212/01.wnl.0000438220.16190.42.

24. Bazarian JJ, Zhu T, Blyth B, Borrino A, Zhong J (2012) Subject-specific changes in brain white matter on diffusion tensor imaging after sports-related concussion. Magnetic Resonance Imaging 30: 171–180.

25. Fujita M, Wei EP, Povlishock JT (2012) Intensity- and interval-specific repetitive traumatic brain injury can evoke both axonal and microvascular damage. Journal of Neurotrauma 29: 2172–2180.

26. Mihalik JP, Bell DR, Marshall SW, Guskiewicz KM (2007) Measurement of head impacts in collegiate football players: an investigation of positional and event-type differences. Neurosurgery 61: 1229–1235; discussion 1235.

27. Corrigan JD, Bogner J (2007) Initial reliability and validity of the Ohio State University TBI Identification Method. Journal of Head Trauma Rehabilitation 22: 318–329.

28. Blumbergs PC, Scott G, Manavis J, Wainwright H, Simpson DA, et al. (1995) Topography of axonal injury as defined by amyloid precursor protein and the sector scoring method in mild and severe closed head injury. J Neurotrauma 12: 565–572.

29. Blumbergs PC, Scott G, Manavis J, Wainwright H, Simpson DA, et al. (1994) Staining of amyloid precursor protein to study axonal damage in mild head injury. Lancet 344: 1055–1056.

30. Buki A, Povlishock JT (2006) All roads lead to disconnection?—Traumatic axonal injury revisited. Acta Neurochirurgica 148: 181-193; discussion 193–184.

31. Bazarian JJ, Blyth B, Cimpello L (2006) Bench to bedside: evidence for brain injury after concussion—looking beyond the computed tomography scan. Academic Emergency Medicine 13: 199–214.

32. Hayes WC, Erickson MS, Power ED (2007) Forensic injury biomechanics. Annual Review of Biomedical Engineering 9: 55–86.

33. Collins MW, Iverson GL, Lovell MR, McKeag DB, Norwig J, et al. (2003) On-field predictors of neuropsychological and symptom deficit following sports-related concussion. Clinical Journal of Sport Medicine 13: 222–229.

34. Riemann B, Guskiewicz K (1997) Assessment of mild head injury using measures of balance and cognition: a case study. Journal of Sport Rehabilitation 6: 283–289.

35. Finnoff JT, Peterson VJ, Hollman JH, Smith J, Finnoff JT, et al. (2009) Intrarater and interrater reliability of the Balance Error Scoring System (BESS). Pm & R 1: 50–54.

36. Clark RA, Bryant AL, Pua Y, McCrory P, Bennell K, et al. (2010) Validity and reliability of the Nintendo Wii Balance Board for assessment of standing balance. Gait & Posture 31: 307–310.

37. Hixson JE, Vernier DT (1990) Restriction isotyping of human apolipoprotein E by gene amplification and cleavage with HhaI. Journal of Lipid Research 31: 545–548.

38. Saczynski JS, White L, Peila RL, Rodriguez BL, Launer IJ (2007) The relation between apolipoprotein A-I and dementia: the Honolulu-Asia aging study. American Journal of Epidemiology 165: 985–992.

39. Merched A, Xia Y, Visvikis S, Serot JM, Siest G (2000) Decreased high-density lipoprotein cholesterol and serum apolipoprotein AI concentrations are highly correlated with the severity of Alzheimer's disease. Neurobiology of Aging 21: 27–30.

40. Craig-Schapiro R, Kuhn M, Xiong C, Pickering EH, Liu J, et al. (2011) Multiplexed immunoassay panel identifies novel CSF biomarkers for Alzheimer's disease diagnosis and prognosis. PLoS ONE [Electronic Resource] 6: e18850.

41. Perrin RJ, Fagan AM, Holtzman DM (2009) Multimodal techniques for diagnosis and prognosis of Alzheimer's disease. Nature 461: 916–922.

42. Cantu R, Nowinski C (February 2012) Sports Legacy Institute, Hit Count Initiative. http://wwwsportslegacyorg/policy/hit-count/ Last accessed Nov. 24, 2013.

43. Marchi N, Bazarian J, Puvenna V, Janigro M, Ghosh C, et al. (2013) Consequences of Repeated Blood-Brain Barrier Disruption in Football Players. PLoS ONE [Electronic Resource] 8: e56805. doi:56810.51371/journal.pone.0056805.

44. Gons RAR, Tuladhar AM, de Laat KF, van Norden AGW, van Dijk EJ, et al. (2013) Physical activity is related to the structural integrity of cerebral white matter. Neurology 81: 971–976.

# 18

# Traumatic Brain Injury in the Netherlands: Incidence, Costs and Disability-Adjusted Life Years

**Annemieke C. Scholten**[1]*, **Juanita A. Haagsma**[1], **Martien J. M. Panneman**[2], **Ed F. van Beeck**[1], **Suzanne Polinder**[1]

1 Department of Public Health, Erasmus University Medical Center, Rotterdam, The Netherlands, 2 Research Department, Consumer and Safety Institute, Amsterdam, The Netherlands

## Abstract

*Objective:* Traumatic brain injury (TBI) is a major cause of death and disability, leading to great personal suffering and huge costs to society. Integrated knowledge on epidemiology, economic consequences and disease burden of TBI is scarce but essential for optimizing healthcare policy and preventing TBI. This study aimed to estimate incidence, cost-of-illness and disability-adjusted life years (DALYs) of TBI in the Netherlands.

*Methods:* This study included data on all TBI patients who were treated at an Emergency Department (ED - National Injury Surveillance System), hospitalized (National Medical Registration), or died due to their injuries in the Netherlands between 2010–2012. Direct healthcare costs and indirect costs were determined using the incidence-based Dutch Burden of Injury Model. Disease burden was assessed by calculating years of life lost (YLL) owing to premature death, years lived with disability (YLD) and DALYs. Incidence, costs and disease burden were stratified by age and gender.

*Results:* TBI incidence was 213.6 per 100,000 person years. Total costs were €314.6 (USD $433.8) million per year and disease burden resulted in 171,200 DALYs (on average 7.1 DALYs per case). Men had highest mean costs per case (€19,540 versus €14,940), driven by indirect costs. 0–24-year-olds had high incidence and disease burden but low economic costs, whereas 25–64-year-olds had relatively low incidence but high economic costs. Patients aged 65+ had highest incidence, leading to considerable direct healthcare costs. 0–24-year-olds, men aged 25–64 years, traffic injury victims (especially bicyclists) and home and leisure injury victims (especially 0–5-year-old and elderly fallers) are identified as risk groups in TBI.

*Conclusions:* The economic and health consequences of TBI are substantial. The integrated approach of assessing incidence, costs and disease burden enables detection of important risk groups in TBI, development of prevention programs that target these risk groups and assessment of the benefits of these programs.

**Editor:** Subhra Mohapatra, University of South Florida, United States of America

**Funding:** These authors have no support or funding to report.

**Competing Interests:** The authors have declared that no competing interests exist.

* Email: a.scholten@erasmusmc.nl

## Introduction

Traumatic brain injury (TBI) – defined as an alteration in brain function, or other evidence of brain pathology, caused by an external cause [1] – is a leading cause of morbidity, disability, and mortality worldwide. In Europe, the annual incidence rate of hospitalized and fatal TBI is about 235 per 100,000 person years [2]. TBI survivors almost all experience some level of impairment or disability [2], which drastically reduces their health-related quality of life (HRQL) [3,4].

In addition to the often long-term impact of TBI on a person's life, the economic consequences of TBI for both individuals and society are substantial [5,6]. TBI patients require specialized pre-hospital care, transport, in-hospital (emergency) care, and often long-term rehabilitation. Survivors of more severe TBI are often unable to return to full employment [7,8]. TBI therefore leads to significant direct healthcare costs in terms of pre-hospital care, emergency care, hospitalization, long-term outpatient care and rehabilitation, and indirect costs due to loss of productivity. The total direct and indirect costs of TBI occurring in Europe were estimated to €33 billion (approximately USD $45.4 billion) [9].

Most efforts on assessing the impact of TBI have been limited to either its epidemiology [2,10,11], costs [5,6,9,12–18] or disease burden [17,19,20]. Integrated knowledge on epidemiology, economic consequences and disease burden of TBI is scarce but essential for optimizing healthcare policy, allocating scarce resources, preventing TBI, and developing effective healthcare and rehabilitation services. Up till now, an insight of the total population impact of TBI is lacking. The purpose of this study was to estimate the incidence, cost-of-illness and disability-adjusted life years (DALYs) of TBI in the Dutch population, and to detect important risk groups in TBI.

## Methods

### Data sources

This surveillance-based study included data on all patients with TBI treated at an ED and/or admitted to hospital in the Netherlands in the period 2010–2012. TBI cases were extracted from the Dutch Injury Surveillance System (LIS) [21] and the National Hospital Discharge Registry (LMR) [22], to include data of TBI patients treated at the ED and hospitalized TBI patients respectively.

LIS is an ongoing monitoring system which records data of all unintentional and intentional injured patients who attend the ED. LIS is based upon the registration of 13 hospitals in the Netherlands (12–15% coverage) that are considered to be representative for the total Dutch injury-related ED visits. To generate national estimates of the injury-related ED visits in the Netherlands, an extrapolation factor was calculated in which the number of ED treatments due to injury registered by the participating hospitals is multiplied by the quotient of the number of hospital admissions due to injury in the Netherlands divided by the number of hospital admissions due to injury registered in the participating hospitals [23]. The required data on the number of hospital admissions due to TBI in the Netherlands is obtained from the LMR, which collects data from all Dutch hospitals regarding patient information from hospital admission to discharge. In this study, data from LIS was used to assess sociodemographic (age at injury and sex), injury (type of injury, external cause of injury, multiple injury), and healthcare related characteristics (hospitalization and length of stay). To avoid double counting, only the LMR was used to obtain data of hospitalized patients on the type of injury (ICD-9-codes) and for costs calculations.

### Definition of TBI

For patients treated at the ED, TBI was defined as having a "Concussion" or "Other skull – brain injury" in at least one of the three injuries that can be recorded in LIS. This study therefore included all cases in which TBI was registered as first, second or third injury. In case of multiple injuries, an hierarchy derived from the literature was used to determine the most severe injuries [24]. This hierarchy prioritized spinal cord injury over skull or brain injury (except concussions), hip fracture, and other lower extremity fractures, respectively. For hospitalized patients, TBI was defined using the International Classification of Diseases, ninth revision (ICD-9-CM). This study included ICD-9-codes related to concussion (850), fractures (800–801, 803, 804), lesion (851–854), late effects (905, 907), nerve injury (950), and unspecified head injury (959).

### Cost-of-illness

Short- and long-term direct costs (e.g., healthcare costs) and indirect costs (e.g., productivity loss) of TBI were calculated with use of the incidence-based Dutch Burden of Injury Model [23,25]. This model calculates patient numbers, healthcare consumption, and related costs for predefined patient groups that are homogenous in terms of health service use. Data on healthcare consumption was obtained from the LIS and LMR database, rehabilitation centers (LIVRE), nursing homes (SIVIS), and a patient follow-up survey conducted in 2007–2008 [23,26,27].

Direct healthcare costs of TBI were calculated by multiplying incidence by healthcare volumes (e.g., length of stay), transition probabilities (e.g., probability of hospital admission), and unit costs (e.g., costs per day in hospital). All unit costs were estimated according to national guidelines for healthcare costing [28],

reflecting real resource use (Table 1). Indirect costs of TBI were calculated for all TBI patients in the working age 15 to 64 years treated at the ED or hospitalized, based on information on work absence and return to work from the patient follow-up questionnaire conducted in 2007–2008 [23,26,27].

In order to compare the costs of TBI in the Netherlands with previous cost studies conducted in other countries and at varying points in time, all costs estimates were adjusted for inflation with use of the Consumer Price Index [29–31] and converted into 2012 Euros (as at 31 December 2012 €1.00 = USD $1.3203).

### Burden of TBI

The national disease burden of TBI was measured using the disability-adjusted life year (DALY), a summary measure of population health [32]. To calculate the burden of disease, information on premature mortality, and morbidity and disability due to non-fatal health outcome is combined into one single number. This number represents the health gap between the current state of a population's health compared to an ideal situation where individuals would live to the standard life expectancy in full health, i.e., free of disease and disability. DALYs are the sum of the years of life lost due to premature mortality (YLLs) and years lived with disability (YLDs). YLLs were calculated by multiplying the number of deaths at each age by a standard life expectancy at that age. The number of deaths at each age were calculated with use of the average European case-fatality rate of 11%; about 3% in-hospital and 8% out-of-hospital [2,33]. To allow for international comparisons, the life expectancy was calculated using the Coale-Demeny model West life tables, with a life expectancy at birth of 80 years for males and 82.5 years for females [34].

YLDs were calculated in three steps [35]. First, data was gathered on the incidence, age and sex distribution of patients treated at the ED or hospitalized due to TBI. Second, the incidence data was divided into the injury categories "Concussion" and "Skull-brain injury" of the EUROCOST classification system [36]. Finally, the grouped incidence data was combined with the disability weights and durations developed within the framework of the European INTEGRIS (Integration of European Injury Statistics) study [35]. Registered cases were multiplied with the 1-year disability weight, the proportion of lifelong consequences (Concussion: 4% ED, 21% hospitalized; Skull-brain injury: 13% ED, 23% hospitalized) and the duration (life expectancy at age of injury, by sex). The mean 1-year disability weights included the temporary and lifelong consequences for cases seen in EDs and those recorded in hospital discharge registers for both concussions (Temporary: 0.015 ED, 0.100 hospitalized; Lifelong: 0.151) and skull-brain injuries (Temporary: 0.090 ED, 0.241 hospitalized; Lifelong: 0.323). To compare the impact of TBI with that of other injuries, YLDs for the other injuries were also calculated with disability weights obtained from the INTEGRIS study. The disability weights were derived from empirical follow-up data on the health-related quality of life of individual trauma patients, and adjusted for population norms, age and gender [35].

### Data and statistical analysis

All statistical analyses were carried out using the statistical package SPSS for Windows, version 21 (IBM SPSS Statistics, SPSS Inc, Chicago, IL). Descriptive statistics were used to provide insight in the characteristics of TBI patients. Continuous variables were described by presenting the median and interquartile range. Incidence rates per 100,000 person years were calculated using population data from Statistics Netherlands [37]. A value of $p < 0.05$ was used to determine statistical significance. All data reported in this article are national estimates.

**Table 1.** Unit costs (2012).

| Resource | Unit costs |
| --- | --- |
| **General Practitioner** | |
| Practice consultation | €33.70 |
| Consultation by telephone | €16.90 |
| Home visit | €67.40 |
| Referral patient treated at the ED | €35.00 |
| Referral hospitalized patient | €44.00 |
| Follow-up care patient treated at the ED | €33.70 |
| Follow-up care hospitalized patient | €37.80 |
| **Ambulance** | |
| Emergency journey | €538.20 |
| Scheduled journey | €206.20 |
| **Hospital** | |
| Attendance of emergency department | Injury specific fees[1] |
| Hospitalization general hospital | €460.40/day |
| Hospitalization academic hospital | €629.00/day |
| Intensive care | €1,751.50/day |
| Day care | €310.30/day |
| Outpatient department visit | €178.10/visit |
| Medical procedures | Reimbursement fees |
| **Long term care** | |
| Nursing home | €264.60/day, 138.80/day care |
| Rehabilitation | €469.10/day |
| Physiotherapy | €38.00/treatment |
| **Home care** | |
| Domestic care | €30.60/h |
| Care | €39.10/h |
| Nursing | €67.60/h |
| Nursing & care | €46.40/h |
| **Labor costs (including VAT)** | |
| 15–19 year | €13.50/hour |
| 20–24 year | €24.70/hour |
| 25–29 year | €32.80/hour |
| 30–34 year | €39.30/hour |
| 35–39 year | €43.30/hour |
| 40–44 year | €45.40/hour |
| 45–49 year | €46.80/hour |
| 50–54 year | €48.50/hour |
| 55–59 year | €49.70/hour |
| 60–64 year | €50.70/hour |
| Overall mean | €40.90/hour |

[1]Unit costs for attendance of emergency department are calculated per type of injury in an annually unit cost study indexing the tariffs per minute of nurses, physicians and specialists.
ED: emergency department; VAT: value added tax.

## Results

### Incidence

In the period 2010–2012, annually 34,681 patients visited the ED due to TBI (Table 2), comprising about 4% of the total injury-related ED visits per year in the Netherlands. The overall incidence rate of ED visits due to TBI was 213.6 per 100,000 person years, 241.9 for males and 175.3 for females respectively. Incidence rates were highest in children (268.2), young adults (271.6) and older patients in the age of 75–84 years (307.6) or 85 and older (578.2). The majority of patients sustained a TBI because of a home and leisure injury (47.9%) or traffic injury (33.5%).

**Table 2.** Incidence and characteristics of traumatic brain injuries in the Dutch population (2010–2012)[1].

| | Dutch Injury Surveillance System N = 3,762 (%) | National estimate N = 34,681 (%) | Incidence (per 100,000) Total: 213.6 |
|---|---|---|---|
| **Gender** | | | |
| Male | 2,162 (57.5) | 19,937 (57.5) | 241.9 |
| Female | 1,600 (42.5) | 14,744 (42.5) | 175.3 |
| **Age** | | | |
| 0–14 | 846 (22.5) | 7,793 (22.5) | 268.2 |
| 15–24 | 601 (16.0) | 5,538 (16.0) | 271.6 |
| 25–44 | 714 (19.0) | 6,584 (19.0) | 148.7 |
| 45–64 | 789 (21.0) | 7,281 (21.0) | 156.1 |
| 65–74 | 332 (8.8) | 3,062 (8.8) | 211.4 |
| 75–84 | 287 (7.6) | 2,648 (7.6) | 307.6 |
| 85+ | 192 (5.1) | 1,775 (5.1) | 578.2 |
| **Accident category and type of road user** | | | |
| Home and leisure | 1,806 (48.0) | 16,628 (47.9) | |
| Traffic | 1,256 (33.4) | 11,616 (33.5) | |
| *Pedestrian* | *66 (5.3)* | *613 (5.3)* | |
| *Bicyclist* | *706 (56.9)* | *6,522 (56.9)* | |
| *Moped occupant* | *151 (12.2)* | *1,406 (12.3)* | |
| *Motor vehicle/scooter occupant* | *63 (5.1)* | *575 (5.0)* | |
| *Passenger vehicle occupant* | *205 (16.5)* | *1,898 (16.5)* | |
| *Other* | *49 (4.0)* | *455 (4.0)* | |
| *Unknown* | *16* | *148* | |
| Sport | 307 (8.2) | 2,824 (8.1) | |
| Occupational | 109 (2.9) | 1,003 (2.9) | |
| Assault | 247 (6.6) | 2,269 (6.5) | |
| Self-mutilation | 18 (0.5) | 171 (0.5) | |
| Other | 19 (0.5) | 172 (0.5) | |
| **Type of brain injury**[2,3] | | | |
| *Concussion* | | 8,983 (44.7) | |
| *Fracture* | | | |
| Vault | | 317 (1.6) | |
| Base | | 1,319 (6.6) | |
| Other/unqualified | | 330 (1.6) | |
| Multiple fractures | | 130 (0.6) | |
| *Lesion* | | | |
| Cerebral laceration/contusion | | 1,977 (9.8) | |
| Subarachnoid/sub-/extradural hemorrhage | | 1,598 (7.9) | |
| Other/NFS intracranial hemorrhage | | 262 (1.3) | |
| Intracranial injury, other/NFS nature | | 5,116 (25.5) | |
| *Late effects* | | | |
| Musculoskeletal and connective tissue | | 46 (0.2) | |
| Nervous system | | 18 (0.1) | |
| *Nerve injury* | | | |
| Optic nerve and pathways | | 3 (<0.1) | |
| Unknown | | 14,581 (42.0) | |
| **Number of injuries** | | | |
| 1 injury | 1,065 (28.3) | 9,766 (28.2) | |
| 2 injuries | 2,033 (54.0) | 18,773 (54.1) | |
| ≥3 injuries | 664 (17.7) | 6,142 (17.7) | |
| **Hospitalization** | | | |

**Table 2.** Cont.

| | Dutch Injury Surveillance System N = 3,762 (%) | National estimate N = 34,681 (%) | Incidence (per 100,000) Total: 213.6 |
|---|---|---|---|
| Not admitted | 1,633 (43.5) | 15,024 (43.4) | |
| Unknown | 8 | 70 | |
| 1–3 days | 1,424 (70.4) | 13,146 (70.4) | |
| ≥4 days | 597 (29.6) | 5,529 (29.6) | |
| N days unknown | 106 | 982 | |

[1]Mean number per year in the period 2010–2012.
[2]Traumatic brain injury diagnoses (ICD-9 codes): *Concussion:* Concussion (850): *Cranial fracture:* Fracture of vault of skull (800); Fracture of base of skull (801); Other and unqualified skull fractures (803); Multiple fractures involving skull or face with other bones (804): *Lesion:* Cerebral laceration and contusion (851); Subarachnoid, subdural, and extradural hemorrhage after injury (852); Other and unspecified intracranial hemorrhage after injury (853); Intracranial injury of other and unspecified nature (854): *Late effects:* Late effects of musculoskeletal and connective tissue injuries (905); Late effects of injuries to the nervous system (907): *Nerve injury:* Injury to optic nerve and pathways (950): *Head injury, unspecified* (959, N = 0).
[3]Data on injury type (ICD) only known for hospitalized patients in the LMR database (National estimate: N = 20,100).

Patients that sustained a TBI due to a traffic accident often concerned bicyclists (56.9%) and passenger vehicle occupants (16.5%). Home and leisure injuries often concerned a fall among 0–5-year-olds and elderly patients (aged 60 years and older). ED visits due to TBI often included the diagnoses concussion (44.7%), intracranial injury of other or unspecified nature (25.5%) and cerebral laceration or contusion (9.8%). Almost one in three TBI patients were treated for more than one injury and more than half of the patients were hospitalized, most frequently for 1 or 2 days (61.7% of the hospitalized patients).

## Cost-of-illness

The estimated total costs of TBI in the Netherlands was €314.6 million per year (Table 3). Total direct healthcare costs (€158.6 million) were comparable to indirect costs (€155.9 million), whereas in the working population per case mean direct healthcare costs were more than 3 times lower than the indirect costs. Overall, the mean total costs per case were €18,030, and were higher for men (€19,540) than for women (€14,940). This difference is mostly driven by the difference in indirect costs per TBI patient (males €15,416; females €10,257; p<0.001). The estimated total amount of omitted work days among TBI patients with paid employment was 44 days per case, and significantly differed between men (mean 46 days) and women (mean 38 days) (p<0.001). Both direct and indirect costs per TBI patient increased with the length of hospital stay.

The average direct costs per case increased with age (Figure 1). Mean direct costs per case were higher (up to €950) for men than for women in the ages up to 74 years, while in individuals aged over 75 years women had much higher mean direct costs per case (up to € 3,210) than men. Indirect costs (applicable to individuals aged 15–64 years old) also increased with age, and were higher (up to €6,280) for men than for women.

## Disability-adjusted life years

TBI resulted in 52,998 YLD and 118,207 YLL respectively, amounting to 171,205 DALYs (on average 7.07 DALYs per TBI patient, Table 4). Overall, 69% of the total burden was caused by premature mortality. The burden due to permanent (lifelong) disability was high compared with temporary (short-term) disability. Men were responsible for 59% of the total burden of TBI, and had higher YLDs, YLLs and DALYs per case than women (YLD per case: 2.29 in men vs 2.05 in women; YLL per case: 4.97 vs 4.76; DALY per case: 7.27 vs 6.81). Mean YLD decreased with age in both men and women, and was highest among 0–14-years-olds (Figure 2).

**Table 3.** Cost-of-illness by hospitalization and gender (2010–2012).

| | Hospitalization | Direct costs per case[1] | Indirect costs per case[1] | Total costs per case[1] | Total costs (€) |
|---|---|---|---|---|---|
| **Total** | 0–7 days | 3,584 | 12,454 | 16,040 | 234,259,230 |
| | >7 days | 9,854 | 21,431 | 31,280 | 64,608,290 |
| | Total | **4,361** | **13,668** | **18,030** | **314,592,930** |
| **Men** | 0–7 days | 3,413 | 14,116 | 17,530 | 149,815,870 |
| | >7 days | 8,809 | 22,216 | 31,020 | 41,805,590 |
| | Total | **4,128** | **15,416** | **19,540** | **202,953,300** |
| **Women** | 0–7 days | 3,812 | 9,479 | 13,290 | 84,443,360 |
| | >7 days | 11,433 | 18,638 | 30,070 | 22,802,690 |
| | Total | **4,680** | **10,257** | **14,940** | **111,639,630** |

[1]Mean costs per case: indirect costs per case are presented as an average of only the working population (15 to 65 years).

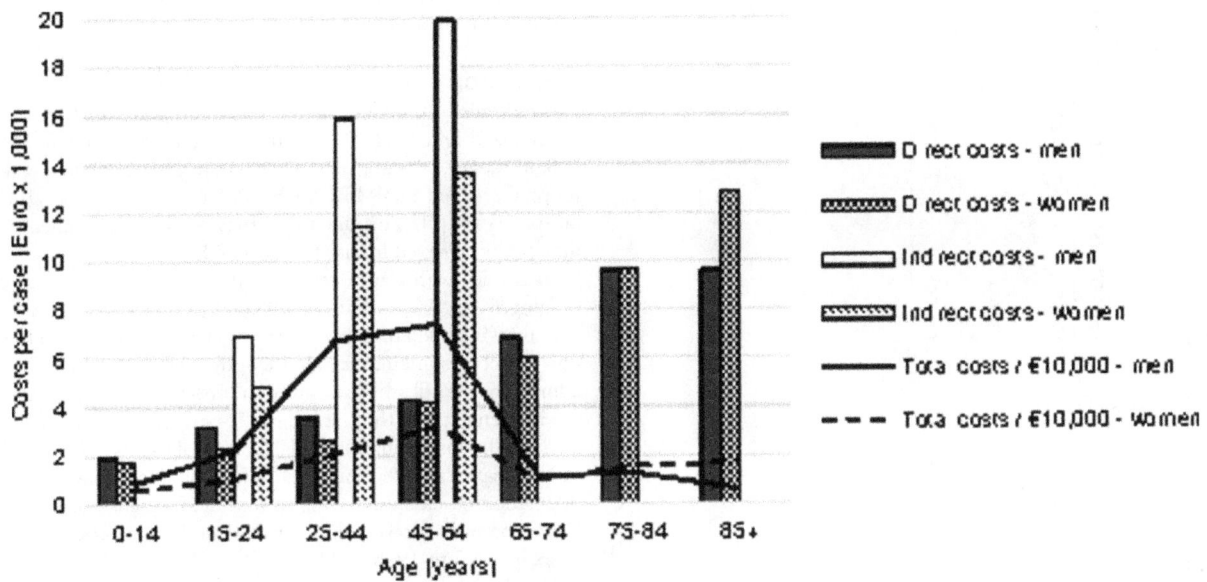

**Figure 1. Mean direct and indirect costs per case and total costs by age and gender (2010–2012).**

## TBI in comparison to other injury categories

In the period 2007–2011, TBI accounted 10% of the total YLDs and 12% of the lifelong YLDs caused by all injuries in the Netherlands (data not shown). Concussion and skull-brain injury both were ranked in the top 5 of injuries with highest total YLDs, after fractures of the knee or lower leg, ankle, and foot or toes (Table 5). Skull-brain injury accounted for the highest YLDs per case after spinal cord injury: 2.89 and 14.68 respectively (data not shown).

## Discussion

The purpose of this paper was to estimate the incidence, cost-of-illness and disability-adjusted life years (DALYs) of TBI in the Netherlands. Our study revealed that TBI imposes a substantial economic and disease burden (on average 7.1 DALYs per TBI patient) on the Dutch population, accounting for more than 4% of injury-related ED visits, 9% of the injury-related costs and 10% of the injury-related YLDs in the Netherlands.

The integrated approach of our study showed that the incidence and burden of disease among children and young adults aged 0–24 years is high, whereas the economic consequences for this group were low due to relatively shorter hospitalization and almost no indirect costs (Figure 3). The reverse is shown in the 25–64-year-olds, who have relatively low incidence and high economic costs, driven by loss of productivity. Older patients aged 65+ had highest

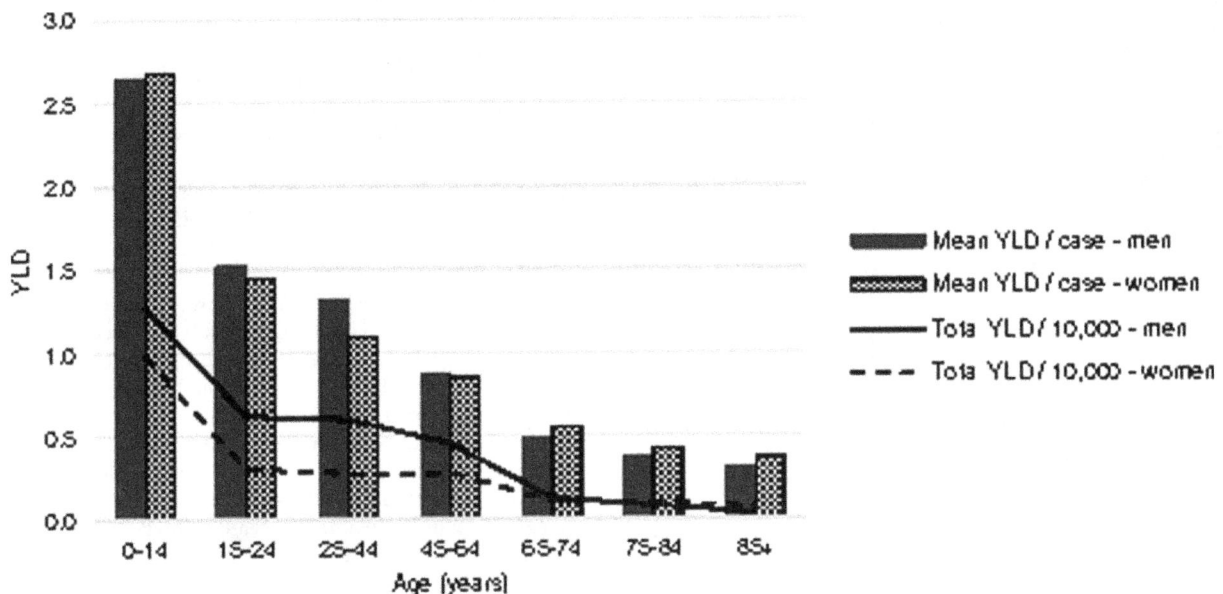

**Figure 2. Mean years lived with disability by age and gender (2010–2012). YLD: years lived with disability.**

**Table 4.** Total temporary and lifelong years lived with disability, years of life lost and disability-adjusted life-years per 1-year interval (2010–2012).

| | N | YLD ED visits | | YLD hospital admission | | YLL | Total DALYs¹ | DALYs per case |
|---|---|---|---|---|---|---|---|---|
| | | Temporary | Lifelong | Temporary | Lifelong | | | |
| Men | 13,877 | 56 | 1,077 | 2,098 | 28,603 | 69,022 | 100,856 | 7.27 |
| Women | 10,330 | 47 | 941 | 1,470 | 18,706 | 49,185 | 70,348 | 6.81 |
| Concussion | 12,580 | 54 | 1,023 | 897 | 13,540 | 118,207 | 171,205 | 7.07 |
| Skull-brain injury | 11,631 | 50 | 995 | 2,670 | 33,769 | | | |
| **Total** | **24,211** | **104** | **2,018** | **3,567** | **47,309** | **118,207** | **171,205** | **7.07** |

¹Disability-adjusted life-years (DALYs) per year.
YLD: years lived with disability; ED: emergency department; YLL: years of life lost.

incidence of TBI, leading to considerable direct healthcare costs, and a relatively low disease burden.

## Comparison of results to other studies

**Incidence.** Our estimated incidence rate of ED treated, hospitalized and fatal TBI for the Netherlands of about 214 per 100,000 person years was lower than the estimated rate of hospitalized and fatal TBI for Europe of about 235 per 100,000 persons years [2]. This difference may partly be explained by the time period covered in the studies. The European rate was derived from studies with data over 1974 to 2000, with incidence rates ranging from 150 to 300 per 100,000 person years [2], whereas our study included data from 2010 to 2012. Compared to the US, the Dutch estimated incidence rates of ED visits, hospital admissions and deaths are considerably lower. It is estimated that the incidence of TBI in the US is 577 per 100,000 person years in 2006 [38], comprising about 1,365,000 ED visits (81%), 275,000 hospitalizations (16%) and 52,000 deaths (3%). However, other population-based studies suggest that the incidence of TBI in the US is somewhat lower, between 180 to 250 per 100,000 person years in 1965 to 1996 [2,11].

Consistent with prior research [2,38], TBI incidence was higher among men than women, and highest among children and older people. Whereas motor vehicle accidents and falls were the most common mechanisms of injury in previous studies in Europe [2] and the US [6,17,38], our sample showed a high number of ED treatments among bicyclists in the traffic setting. Cycling is a very popular form of transport and recreation in the Netherlands, as up to 28% of all trips nationwide are made by bicycle [39]. The popularity of cycling however also imposes a high burden on society, due the large number of (brain) injuries among cyclist [40–42]. Bicycle helmets are not compulsory in the Netherlands and are only commonly used among road cyclist, mountain bikers and young children.

**Cost-of-illness.** TBI accounted for 9% of total costs of all injuries in the Netherlands (about €3.5 billion). The direct healthcare costs of TBI are on average €4,300 per case. This is in line with the outcomes of a previous study on the costs of all types of injuries in the Netherlands in 2004 that estimated the average direct healthcare costs of skull and brain injury cases at €3,100 [12]. This is approximately €4,100 when converting 2004 Euros to 2012 Euros using consumer price index.

Compared to other European countries our estimation of direct healthcare costs of TBI are somewhat higher [5]: from €2,700 in whole Europe, to €2,930 in Germany, €3,490 in Spain and €3,453 in Sweden after adjustment for inflation up to 2012. Estimates from the US are however more than two times the estimates in our present study: about €23,500 acute hospital charges per TBI [15], €6,200 per TBI in Missouri [17], and €8,500 to €35,000 for mild to severe hospitalized patients [6] - all scaled to 2012 price levels and 2012 Euro. These differences can partly be explained by differences in cost calculations. The European cost calculations were limited to inpatient costs while the current study included also extramural healthcare costs, and most US studies used charges instead of unit costs. Although the methodology of cost calculations varied considerably, our study confirms that indirect costs of TBI are far higher than direct healthcare costs of TBI [9,17,43,44], costs of TBI are higher among men than women and increase with age [5] and that the costs increase with the length of hospital stay [6]. The latter suggests that the economic burden of TBI varies considerably by TBI severity.

Overall, TBI imposes a high economic burden on society and, together with hip fracture, is a leading source of hospital costs [13]

**Table 5.** Top ten injuries with highest disability in the Netherlands by accident category (2007–2011)[1].

| Rank | Home and leisure | Traffic | Sport | Occupational | Total |
|---|---|---|---|---|---|
| 1 | Fracture ankle | Fracture knee/lower leg | Fracture knee/lower leg | Fracture foot/toes | Fracture knee/lower leg |
| 2 | Fracture foot/toes | **Skull-brain injury** | Fracture ankle | Fracture knee/lower leg | Fracture ankle |
| 3 | Fracture knee/lower leg | **Concussion** | Fracture foot/toes | Fracture ankle | Fracture foot/toes |
| 4 | **Concussion** | Fracture ankle | Lux/dist ankle/foot | Spinal cord injury | **Skull-brain injury** |
| 5 | **Skull-brain injury** | Spinal cord injury | Lux/dist knee | **Skull-brain injury** | **Concussion** |
| 6 | Hip fracture | Fracture foot/toes | **Concussion** | Complex soft tissue arm/hand | Spinal cord injury |
| 7 | Spinal cord injury | Hip fracture | Fracture wrist | Lux/dist ankle/foot | Hip fracture |
| 8 | Fracture upper arm | Fracture shoulder | **Skull-brain injury** | **Concussion** | Lux/dist ankle/foot |
| 9 | Lux/dist ankle/foot | Fracture upper arm | Fracture upper arm | Lux/dist knee | Fracture upper arm |
| 10 | Fracture wrist | Fracture upper leg | Fracture shoulder | Open wound | Lux/dist knee |

[1]Ranked by total years lived with disability (YLD) for short- and long-term disability.
Lux/dist: luxation/distortion.

and direct healthcare costs [12] in the Netherlands due to high healthcare costs per patient.

**Disability-adjusted life years.** TBI accounted for 10% of total YLD and 12% of the lifelong YLD caused by all injuries in the Netherlands, due to lifelong consequences in a relative young patient group. TBI resulted in both high temporary and lifelong YLD among road traffic injuries and home and leisure injuries, as confirmed in the literature [19,45]. TBI is one of the leading causes of disease burden compared to other injuries and diseases in the Netherlands. TBI imposes a disease burden comparable to that of depression, diabetes, and lung cancer, which are all in the top 10 diseases with highest total DALY in the Netherlands [46]. Mean YLD decreased with age and was highest among children (0–14 years). This can partly be explained by the use of the expected number of years of life remaining as the duration of TBI in the YLD calculation. This method assumes that a proportion of the TBI patients will live with disability outcomes for the remainder of their expected lifetime. Therefore the duration used

in the YLD calculation equaled the life expectancy at age based on the Coale-Demeny model West life tables [34]; in our sample on average 45 years in men and 43 in women. This may have led to a higher estimate of the years lived with disability after TBI in comparison to the use of a fixed average duration for TBI.

## Limitations

The number of deaths due to TBI in the Netherlands could not be generated from national death statistics, because these are only available for specific diseases (e.g., type of cancer, cardiovascular diseases) or injuries specified by cause (e.g., traffic accidents, falls, drowning, self-mutilation). Therefore, the YLL component of the total DALY was estimated with use of the European average case fatality rate of TBI, derived from 18 studies. This overall case fatality rate was on average about 11 per 100 persons with TBI; about 3% in-hospital and 8% out-of-hospital deaths among patients with TBI [2,33]. Due to the use of the average European overall case fatality rate, the number of YLLs and thereby the

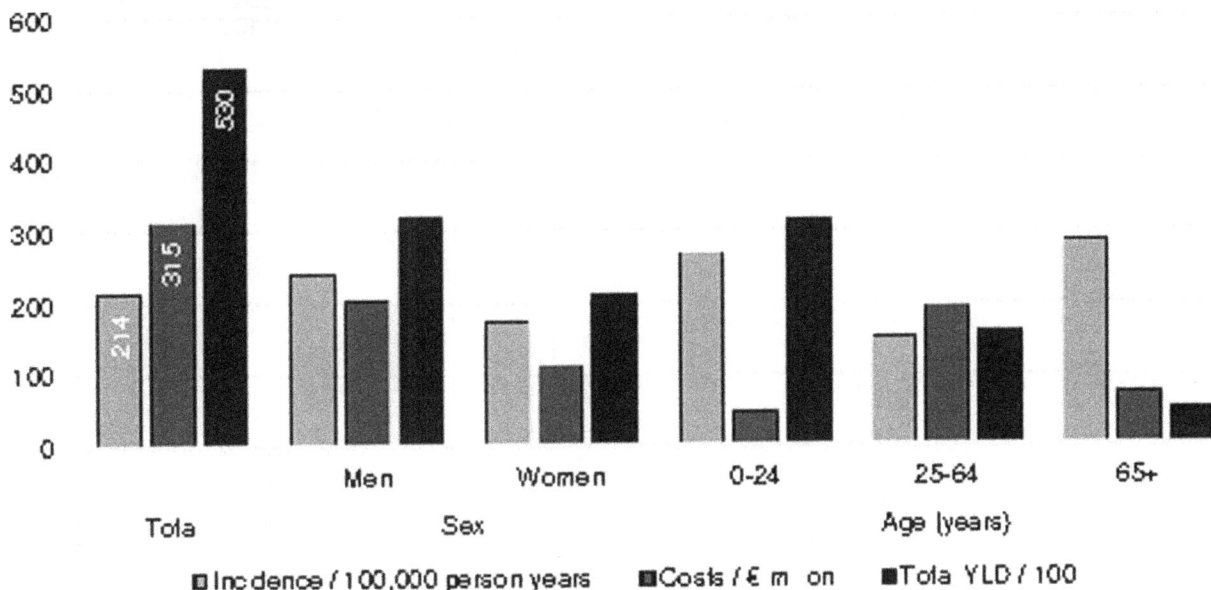

Figure 3. Economic and disease burden of traumatic brain injury in the Netherlands (2010–2012). YLD: years lived with disability.

disease burden of TBI may be over- or underestimated. However, actual case fatality rates and disease burden of TBI may be even higher due to higher excess mortality in the long-term [47–49]. In order to improve the YLL and disease burden estimates of TBI and other injuries and diseases in the Netherlands, specific (long-term) mortality data should be registered and available for future research.

Other limitations concern the classification of TBI and the calculation of costs. TBI patients treated at the ED were registered as having a "Concussion" or "Other skull – brain injury". No additional data was available on ICD-codes, AIS-codes or a Glasgow Outcome Scale to uniformly determine TBI; data that was available for the majority of the hospitalized patients.

The ICD-9 codes used to determine the type of TBI among hospitalized patients slightly differed from those recommended by the Center for Disease Control (CDC) [50], in that this study also included the late effects of TBI (ICD-9 codes 905, 907, 950). These late effects however comprise far less than 1% of all hospitalized traumatic brain injuries in the Netherlands, and therefore will not complicate comparison of our results to those of other studies in which the CDC ICD-9 codes for TBI were used.

The cost-of-illness of TBI may have been overestimated because of the use of a patient follow-up survey to obtain information on healthcare consumption and labor status. Comparison of the hospital discharge data and the patient follow-up data indicated that there is a higher response among the more severe injured patients. This may lead to an overestimation of the costs and disease burden of TBI.

On the other hand, our estimation of indirect costs of TBI comprised only costs of lost work productivity for TBI patients of working age. Other potential sources of indirect costs, such as the work productivity and finances of families and caregivers were not incorporated in this study. Previous research showed that TBI imposes a significant level of financial burden on families and caregivers [51,52], which is directly related to the severity of TBI [51]. Total indirect costs of TBI will therefore be far higher than estimated in this study, particularly among children and elderly with caregivers in the working age.

Our study is limited to TBI patients that were treated at the ED or admitted to hospital. Patients who consulted a GP were not included in our overview. Hence, incidence rates, cost-of-illness and burden of TBI may be even higher [53]. According to registries from Dutch general practice, in 2012 about 7,600 persons contacted their General Practitioner (GP) or after-hours General Practitioner Co-operation (GPC) due to TBI [54]. Assuming that direct healthcare costs of GP visits are on average €39 per contact (Table 1; mean costs for practice or telephone

consultation, and home visit), and the indirect costs and disease burden of TBI will not be larger than that of ED-treated patients, they will add about 7–8% only to our cost estimate and about 1–2% only to our DALY estimate.

## Recommendation for future research

The results of our study reveal that TBI imposes a relatively high economic and health impact compared to all injuries and diseases in the Netherlands. TBI is a growing worldwide problem, as recent reports suggest a rapid increase in ED visits and hospitalizations resulting from traumatic brain injury, especially fall-related TBI in older adults [55–57] and traffic-related TBI [58,59]. There is a need for prevention programs targeting on the reduction of incidence and severity of TBI. On the bases of our study, we conclude that especially children and young adults aged 0–24 years, men aged 25–64 years and traffic injury victims (in the Netherlands especially bicyclists) and home and leisure injury victims are an important target for intervention. In the working population, screening for risk of problems to return to work and immediate rehabilitation after TBI may help to minimize lost productivity [60].

Future research should examine how helmet use among cyclists can be increased. Bicycle helmets have shown to be highly effective in preventing head, brain, and facial injuries to cyclist [61,62]. Previous research in Canada showed that helmet legislation may be an effective tool in the prevention of childhood bicycle-related head injuries [63]. Overall, future research on the population impact of TBI in terms of costs and disease burden should also include patients who receive no treatment or out-of-hospital treatment (e.g., from a GP or by sports trainers).

## Conclusions

This study provided comprehensive population-based estimates on the epidemiology, costs and disease burden (in DALYs) of ED-treated and hospitalized persons with TBI over 2010–2012 in the Netherlands. The study included all age groups, all TBI severities, and both patients treated at the ED and hospitalized patients. The economic and health consequences of TBI are substantial. Prevention programs are needed to reduce incidence and severity of TBI. The integrated approach of assessment of incidence, costs and disease burden (in DALYs) of TBI enables the detection of all important risk groups in TBI.

## Author Contributions

Analyzed the data: AS MP. Contributed reagents/materials/analysis tools: MP. Wrote the paper: AS JH SP EvB.

## References

1. Menon DK, Schwab K, Wright DW, Maas AI (2010) Demographics and Clinical Assessment Working Group of the International Interagency Initiative toward Common Data Elements for Research on Traumatic Brain Injury Psychological Health. Position statement: definition of traumatic brain injury. Arch Phys Med Rehabil 91: 1637–1640.

2. Tagliaferri F, Compagnone C, Korsic M, Servadei F, Kraus J (2006) A systematic review of brain injury epidemiology in Europe. Acta Neurochir (Wien) 148: 255–268; discussion 268.

3. Andelic N, Hammergren N, Bautz-Holter E, Sveen U, Brunborg C, et al. (2009) Functional outcome and health-related quality of life 10 years after moderate-to-severe traumatic brain injury. Acta Neurol Scand 120: 16–23.

4. Dijkers MP (2004) Quality of life after traumatic brain injury: a review of research approaches and findings. Arch Phys Med Rehabil 85: S21–35.

5. Berg J, Tagliaferri F, Servadei F (2005) Cost of trauma in Europe. Eur J Neurol 12 Suppl 1: 85–90.

6. McGarry LJ, Thompson D, Millham FH, Cowell L, Snyder PJ, et al. (2002) Outcomes and costs of acute treatment of traumatic brain injury. J Trauma 53: 1152–1159.

7. Radford K, Phillips J, Drummond A, Sach T, Walker M, et al. (2013) Return to work after traumatic brain injury: cohort comparison and economic evaluation. Brain Inj 27: 507–520.

8. Holtslag HR, Post MW, van der Werken C, Lindeman E (2007) Return to work after major trauma. Clin Rehabil 21: 373–383.

9. Olesen J, Gustavsson A, Svensson M, Wittchen HU, Jönsson B, et al. (2012) The economic cost of brain disorders in Europe. Eur J Neurol 19: 155–162.

10. Feigin VL, Theadom A, Barker-Collo S, Starkey NJ, McPherson K, et al. (2013) Incidence of traumatic brain injury in New Zealand: a population-based study. Lancet Neurol 12: 53–64.

11. Bruns J, Hauser WA (2003) The epidemiology of traumatic brain injury: a review. Epilepsia 44 Suppl 10: 2–10.

12. Meerding WJ, Mulder S, van Beeck EF (2006) Incidence and costs of injuries in The Netherlands. Eur J Public Health 16: 272–278.

13. Polinder S, Meerding WJ, van Baar ME, Toet H, Mulder S, et al. (2005) Cost estimation of injury-related hospital admissions in 10 European countries. J Trauma 59: 1283–1290; discussion 1290–1281.

14. McGregor K, Pentland B (1997) Head injury rehabilitation in the U.K.: an economic perspective. Soc Sci Med 45: 295–303.

15. Schootman M, Buchman TG, Lewis LM (2003) National estimates of hospitalization charges for the acute care of traumatic brain injuries. Brain Inj 17: 983–990.
16. Humphreys I, Wood RL, Phillips CJ, Macey S (2013) The costs of traumatic brain injury: a literature review. Clinicoecon Outcomes Res 5: 281–287.
17. Kayani NA, Homan S, Yun S, Zhu BP (2009) Health and economic burden of traumatic brain injury: Missouri, 2001–2005. Public Health Rep 124: 551–560.
18. Farhad K, Khan HM, Ji AB, Yacoub HA, Qureshi AI, et al. (2013) Trends in outcomes and hospitalization costs for traumatic brain injury in adult patients in the United States. J Neurotrauma 30: 84–90.
19. Polinder S, Meerding WJ, Mulder S, Petridou E, van Beeck E, et al. (2007) Assessing the burden of injury in six European countries. Bull World Health Organ 85: 27–34.
20. Olesen J, Leonardi M (2003) The burden of brain diseases in Europe. Eur J Neurol 10: 471–477.
21. Meerding WJ, Polinder S, Lyons RA, Petridou ET, Toet H, et al. (2010) How adequate are emergency department home and leisure injury surveillance systems for cross-country comparisons in Europe? Int J Inj Contr Saf Promot 17: 13–22.
22. Van der Stegen RHM, Ploemacher J (2009) Discription of methods for statistics by diagnoses in time by using the LMR (1981–2005). The Hague: Statistics Netherlands.
23. Consumer and Safety Institute (2005) The Dutch Burden of Injury Model. Amsterdam: Consumer and Safety Institute.
24. MacKenzie EJ, Siegel JH, Shapiro S, Moody M, Smith RT (1988) Functional recovery and medical costs of trauma: an analysis by type and severity of injury. J Trauma 28: 281–297.
25. Mulder S, Meerding WJ, Van Beeck EF (2002) Setting priorities in injury prevention: the application of an incidence based cost model. Inj Prev 8: 74–78.
26. Polinder S, van Beeck EF, Essink-Bot ML, Toet H, Looman CW, et al. (2007) Functional outcome at 2.5, 5, 9, and 24 months after injury in the Netherlands. J Trauma 62: 133–141.
27. Haagsma JA, Polinder S, Olff M, Toet H, Bonsel GJ, et al. (2012) Posttraumatic stress symptoms and health-related quality of life: a two year follow up study of injury treated at the emergency department. BMC Psychiatry 12: 1.
28. Oostenbrink JB, Koopmanschap MA, Rutten FF (2002) Standardisation of costs: the Dutch Manual for Costing in economic evaluations. Pharmacoeconomics 20: 443–454.
29. Eurostat (2014) HICP - inflation rate.
30. Statistics Netherlands (CBS) (2014) [Consumer prices; inflation from 1963]. The Hague: Statistics Netherlands.
31. US Inflation Calculator (2014) US Inflation Calculator.
32. Murray CJL, Lopez AD, Harvard School of Public Health, World Health Organization, World Bank. (1996) The global burden of disease: a comprehensive assessment of mortality and disability from diseases, injuries, and risk factors in 1990 and projected to 2020. Cambridge, MA: Published by the Harvard School of Public Health on behalf of the World Health Organization and the World Bank; Distributed by Harvard University Press. xxxii, 990 p. p.
33. World Health Organization (2006) Neurological disorders: public health challenges: World Health Organization.
34. Murray CJ (1994) Quantifying the burden of disease: the technical basis for disability-adjusted life years. Bull World Health Organ 72: 429–445.
35. Haagsma JA, Polinder S, Lyons RA, Lund J, Ditsuwan V, et al. (2012) Improved and standardized method for assessing years lived with disability after injury. Bull World Health Organ 90: 513–521.
36. Polinder S, Meerding W, Toet H, van Baar M, Mulder S, et al. (2004) A surveillance based assessment of medical costs of injury in Europe: phase 2. Amsterdam: Consumer and Safety Institute.
37. Statistics Netherlands (CBS) (2014) [Population data]. The Hague: Statistics Netherlands.
38. Faul M, Xu L, Wald MM, Coronado VG (2010) Traumatic brain injury in the United States: emergency department visits, hospitalizations and deaths 2002–2006. Atlanta, GA: Centers for Disease Control and Prevention, National Center for Injury Prevention and Control. 2–70 p.
39. Statistics Netherlands (CBS) (2014) [Mobility in the Netherlands]. The Hague: Statistics Netherlands.
40. Consumer and Safety Institute (2011) [Fact sheet: bicycle accidents]. Amsterdam.
41. Consumer and Safety Institute (2011) [Fact sheet: sports injuries]. Amsterdam.
42. Consumer and Safety Institute (2012) [Fact sheet: sports injuries]. Amsterdam.
43. Schulman J, Sacks J, Provenzano G (2002) State level estimates of the incidence and economic burden of head injuries stemming from non-universal use of bicycle helmets. Inj Prev 8: 47–52.
44. Gustavsson A, Svensson M, Jacobi F, Allgulander C, Alonso J, et al. (2011) Cost of disorders of the brain in Europe 2010. Eur Neuropsychopharmacol 21: 718–779.
45. Hyder AA, Wunderlich CA, Puvanachandra P, Gururaj G, Kobusingye OC (2007) The impact of traumatic brain injuries: a global perspective. NeuroRehabilitation 22: 341–353.
46. Gommer A, Poos M, Hoeymans N (2010) [Years of life lost, morbidity and disease burden for 56 selected disorders]. Bilthoven: Rijksinstituut voor Volksgezondheid en Milieu (RIVM).
47. McMillan TM, Teasdale GM (2007) Death rate is increased for at least 7 years after head injury: a prospective study. Brain 130: 2520–2527.
48. Baguley IJ, Nott MT, Howle AA, Simpson GK, Browne S, et al. (2012) Late mortality after severe traumatic brain injury in New South Wales: a multicentre study. Med J Aust 196: 40–45.
49. Flaada JT, Leibson CL, Mandrekar JN, Diehl N, Perkins PK, et al. (2007) Relative risk of mortality after traumatic brain injury: a population-based study of the role of age and injury severity. J Neurotrauma 24: 435–445.
50. Thurman D.J SJE, Johnson D., Greenspan A., Smith S.M. (1995) Guidelines for surveillance of central nervous system injury. Atlanta, GA: US Department of Health and Human Services, Public Health Service, CDC.
51. Hoang HT, Pham TL, Vo TT, Nguyen PK, Doran CM, et al. (2008) The costs of traumatic brain injury due to motorcycle accidents in Hanoi, Vietnam. Cost Eff Resour Alloc 6: 17.
52. Hall KM, Karzmark P, Stevens M, Englander J, O'Hare P, et al. (1994) Family stressors in traumatic brain injury: a two-year follow-up. Arch Phys Med Rehabil 75: 876–884.
53. Consumer and Safety Institute (2013) [Fact sheet: traumatic brain injury]. Amsterdam.
54. Nielen M, Spronk I, Davids R, Zwaanswijk M, Verheij R, et al. (2014) [Incidence and prevalence rates of health problems in Dutch general practice in 2012]. NIVEL Zorgregistraties eerste lijn: Netherlands institute for health services research (NIVEL).
55. Hartholt KA, Van Lieshout EM, Polinder S, Panneman MJ, Van der Cammen TJ, et al. (2011) Rapid increase in hospitalizations resulting from fall-related traumatic head injury in older adults in The Netherlands 1986–2008. J Neurotrauma 28: 739–744.
56. Kannus P, Niemi S, Parkkari J, Palvanen M, Sievänen H (2007) Alarming rise in fall-induced severe head injuries among elderly people. Injury 38: 81–83.
57. Coronado VG, McGuire LC, Sarmiento K, Bell J, Lionbarger MR, et al. (2012) Trends in Traumatic Brain Injury in the U.S. and the public health response: 1995–2009. J Safety Res 43: 299–307.
58. World Health Organization (2004) World report on road traffic injury prevention Geneva: World Health Organization.
59. Murray CJ, Vos T, Lozano R, Naghavi M, Flaxman AD, et al. (2012) Disability-adjusted life years (DALYs) for 291 diseases and injuries in 21 regions, 1990–2010: a systematic analysis for the Global Burden of Disease Study 2010. Lancet 380: 2197–2223.
60. Boake C, McCauley SR, Pedroza C, Levin HS, Brown SA, et al. (2005) Lost productive work time after mild to moderate traumatic brain injury with and without hospitalization. Neurosurgery 56: 994–1003; discussion 1994–1003.
61. Thompson RS, Rivara FP, Thompson DC (1989) A case-control study of the effectiveness of bicycle safety helmets. N Engl J Med 320: 1361–1367.
62. Rivara FP, Thompson DC, Patterson MQ, Thompson RS (1998) Prevention of bicycle-related injuries: helmets, education, and legislation. Annu Rev Public Health 19: 293–318.
63. Macpherson AK, To TM, Macarthur C, Chipman ML, Wright JG, et al. (2002) Impact of mandatory helmet legislation on bicycle-related head injuries in children: a population-based study. Pediatrics 110: e60.

# 19

# Gender-Based Comorbidity in Benign Paroxysmal Positional Vertigo

**Oluwaseye Ayoola Ogun[1], Kristen L. Janky[1], Edward S. Cohn[1], Bela Büki[2], Yunxia Wang Lundberg[1]***

**1** Boys Town National Research Hospital, Omaha, Nebraska, United States of America, **2** Department of Otolaryngology, Karl Landsteiner University Hospital Krems, Krems an der Donau, Austria

## Abstract

It has been noted that benign paroxysmal positional vertigo (BPPV) may be associated with certain disorders and medical procedures. However, most studies to date were done in Europe, and epidemiological data on the United States (US) population are scarce. Gender-based information is even rarer. Furthermore, it is difficult to assess the relative prevalence of each type of association based solely on literature data, because different comorbidities were reported by various groups from different countries using different patient populations and possibly different inclusion/exclusion criteria. In this study, we surveyed and analyzed a large adult BPPV population (n = 1,360 surveyed, 227 completed, most of which were recurrent BPPV cases) from Omaha, NE, US, and its vicinity, all diagnosed at Boys Town National Research Hospital (BTNRH) over the past decade using established and consistent diagnostic criteria. In addition, we performed a retrospective analysis of patients' diagnostic records (n = 1,377, with 1,360 adults and 17 children). The following comorbidities were found to be significantly more prevalent in the BPPV population when compared to the age- and gender-matched general population: ear/hearing problems, head injury, thyroid problems, allergies, high cholesterol, headaches, and numbness/paralysis. There were gender differences in the comorbidities. In addition, familial predisposition was fairly common among the participants. Thus, the data confirm some previously reported comorbidities, identify new ones (hearing loss, thyroid problems, high cholesterol, and numbness/paralysis), and suggest possible predisposing and triggering factors and events for BPPV.

**Editor:** Pedro Gonzalez-Alegre, University of Iowa Carver College of Medicine, United States of America

**Funding:** This work was supported by grants from the National Institutes of Health, R01DC008603, R01DC008603-S1, and P20GM103471 (formerly P20RR018788) pilot funding to YWL; postdoctoral training grant T32DC000013 to OAO; and P20GM103471 pilot funding to ESC. The funders had no role in study design, data collection and analysis, decision to publish, or preparation of the manuscript.

**Competing Interests:** The authors have declared that no competing interests exist.

* Email: Yesha.Lundberg@boystown.org

## Introduction

The peripheral vestibular organ consists of miniature inertial accelerometers: the semicircular canals (SCCs) specialized in detecting angular acceleration, and the otolithic organs in sensing linear acceleration including gravitational changes. In benign paroxysmal positional vertigo (BPPV), according to the accepted theory, utricular otoconia break apart from the mass and become dislocated into the semicircular canals. Thereby, the canals are sensitized to gravity and generate false information of angular acceleration in response to head position changes with respect to gravity.

BPPV is the most common cause of vertigo. In young people, one third to one half of BPPV cases can be attributed to some type of head trauma/injury [1–5]. A number of surgery-induced BPPV cases, especially inner ear and dental surgeries, have also been reported [6–10]. In the absence of head trauma or mechanical impact (e.g. surgical drilling) to cause otoconia dislocation, BPPV is categorized as unknown origin or idiopathic. In middle aged and older people, idiopathic BPPV cases are much more common. It is becoming increasingly evident that idiopathic BPPV cases can be associated with other illnesses such as migraine [9,11–16],

vestibular neuritis [17,18], Meniere's disease [9,19–21], sudden hearing loss [19,22–27], diabetes [28,29], and autoimmune thyroiditis [31]. BPPV has also been linked with reduced bone mineral density [32–34], suggesting that the spontaneous release of otoconia may parallel bone demineralization (for review see [30]).

Unfortunately, the methods of the reported epidemiological studies were not standardized, and possibly used different diagnostic and inclusion/exclusion criteria. Sometimes there is disagreement between reports whether BPPV is associated with some diseases/conditions. For example, Warninghoff et al [35] did not detect an increased prevalence of diabetes mellitus, arterial hypertension, migraine, other headaches or obesity in the BPPV patients compared to the control population, likely due to a small sample size (n = 19 BPPV patients). Given some inconsistencies in the comorbidity findings and the scarcity of epidemiological studies in the US, we surveyed and reviewed the medical records of a large BPPV patient population diagnosed and treated at BTNRH in the current study, and identified predisposing and triggering factors and events. Our long-term goal is to use the information as a starting point to study the pathophysiology of BPPV, as well as help improve or modify treatment and prevention strategies.

## Materials and Methods

### Study design and subjects

Diagnostic records of BPPV patients at the BTNRH Vestibular Clinic between 2002–2011 (n = 1,377, with 1360 adults and 17 children) were analyzed after patients' information was de-identified and anonymized. The quoted numbers of patients in this study excluded a small subset that also had other types of vertigo/dizziness in addition to BPPV. Then, adult patients (n = 1,360) were directly surveyed using an anonymous questionnaire. Only the participants who completed the questionnaire in its entirety with evaluable data were included. A positive diagnosis of BPPV was the presence of nystagmus elicited in either the Dix-Hallpike or roll maneuver. The current study did not differentiate or exclude sub-types of BPPV, such as subjective BPPV [36] or BPPV sub-typed by location (posterior, lateral or superior canal) [37]. Our purpose was to investigate comorbidities that predispose an individual to freeing otoconia and not location of otoconia displacement; sub-typing would result in very small numbers in some sub-groups for statistical analysis.

All aspects of the study, including the retrospective analysis, the content of the survey, the invitation letter and the survey procedures, were reviewed and approved by the Institutional Review Board at BTNRH in accordance with institutional, federal and international guidelines (approval number 11-11-X). As described above, patients' information was de-identified and anonymized prior to analysis. Since the retrospective analysis and the adult-only survey were done anonymously, no consent was necessary.

### Procedures

Initially, a retrospective review of the medical records of the stated BPPV patient population was conducted, which provided preliminary information on comorbidities of BPPV and the rate of BPPV recurrence.

Then, a survey was created and administered through Survey Monkey (www.surveymonkey.com). Most questions required the participant to select one answer from two to several choices, with additional lines to add other information or explanation by the participant. When applicable, the choices included "I am not sure", "I cannot remember" or "Does not apply". The survey was divided into the following sub-sections:

(1) Demographic information, including age (in years), sex, race, ethnicity, and general area of residence (urban/suburban or rural).

(2) BPPV recurrence, family history, season of onset. Recurrence was defined in the survey as experiencing an additional episode of BPPV after being symptom-free for at least 30 days.

(3) Events/illnesses immediately preceding BPPV onset, medical history, medications and diet. A table (see Results) contained a list of events/illnesses and asked whether the participant experienced them prior to BPPV. The "prior to" was arbitrarily defined as "less than 6 months before". With the exception of head trauma, we speculated that other events/illnesses would not immediately result in BPPV, so we were looking for associations in a more loose time-locked fashion. The survey questions were asked as listed in the tables in the Results, except that the phrase "Did you experience xxx prior to your first BPPV symptom (or during your BPPV symptoms)" was included in each line item for each condition/disease in the survey. In the table, this phrase is summarized in the legend to save space.

In the medical history section, participants were given a comprehensive list of medical conditions to select from and blank lines to fill in any other medical conditions. Participants were asked to list their current medications, and to indicate whether their medical conditions and medication taken co-occurred with BPPV onset. Some questions regarding events/illnesses immediately preceding BPPV onset somewhat overlapped questions in the medical history section, thus serving as confirmation.

Frequency of consumption of alcohol, tobacco, caffeine, tea or carbonated beverages, high fat/sugary/salty foods, fresh fruits/vegetables, and meat/fish was filed as never, less than once a week, 2–3 times a week, or more than 3 times a week for each stated item. Consumption of special diet (e.g. vegetarian) was also asked.

An invitation letter to participate in the study was mailed to 1,360 adult BPPV patients. Participants had the option of completing the survey online or on paper. Some surveys were also distributed to new patients at the time when BPPV was diagnosed at BTNRH. All responses were downloaded into Excel, which served as the database for review and analysis.

For comparison, age- and gender-matched prevalence data on the general US population were obtained from the Center for Disease Control (CDC), the National Institute of Health (NIH), and peer-reviewed published papers. With a few diseases, control data on the general US population stratified by age and gender were not available, so European gender-based data on similar age groups were used. Such cases are indicated in the tables in the Results section.

### Statistical analysis

The total number of participants who answered each question and the subtotals who gave one type of answer were tallied. When calculating the percentage of each subtotal over the total, those who answered "I am not sure", "I cannot remember" or "It does not apply" were not included in the total or subtotal. The control statistics usually consisted of thousands to hundreds of thousands of people. To provide an estimate of the statistical significance of the difference in the disease prevalence between BPPV patients and the general population, p values were calculated for each comorbid disease using Fisher's exact test. To simplify the analysis and to provide a conservative estimate of statistical significance, the control population size was set at 1,000 for all comorbidities, and the mean values from meta-analysis (if available) or the highest prevalence data available were used in the analysis.

The ages of the survey participants (n = 227) and the entire adult BPPV population (n = 1,360) were compared using Student's t-test, and statistical significance of the effects of comorbid conditions on BPPV recurrence was evaluated using Fisher's exact test. Familial cases of BPPV (a 2nd, 3rd and more cases of BPPV in blood relatives in a family) were compared with the highest reported prevalence (life-time prevalence) of BPPV in the general population using Fisher's exact test.

## Results

### Demographics

Of the 1,360 total adult patients, 227 (164:63 or 2.6:1 female to male) completed the survey in its entirety. Characteristics of the two groups are summarized in **Table 1**. The survey participants had an age and gender distribution similar to the entire patient population under invitation (**Figure 1**), except that the former had slightly fewer people above 70 years old.

Among the survey participants, the ethnicity distribution was 80.9% "Not Hispanic or Not Latino", and 19.1% "Hispanic or Latino". The racial distribution was 95.8% White, 2.5% African

**Table 1.** Demographics of the study population.

| | BPPV adult patient population | | | | BPPV survey participants | | | |
|---|---|---|---|---|---|---|---|---|
| | N | Age range (years) | Mean age (years) | P | N | Age range (years) | Mean age (years) | P |
| Female | 923 | 18–94 | 58.3±16.0 | | 164 | 19–84 | 56.1±13.0 | 0.04 |
| Male | 437 | 18–91 | 60.2±15.7 | | 63 | 30–86 | 56.4±15.2 | 0.0007 |
| Gender mixed | 1,360 | 18–94 | 58.9±15.9 | | 227 | 19–86 | 56.2±13.6 | 0.006 |

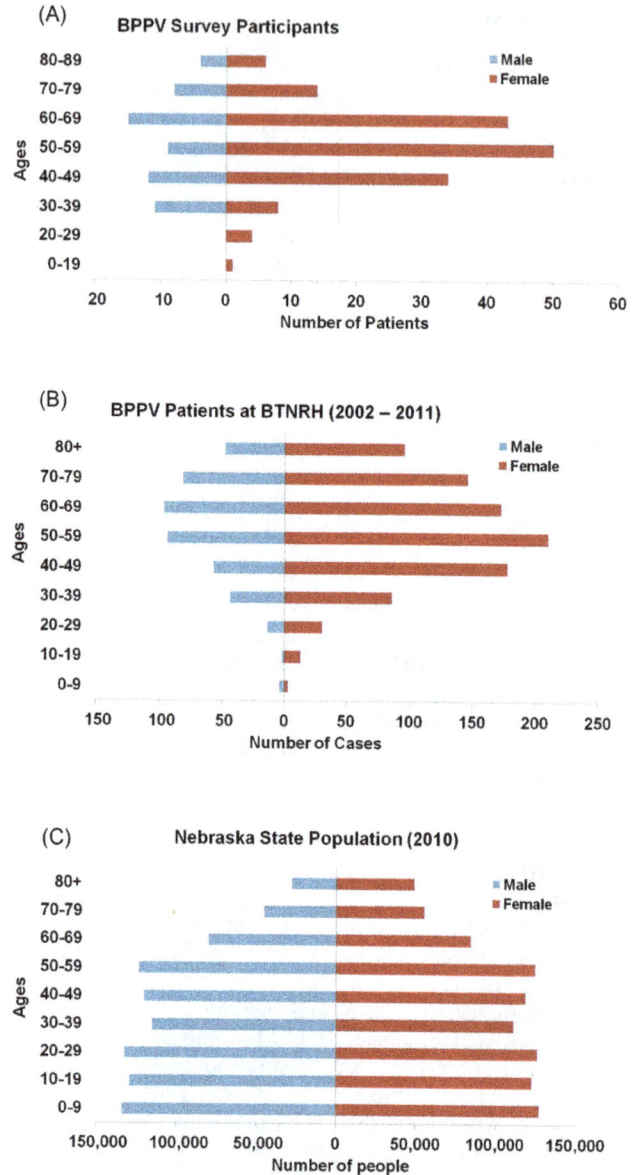

Figure 1. Age and gender distribution of BPPV survey participants (n = 227 total) (A), BPPV cases diagnosed at BTNRH in 2002–2011 (n = 1,377 total) (B), and Nebraska population in year 2010 (n = 1,826,341 total) [73] (C). Recurrent cases are counted only once (the first occurrence).

American or Black, 1.3% Asian and 0.4% American Indian or Alaskan. Of the participants, 69.9% live in urban and suburban areas, 28.0% live in rural areas and 2.1% were not sure.

## Recurrence of BPPV

In the BPPV survey population (n = 227), 174 participants (131 females and 43 males) reported recurrence of BPPV (53 non-recurrent cases), resulting in a recurrence rate of 76.3%. This is higher than the recurrence rates (27%–50%) reported by others [38,39,40], suggesting that recurrence may have been a strong motivation for participation.

Among the entire BPPV population from 2002–2011 (n = 1,377), female recurrent and non-recurrent BPPV cases had a similar age distribution (**Figure 2**), but male recurrent cases had an even greater age-related increase in the 70s group when compared to male non-recurrent cases. There were no recurrent female cases in the first 2 decades of life, and no recurrent male cases in the first 3 decades of life. In terms of recurrence, there was no significant difference between urban and rural dwellers, or in the frequencies of different types of diets or vitamin use. It could not be determined in the current study whether medication could have been a factor in BPPV occurrence or recurrence.

## Family history and other information

Among the survey participants, 23.8% (n = 54) reported having a known family member diagnosed with BPPV, 64.8% (n = 147) reported not having a family member with BPPV, and 11.4% (n = 26) did not know if any family member had BPPV. The affected family members were all blood-related except for 3 cases of non-genetic family members (spouses) who also had BPPV (**Table 2**). The frequency of having a blood relative diagnosed with BPPV is significantly higher (p<0.0001) than the 2.4% life-time prevalence reported for the general population [41].

Among the 68.4% (n = 227) of survey participants who remembered with certainty the season of BPPV onset, a higher percentage of participants had BPPV symptoms in the spring and fall: 28.2% in the spring, 18.0% in the summer, 28.9% in the fall, and 24.9% in the winter. Medical records showed that in the entire BPPV population, April and August had the highest number of cases at 11.0% and 10.7%, respectively. The higher incidences in the spring and fall implicate allergy in facilitating BPPV onset, which is supported by patients' self-reported problems with allergy (see below).

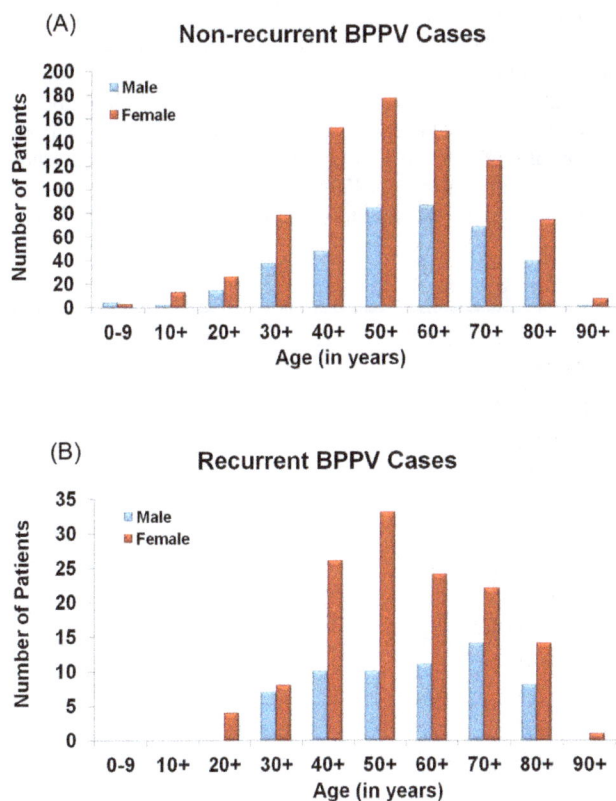

**(A)** **Non-recurrent BPPV Cases**

**(B)** **Recurrent BPPV Cases**

**Figure 2. Age and gender distribution of non-recurrent (A, n = 1,185 total) and recurrent (B, 192 total) BPPV cases diagnosed at BTNRH from 2002–11.**

## Possible triggers and comorbidities of BPPV

When asked about incidents and conditions immediately preceding BPPV symptoms, most participants reported hearing loss (**Table 3**). The next most common problem was headache associated with light and/or sound sensitivity and migraine, followed by infection. Most common infection was ear infection (28.6%, n = 10), sinus infection (28.6%, n = 10), and both (17.1%, n = 6).

In the Medical History section, the comprehensive list provided information on possible comorbidities and whether they co-occurred with BPPV, and confirmed those of the previous section in the survey (**Tables 4 & 5**). Some differences in the answers may not be inconsistencies but may be the result of how the questions are phrased: one seeks information about the incidents/illnesses immediately preceding the first BPPV symptoms (**Table 3**), while the second seeks information about their chronic situations that may or may not accompany the vertigo attacks (**Tables 4 & 5**). Given the gender differences in comorbidities, male and female data were analyzed separately.

Among the 3 dozen listed categories of diseases and medical conditions, about a dozen had a different prevalence than that of the general population, with only some reaching significance (**Tables 4 & 5**). Problems with the ear/hearing were again among the most common complaints in both genders. Incidences of headaches/migraine and head injury were also consistent with the previous question, and were common in females and males (especially young males), respectively. With male participants, the listed decades of life (1–9) had 0%, 0%, 0%, 45.5%, 23.1%, 36.4%, 21.4%, 0%, 25%, respectively, of head injury cases. With females, each decade had 0%, 0%, 1.7%, 20.0%, 6.0%, 5.4%, 15.8%, 0%, 0%, respectively, of head injury cases. When all age groups and genders were combined, the percentage of BPPV cases with head trauma was 12.4%, comparable to the reported range of 14%–18% in other BPPV populations [4,29,42,43]. Because it has not been established that head and physical trauma in these patients were actually the cause of their BPPV (e.g. someone may have had head trauma and hearing loss at the same time), these participants were not excluded in the analysis of other comorbidities.

In both genders, problems with thyroid and high cholesterol were significantly more prevalent in the BPPV population (**Tables 4 & 5**), although the comparison for thyroid diseases was made with control data from a large study conducted in the United Kingdom (UK) as age- and gender-matched data were not available on the US population.

In the BPPV female population, complaints of allergies and headaches were significantly more prevalent than in the control population. The former is consistent with above mentioned trend of BPPV occurring more frequently during allergy season. Musculoskeletal disorders (28.3%) were not more common in BPPV patients than the general population; however, it is unclear if the survey participants have had a bone scan, therefore, a negative answer to the question whether they had osteoporosis/osteopenia may not exclude the presence of the condition in some people.

Among the conditions that had a significantly higher prevalence in the BPPV population, some also appeared to increase disease recurrence (**Table 6**); however, only numbness/paralysis reached statistical significance. Neither ear surgery nor head injury impacted BPPV recurrence significantly. Gender-separated analysis did not significantly improve the p values; it increased the p values with most of the comorbidities.

In the medical records of BPPV cases in 2002–2011 (n = 1,377), there were 67 cases of hearing loss (60 sensorineural hearing loss, 6

**Table 2.** Family history of BPPV.

| Family member | % of yes (n = 54 total) |
| --- | --- |
| Parents | 29.6% (n = 16) |
| Children | 14.8% (n = 9) |
| Siblings | 27.8% (n = 16) |
| Siblings and children | 1.9% (n = 1) |
| Parents & siblings | 11.1% (n = 6) |
| Grandparents/uncles/aunts/cousins | 7.4% (n = 4) |
| Spouse | 5.6% (n = 3) |
| No response | 1.9% (n = 1) |

conductive, 1 unspecified sudden hearing loss), 20 hypoactive labyrinth, 10 migraine, 8 Meniere's disease, 7 allergic rhinitis, 5 infective otitis externa, and 2 viral labyrinthitis. These comorbidities were reportedly co-occurring with BPPV at the time of the clinical visits, making them appear less prevalent than hearing loss reported in the survey. It is also possible that many patients did not mention their other medical conditions as vertigo was their primary concern during the clinical visits, or other diagnoses were not recorded.

## Discussion

Due to the high prevalence and potentially incapacitating nature of BPPV, the present study examined factors that may predispose an individual to BPPV. We found a few significant comorbidities and familial predisposition for BPPV.

Notably, the number of cases with hearing loss is quite high among our BPPV patients, whereas previously reported numbers were quite low (less than 1%) [19,44] except for incidences of sudden hearing loss. Sudden hearing loss has commonly been reported in BPPV patients, ranging from 9–51% [24–27,45]; however, sudden hearing loss was rare among the BTNRH BPPV

cases in the medical records (n = 1,377). Given that most of our BPPV patients are beyond middle age, we postulate that their hearing loss associated with BPPV is more likely caused by age-related degeneration, rather than by immune or inflammatory responses proposed as the cause of some cases of sudden hearing loss. This hypothesis would be in agreement with the observed effects of aging on BPPV in this population [46] and in other BPPV populations as well (for references see Introduction).

Nevertheless, our survey suggests that ear infection and inflammatory processes (infection and allergy) may also trigger BPPV. Increased incidences of sinus infections in other BPPV populations in the US have been noted [47]. Nasal allergies have also been associated with increased inner ear pathology [48]. The data suggest a possible association between allergies and BPPV onset, especially in women. Although our survey does not specify the type of allergies, nasal allergy is the most common type of allergies in the general population.

We also identified thyroid problems as a possible predisposing factor for BPPV occurrence. Thyroid problems disrupt the homeostasis of calcium and chloride [49], both of which affect otoconia in animal studies [50–52]. In addition, hypothyroidism delays the onset of inhibitory neurotransmission [49] during

**Table 3.** Incidents and conditions immediately preceding the first BPPV symptoms.

| Answers | Yes (n, %) | No (n, %) |
| --- | --- | --- |
| Hearing loss | 93 (41.9%) | 129 (58.1%) |
| Any other ear problems | 14 (6.2%) | 211 (93.8%) |
| Current ear problems | 55 (24.3%) | 171 (75.7%) |
| Tinnitus | 6 (4.0%) | 144 (96.0%) |
| Headaches associated with increased light/sound sensitivity | 47 (20.9%) | 178 (79.1%) |
| Migraine | 28 (12.4%) | 197 (87.6%) |
| Any infection | 37 (16.5%) | 187 (83.5%) |
| Any illness | 32 (14.3%) | 192 (85.7%) |
| Head injury | 27 (12.0%) | 198 (88.0%) |
| Other physical trauma | 13 (5.8%) | 212 (94.2%) |
| Any ear surgery | 13 (5.8%) | 212 (94.2%) |
| Any other surgery | 32 (14.3%) | 192 (85.7%) |
| Any other symptoms | 60 (27.0%) | 162 (73.0%) |

Only those who answered "yes" or "no" were included in the total or subtotal to obtain the percentages. Those who answered "does not apply" or "do not know/remember" were not included in the presented percentages.

**Table 4.** Factors associated with BPPV in females.

| Comorbidities | Female BPPV patients yes% (n out of 164 total) | General female population (set at n = 1,000) | P | References and notes for control data |
|---|---|---|---|---|
| **Allergies** | 50% (82) | 32.3%–35% (350) | **0.0003** | [56,57] |
| Blood pressure | 38.4% (63) | 26.4–32.8% (328) | 0.18 | [58] |
| **Ear/Hearing** | 33.5% (55) | 12.7–14.4% (144) | **<0.0001** | [58] Estimated based on gender ratio and data in 45–64 age group |
| **Head injury** | 8.5% (14) | 3.0% (30) | **0.003** | [59] Annual occurrence (0.3%) x 10 years |
| **Headaches** | 38.4% (63) | 17.0–38.0% (275) | **0.005** | [60,61] Mean from meta-analysis; Chronic or repeated headaches were assumed |
| **Heart** | 17.7% (29) | 12.0% (120) | **0.058** | [58] Estimated from gender ratio |
| **High cholesterol** | 39.0% (64) | 31.0% (310) | **0.047** | [62] |
| Kidney/bladder | 10.4% (17) | 6.6% (66) | 0.10 | [58,63] 1.8% chronic kidney diseases + 4.8% chronic bladder problems |
| **Migraine** | 26.2% (43) | 19.7% (197) | **0.06** | [64] |
| Numbness/Paralysis | 9.2% (15) | 5.6% (56) | 0.11 | [65,66] Control on numbness (3.8%) only had stroke data (including mild stroke); on paralysis (1.8%) included injury cases |
| **Thyroid** | 21.3% (35) | 13.2% (132) | **0.008** | [67–69] Data on UK population |

The age- and gender-matched control statistics are on the general population in the size of thousands to hundreds of thousands. To simplify the analysis and to provide a conservative estimate of statistical significance, the control population size is set at 1,000 for all diseases for Fisher's exact test in the table. If no mean prevalence data by meta-analysis are available, the highest prevalence data available for each disease in the control population is used to obtain the two-tailed p values. Significant (or nearly significant) comorbidities are bolded.

development. Although not yet examined in adults, if hypothyroidism also negatively affects inhibitory transmission in adulthood, it can lead to an imbalance of excitatory/inhibitory transmission. Indeed, autoimmune thyroiditis has been associated with BPPV [19,30,31].

Other previously unknown factors that we identified to be associated with BPPV include high cholesterol and numbness/

paralysis. It is not clear how these and other factors in Tables 4 & 5 could be biologically linked to BPPV, but immobility may be a factor. For example, there are reports of BPPV possibly arising from bed-rest after surgeries which do not have mechanic impact on the ear or head [53].

In a concurrent study [46], we found that menopause is a major trigger of BPPV. Another common menopausal disease is

**Table 5.** Factors associated with BPPV in males.

| Comorbidities | Male BPPV patients yes% (n out of 63 total) | General male population (set at n = 1,000 total) | P | References and notes for control data |
|---|---|---|---|---|
| Allergies | 38.1% (24) | 27.6% (276) | 0.08 | [57] Control are non-US population |
| Blood pressure | 44.4% (28) | 33.9% (339) | 0.10 | [58] |
| Cancer | 14.3% (9) | 9.5% (95) | 0.27 | [58] Estimated based on gender ratio and data in 45–64 age group |
| **Ear/Hearing** | 47.6% (30) | 23.4% (234) | **<0.0001** | [58] Estimated based on gender ratio and data in 45–64 age group. |
| **Head injury** | 25.4% (16) | 4.0% (40) | **<0.0001** | [59] Annual occurrence (0.4%) x 10 years |
| Headaches | 20.6% (13) | 12.5–31.0% (218) | 1.00 | [60] Mean from meta-analysis; Chronic or repeated headaches were assumed |
| **High cholesterol** | 50.8% (32) | 32.5% (325) | **0.004** | [62] |
| Kidney/bladder | 12.7% (8) | 6.8% (68) | 0.12 | [58,63,70,71] 2.0% chronic kidney diseases + 4.8% chronic bladder problems |
| Migraine | 11.1% (7) | 7.0% (70) | 0.21 | [64] |
| **Numbness/Paralysis** | 14.3% (9) | 5.1% (51) | **0.007** | [65,66] Control on numbness (3.0%) only had stroke data (including mild stroke); on paralysis (2.1%) included injury cases |
| Seizures | 4.8% (3) | 1.7% (17) | 0.11 | [72] |
| **Thyroid** | 11.1% (7) | 1.5% (15) | **0.0002** | [67–69] Data on UK population |

See Table 4 legend.

**Table 6.** Effects of comorbid conditions on BPPV recurrence.

| Comorbidities | RR | OR | P | N |
|---|---|---|---|---|
| Allergies | 0.94 | 0.77 | 0.43 | 76/27:91/25 |
| Ear/Hearing problems | 1.12 | 1.64 | 0.15 | 74/17:93/35 |
| High cholesterol | 1.10 | 1.54 | 0.20 | 75/18:92/34 |
| Headaches | 0.98 | 0.93 | 0.87 | 55/18:112/34 |
| Migraine | 1.08 | 1.41 | 0.44 | 38/9:129/43 |
| **Numbness/Paralysis** | 1.29 | 7.34 | **0.03** | 21/1:146/51 |
| Thyroid disease | 1.14 | 1.96 | 0.22 | 34/6:133/46 |
| Physical trauma | 1.23 | 3.95 | 0.30 | 12/1:155/51 |

The relative risk (RR) and odds ratio (OR) of BPPV recurrence in the presence vs. absence of a comorbid condition were calculated. The actual case numbers (N) are also presented in the order of recurrent/non-recurrent cases with and without the comorbid condition. Fisher's exact test was used to obtain the two-tailed p values.

osteoporosis and osteopenia. Although our data do not provide a definitive conclusion regarding the association of BPPV with osteoporosis or osteopenia, several other independent groups from different countries have reported significantly reduced bone mineral density and increased incidences of osteoporosis/osteopenia in BPPV patients [32–34]. Many other diseases can also be triggered or aggravated by menopause, such as allergies, high blood pressure, high cholesterol, headaches, migraine, heart diseases, and hearing loss [54], whether or not the condition shows a female preponderance in the overall prevalence. Most of these conditions showed a significantly higher prevalence in the BPPV patients than the age- and gender- matched controls (Table 4). Our survey data showed a possible association between migraine and BPPV when compared to the general population, and a strong association between generalized headache and BPPV. It is not clear if the higher migraine prevalence in BPPV patients reported by other investigators [16]; [12] reached statistics significance. Ishiyama et al. [12] noted a younger average age of onset and a higher recurrence rate of BPPV in patients with migraine than those without. Our migraine prevalence in BPPV patients may have been underestimated, because our survey invitation letter and an earlier part of the questionnaire emphasized a disease as "diagnosed", so the participants likely only selected "yes" to migraine if they have been diagnosed. Also, BTNRH does not have a neurology specialty, and some patients with migraine may ignore their BPPV symptoms or not come to BTNRH clinics.

Our data confirm the previously noted familial predisposition in BPPV occurrence [55]. With the exception of 3 spousal cases, the affected family members are all genetic relatives. Anecdotally, vestibular clinicians have encountered twins who have lived apart but all have suffered BPPV (Janet O Helminski, personal communication). All these facts implicate a genetic contribution, not similar life styles or environment, in causing these familial BPPV incidences.

The survey response rate of 16% (18.5% when incomplete responses are counted) is reasonable because we had a long questionnaire, and the invitation letter was mailed on paper rather than emailed with a link (email is more convenient and could improve the response rate). As shown in Figure 1, the response is good representation of the entire BPPV population at BTNRH except for those above 70 years of age. Although comorbid diseases in very old patients may be missed, our findings may be more specific to BPPV rather than as a non-specific coincidence of aging. It should be noted that the majority of the participants were

recurrent BPPV sufferers, therefore, the observed comorbidities may be somewhat biased toward BPPV recurrence even though most of the effects did not reach statistical significance (Table 6). Another potential bias of the study is that BTNRH is primarily an otolaryngology and pediatrics facility, and the patient data may over- or under-represent some comorbidities, such as hearing loss (possibly over), migraine (under), and high blood pressure (under). We anticipate such possibility to be small because these clinical visits at BTNRH were sought by patients for BPPV symptoms. Furthermore, certain conditions that showed a significantly higher prevalence in BPPV patients were also reported to occur shortly before the onset of BPPV (Table 3). When BPPV is consistently associated with certain diseases in studies done by independent groups using different patient populations, it would be important to conduct future studies to examine the biological mechanism and genetic predisposition to explain the link between these comorbidities and BPPV.

## Conclusion

Our data show a significant effect of gender, familial predisposition, and certain conditions/diseases in BPPV etiology. Some of these associations (hearing loss, thyroid problems, high cholesterol, and numbness/paralysis) were previously unknown or are much higher than previously reported. When other investigators' findings are also considered, it may be beneficial to the patients if clinicians diagnosing BPPV are alerted about potential comorbid conditions and consider screening these patients or checking their medical history for the following conditions: hearing loss, head injury, thyroid, lipid, allergies, headaches, diabetes, bone density, and family history.

## Acknowledgments

We thank Kendra K. Schmid for statistical consultation, Walt Jesteadt for feedback on the manuscript, Susan J. Grennan and Hongyang Tan for help with some Excel analysis, and Rebecca Cash for help with the IRB application process.

## Author Contributions

Conceived and designed the experiments: OAO YWL KLJ ESC. Performed the experiments: OAO YWL KLJ ESC. Analyzed the data: OAO YWL BB. Contributed to the writing of the manuscript: YWL OAO KLJ BB ESC.

# References

1. Ahn SK, Jeon SY, Kim JP, Park JJ, Hur DG, et al. (2011) Clinical characteristics and treatment of benign paroxysmal positional vertigo after traumatic brain injury. J Trauma 70: 442–446.

2. Blessing R, Strutz J, Beck C (1986) Epidemiology of benign paroxysmal positional vertigo. Laryngol Rhinol Otol (Stuttg) 65: 455–458.

3. Dispenza F, De SA, Mathur N, Croce A, Gallina S (2011) Benign paroxysmal positional vertigo following whiplash injury: a myth or a reality? Am J Otolaryngol 32: 376–380.

4. Katsarkas A (1999) Benign paroxysmal positional vertigo (BPPV): idiopathic versus post-traumatic. Acta Otolaryngol 119: 745–749.

5. Suarez H, Alonso R, Arocena M, Suarez A, Geisinger D (2011) Clinical characteristics of positional vertigo after mild head trauma. Acta Otolaryngol 131: 377–381.

6. Viccaro M, Mancini P, La GR, De SE, Covelli E, et al. (2007) Positional vertigo and cochlear implantation. Otol Neurotol 28: 764–767.

7. Andaz C, Whittet HB, Ludman H (1993) An unusual cause of benign paroxysmal positional vertigo. J Laryngol Otol 107: 1153–1154.

8. Atacan E, Sennaroglu L, Genc A, Kaya S (2001) Benign paroxysmal positional vertigo after stapedectomy. Laryngoscope 111: 1257–1259.

9. Hughes CA, Proctor L (1997) Benign paroxysmal positional vertigo. Laryngoscope 107: 607–613.

10. Kaplan DM, Hehar SS, Tator C, Guha A, Laperriere N, et al. (2003) Hearing loss in acoustic neuromas following stereotactic radiotherapy. J Otolaryngol 32: 23–32.

11. Lanzi G, Balottin U, Fazzi E, Tagliasacchi M, Manfrin M, et al. (1994) Benign paroxysmal vertigo of childhood: a long-term follow-up. Cephalalgia 14: 458–460.

12. Ishiyama A, Jacobson KM, Baloh RW (2000) Migraine and benign positional vertigo. Ann Otol Rhinol Laryngol 109: 377–380.

13. Thakar A, Anjaneyulu C, Deka RC (2001) Vertigo syndromes and mechanisms in migraine. J Laryngol Otol 115: 782–787.

14. Uneri A (2004) Migraine and benign paroxysmal positional vertigo: an outcome study of 476 patients. Ear Nose Throat J 83: 814–815.

15. Marcelli V, Piazza F, Pisani F, Marciano E (2006) Neuro-otological features of benign paroxysmal vertigo and benign paroxysmal positioning vertigo in children: a follow-up study. Brain Dev 28: 80–84.

16. Von Brevern M, Radtke A, Lezius F, Feldmann M, Ziese T, et al. (2007) Epidemiology of benign paroxysmal positional vertigo: a population based study. J Neurol Neurosurg Psychiatry 78: 710–715.

17. Mandala M, Santoro GP, Awrey J, Nuti D (2010) Vestibular neuritis: recurrence and incidence of secondary benign paroxysmal positional vertigo. Acta Otolaryngol 130: 565–567.

18. Parnes LS, Agrawal SK, Atlas J (2003) Diagnosis and management of benign paroxysmal positional vertigo (BPPV). CMAJ 169: 681–693.

19. Karlberg M, Hall K, Quickert N, Hinson J, Halmagyi GM (2000) What inner ear diseases cause benign paroxysmal positional vertigo? Acta Otolaryngol 120: 380–385.

20. Wu ZM, Zhang SZ, Liu XJ, Chen X, Ji F, et al. (2007) Benign paroxysmal positioning vertigo related to inner ear disorders. Zhonghua Er Bi Yan Hou Tou Jing Wai Ke Za Zhi 42: 821–825.

21. Gross EM, Ress BD, Viirre ES, Nelson JR, Harris JP (2000) Intractable benign paroxysmal positional vertigo in patients with Meniere's disease. Laryngoscope 110: 655–659.

22. Rambold H, Heide W, Helmchen C (2004) Horizontal canal benign paroxysmal positioning vertigo with ipsilateral hearing loss. Eur J Neurol 11: 31–35.

23. Mizukoshi K, Watanabe Y, Shojaku H, Okubo J, Watanabe I (1988) Epidemiological studies on benign paroxysmal positional vertigo in Japan. Acta Otolaryngol Suppl 447: 67–72.

24. Park HM, Jung SW, Rhee CK (2001) Vestibular diagnosis as prognostic indicator in sudden hearing loss with vertigo. Acta Otolaryngol Suppl 545: 80–83.

25. Kim MB, Ban JH (2012) Benign paroxysmal positional vertigo accompanied by sudden sensorineural hearing loss: a comparative study with idiopathic benign paroxysmal positional vertigo. Laryngoscope 122: 2832–2836.

26. Song JJ, Yoo YT, An YH, Yoo JC, Kim JS, et al. (2012) Comorbid benign paroxysmal positional vertigo in idiopathic sudden sensorineural hearing loss: an ominous sign for hearing recovery. Otol Neurotol 33: 137–141.

27. Lee NH, Ban JH, Lee KC, Kim SM (2010) Benign paroxysmal positional vertigo secondary to inner ear disease. Otolaryngol Head Neck Surg 143: 413–417.

28. Papi G, Guidetti G, Corsello SM, Di DC, Pontecorvi A (2010) The association between benign paroxysmal positional vertigo and autoimmune chronic thyroiditis is not related to thyroid status. Thyroid 20: 237–238.

29. Cohen HS, Kimball KT, Stewart MG (2004) Benign paroxysmal positional vertigo and comorbid conditions. ORL J Otorhinolaryngol Relat Spec 66: 11–15.

30. Lee SH, Kim JS (2010) Benign paroxysmal positional vertigo. J Clin Neurol 6: 51–63.

31. Modugno GC, Pirodda A, Ferri GG, Montana T, Rasciti L, et al. (2000) A relationship between autoimmune thyroiditis and benign paroxysmal positional vertigo? Med Hypotheses 54: 614–615.

32. Vibert D, Kompis M, Hausler R (2003) Benign paroxysmal positional vertigo in older women may be related to osteoporosis and osteopenia. Ann Otol Rhinol Laryngol 112: 885–889.

33. Jang YS, Kang MK (2009) Relationship between bone mineral density and clinical features in women with idiopathic benign paroxysmal positional vertigo. Otol Neurotol 30: 95–100.

34. Jeong SH, Choi SH, Kim JY, Koo JW, Kim HJ, et al. (2009) Osteopenia and osteoporosis in idiopathic benign positional vertigo. Neurology 72: 1069–1076.

35. Warninghoff JC, Bayer O, Ferrari U, Straube A (2009) Co-morbidities of vertiginous diseases. BMC Neurol 9: 29.

36. Buki B, Simon L, Garab S, Lundberg YW, Junger H, et al. (2011) Sitting-up vertigo and trunk retropulsion in patients with benign positional vertigo but without positional nystagmus. J Neurol Neurosurg Psychiatry 82: 98–104.

37. Cambi J, Astore S, Mandala M, Trabalzini F, Nuti D (2013) Natural course of positional down-beating nystagmus of peripheral origin. J Neurol 260: 1489–1496.

38. Hain TC, Helminski JO, Reis IL, Uddin MK (2000) Vibration does not improve results of the canalith repositioning procedure. Arch Otolaryngol Head Neck Surg 126: 617–622.

39. Nunez RA, Cass SP, Furman JM (2000) Short- and long-term outcomes of canalith repositioning for benign paroxysmal positional vertigo. Otolaryngol Head Neck Surg 122: 647–652.

40. Perez P, Franco V, Cuesta P, Aldama P, Alvarez MJ, et al. (2012) Recurrence of benign paroxysmal positional vertigo. Otol Neurotol 33: 437–443.

41. Fife TD (2009) Benign paroxysmal positional vertigo. Semin Neurol 29: 500–508.

42. Baloh RW, Honrubia V, Jacobson K (1987) Benign positional vertigo: clinical and oculographic features in 240 cases. Neurology 37: 371–378.

43. Froehling DA, Silverstein MD, Mohr DN, Beatty CW, Offord KP, et al. (1991) Benign positional vertigo: incidence and prognosis in a population-based study in Olmsted County, Minnesota. Mayo Clin Proc 66: 596–601.

44. Celebisoy N, Polat F, Akyurekli O (2008) Clinical features of benign paroxysmal positional vertigo in Western Turkey. Eur Neurol 59: 315–319.

45. Kim YH, Kim KS, Choi H, Choi JS, Han CD (2012) Benign Paroxysmal Positional Vertigo Is Not a Prognostic Factor in Sudden Sensorineural Hearing Loss. Otolaryngol Head Neck Surg 146: 279–82.

46. Ogun OA, Buki B, Cohn ES, Janky KL, Lundberg YW (2014) Menopause and benign paroxysmal positional vertigo. Menopause 21: 886–889.

47. Cohen HS, Stewart MG, Brissett AE, Olson KL, Takashima M, et al. (2010) Frequency of sinus disease in normal subjects and patients with benign paroxysmal positional vertigo. ORL J Otorhinolaryngol Relat Spec 72: 63–67.

48. Lasisi AO, Abdullahi M (2008) The inner ear in patients with nasal allergy. J Natl Med Assoc 100: 903–905.

49. Friauf E, Wenz M, Oberhofer M, Nothwang HG, Balakrishnan V, et al. (2008) Hypothyroidism impairs chloride homeostasis and onset of inhibitory neurotransmission in developing auditory brainstem and hippocampal neurons. Eur J Neurosci 28: 2371–2380.

50. Dror AA, Politi Y, Shahin H, Lenz DR, Dossena S, et al. (2010) Calcium oxalate stone formation in the inner ear as a result of an Slc26a4 mutation. J Biol Chem 285: 21724–21735.

51. Everett LA, Belyantseva IA, Noben-Trauth K, Cantos R, Chen A, et al. (2001) Targeted disruption of mouse Pds provides insight about the inner-ear defects encountered in Pendred syndrome. Hum Mol Genet 10: 153–161.

52. Kozel PJ, Friedman RA, Erway LC, Yamoah EN, Liu LH, et al (1998) Balance and hearing deficits in mice with a null mutation in the gene encoding plasma membrane Ca2+-ATPase isoform 2. J Biol Chem 273: 18693–18696.

53. Gyo K (1988) Benign paroxysmal positional vertigo as a complication of postoperative bedrest. Laryngoscope 98: 332–333.

54. Hederstierna C, Hultcrantz M, Collins A, Rosenhall U (2007) Hearing in women at menopause. Prevalence of hearing loss, audiometric configuration and relation to hormone replacement therapy. Acta Otolaryngol 127: 149–155.

55. Gizzi M, Ayyagari S, Khattar V (1998) The familial incidence of benign paroxysmal positional vertigo. Acta Otolaryngol 118: 774–777.

56. Meggs WJ, Dunn KA, Bloch RM, Goodman PE, Davidoff AL (1996) Prevalence and nature of allergy and chemical sensitivity in a general population. Arch Environ Health 51: 275–282.

57. Chen W, Mempel M, Schober W, Behrendt H, Ring J (2008) Gender difference, sex hormones, and immediate type hypersensitivity reactions. Allergy 63: 1418–1427.

58. Schiller JS, Lucas JW, Ward BW, Peregoy JA (2012) Summary health statistics for U.S. adults: National Health Interview Survey, 2010. National Center for Health Statistics. Vital Health Stat 10: 252.

59. Faul M, Xu L, Wald MM, Coronado VG (2010) Traumatic Brain Injury in the United States: Emergency Department Visits, Hospitalizations and Deaths 2002–2006. Atlanta (GA): Center for Disease Control and Prevention, National Center for Injury prevention and Control.

60. MacGregor EA, Rosenberg JD, Kurth T (2011) Sex-related differences in epidemiological and clinic-based headache studies. Headache 51: 843–859.

61. Scher AI, Stewart WF, Liberman J, Lipton RB (1998) Prevalence of frequent headache in a population sample. Headache 38: 497–506.

62. CDC (2012) Cholesterol facts. Available: http://www.cdc.gov/cholesterol/facts. htm. Accessed 2013 February 6.

63. NIDDK (2012) National Kidney and Urologic Diseases Information Clearinghouse (NKUDIC). Available: http://kidney.niddk.nih.gov/KUDiseases/pubs/kustats/index.aspx. Accessed 2013 February 6.

64. Lipton RB, Stewart WF, Diamond S, Diamond ML, Reed M (2001) Prevalence and burden of migraine in the United States: data from the American Migraine Study II. Headache 41: 646–657.

65. Christopher and Dana Reeve Foundation (2013) One Degree of Separation: Paralysis and Spinal Cord Injury in the United States. Available: http://www.christopherreeve.org/site/c.ddJFKRNoFiG/b.5091685. Accessed 2013 February 6.

66. NHLBI (2012) Morbidity & Mortality: 2012 Chart Book on Cardiovascular, Lung, and Blood Diseases. Available: http://www.nhlbi.nih.gov/resources/docs/2012_ChartBook_508.pdf, NIH NHLBI. Accessed 2013 February 6.

67. Tunbridge WM, Evered DC, Hall R, Appleton D, Brewis M, et al. (1977) The spectrum of thyroid disease in a community: the Whickham survey. Clin Endocrinol (Oxf) 7: 481–493.

68. Tunbridge WM, Evered DC, Hall R, Appleton D, Brewis M, et al. (1977) Lipid profiles and cardiovascular disease in the Whickham area with particular reference to thyroid failure. Clin Endocrinol (Oxf) 7: 495–508.

69. Vanderpump MP, Tunbridge WM, French JM, Appleton D, Bates D, et al. (1995) The incidence of thyroid disorders in the community: a twenty-year follow-up of the Whickham Survey. Clin Endocrinol (Oxf) 43: 55–68.

70. Blackwell DL, Collins JG, Coles R (2002) Summary health statistics for U.S. adults: National Health Interview Survey, 1997. Vital Health Stat 10: 1–109.

71. Blackwell DL, Tonthat L (2002) Summary health statistics for the U.S. population: National Health Interview Survey, 1997. Vital Health Stat 10: 1–92.

72. Kobau R, Zahran H, Thurman DJ, Zack MM, Henry TR, et al. (2008) Epilepsy surveillance among adults–19 States, Behavioral Risk Factor Surveillance System, 2005. MMWR Surveill Summ 57: 1–20.

73. U.S.Census Bureau (2010) 2010 Demographic Profile Data - Nebraska. Available: http://quickfacts.census.gov/qfd/states/31000.html. Accessed 2013 February 8.

# 20

# DVT Surveillance Program in the ICU: Analysis of Cost-Effectiveness

Ajai K. Malhotra[1]*, Stephanie R. Goldberg[1], Laura McLay[2¤a], Nancy R. Martin[1], Luke G. Wolfe[1], Mark M. Levy[1], Vishal Khiatani[1¤b], Todd C. Borchers[1], Therese M. Duane[1], Michel B. Aboutanos[1], Rao R. Ivatury[1]

1 Department of Surgery, Virginia Commonwealth University, Richmond, Virginia, United States of America, 2 Department of Biostatistics, Virginia Commonwealth University, Richmond, Virginia, United States of America

## Abstract

**Background:** Venous Thrombo-embolism (VTE – Deep venous thrombosis (DVT) and/or pulmonary embolism (PE) – in traumatized patients causes significant morbidity and mortality. The current study evaluates the effectiveness of DVT surveillance in reducing PE, and performs a cost-effectiveness analysis.

**Methods:** All traumatized patients admitted to the adult ICU underwent twice weekly DVT surveillance by bilateral lower extremity venous Duplex examination (48-month surveillance period – SP). The rates of DVT and PE were recorded and compared to the rates observed in the 36-month pre-surveillance period (PSP). All patients in both periods received mechanical and pharmacologic prophylaxis unless contraindicated. Total costs – diagnostic, therapeutic and surveillance – for both periods were recorded and the incremental cost for each Quality Adjusted Life Year (QALY) gained was calculated.

**Results:** 4234 patients were eligible (PSP – 1422 and SP – 2812). Rate of DVT in SP (2.8%) was significantly higher than in PSP (1.3%) – $p < 0.05$, and rate of PE in SP (0.7%) was significantly lower than that in PSP (1.5%) – $p < 0.05$. Logistic regression demonstrated that surveillance was an independent predictor of increased DVT detection (OR: 2.53 – CI: 1.462–4.378) and decreased PE incidence (OR: 0.487 – CI: 0.262–0.904). The incremental cost was $509,091/life saved in the base case, translating to $29,102/QALY gained. A sensitivity analysis over four of the parameters used in the model indicated that the incremental cost ranged from $18,661 to $48,821/QALY gained.

**Conclusions:** Surveillance of traumatized ICU patients increases DVT detection and reduces PE incidence. Costs in terms of QALY gained compares favorably with other interventions accepted by society.

**Editor:** Natalie Walker, The National Institute for Health Innovation, New Zealand

**Funding:** The authors have no support or funding to report.

**Competing Interests:** The authors have declared that no competing interests exist.

* Email: akmalhot@vcu.edu

¤a Current address: University of Wisconsin, Madison, Wisconsin, United States of America
¤b Current address: Coastal Radiology Associates PLLC, New Bern, North Carolina, United States of America

## Introduction

Venous thrombo-embolism (VTE), encompassing deep vein thrombosis (DVT) and pulmonary embolism (PE) causes significant morbidity and mortality among traumatized patients. Without prophylaxis, the incidence of DVT is estimated to be 60% [1] dropping to 6–21% with adequate mechanical and/or pharmacologic prophylaxis. [2–8] In view of this, prophylaxis against VTE is standard of care for traumatized patients at high risk of VTE. With or without prophylaxis, patients that do develop DVT are at risk of short term complications (limb threatening phlegmasia, and life threatening PE) and long term complications (post-phlebetic limb, and pulmonary hypertension). Thus the total burden of VTE in traumatized patients is significant both in terms of cost and suffering.

Despite adequate prophylaxis, [9] DVT does occur and can be silent with the first manifestation being a PE that is fatal in 5–10%. [10,11] Surveillance screening for DVT in high risk patients may be an effective strategy to diagnose and treat DVT and thus reduce both short and long term morbidity and mortality. The current study evaluates the cost effectiveness of such a surveillance program on traumatized patients at high risk of VTE, with a particular focus on the quality adjusted life years (QALY) gained from any reduction in PE.

## Materials and Methodology

The study was performed at the level-I trauma center at the Virginia Commonwealth University (VCU) Medical Center. The trauma center is a state designated and American College of

Surgeons verified level-I center in central Virginia serving a population of two million, with annual trauma admissions of >4,000. The study was approved by the Institutional Review Board (IRB) of VCU. The study was exempt from informed consent since 1. all the data was already gathered in the registry of the trauma center prior to the conception of the study and 2. data from the registry was de-identified.

All adult traumatized patients admitted to an intensive care unit (ICU) were included. During the 36-month pre-surveillance period, patients received mechanical prophylaxis (thigh-high sequential compression device) *and* pharmacologic prophylaxis [low molecular weight (LMW) heparin], unless contraindicated. Prophylaxis was initiated within 24 hours of admission. In the year 2000 the institution adopted the policy of initiating un-fractionated heparin for all head injured patients within 24 hours of admission unless the patient had an expanding head bleed and this policy was continued throughout the study period. The prophylaxis protocol did not change over the time course of the study, and the non-compliance rate was <10%. During the 48-month surveillance period, in addition to pharmacologic prophylaxis, patients underwent twice weekly DVT surveillance of both lower extremities by bedside venous Duplex examination, till discharged from the unit. Surveillance was performed on the lower extremities since 90% of the PEs originate in the lower extremity, [12] and the focus of the study was to examine the reduction in PEs by early detection and prompt therapy of DVT. Patients diagnosed with clinically significant (popliteal vein or higher) DVT were initially treated with therapeutic heparin (unfractionated or LMW) and later either maintained on LMW heparin or changed to oral anti-coagulation. In instances where therapeutic anti-coagulation was contra-indicated, or there was progression of VTE despite adequate anti-coagulation, inferior vena-caval filter was inserted to prevent PE. Anti-coagulant therapy was continued for at least six months. DVTs that involved only the infra-popliteal calf veins were not treated, however prophylaxis and surveillance was continued.

Each incidence of DVT and PE was recorded. Cost determinations were based on the following: Diagnosis/surveillance for DVT = $200/duplex study; diagnosis of PE by contrast enhanced computed tomography (CECT) of chest = $500; VTE therapy cost = $6,000. [13] During PSP, total cost was calculated by adding the diagnostic cost of each incidence of DVT (single venous duplex examination) and PE (single CECT of chest) and the therapeutic cost of all VTE requiring therapy. For SP surveillance costs were calculated by multiplying the cost of a single Duplex study by the average number of studies per ICU patient under surveillance. The average number of studies per patient was determined by dividing the average ICU length of stay in days by 3.5 since surveillance studies were performed twice in one week. To the surveillance cost was added the diagnostic cost of each incidence of PE, and the therapeutic cost of all VTE requiring therapy. For cost calculations in SP, it was assumed that all DVT detected was via surveillance, hence there are no separate diagnostic cost for DVT.

## Statistical and Cost benefit analysis

Uni-variate comparisons were performed using the appropriate tests – Chi-square, with Fisher's exact correction where required, for discrete variables, and Student's t-test for parametric and Wilcoxson rank sum test for non-parametric continuous variables. Regression analysis was performed to evaluate the independent predictors of DVT and PE including the role of surveillance. Significance was set at $p < 0.05$. For cost benefit analysis, the total cost of the program was calculated as detailed above. This cost was used to calculate the cost per life saved if the program led to a decrease in number of PEs. All costs were computed in US dollars. All calculations were performed using Statview software (SAS Institute Inc Cary NC, USA). All continuous data is presented as Mean±Standard Error of Mean (SEM).

## Results

There were 4234 trauma patients admitted to the ICU during the 84-month study period (Table 1). The overall characteristics of the population were similar to most trauma populations with a relatively young age, and male preponderance. Of these, 1422 were during PSP and 2812 during SP.

### VTE

There were 139 incidents of VTE (DVT-96; PE-43) among 129 patients. The characteristics of patients that developed VTE and those that did not are presented in Table 2. Patients developing VTE were older with a higher injury severity score (ISS) – $p < 0.05$ for both. VTE was more common in males, and those that suffered blunt trauma, though these differences were not statistically significant – $p > 0.05$ for both. VTE was also more common in patients sustaining injuries to face, chest and extremity as evidenced by the higher abbreviated injury scale (AIS) for these body regions – $p < 0.05$ for all. Older age and higher ISS was observed in the DVT patients ($p < 0.05$), but only ISS was significantly higher in the PE patients ($p < 0.05$). Like VTE in general, both DVT and PE patients demonstrated a male preponderance and more blunt mechanism, however these differences were not statistically significant ($p > 0.05$). Among the 96 DVTs, 18 were in PSP, and of these nine (50%) were clinically significant, requiring therapy as per protocol. The remaining 78 DVTs were in SP, and of these 47 (60%) were clinically significant. Five of these 47 were in patients in whom surveillance had previously detected calf vein DVT, and with continued surveillance the DVT was observed to progress. Of the 43 PEs, 22 were in PSP and 21 in SP.

The rate of DVT increased while the rate of PE decreased between PSP and SP. The overall rate of DVT was 2.2% (96/4234). The rate during PSP was 1.3% (18/1422), and with surveillance, the rate increased by 115% to 2.8% (78/2812). The overall rate of PE was 1% (43/4234). The rate of PE during SP (0.7% – 21/2812) was 50% lower than in PSP (1.5% – 22/1422). The differences in the rates of both DVT and PE during PSP vs SP, were statistically significant – $p < 0.05$ for both (Fig. 1). Since there were some differences in the patient population and injury characteristics between the two periods (Table 1), a logistic regression model was constructed to identify independent predictors of DVT and PE (Table 3). Among the patient and injury characteristics, age, ISS and AIS of extremity were independently predictive of DVT, and AIS of chest and extremity were independently predictive of PE. After controlling for all variables identified, surveillance was an independent predictor of increased DVT detection (OR 2.53 with 95% CI of 1.462–4.378) and of decreased PE incidence (OR 0.487 with 95% CI of 0.262–0.904).

## Outcomes

Occurrence of VTE significantly worsened outcomes in terms of increased mortality and longer lengths of stay in the ICU and the hospital – $p < 0.05$ for all (Table 2). These differences remained when the VTE group was separated into those with DVT and those with PE (Table 2). Overall mortality in PSP was 9.1% and in SP was 8.9% ($p > 0.05$).

**Table 1.** Patient populations in the two periods of study.

| | PSP (n = 1422) | SP (n = 2812) |
|---|---|---|
| Age (years) | 40.76±0.50 | 40.69±0.36 |
| Gender (% male:female) | 72:28 | 73:27 |
| Mechanism (% blunt:penetrating)* | 81:19 | 84:16 |
| ISS* | 19.37±0.33 | 20.89±0.25 |
| RTS | 6.95±0.05 | 6.89±0.04 |
| AIS | | |
| Head* | 2.93±0.04 | 3.14±0.03 |
| Face* | 1.42±0.03 | 1.95±0.03 |
| Chest* | 3.05±0.04 | 3.29±0.02 |
| Abdomen | 2.74±0.04 | 2.66±0.03 |
| Extremity* | 2.28±0.03 | 2.55±0.02 |
| External* | 1.12±0.04 | 1.04±0.01 |
| Inferior Vena Caval filter* | 34 (2%) | 28 (1%) |
| Mortality | 129 (9.1%) | 250 (8.9%) |

*$p < 0.05$: PSP vs SP. PSP: pre-surveillance period, SP: surveillance period, ISS: injury severity score, RTS: revised trauma score, AIS: Abbreviated Injury Scale.

## Data assumptions, and Cost calculations

To compute the incremental cost/QALY gained, the following assumptions were made:

1. Attention was restricted to men aged 50 and older to be consistent with the cohort studied. Survival for men up to age 99 was computed using CDC data. [14]

2. The base case health utility for all patients was 0.9, which is consistent with publicly reported values associated with DVT. [15] For sensitivity analysis, this was varied from 0.8–1.0.

3. All health effects were discounted at 3% which is also standard in terms of reduction in quality of life with age. For sensitivity analysis the discount rate was varied from 0–5%.

4. To calculate cost per life saved, it was assumed that the main difference between SP and PSP was a reduction in PEs. The difference in PE incidence rate between PSP and SP was computed using the observations from the study – an absolute reduction of 0.8% (1.5% in PSP to 0.7% in SP). For sensitivity analysis 95% confidence interval for the reduction in the PE rate was utilized. This, using the normal approximation to the binomial distribution, is 0.2%–1.4%.

**Table 2.** Details and outcomes of patients developing venous thrombo-embolism (VTE) or not.

| | No VTE (n = 4105) | VTE (n = 129) | DVT (n = 96) | PE (n = 43) |
|---|---|---|---|---|
| Age (years)*# | 40.52±0.3 | 47.11±1.62 | 48.51±1.99 | 42.90±2.30 |
| Gender (% male:female) | 72:28 | 78:22 | 78:22 | 84:16 |
| Mechanism (%blunt:penetrating) | 83:17 | 87:13 | 85:15 | 93:7 |
| ISS*#^ | 20.09±0.20 | 28.46±1.13 | 29.67±0.20 | 25.66±1.81 |
| RTS | 6.91±0.03 | 6.72±0.18 | 6.82±0.19 | 6.54±0.42 |
| AIS | | | | |
| Head | 3.07±0.02 | 3.22±0.13 | 3.07±0.02 | 3.23±0.26 |
| Face* | 1.70±0.02 | 1.92±0.12 | 1.86±0.14 | 2.00±0.22 |
| Chest*# | 3.21±0.02 | 3.44±0.10 | 3.60±0.11 | 3.19±0.19 |
| Abdomen | 2.69±0.02 | 2.78±0.12 | 2.79±0.13 | 2.76±0.25 |
| Extremity*# | 2.44±0.02 | 2.64±0.08 | 2.70±0.08 | 2.50±0.14 |
| External | 1.04±0.01 | 1.06±0.06 | 1.08±0.08 | 1.00±0.00 |
| ICULOS (days)*#^ | 5.59±0.14 | 20.15±1.67 | 22.03±2.02 | 13.19±2.12 |
| HLOS (days)*#^ | 11.78±0.23 | 35.88±2.76 | 36.90±3.09 | 30.79±4.87 |
| Mortality*#^ | 356 (8.3%) | 23 (17.8%) | 16 (16.7%) | 8 (18.6%) |

Among those developing VTE, details of those developing deep vein thrombosis (DVT), or pulmonary embolism (PE). $p < 0.05$: *No VTE vs VTE, #No DVT vs DVT, ^No PE vs PE. ISS: injury severity score, RTS: revised trauma score, AIS: abbreviated injury scale, ICULOS: Intensive Care Unit Length of Stay, HLOS: Hospital Length of Stay.

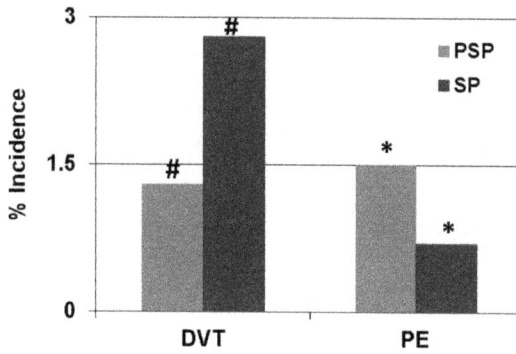

**Figure 1. Figure showing the rates of deep vein thrombosis (DVT) and pulmonary embolism (PE) during the pre-surveillance period (PSP: 2001–03) and the surveillance period (SP: 2004–07).** #p<0.05 – DVT (PSP vs SP); *p<0.05 – PE (PSP vs SP).

5. The PE fatality rate for the base case was assumed to be 7.5%, and a range from 5–10% was considered for sensitivity analysis. [10,11]

6. Those who survive PE suffer from a short-term loss in 0.0115 QALYs due to short-term hospitalization. [16]

The total VTE related patient care cost during PSP (diagnostic and therapeutic) was $194,600/1422 patients – $136,850/1000 patients and during SP (diagnostic, therapeutic and surveillance) was $1,244,100/2812 patients – $442,425/1000 patients. Thus, the total additional cost of the surveillance program was $305,575/1000 patients. During this period the PE rate decreased from 1.5% to 0.7% or, eight PEs were prevented per 1000 patients placed under surveillance. Assuming a base case PE fatality rate of 7.5%, it is necessary to prevent 13.33 PEs in order to save one life. This translates to 1666 patients placed under surveillance at a cost of $509,091 per life saved.

The incremental cost per QALY saved was computed as follows. Future expected life years were computed using CDC mortality data for men aged 50 and over to be consistent with the cohort studied. [14] Given these assumptions, patients not experiencing a PE fatality would live an additional 30.31 expected life years, which translates to an additional 17.49 quality-adjusted/discounted life years with a health state utility of 0.9. This yielded an incremental cost of $29,102/QALY gained for the base case.

## Discussion

VTE is a major problem for high risk trauma patients. A large body of literature has established that trauma patients are at higher risk of developing DVT that can lead to mortality from PE, and both short and long term morbidity. Without prophylaxis the incidence of DVT in trauma patients has been reported to be as high as 60%. [1] This has resulted in some form of prophylaxis becoming a standard of care for all high risk trauma patients. [17]

Despite prophylaxis, DVT occurs in 6–12% of trauma patients. [8] Oftentimes the DVT itself is silent, with the first sign of VTE being a pulmonary embolism that is fatal in 5–10% of instances. [10,11] Routine surveillance for DVT maybe a method to diagnose DVT at an asymptomatic stage, with the hope that by therapy and/or placement of a protective inferior vena-caval filter, a large hemodynamically compromising or fatal PE will be prevented. The value and cost-effectiveness of this approach is debated. In an early prospective study, Piotrowski et al reported on 343 high-risk trauma patients placed on DVT surveillance and concluded that since with prophylaxis the risk of DVT was low, the cost of detecting a single DVT by surveillance was extremely high. [18] They did however suggest that routine DVT surveillance may reduce the risk of PE. [18] In a retrospective study Meyer et al reported on traumatized ICU patients and concluded that at US$ 6688/DVT detected, the cost was too high to recommend routine surveillance, but it should be considered in patients at the highest risk. [19] Major et al reported on 726 patients admitted to the surgical ICU (majority due to trauma) of which some underwent routine DVT surveillance and concluded that with adequate prophylaxis the incidence of both DVT and PE were low and hence, surveillance was not indicated. [20] Similar doubts regarding the utility and cost-effectiveness of surveillance have been reported by others. [21–24] Based on the results of these studies, the latest edition (9th) of the American College of Chest Physicians (ACCP) evidenced based guidelines on DVT prevention state that the benefit of DVT surveillance by duplex sonography in reducing the incidence of PE and mortality is unclear. Additionally, since up to 30% of screen positives maybe false, [25] there is potential harm in that the falsely positive patients may get unnecessary anticoagulation therapy with its attendant risks. [9] On the other hand, Napolitano et al reported on 458 high-risk traumatized patients that underwent routine surveillance, and found a significant incidence of asymptomatic DVT concluding that for the high-risk trauma patient, surveillance is justified. [26] Adams et al, in a large recent study involving> 4,000 traumatized patients of whom 982 high-risk patients were placed on DVT surveillance, reported that 86% of the lower extremity DVTs were clinically silent and detected by surveillance. They concluded that surveillance was justified in this patient population. [27] In light of these conflicting conclusions, the CDC convened a panel of experts to examine and advise about the utility of DVT surveillance in hospitalized patients. The panel recommended that surveillance can provide robust data on the

**Table 3.** Results of logistic regression showing the independent predictors of Deep Vein Thrombosis (DVT) and Pulmonary Embolism (PE).

|  | DVT | | PE | |
|---|---|---|---|---|
|  | OR | 95% CI | OR | 95%CI |
| Age | 1.022 | 1.011–1.032 | - | - |
| ISS | 1.039 | 1.023–1.055 | - | - |
| AIS Chest | - | - | 1.318 | 1.094–1.587 |
| AIS Extremity | 1.379 | 1.168–1.627 | 1.297 | 1.025–1.641 |

OR: odds ratio, CI: confidence interval, ISS: injury severity score, AIS: abbreviated injury scale.

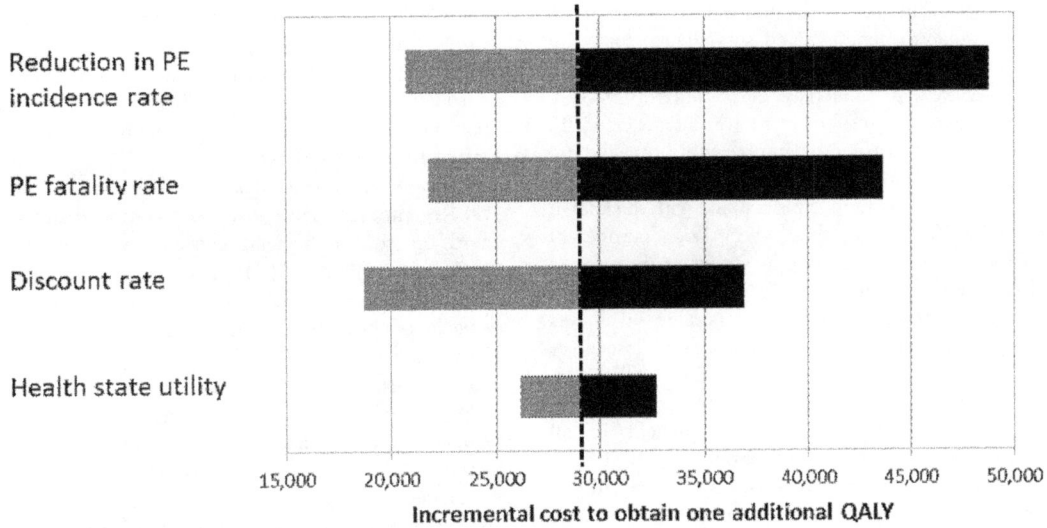

**Figure 2. Figure showing a sensitivity analysis on the incremental cost to obtain one additional QALY.** The bars represent upper and lower bounds on the incremental cost relative to the base case of $29,102 (dashed line) with respect to the bounds on each parameter value. In this figure, the discount rate ranges from 0% to 5%, the difference in the PE incidence rate between PSP and SP ranges from 0.2% to 1.4%, the PE fatality rate ranges from 5% to 10%, and the health state utility ranges from 0.8 to 1.0.

epidemiology of VTE and effectiveness of prevention programs however more data was needed regarding the utility of surveillance itself in improving patient outcomes. [28] The current study reports on a surveillance program at a busy level-I trauma center, and aims at performing a detailed cost effectiveness analysis of such a program. In the current economic and healthcare environment, merely demonstrating a medical benefit may no longer be enough to support an intervention. The direct cost and the resultant benefit has to be at a level that society is willing and able to afford. Past DVT surveillance studies have focused on establishing the incidence and risk factors for VTE, however, to the best of our knowledge, this is the first report of QALY based

cost effectiveness analysis of such a program in an acute care setting.

VTE was seen more often in older patients with a higher ISS and those with injuries to extremity and the chest regions. This is similar to what has been reported in many studies. [1,6,7,18,27] Unlike other studies, the current study failed to demonstrate a higher incidence of VTE in head injured patients. This may be related to the very aggressive prophylaxis program instituted at our institution in 2000 where all head injured patients received unfractionated heparin within 24 hours of admission, unless the repeat CT demonstrated expansion of intra-cranial hemorrhage. Surveillance resulted in higher numbers of DVTs being diagnosed

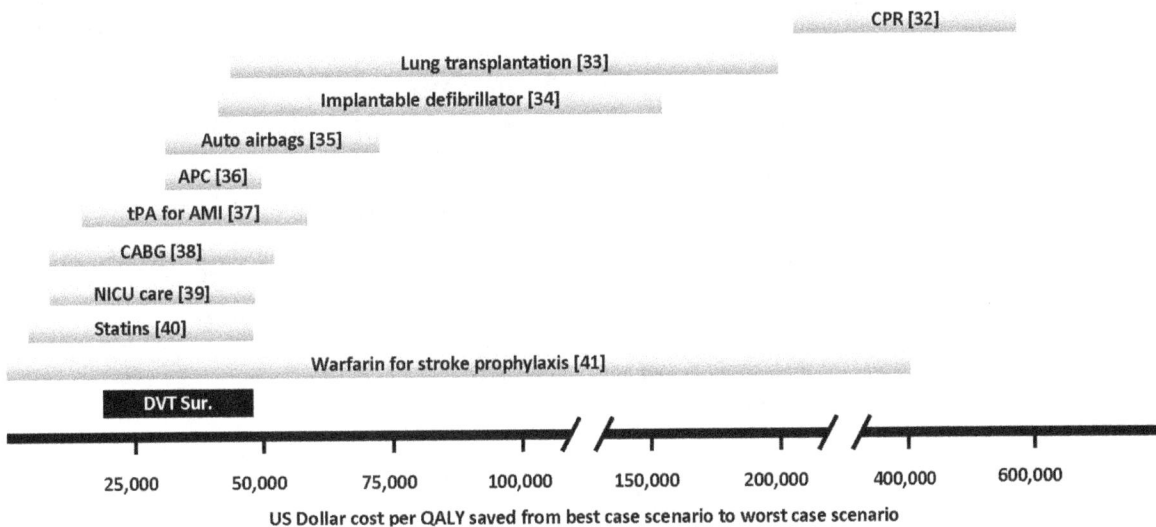

**Figure 3. Incremental dollar cost per quality adjusted life year (QALY) saved for selected interventions as compared to the cost of deep venous thrombosis surveillance (DVT Sur.).** The bars represent range of cost from the best case scenario (most cost effective) to the worst case scenario (least cost effective) for each intervention. CPR: cardio-pulmonary resuscitation, APC: activated protein C for sepsis, tPA for AMI: tissue plasminogen activator for acute myocardial infarction, CABG: coronary artery bypass grafting, NICU: neonatal intensive care unit. The bracketed number represents the reference the data is derived from.

and treated, and at the same time, lowering the incidence of PE (Fig. 1). Regression analysis demonstrated surveillance to be an independent predictor of increased DVT detection and decreased PE incidence. We believe that the increase in the numbers of DVT diagnosed, and treated directly resulted in a lower incidence of PE. While clearly effective in decreasing the number of PEs, we did not see a significant decrease in mortality. The total incidence of PE was 43 or 1% of the total population. This coupled with the known PE fatality rate of 5–10% means that a very large number of patients will be required to demonstrate a significant decrease in the PE related mortality by such a surveillance program.

In the current study, the incremental cost per life saved was $509,091. In comparison, post-exposure prophylaxis against rabies is estimated to cost>$500,000 per life saved. [29] In the non-disease arena, in 2002, The National Highway Traffic Safety Administration (NHTSA) evaluated the cost benefit of all mandated Federal Motor Vehicle Safety Standards (FMVSS). The report concluded that these standards helped save 20,851 lives in 2002 at a cost of $544,482 per life saved. [30] There was only one study that directly evaluated cost-effectiveness of DVT surveillance. In that 1996 study on traumatic and non-traumatic brain injured patients, that underwent a single screening duplex examination at the time of admission to the rehabilitation unit, the cost per life saved was $129, 527. [31] The cost in the current study is much higher. The reasons for that are likely twofold: first is medical care cost inflation, with the current study basing all costs of 2004 estimates as compared to the cited study on 1996 estimates, and secondly, the current study bases costs on twice weekly surveillance examinations, while the brain injury study had a single screening examination at the time of admission only. Cost per life saved however, is a very crude measure of cost benefit evaluation since the method treats each life saved as equivalent irrespective of the future life expectancy at the age death was prevented.

In the current study, to account for the difference in the quantity and quality of life saved, the incremental cost per QALY was computed at $29,102/QALY gained. To further analyze this value, a uni-variate sensitivity analysis was performed over four of the parameters used in the cost-effectiveness analysis: the discount rate (base case 3% with range of 0%–5%), the difference in the PE incidence rate between PSP and SP (base case 0.8% with range of 0.2%–1.4%), the PE fatality rate (base case 7.5% with range of 5%–10%), and the health state utility (base case 0.9 with range of 0.8–1.0). The resulting incremental costs per QALY saved in the uni-variate sensitivity analysis are illustrated in Fig. 2. The results show that the incremental costs are relatively insensitive to the health state utility ($26,191 – $32,739). The results are somewhat more sensitive to the PE fatality rate, the reduction in the PE rate, and the discount rate, which result in incremental costs per QALY saved of $21,829 – $43,652, $20,729 – $48,821, and $18,661 – $36,905, respectively. The sensitivity analysis results suggests that in all scenarios, the incremental costs compares well with a number of other life saving interventions that are accepted by

society in the medical and non-medical arenas as shown in Fig. 3 (compiled from references [32–41].

The question as to how much a society is able and willing to afford for each QALY saved is a difficult one. The answer depends upon the societal values and the economic status of an individual society. In the United States a figure of $50,000 per QALY saved is oftentimes utilized to make decisions about resource allocation. [42] Recently that figure has been questioned and it is argued that based on current societal expectations, the figure should be significantly higher. [30] However, even by the traditional model of $50,000 per QALY saved as cost effective, the DVT surveillance program is cost effective under nearly all of the scenarios considered.

There are some limitations to this study. Firstly, it is a retrospective analysis. Due to this, we cannot be sure of the compliance with surveillance. Second, it is not powered to demonstrate a difference in mortality. Since with prophylaxis, the incidence of PE is low (∼1%) and the mortality from PE is < 10%, only a very large multi-institutional study could have enough power to demonstrate a difference in PE related mortality. Third, even though the prophylaxis protocol has not changed over the study period, some other subtle changes may have occurred that are missed in a study spanning seven years. Finally, probably the most significant limitation of the study is that while the increased DVT detection and decreased PE incidence were directly observed (measured) and are likely due to surveillance, all the cost calculations leading to the dollar cost/QALY gained, are extrapolations of the data and represent *potential* estimates per QALY gained, if the observations of this study true. As mentioned above, the study is not large enough to demonstrate an actual difference in mortality that maybe attributable to surveillance. Despite these limitations, the study demonstrates that DVT surveillance among traumatized ICU patients increases DVT detection, decreases PE incidence and is cost-effective.

## Conclusions

A DVT surveillance program for trauma patients admitted to the ICU at high risk for VTE, is effective in reducing the incidence of PE, and cost effective in terms of preventing fatal PE.

## Acknowledgments

Podium presentation: 67th annual meeting of America Association for the Surgery of Trauma (AAST), Maui, HI.

## Author Contributions

Conceived and designed the experiments: AKM SG LM NRM VK TCB RRI. Performed the experiments: AKM SG NRM LGW MML VK TCB TMD MBA. Analyzed the data: AKM SG LM NRM LGW MML TMD MBA RRI. Contributed reagents/materials/analysis tools: AKM LM LGW. Wrote the paper: AKM SG LML LGW MML VK TCB TMD MBA RRI.

## References

1. Geerts WH, Code KI, Jay RM, Chen E, Szalai JP (1994) A prospective study of venous thromboembolism after major trauma. N Eng J Med. 331: 1601–1606.

2. Shackford SR, Davis JW, Hollingsworth-Fridlund P, Brewer NS, Hoyt DB, et al. (1990) Venous thromboembolism in patients with major trauma. Am J Surg. 159: 365–369.

3. Kudsk KA, Fabian TC, Baum S, Gold RE, Mangiante E, et al. (1989) Silent deep vein thrombosis in immobilized multiple trauma patients. Am J Surg. 158: 515–519.

4. Dennis JW, Menawat S, Von Thorn J, Fallon WF Jr, Vinsant GO, et al. (1993) Efficacy of deep venous thrombosis prophylaxis in trauma patients and identification of high-risk groups. J Trauma. 35: 132–139.

5. Burns GA, Cohn SM, Frumento RJ, Degutis LC, Hammers L (1993) Prospective ultrasound evaluation of deep venous thrombosis in high-risk trauma patients. J Trauma. 35: 405–408.

6. Knudson MM, Collins JA, Goodman SB, McCrory DW (1992) Thromboembolism following multiple trauma. J Trauma. 32: 2–11.

7. Knudson MM, Lewis FR, Clinton A, Atkinson K, Megerman J (1994) Prevention of venous thromboembolism in trauma patients. J Trauma. 37: 480–487.

8. Geerts WH, Jay RM, Code KI, Chen E, Szalai JP, et al. (1996) A comparison of low-dose heparin with low-molecular weight heparin as prophylaxis against venous thromboembolism after major trauma. N Engl J Med. 335: 701–707.

9.  Gould MK, Garcia DA, Wren SM, Karanicolas PJ, Arcelus JI, et al. (2012) Prevention of VTE in nonorthopedic surgical patients: Antithrombotic therapy and prevention of thrombosis, 9th ed: American College of Chest Physicians Evidence-Based Clinical Practice Guidelines. Chest. 141(2 Suppl): e227S–e277S.

10. Sharma OP, Oswanski MF, Joseph RJ, Tonui P, Westrick L, et al. (2007) Venous thromboembolism in trauma patients. Am Surg. 73: 1173–1180.

11. Grigorakos L, Sotiriou E, Myriantheís P, Michail A, Koulendi D, et al. (2008) Approach to patients with pulmonary embolism in a surgical intensive care unit. Hepatogastroenterology. 55: 887–890.

12. Moser KM, Lemoine JR (1981) Is embolic risk conditioned by the location of the deep-venous thrombosis? Ann Int Med. 94: 439–444.

13. Doyle NM, Ramirez MM, Mastrobattista JM, Monga M, Wagner LK, et al. (2004) Diagnosis of pulmonary embolism: a cost-effectiveness analysis. Am J Obstet Gynecol. 191: 1019–1023.

14. Arias E (2011) United States life tables, 2007. National vital statistics reports; vol 59 no 9. Hyattsville, MD: National Center for Health Statistics.

15. Gould MK, Dembitzer AD, Sanders GD, Garber AM (1999) Low-molecular-weight heparins compared with unfractionated heparin for treatment of acute deep venous thrombosis. Ann Int Med. 130: 789–799.

16. Perlroth DJ, Sanders GD, Gould MK (2007) Effectiveness and cost-effectiveness of thrombolysis in submassive pulmonary embolism. Arch Intern Med. 167: 74–80.

17. Rogers FB, Cipolle MD, Velmahos G, Rozycki G, Luchette FA (2002) Practice management guidelines for the prevention of venous thromboembolism in trauma patients: the EAST practice management guidelines work group. J Trauma. 53: 142–164.

18. Piotrowski JJ, Alexander JJ, Brandt CP, McHenry CR, Yuhas JP, et al. (1996) Is deep vein thrombosis surveillance warranted in high-risk trauma patients? Am J Surg. 172: 210–213.

19. Meyer CS, Blebea J, Davis K Jr, Fowl RJ, Kempczinski RF (1995) Surveillance venous scans for deep venous thrombosis in multiple trauma patients. Ann Vasc Surg. 9: 109–114.

20. Major KM, Wilson M, Nishi GK, Farber A, Chopra R, et al. (2003) The incidence of thromboembolism in surgical intensive care unit. Am Surg. 69: 857–861.

21. Spain DA, Richardson D, Polk HC, Bergamini TM, Wilson MA, et al. (1997) Venous thromboembolism in high-risk trauma patient: do risks justify aggressive screening and prophylaxis? J Trauma. 42: 463–469.

22. Schwartz TH, Quick RC, Minion DH, Kearney PA, Kwolek CJ, et al. (2001) Enoxiparin treatment in high-risk trauma patients limis the utility of surveillance venous duplex scanning. J Vasc Surg. 34: 447–452.

23. Satiani B, Falcone R, Shook L, Price J (1997) Screening for major deep vein thrombosis in seriously injured patients: a prospective study. Ann Vasc Surg. 11: 626–629.

24. Cipolle MD, Wojcik R, Seislove E, Wasser TE, Pasquale MD (2002) The role of surveillance duplex scanning in preventing venous thromboembolism in trauma patients. J Trauma. 52: 453–462.

25. Spinal Cord Injury Thromboprophylaxis Investigators. (2003) Prevention of venous thromboembolism in the acute treatment phase after spinal cord injury: a randomized trial comparing low-dose heparin plus intermittent pneumatic compression with enoxaparin. J Trauma. 54: 1116–1124.

26. Napolitano LM, Garlapati VS, Heard SO, Silva WE, Cutler BS, et al. (1995) Asymptomatic deep venous thrombosis in the trauma patient: Is an aggressive screening protocol justified? J Trauma. 39: 651–659.

27. Adams RC, Hamrick M, Berenguer C, Senkowski C, Ochsner G (2008) Four years of aggressive prophylaxis and screening for venous thromboembolism in a large trauma population. J Trauma. 65: 300–308.

28. Raskob GE, Silverstein R, Bratzler DW, Heit JA, White RH (2010) Surveillance for deep vein thrombosis and pulmonary embolism: recommendations from a national workshop. Am J Prev Med. 38(4 suppl): s502–509.

29. Dhankhar P, Vaidya SA, Fishbien DB, Meltzer MI (2008) Cost effectiveness of rabies post exposure prophylaxis in the United States. Vaccine. 26: 4251–4255.

30. Kahane CJ (2004) Cost per life saved by the Federal Motor Vehicle Safety Standards (DOT HS 809 835). Available: www.nhtsa.dot.gov

31. Meythaler JM, DeVivo MJ, Hayne JB (1996) Cost-effectiveness of routine screening for proximal deep venous thrombosis in acquired brain injury patient admitted to rehabilitation. Arch Phys Med Rehabil. 77: 1–5.

32. Lee KH, Angus DC, Abromson NS (1996) Cardiopulmonary resuscitation: What cost to cheat death? Crit Care Med. 24: 2046–2052.

33. Ramsey SD, Patrick DL, Albert RK, Larson EB, Wood DE, et al. (1995) The cost-effectiveness of lung transplantation: A pilot study. University of Washington Medical Center Lung Transplant Study Group. Chest. 108: 1594–1601.

34. Owens DK, Sanders GD, Harris RA, McDonald KM, Heidenreich PA, et al. (1997) Cost-effectiveness of implantable cardioverter defibrillators relative to amiodarone for prevention of sudden cardiac death. Ann Intern Med. 126: 1–12.

35. Graham JD, Thompson KM, Goldie SJ, Segui-Gomez M, Weinstein MC (1997) The cost-effectiveness of airbags by seating position. JAMA. 278: 1418–1425.

36. Angus DC, Linde-Zwirble WT, Clermont G, Ball DE, Basson BR, et al; PROWESS investigators. (2003) Cost-effectiveness of drotrecogin alfa (activated) in the treatment of severe sepsis. Crit Care Med. 31: 1–11.

37. Kalish SC, Gurwitz J, Krumholz HM, Avorn J (1995) A cost-effectiveness model of thrombolytic therapy for acute myocardial infarction. J Gen Intern Med. 10: 321–330.

38. Weinstein MC, Stason WB (1982) Cost-effectiveness of coronary artery bypass grafting. Circulation. 66: III56–III66.

39. Boyle MH, Torrence GW, Sinclair JC, Horwood SP (1983) Economic analysis of neonatal intensive care for very-low-birth-weight-infants. N Eng J Med. 308: 1330–1337.

40. Stinett AA, Mittleman MA, Weinstein MC (1996) Cost-effectiveness of dietary and pharmacologic therapy for cholesterol reduction in adults. In: Gold MR, Siegel JE, Russell LB, Weinstein MC, editors. Cost-Effectiveness in Health and Medicine. New York, NY: Oxford University Press. pp. 349–391.

41. Gage BF, Cardinalli AB, Albers GW, Owens DK (1995) Cost-effectiveness of warfarin and aspirin for prophylaxis of stroke in patients with non-valvular atrial fibrillation. JAMA. 274: 1839–1845.

42. Braithwaite RS, Meltzer DO, King JT Jr, Leslie D, Roberts MS (2008) What does the value of modern medicine say about the $50,000 per quality-adjusted life-year decision rule? Med Care. 46: 349–346.

# 21

# Traumatic Intracranial Hemorrhage Correlates with Preinjury Brain Atrophy, but not with Antithrombotic Agent use

**C. Michael Dunham**[1]*, **David A. Hoffman**[2], **Gregory S. Huang**[1], **Laurel A. Omert**[3], **David J. Gemmel**[4], **Renee Merrell**[1]

1 Trauma/Critical Care Services, St. Elizabeth Health Center, Youngstown, Ohio, United States of America, 2 Division of Cardiology, St. Elizabeth Health Center, Youngstown, Ohio, United States of America, 3 CSL Behring, King of Prussia, Pennsylvania, United States of America, 4 Medical Education and Statistics, St. Elizabeth Health Center, Youngstown, Ohio, United States of America

## Abstract

*Background:* The impact of antithrombotic agents (warfarin, clopidogrel, ASA) on traumatic brain injury outcomes is highly controversial. Although cerebral atrophy is speculated as a risk for acute intracranial hemorrhage, there is no objective literature evidence.

*Materials and Methods:* This is a retrospective, consecutive investigation of patients with signs of external head trauma and age ≥60 years. Outcomes were correlated with antithrombotic-agent status, coagulation test results, admission neurologic function, and CT-based cerebral atrophy dimensions.

*Results:* Of 198 consecutive patients, 36% were antithrombotic-negative and 64% antithrombotic-positive. ASA patients had higher arachidonic acid inhibition (p = 0.04) and warfarin patients had higher INR (p<0.001), compared to antithrombotic-negative patients. Antithrombotic-positive intracranial hemorrhage rate (38.9%) was similar to the antithrombotic-negative rate (31.9%; p = 0.3285). Coagulopathy was not present on the ten standard coagulation, thromboelastography, and platelet mapping tests with intracranial hemorrhage and results were similar to those without hemorrhage (p≥0.1354). Hemorrhagic-neurologic complication (intracranial hemorrhage progression, need for craniotomy, neurologic deterioration, or death) rates were similar for antithrombotic-negative (6.9%) and antithrombotic-positive (8.7%; p = 0.6574) patients. The hemorrhagic-neurologic complication rate was increased when admission major neurologic dysfunction was present (63.2% versus 2.2%; RR = 28.3; p<0.001). Age correlated inversely with brain parenchymal width (p<0.001) and positively with lateral ventricular width (p = 0.047) and cortical atrophy (p<0.001). Intracranial hemorrhage correlated with cortical atrophy (p<0.001) and ventricular width (p<0.001).

*Conclusions:* Intracranial hemorrhage is not associated with antithrombotic agent use. Intracranial hemorrhage patients have no demonstrable coagulopathy. The association of preinjury brain atrophy with acute intracranial hemorrhage is a novel finding. Contrary to antithrombotic agent status, admission neurologic abnormality is a predictor of adverse post-admission outcomes. Study findings indicate that effective hemostasis is maintained with antithrombotic therapy.

**Editor:** Anna-Leena Sirén, University of Wuerzburg, Germany

**Funding:** The authors have no support or funding to report.

**Competing Interests:** Dr. Omert is a former employee of the Haemonetics Corporation and a current employee of CSL Behring. Dr. Hoffman is on the advisory boards of CardioDX and AstraZeneca. The authors declare that these affiliations have not caused any bias in conception and design of the study, data interpretation, content of the original submitted manuscript, or any statement in the revised manuscript.

* Email: dunham.michael@sbcglobal.net

## Introduction

Among the elderly in the United States, there are 155,000 cases of traumatic brain injury annually, leading to 12,000 deaths [1]. Chronic oral anticoagulation or antiplatelet agents have been used with increasing frequency for reducing the risk of venous thromboembolism, preventing clot formation and stroke development with atrial fibrillation, and reducing coronary artery thrombosis in patients with atherosclerosis and cardiac stents [2,3]. The prevalence of warfarin use in the United States is unknown, but the Food and Drug Administration estimates that more than 31 million prescriptions for warfarin were written in 2004 [4]. A publication by Dossett et al. indicates that warfarin use is common among injured patients and its prevalence has increased each year since 2002 [5].

Numerous studies assessing the impact of antithrombotic (AT) agents on traumatic brain injury reveal conflicting results. Some investigations indicate that AT drugs are associated with increased brain-injury mortality [6–12], while others suggest that this is not the case [13–19]. Although certain studies demonstrate that AT medications increase intracranial hemorrhage (ICH) rates [6,7,10,12,15], others differ [8,19]. Also at odds are findings that AT agents are associated with increased ICH progression [16], while some studies observed contrary findings [19,20].

Recent meta-analyses objectively summarize the controversy that exists regarding the impact of AT-agents on traumatic brain injury (TBI) outcomes. The meta-analysis performed for ASA and the separate meta-analysis for clopidogrel demonstrated that the tests for data result heterogeneity were statistically significant and the overall mortality rates, with and without the respective AT-agent, were not statistically different [21]. A separate meta-analysis for warfarin also showed that the statistic for data results heterogeneity was significant [22]. A significant meta-analysis test for heterogeneity indicates that there was substantial variance among the studies, relative to AT-positive and AT-negative mortality rate differences. The significant test for heterogeneity in each of the 3 meta-analyses (ASA, clopidogrel, and warfarin) clearly demonstrates that the impact of these AT-agents on TBI mortality is controversial.

Several publications have included comments suggesting that preinjury cerebral atrophy predisposes to acute ICH [23–27]. The relevant statement in each publication had a referenced citation. However, a review of the referenced material failed to describe any objective evidence that preinjury cerebral atrophy engenders acute ICH.

Due to the controversial results in the literature regarding the impact of AT agents on brain-injury outcomes, the authors undertook a retrospective investigation of consecutive patients to further examine this issue. First, we hypothesized AT-positive patients would not have an increased hemorrhage rate, higher rate of hemorrhagic complications, or worse neurologic outcomes. Second, we hypothesized that admission neurological function would better predict brain injury outcomes, than would a history of AT agent use. Third, we conjectured that intracranial hemorrhage would correlate with the degree of preinjury brain atrophy.

## Materials and Methods

This study was approved by the Humility of Mary Health Partners Institutional Review Board for Human Investigations. The Institutional Review Board waived the need for written informed consent from the patients, due to the retrospective nature of the investigation. Inclusion criteria utilized: age ≥60 years, fall from standing height or motor vehicular crash, physical evidence for head trauma (facial fracture, skull fracture, scalp soft tissue injury, facial soft tissue injury, or cervical spine injury), and trauma center admission. An Abbreviated Injury Scale score (AIS) for each body region was determined by the trauma registrar after receiving input from radiographic reports, operative records, Advanced Practice Nurses, and attending trauma surgeons. Regional AIS values were stored in the trauma registry and a standardized process was used to compute Injury Severity Scores.

## Patient outcomes

Admission major neurologic dysfunction was defined as patients with Glasgow Coma Score 3–12 and/or the presence of speech aphasia or severe agitation. Patients who were prescribed ASA, clopidogrel, warfarin, or rivaroxaban preinjury were classified as AT-positive. Those who were not prescribed these agents were classified as AT-negative. ICH was determined to be absent or present and subcategorized as creating or not creating brain compression. ICH complications were the need for craniotomy or ICH progression. Neurologic complications were hospital death, transfer to hospice, or a decrease in discharge Glasgow Coma Score ≥ three points below the admission value.

The Glasgow Outcome Score (GOS) was determined at 3 months following trauma center discharge. The electronic medical record was reviewed for patient follow-up, which included re-hospitalization, clinic and office visits, and telephone conversations. The 3-month GOS was dichotomized into a good-outcome (moderate or minimal-to-no disability) or bad-outcome (death, vegetative state, or severe disability). When the data were insufficient to categorize a patient, the GOS category was considered unknown.

## Coagulation profile

Standard coagulation testing results included partial thromboplastin time, International Normalized Ratio (INR), and platelet count. Thromboelastography results included R-Time, K-Time, alpha-angle, maximum amplitude, and Coagulation Index. Thromboelastography platelet mapping included arachidonic acid and adenosine diphosphate percent inhibition. A coagulation intervention included the administration of platelets, desmopressin, plasma, and/or intravenous vitamin K. Policy dictated that a Trauma Service Advanced Practice Nurse must document, within 48 hours, the use of all preinjury AT agents for each patient admitted to the trauma center. Standard coagulation, thromboelastography, and platelet mapping tests were performed by the Central Laboratory Services.

## Preinjury brain atrophy

Brain CT reports were reviewed to determine how often the radiologist commented on the presence of brain atrophy. Axial views of the brain CT were reviewed to locate and measure the maximal transverse width of the left and right lateral ventricular bodies. A brain parenchymal width (right and left transverse distance from cortical surface to ipsilateral ventricular margin) was measured at the axial level of the maximal lateral ventricular body width. At the level of the maximal lateral ventricular body width, the cortical sulci were scored to assess cortical atrophy [28]. Cortical atrophy was considered insignificant with a score of 0 or 1 and was considered present with a score of 2 or 3.

## Statistical analysis

Data were entered into a Microsoft Excel 2010 spreadsheet and imported into a SAS System for Windows, release 9.2 (SAS Institute Inc., Cary, NC, USA), for statistical analyses. For continuous variable cohort data, standard deviation was used to complement the mean. Non-parametric analysis was used to compare continuous data results between two groups. Fischer's exact testing was used to assess the relationship of two dichotomous variables. Multivariate logistic regression analysis was performed to assess independent variable relationships with a dependent variable that was dichotomous.

## Results

### Patient traits

In this consecutive series, there were 198 patients with an age of 78.4±10 years. All patients had an admission brain CT scan and 71 of 72 with ICH had a repeat brain CT (one rapidly progressed to brain death). Patient injury traits are summarized in **Table 1** and preexisting medical conditions according to AT status are in **Table 2**.

**Table 1.** Patient Traits and Outcomes.

| | | Number | Percent |
|---|---|---|---|
| Number | | 198 | 100% |
| Admission Glasgow Coma Score 3-12 | | 15 | 7.6% |
| Admission Major Neurologic Dysfunction | | 19 | 9.6% |
| Fall from Standing Height | | 162 | 81.8% |
| Motor Vehicular Collision | | 36 | 18.2% |
| Antithrombotic-Negative | | 72 | 36.4% |
| Antithrombotic-Positive | | 126 | 63.6% |
| | ASA | 89 | 45.0% |
| | Clopidogrel | 18 | 9.1% |
| | ASA and/or Clopidogrel (no anticoagulant) | 76 | 38.4% |
| | Warfarin | 46 | 23.2% |
| | Rivaroxaban | 4 | 2.0% |
| Preinjury Brain Atrophy | | 98 | 49.5% |
| Intracranial Hemorrhage | | 72 | 36.4% |
| Intracranial Hemorrhage with Brain Compression | | 12 | 6.1% |
| Intracranial Hemorrhage Complication | | 8 | 4.0% |
| Neurologic Complication | | 13 | 6.6% |
| Intracranial Hemorrhage-Neurologic Complication | | 16 | 8.1% |

## Coagulation profile

Of the 198 patients, standard coagulation testing was partial thromboplastin time in 166 (83.8%), INR in 184 (92.9%), and platelet count in 187 (94.4%). Of the 72 AT-negative patients, 21 (29.2%) had thromboelastography and 14 (19.4%) platelet mapping. Of the 126 AT-positive patients, 97 (77.0%) had thromboelastography and 83 (65.9%) platelet mapping. The coagulation profile, according to AT status, is displayed in **Table 3**. ASA patients had a higher arachidonic acid percent inhibition and lower Coagulation Index, compared to the AT-negative group. Warfarin patients had higher INR and R-Time values and lower Coagulation Index, compared to the AT-negative group. Of the 126 patients in the AT-positive group, ASA and/or warfarin patients accounted for 121 (96.0%).

## Preinjury brain atrophy

The CT report included a statement that age-related changes were present in 170 (87.4%). Of the 12 with ICH mass effect,

seven had a brain CT within the prior 12 months and were scored. Scoring was not performed for the other five. Because one Glasgow Coma Score 15 patient had a normal brain CT at a referring facility, the scan was not archived and available for scoring. Thus, 192 of the 198 (97.0%) patients underwent CT grading to evaluate evidence of atrophy. Dimension results were: ventricular diameter $31.4 \pm 5.6$ mm; brain diameter $90.6 \pm 8.3$ mm; and cortical atrophy (sulcus score of 2 or 3) in 31.8%. Ventricular width was higher in patients with cortical atrophy ($34.1 \pm 4.7$ mm), when compared to no atrophy ($30.1 \pm 5.5$ mm; $p < 0.001$). Composite brain atrophy (cortical atrophy or ventricular width $> 30$ mm) was found in 51.0% (n = 98). Increasing age had an inverse correlation with brain width ($p < 0.001$) and positive associations with ventricular width ($p = 0.0465$) and ventricular width $\div$ brain width ($p = 0.0014$). Age was higher in patients with cortical atrophy ($83.0 \pm 8.2$ years), compared to no atrophy ($76.2 \pm 10.1$ years; $p < 0.001$).

**Table 2.** Pre-existing Medical Conditions by Antithrombotic Status.

| Condition | Antithrombotic (−) | Antithrombotic (+) | P-value |
|---|---|---|---|
| Cerebrovascular Accident | 4.3% | 6.5% | 0.5227 |
| Cardiac Disease | 20.0% | 58.5% | <0.001 |
| Diabetes Mellitus | 24.3% | 34.2% | 0.1528 |
| Dementia | 22.9% | 19.5% | 0.5815 |
| Hypertension | 64.3% | 79.7% | 0.0190 |
| Psychiatric Disorder | 15.7% | 13.8% | 0.7196 |
| Pulmonary Disease | 12.9% | 17.9% | 0.3603 |
| Smoker (Active) | 15.7% | 4.1% | 0.0048 |

**Table 3.** Coagulation Profile According to Pre-Injury Antithrombotic Status.

| | AT (−) | Aspirin | Clopidogrel | Warfarin | Rivaroxaban |
|---|---|---|---|---|---|
| Number | 72 | 89 | 18 | 46 | 4 |
| International Normalized Ratio | 1.2±0.2 | 1.4±0.8 | 1.3±0.7 | 2.8±0.9** | 1.5±0.6 |
| Partial Thromboplastin Time | 29±5 | 31±7 | 28±7 | 38±8** | 29±6 |
| Platelet Count | 211±64 | 215±75 | 215±64 | 199±60 | 215±71 |
| R-Time | 4.1±1.3 | 5.5±2.1 | 4.8±1.3 | 6.4±2.2** | 3.8±1.8 |
| K-Time | 1.2±0.4 | 1.4±0.6 | 1.3±0.3 | 1.5±0.5 | 1.1±0.4 |
| Alpha Angle | 72±5 | 69±9 | 71±4 | 69±7 | 64±22 |
| Maximum Amplitude | 65±6 | 67±5 | 66±5 | 67±4 | 65±9 |
| Coagulation Index | 2.6±1.6 | 1.5±2.4** | 2.2±1.3 | 1.0±2.2** | 2.1±3.4 |
| Arachidonic Acid % inhibition | 41±42 | 62±31** | 52±37 | 35±39 | 29±50 |
| Adenosine Diphosphate % inhibition | 44±23 | 48±33 | 49±30 | 40±26 | 50±27 |

AT (−), Antithrombotic-negative;
**: P<0.05, compared to Antithrombotic-negative group

## Intracranial hemorrhage correlations

The ICH rates, according to each head trauma risk condition, were cervical spine injury 12.5% (3/24), facial fracture 21.6% (8/37), skull fracture 31.6% (6/19), facial soft tissue injury 43.5% (10/23), and scalp soft tissue injury 35.6% (53/149). The frequency of each head trauma ICH risk condition, by AT-negative and AT-positive grouping, is depicted in **Table 4**; risk conditions for the two groups are clinically and statistically similar.

Of the 198 patients, ICH was present in 72 (36.4%) and caused major brain compression in 12 (6.1%). The ICH rate was higher with cortical atrophy (60.7%), compared to no atrophy (22.9%; p<0.001; OR = 5.2). Ventricular width was higher with ICH (33.7±5.4), compared to no ICH (30.1±5.3; p<0.001). Ventricular width ÷ brain width was higher with ICH (37.7±7.1%), when compared to no ICH (33.5±6.9%; p<0.001). ICH rate was higher with ventricular width>30 mm (57.0%), versus width ≤ 30 mm (19.5%; p<0.001; OR = 5.5). The ICH rate was higher with composite brain atrophy (54.1%), compared to no brain atrophy (14.9%; p<0.001; OR = 6.7).

The AT-positive ICH rate (38.9% [49/126]; [ASA - 42.7%; clopidogrel - 50.0%; warfarin or rivaroxaban - 28.0%]) was similar to the AT-negative ICH rate (31.9% [23/72]; p = 0.3285; Lambda proportional reduction in error = 0.000). ICH was similar for warfarin-positive (28.3% [13/46]) and AT negative (31.9% [23/72]; p = 0.8378; lambda proportional reduction in error = 0.0000) patients. ICH is insignificantly higher for platelet inhibitor-positive (46.1% [35/76]), compared to AT negative (31.9% [23/72]; p = 0.0932; lambda proportional reduction in error = 0.1111) patients. Relative to the ICH that created brain deformation, the AT-positive rate (7.1%) was similar to the AT-negative rate (4.2%; p = 0.5415). The ISS and highest regional AIS values, according to AT-positive and AT-negative status, are displayed in **Table 5**. The Injury Severity Scores and AIS values for the AT-positive and AT-negative patients were not statistically different. Head AIS scores for ICH-positive patients were similar according to AT-negative (3.6±0.8) and AT-positive (3.4±1.1; p = 0.4265) status.

Standard coagulation, thromboelastography, and platelet mapping results demonstrated no coagulopathy in ICH-positive patients and were similar to the ICH -negative patients (**Table 6**). Of the 89 patients receiving preinjury ASA, the ICH-negative arachidonic acid percent inhibition (62±31) and Coagulation Index (1.9±1.8) (n = 51) were similar to the ICH-positive arachidonic acid percent inhibition (62±32) and Coagulation Index (1.2±3.0) (n = 38) (p≥0.2657). For the 18 patients receiving preinjury clopidogrel, the ICH-negative adenosine diphosphate percent inhibition (49±34) and Coagulation Index (2.6±1.2) (n = 9) were similar to the ICH-positive adenosine diphosphate percent inhibition (49±26) and Coagulation Index (1.6±0.4) (n = 9) (p≥0.1043). In the 46 patients receiving preinjury warfarin, the ICH-negative INR (2.8±1.0), R-Time (6.1±2.2), and K-Time (1.5±0.6) (n = 33) were similar to the ICH-positive INR (2.8±0.5), R-Time (7.1±2.1), and K-Time (1.5±0.3) (n = 13) (p≥0.2829).

**Table 4.** Head Trauma ICH Risk Conditions by Antithrombotic Status.

| | AT-negative | AT-positive | P-value |
|---|---|---|---|
| Number | 72 | 126 | |
| Cervical spine injury | 11 (15.3%) | 13 (10.3%) | 0.3663 |
| Facial fracture | 17 (23.6%) | 20 (15.9%) | 0.1895 |
| Skull fracture | 10 (13.9%) | 9 (7.1%) | 0.1371 |
| Facial soft tissue injury | 9 (12.5%) | 14 (11.1%) | 0.8193 |
| Scalp soft tissue injury | 54 (75.0%) | 95 (75.4%) | 0.9504 |

ICH, intracranial hemorrhage; AT, antithrombotic.

**Table 5.** Injury Severity Score and AIS Values by Antithrombotic Status.

| | AT-negative | AT-positive | P-value |
|---|---|---|---|
| **Number** | 72 | 126 | |
| **Injury Severity Score** | 11.9±7.6 | 10.6±7.5 | 0.2391 |
| **Head AIS** | 1.9±1.6 | 1.9±1.6 | 0.9452 |
| Head AIS ≥3 | 27 (37.5%) | 41 (32.5%) | 0.5347 |
| **Chest AIS ≥1** | 10 (13.9%) | 19 (15.1%) | 0.8197 |
| Abdominal-pelvis AIS ≥1 | 1 (1.4%) | 5 (4.0%) | 0.4196 |
| **Extremity-pelvic AIS ≥1** | 17 (23.6%) | 31 (24.6%) | 0.8755 |

AIS, Abbreviated Injury Scale score; AT, antithrombotic.

Composite brain atrophy was more common for AT-positive (56.9% [70/123]) compared to AT negative (40.6% [28/69]; p = 0.0355) patients. Brain atrophy occurrence was 56.8% for platelet inhibitor-positive patients and 55.6% for warfarin-positive patients. Multivariate analysis showed that ICH correlated with composite brain atrophy (p<0.0001), but not AT agent status (p = 0.9293) (n = 192 AT-positive or AT-negative patients). ICH correlated with composite brain atrophy (p<0.0001), but not platelet inhibitor agent status (p = 0.3205) (n = 143 AT-negative or platelet inhibitor-positive patients). ICH correlated with composite brain atrophy (p<0.0001), but not warfarin status (p = 0.2733) (n = 114 AT-negative or warfarin-positive patients). ICH had an independent association with composite brain atrophy (p<0.001) and admission major neurologic dysfunction (p<0.001), but not AT status (p = 0.9774) or age (p = 0.8566).

## Admission neurologic function and complication correlations

Admission major neurologic dysfunction rates were comparable for the AT-negative (8.3%) and AT-positive (10.3%; p = 0.6484) patients. The admission major neurologic dysfunction rate was greater for ICH-positive patients (20.8%) versus ICH-negative patients (3.2%; OR = 8.0; p<0.001). Of the 198 patients, 16 (8.1%) had an ICH-neurologic complication. Of those 16, 12 (75.0%) died or were transferred to hospice, with an age of 79.1±9.4 (65–95). ICH expansion occurred or a craniotomy was

needed in 3 of the 4 survivors. The other survivor was GCS 15 on admission and GCS 12 at hospital discharge.

The ICH-neurologic complication rate was similar for AT-positive patients (8.7% [11/126]) and AT-negative patients (6.9% [5/72]; p = 0.6574). The ICH-neurologic complication rate was similar for platelet inhibitor-positive (7.9% [6/76]) and AT-negative (6.9% [5/72] p = 0.6574) patients (total n = 148). The ICH-neurologic complication rate was similar for warfarin-positive (10.9% [5/46]) and AT-negative (6.9% [5/72] p = 0.5089) patients (total n = 118).

The ICH-neurologic complication rate was substantially increased when admission major neurologic dysfunction was present (63.2% [12/19]), compared to absent (2.2% [4/179]; RR = 28.3; p<0.001). The ICH-neurologic complication rate was substantially increased when ICH was present (19.4% [14/72]), compared to absent (1.6% [2/126]; RR = 12.3; p<0.001). Multivariate logistic regression analysis indicated that ICH-neurologic complications were independently associated with admission major neurologic dysfunction (p<0.001) and ICH (p = 0.0218), but not AT status (p = 0.8953). ICH-neurologic complications were independently associated with admission major neurologic dysfunction (p<0.001) and ICH (p = 0.0202), but not with platelet inhibitor-status (p = 0.7055). ICH-neurologic complications were independently associated with admission major neurologic dysfunction (p<0.001) and ICH (p = 0.0209), but not with warfarin-status (p = 0.7219). In the 72 patients with

**Table 6.** Coagulation Profile According to Intracranial Hemorrhage Status.

| | Hemorrhage (−) | Hemorrhage (+) | P-Value |
|---|---|---|---|
| **Number** | 126 | 72 | — |
| **International Normalized Ratio** | 1.6±0.9 | 1.4±0.7 | 0.1354 |
| **Partial Thromboplastin Time** | 31±6 | 32±9 | 0.5472 |
| **Platelet count** | 207±61 | 213±79 | 0.5657 |
| **R-Time** | 5.2±1.9 | 5.6±2.3 | 0.3840 |
| **K-Time** | 1.3±0.4 | 1.5±0.7 | 0.2310 |
| **Alpha-Angle** | 70±8 | 70±8 | 0.9950 |
| **Maximum Amplitude** | 67±4 | 66±7 | 0.3759 |
| **Coagulation Index** | 1.8±2.0 | 1.4±2.7 | 0.3884 |
| **Arachidonic Acid % inhibition** | 46±38 | 49±37 | 0.7090 |
| **Adenosine Diphosphate % inhibition** | 44±31 | 48±32 | 0.5047 |

(−), negative; (+), positive.

ICH, the ICH-neurologic complication rate was similar for the AT-negative (17.4% [4/23]) and AT-positive (20.4% [10/49]; p = 1.0) groups.

Of the 186 patients discharge alive from the trauma center, only one patient was unable to be adequately categorized according to the GOS classification. Of the 185 patients, a 3-month bad-outcome occurred in 18.9% (35/185) and a good-outcome in 81.1% (150/185). The 3-month bad-outcome rate was similar for the AT-negative (20.9% [14/67]) and AT-positive (17.8% [21/118]; p = 0.6050) patients. Univariate analysis showed that 3-month bad-outcome had a positive association with Injury Severity Score (p = 0.0130) and number of preinjury medical conditions (p = 0.0047) and an inverse association with admission GCS (p<0.0001). Multivariate analysis demonstrated that bad-outcome was independently associated with number of preinjury medical conditions (p = 0.0159) and admission GCS (p = 0.0088). Another analysis showed that bad-outcome was independently associated with number of preinjury medical conditions (p = 0.0098) and Injury Severity Score (p = 0.0632).

A summary of outcomes and their relationships with AT status and admission major neurologic dysfunction status is displayed in **Table 7**. The table demonstrates that admission major neurologic dysfunction status correlated with ICH, head AIS, ICH-neurologic complications, and GOS outcome. The table also indicates that AT status had no association with admission major neurologic dysfunction, ICH, head AIS, ICH-neurologic complications, or GOS outcome.

## Coagulation interventions

Coagulation interventions occurred in 28/198 (14.1%) select ICH-positive patients, who were AT-positive. Of the ICH-positive warfarin patients receiving coagulation intervention, all 13 received plasma transfusion and 12 Vitamin K. The mean time from initial therapeutic INR until the INR decreased to <2.0 was 10.6 hours. In ICH-positive patients receiving desmopressin and/or platelet transfusion, 16/18 had preinjury ASA and 3/18 had preinjury clopidogrel. The admission major neurologic dysfunction rate was greater in the 28 patients undergoing coagulation intervention (28.6%), compared to 170 without intervention (6.5%; p<0.001). Using multivariate logistic regression analysis, ICH-neurologic complication was independently associated with admission major neurologic dysfunction (p<0.001) and ICH (p = 0.0216), but not with AT-positive status (p = 0.9966) or coagulation intervention (p = 0.4160).

## Discussion

### Intracranial hemorrhage and antithrombotic agents

The current study focused on patients with documented signs of external head trauma or acute cervical spine injury to demonstrate that trauma to the craniofacial region existed, thus creating a risk for ICH. The similarity of the head trauma risk conditions for the AT-negative and AT-positive patients indicates that patient risk for developing an ICH is comparable. The coagulation studies demonstrate that most AT-positive patients had an objective measurable effect and therefore were taking their medications. The AT-positive and AT-negative ICH rates were similar, suggesting AT agents do not impede effective hemostasis. Further, there was no statistically significant variation according to the specific AT agent. The Injury Severity Score and AIS values indicate that the AT-positive and AT-negative patients had similar intracranial and extra-cranial injuries. Because head AIS values largely reflect the presence and magnitude of ICH, the similarity of these values for the AT-positive and AT-negative patients supports the comparable ICH rates, as determined by the investigator's review of each patient's brain CT. The similarity of AT-negative and AT-positive head AIS values in patients with ICH further demonstrates that AT agents are not associated with adverse TBI outcomes. Another study of elderly patients, sustaining an acute fall, has also demonstrated that there was no increased ICH rate with either warfarin, ASA, or clopidogrel [26].

The similarity of standard coagulation test, thromboelastography, and platelet mapping results for ICH-negative and ICH-positive patients indicates that a mechanism other than altered hemostasis is responsible for developing ICH. In addition, the relevant coagulation test results within each of the ASA, clopidogrel, and warfarin groups were comparable for ICH-negative and ICH-positive cohorts. Other investigators have found similar warfarin-associated ICH rates of 23.2% [29] and 26.6% [11] with external head trauma.

### Intracranial hemorrhage and preinjury brain atrophy

The current study demonstrates that preinjury composite brain atrophy is associated with the occurrence of acute post-traumatic brain injury. The higher atrophy rate in the platelet inhibitor-positive patients is likely to have contributed to its insignificantly higher ICH rate, when compared to AT-negative patients. This is strongly suggested by the multivariate analysis that showed ICH was associated with preinjury composite atrophy, but clearly not related to platelet inhibitor status. The other multivariate analyses

**Table 7.** Outcomes According to Antithrombotic and Admission Major Neurologic Dysfunction Status.

|  | AT (−) | AT (+) | P-value | AMND (−) | AMND (+) | P-value |
|---|---|---|---|---|---|---|
| **Number** | 72 | 126 | — | 179 | 19 | — |
| **AMND** | 8.3% | 10.3% | 0.6484 | — | — | — |
| **ICH** | 31.9% | 38.9% | 0.3285 | 31.8% | 79.0% | <0.001 |
| **Head AIS** | 1.9±1.6 | 1.9±1.6 | 0.9509 | 1.7±1.5 | 3.6±1.3 | <0.001 |
| **ICH Complication** | 1.4% | 5.6% | 0.2623 | 0.0% | 42.1% | <0.001 |
| **Neurologic Complication** | 6.9% | 6.4% | 0.8708 | 2.2% | 47.4% | <0.001 |
| **ICH-Neurologic Complication** | 6.9% | 8.7% | 0.6574 | 2.2% | 63.2% | <0.001 |
| **Bad 3-Month Outcome** | 20.9% | 17.8% | 0.6050 | 16.5% | 66.7% | 0.0017 |

AT, antithrombotic; (−), negative; (+), positive; AMND, Admission Major Neurologic Dysfunction; ICH, intracranial hemorrhage; AIS, Abbreviated Injury Scale score.

also compellingly indicate that ICH correlates with brain atrophy, but not with AT agent status.

As age progressed, brain parenchyma width decreased and ventricular width, ventricular-to-brain parenchymal width, and cortical atrophy increased. At least six investigations of non-demented patients indicate that with advancing age, ventricular or intracranial CSF volume increases [30–34] and brain volume decreases [30–32,34,35]. A recent investigation used axial CT images and found that lateral ventricular volume-to-total brain volume markedly increased with aging [33]. Because multiple atrophy estimates in the current study correlate with age, this supports validity of the CT scoring. Also, the correlation of cortical atrophy with lateral ventricular width further enhances internal validity of the scoring methodology. Matsumae et al. concluded that "expansion of CSF volume with age provides a good index of brain shrinkage" [35]. ICH correlated with increased lateral ventricular body width, cortical sulcus atrophy, and composite brain atrophy. These new findings indicate that preinjury brain atrophy is a factor influencing the development of ICH, following head trauma.

Apropos to the current study, we found an interesting study by Ronty et al. that describes the use of linear CT measurements, that were related to brain atrophy [36]. These measures included linear assessment of the lateral ventricles, brain mass width, and cortical sulci. The study demonstrated that as brain atrophy volume increased, there were concomitant changes in these linear dimensions.

As stated earlier, speculation exists that preinjury cerebral atrophy fosters the development of acute post-traumatic ICH; however, we have been unable to find credible evidence to support this notion. The citation in one publication [27] referenced a textbook by Jennett and Teasdale [37]. Jennett and Teasdale, two prolific and revered neurosurgical investigators in TBI, provided no objective evidence to support their statement. In essence, the relationship between cerebral atrophy and intracranial hemorrhage, heretofore, is derived from expert opinion. Although traumatic ICH and acute CT findings increase with age [23,38], as does cerebral atrophy, a direct association between preinjury atrophy and acute ICH has not been established. The current study is the first to objectively document that acute post-traumatic ICH is associated with preinjury cerebral atrophy.

## ICH-Neurologic complications and 3-month outcomes

Admission major neurologic dysfunction rates were similar for the AT-negative and AT-positive patients. A study of trauma patients by Mina et al. also found that warfarin did not decrease neurologic-function in patients with ICH [11]. These observations provide additional evidence that AT agents do not impact brain-injury. An ICH-neurologic complication was likely to be found in patients with major neurologic dysfunction on admission or with the presence of ICH. Importantly, none of the three conditions had an association with the preinjury use of AT agents. Other investigators have also demonstrated that AT agents are not associated with ICH progression [19,20]. These findings mitigate the notion that AT agents substantially attenuate hemostatic function.

Accordingly, it is imperative to determine discriminate clinical findings that more focally portend the subset that will develop major complications. Apropos, the ICH-neurologic complication rate was substantially greater with admission major neurologic dysfunction, when compared to its absence. Multivariate logistic regression analysis provides evidence that admission neurologic status and ICH, but not AT use, forecasts the probability of developing an ICH-neurologic complication. Other investigators

have also found that mortality is not increased for brain-injury patients receiving preinjury AT agents [13–17]. Ivascu et al. also demonstrated that presenting neurologic-function was predictive of death in trauma patients with ICH and receiving ASA and/or clopidogrel [39]. Peck et al., in a study assessing the influence of AT agents on ICH outcomes, showed that admission neurologic-function had the most statistically significant association with mortality [16]. The investigation by Gaetani et al. also demonstrated that presence of ICH increased mortality in a study of AT agents and brain-injury [9].

A warfarin TBI study by Wojcik et al. [17], included in a recent meta-analysis [22], is of particular interest. It is one of the better quality studies in that 416 TBI warfarin patients were compared to 416 case-controlled, non-warfarin patients. Age, ISS, and admission GCS were virtually identical for the 2 groups, as was mortality, ICU LOS, and hospital LOS (p≥0.70). In concert with our study findings are the two recent meta-analyses indicating that ASA and clopidogrel do not increase TBI mortality [21].

The 3-month GOS scores indicated that AT-negative and AT-positive patients had similar outcomes. It seems reasonable that post-discharge functional outcomes might be affected by preinjury medical conditions and/or severity of acquired traumatic conditions. This is suggested by the associations of post-discharge outcomes with the Injury Severity Score, admission GCS, and number of preinjury medical conditions. Together, the data results indicate that the preinjury use of AT-agents do not alter outcomes in patients who have sustained traumatic injury to the head. Further, these findings are in-concert with the study observations that post-traumatic ICH rates and acute, hospital outcomes were not worse in AT-positive patients.

## Coagulation interventions

Coagulation interventions occurred in select ICH-positive and AT-positive patients, who tended to have admission major neurologic dysfunction. Multivariate logistic regression analysis indicated that adverse outcomes occurred with admission major neurologic dysfunction and ICH, but not with coagulation interventions. Other studies have also documented that coagulation interventions did not alter outcomes [39,40].

It seems reasonable that any AT-positive patient with external signs of head trauma should undergo prompt brain CT scanning and coagulation function testing. For a patient with ICH and no major neurologic dysfunction, it appears sensible to closely monitor the patient and initially only treat with a supratherapeutic coagulopathy. When an AT-positive patient with ICH has admission major neurologic dysfunction, there is uncertainty as to whether a coagulation intervention will mitigate subsequent adverse outcomes; although coagulation intervention would seem to be reasonable. It is important to recognize that acute or sub-acute AT age withdrawal, with or without reversal, can lead to adverse thrombotic events [41,42].

## Evidence hemostasis is effective with antithrombotic therapy

Multiple non-trauma-related investigations demonstrate that ASA and warfarin do not routinely mitigate effective hemostasis. In particular, substantial literature evidence exists to indicate that ASA is not associated with major bleeding complications for surgery [43–48] and other invasive procedures [45,49]. The literature also demonstrates that warfarin does not routinely create increased bleeding with operative procedures [50–53] and other invasive interventions [49,54–56]. These findings suggest that ASA and warfarin do not usually attenuate clinically-relevant functional hemostasis following tissue injury.

## Study Quality

Although the study is retrospective, the following evidence indicates that common study weaknesses have been mitigated. Virtually all the relevant data is available for all patients and the quality is typically reliable; however, results for a few variables were not accessible for a minority of patients. Much of the data results emanate from the trauma registry, where information is obtained from the Trauma History and Physical form, the Trauma Tertiary Survey form, the trauma service Advanced Practice Nurses' daily work-sheet documentation, operative records, radiography reports, and discharge summaries. The Trauma History and Physical form is a comprehensive database completed at the time of patient admission by the trauma resident and verified by the attending trauma surgeon. At 24 hours following admission, a comprehensive Trauma Tertiary Survey form is completed by a trauma service resident and confirmed by the attending trauma surgeon. Each day, an Advanced Practice Nurse updated a work-sheet that captures initial injuries, all preinjury medications, including AT agents, injuries with a delay in diagnosis, and complications. Further, the Advanced Practice Nurses met weekly with the surgical attending staff to discuss patient deaths and all complications. This provides an opportunity to clarify ongoing patient conditions and outcomes in the nurses' daily work-sheet. Accordingly, mechanism of injury, admission and discharge GCS, preinjury AT agent use, preinjury medical conditions, patient injuries, and complications are prospectively documented and subsequently stored in the trauma registry. From injury data, trauma registry personnel compute Abbreviated Injury Scale and Injury Severity Score values. On multiple occasions, American College of Surgeons' Trauma Quality Improvement Program personnel have assessed trauma registry data and found it to be accurate and reliable, with compliance at all levels. Further, the State of Ohio Department of Public Safety has also appraised the trauma registry data and found it to be reliable. ICH status, ICH progression, and preinjury atrophy measurements were made by the first-author after reviewing CT scans for the 198 study patients. As an attending trauma surgeon with board certification in surgical critical care and an extensive history of collaboration with neurosurgeons and neuroradiologists, the first-author has interpreted brain CT images for 30 years. The presence of slurred speech and severe agitation in admission GCS 13–15 patients was made by the first-author after interrogating the Trauma History and Physical form, the neurosurgical consultation note, and nursing notes. The Trauma Service has long-standing and comprehensive policies regarding assessment and management of ASA, clopidogrel, and warfarin patients with signs of external head trauma or altered neurologic function. These policies, in large part, dictated coagulation testing and considerations for coagulation interventions.

We believe that information bias, improper classification of AT-exposure or outcomes, is minimal, because the data quality is creditable. The 3-month GOS designation was assigned following an extensive review of the electronic medical record, where virtually all patients could be readily classified into a bad-outcome or good-outcome category. We also think that selection bias has been minimized by using the trauma registry to identify all patients who were age ≥60 and with signs of external head trauma or cervical spine injury. Minimal selection bias is supported by finding a similarity in the AT-negative and AT-positive patient Injury Severity Score, ICH-risk condition rates, extra-cranial injury severity, and admission major neurologic dysfunction rates.

## Conclusions

The similarity of AT-negative and AT-positive group major admission neurologic dysfunction rates, ICH rates, head AIS scores, hospital complication rates, and 3-month neurologic function rates indicate that AT-agents do not adversely affect brain injury outcomes in patients with signs of external head trauma. Current study outcomes and coagulation test results and the procedural intervention literature suggest that AT agents do not routinely impede effective post-injury hemostasis. It is likely that our study findings will stimulate trauma services to review, and potentially refine, policies regarding management of AT-positive patients with head trauma. Clearly, admission neurologic function is useful for forecasting adverse outcomes in patients with external head trauma, whether or not they receive a preinjury AT agent. For AT-positive patients with ICH, but without major neurologic dysfunction, we recommend close patient monitoring and coagulation interventions for those with supratherapeutic coagulopathy. When an AT-positive patient with ICH has admission major neurologic dysfunction, coagulation intervention seems reasonable; however, there is uncertainty as to whether this course of action will mitigate subsequent adverse outcomes. Considering the substantial activity in developing AT-drug reversal agents, it is imperative that criteria be created to stipulate which patients are likely to benefit from such interventions. The correlation of ICH with atrophy is the first objective evidence that acute post-traumatic ICH is associated with preinjury cerebral atrophy. It seems reasonable that radiologists should begin to assess the magnitude of brain atrophy in patients with an age ≥60 years. If the lateral ventricular body width is >30 mm and/or the cortical sulci score is 2 or 3, the radiologist should indicate that significant brain atrophy is likely present. Accordingly, the treating physician should assess the patient using one of the standard fall-risk assessment tools. If the risk for falling is substantial, the healthcare provider should institute appropriate measures that mitigate the risk of falling.

## Acknowledgments

The authors want to thank Barbara M. Hileman and Marina Hanes for copy editing the manuscript.

## Author Contributions

Conceived and designed the experiments: CMD DAH GSH RM. Performed the experiments: CMD RM. Analyzed the data: CMD DAH GSH LAO DJG RM. Contributed reagents/materials/analysis tools: CMD. Wrote the paper: CMD DAH GSH LAO DJG RM.

## References

1. Richmond R, Aldaghlas TA, Burke C, Rizzo AG, Griffen M, et al. (2011) Age: is it all in the head? Factors influencing mortality in elderly patients with head injuries. J Trauma 71: E8–E11.

2. Yelon JA (2013) The geriatric patient. In: Mattox, Moore, Feliciano, editors. Trauma, Seventh Edition: McGraw Hill. pp. 874–885.

3. Furie KL, Goldstein LB, Albers GW, Khatri P, Neyens R, et al. (2012) Oral antithrombotic agents for the prevention of stroke in nonvalvular atrial fibrillation: a science advisory for healthcare professionals from the American Heart Association/American Stroke Association. Stroke 43: 3442–3453.

4. Wysowski DK, Nourjah P, Swartz L (2007) Bleeding complications with warfarin use: a prevalent adverse effect resulting in regulatory action. Arch Intern Med 167: 1414–1419.

5. Dossett LA, Riesel JN, Griffin MR, Cotton BA (2011) Prevalence and implications of preinjury warfarin use: an analysis of the National Trauma Databank. Arch Surg 146: 565–570.

6. Bonville DJ, Ata A, Jahraus CB, Arnold-Lloyd T, Salem L, et al. (2011) Impact of preinjury warfarin and antiplatelet agents on outcomes of trauma patients. Surgery 150: 861–868.

7.  Franko J, Kish KJ, O'Connell BG, Subramanian S, Yuschak JV (2006) Advanced age and preinjury warfarin anticoagulation increase the risk of mortality after head trauma. J Trauma 61: 107–110.

8.  Gage BF, Birman-Deych E, Kerzner R, Radford MJ, Nilasena DS, et al. (2005) Incidence of intracranial hemorrhage in patients with atrial fibrillation who are prone to fall. Am J Med 118: 612–617.

9.  Gaetani P, Revay M, Sciacca S, Pessina F, Aimar E, et al. (2012) Traumatic brain injury in the elderly: considerations in a series of 103 patients older than 70. J Neurosurg Sci 56: 231–237.

10. Moore MM, Pasquale MD, Badellino M (2012) Impact of age and anticoagulation: need for neurosurgical intervention in trauma patients with mild traumatic brain injury. J Trauma Acute Care Surg 73: 126–130.

11. Mina AA, Bair HA, Howells GA, Bendick PJ (2003) Complications of preinjury warfarin use in the trauma patient. J Trauma 54: 842–847.

12. Pieracci FM, Eachempati SR, Shou J, Hydo LJ, Barie PS (2007) Degree of anticoagulation, but not warfarin use itself, predicts adverse outcomes after traumatic brain injury in elderly trauma patients. J Trauma 63: 525–530.

13. Ahmed N, Bialowas C, Kuo YH, Zawodniak L (2009) Impact of preinjury anticoagulation in patients with traumatic brain injury. South Med J 102: 476–480.

14. Fortuna GR, Mueller EW, James LE, Shutter LA, Butler KL (2008) The impact of preinjury antiplatelet and anticoagulant pharmacotherapy on outcomes in elderly patients with hemorrhagic brain injury. Surgery 144: 598–603; discussion 603–595.

15. Jones K, Sharp C, Mangram AJ, Dunn EL (2006) The effects of preinjury clopidogrel use on older trauma patients with head injuries. Am J Surg 192: 743–745.

16. Peck KA, Calvo RY, Schechter MS, Sise CB, Kahl JE, et al. (2014) The impact of preinjury anticoagulants and prescription antiplatelet agents on outcomes in older patients with traumatic brain injury. J Trauma Acute Care Surg 76: 431–436.

17. Wojcik R, Cipolle MD, Seislove E, Wasser TE, Pasquale MD (2001) Preinjury warfarin does not impact outcome in trauma patients. J Trauma 51: 1147–1151; discussion 1151–1142.

18. Ott MM, Eriksson E, Vanderkolk W, Christianson D, Davis A, et al. (2010) Antiplatelet and anticoagulation therapies do not increase mortality in the absence of traumatic brain injury. J Trauma 68: 560–563.

19. Spektor S, Agus S, Merkin V, Constantini S (2003) Low-dose aspirin prophylaxis and risk of intracranial hemorrhage in patients older than 60 years of age with mild or moderate head injury: a prospective study. J Neurosurg 99: 661–665.

20. Velmahos GC, Gervasini A, Petrovick L, Dorer DJ, Doran ME, et al. (2006) Routine repeat head CT for minimal head injury is unnecessary. J Trauma 60: 494–499; discussion 499–501.

21. Batchelor JS, Grayson A (2013) A meta-analysis to determine the effect of preinjury antiplatelet agents on mortality in patients with blunt head trauma. Br J Neurosurg 27: 12–18.

22. Batchelor JS, Grayson A (2012) A meta-analysis to determine the effect of anticoagulation on mortality in patients with blunt head trauma. Br J Neurosurg 26: 525–530.

23. Holmes JF, Hendey GW, Oman JA, Norton VC, Lazarenko G, et al. (2006) Epidemiology of blunt head injury victims undergoing ED cranial computed tomographic scanning. Am J Emerg Med 24: 167–173.

24. Ellis GL (1990) Subdural hematoma in the elderly. Emerg Med Clin North Am 8: 281–294.

25. Hanif S, Abodunde O, Ali Z, Pidgeon C (2009) Age related outcome in acute subdural haematoma following traumatic head injury. Ir Med J 102: 255–257.

26. Gangavati AS, Kiely DK, Kulchycki LK, Wolfe RE, Mottley JL, et al. (2009) Prevalence and characteristics of traumatic intracranial hemorrhage in elderly fallers presenting to the emergency department without focal findings. J Am Geriatr Soc 57: 1470–1474.

27. Doherty DL (1988) Posttraumatic cerebral atrophy as a risk factor for delayed acute subdural hemorrhage. Arch Phys Med Rehabil 69: 542–544.

28. Pasquier F, Leys D, Weerts JG, Mounier-Vehier F, Barkhof F, et al. (1996) Inter- and intraobserver reproducibility of cerebral atrophy assessment on MRI scans with hemispheric infarcts. Eur Neurol 36: 268–272.

29. Ivascu FA, Howells GA, Junn FS, Bair HA, Bendick PJ, et al. (2005) Rapid warfarin reversal in anticoagulated patients with traumatic intracranial hemorrhage reduces hemorrhage progression and mortality. J Trauma 59: 1131–1137; discussion 1137–1139.

30. Gur RC, Mozley PD, Resnick SM, Gottlieb GL, Kohn M, et al. (1991) Gender differences in age effect on brain atrophy measured by magnetic resonance imaging. Proc Natl Acad Sci U S A 88: 2845–2849.

31. Pfefferbaum A, Mathalon DH, Sullivan EV, Rawles JM, Zipursky RB, et al. (1994) A quantitative magnetic resonance imaging study of changes in brain morphology from infancy to late adulthood. Arch Neurol 51: 874–887.

32. Resnick SM, Pham DL, Kraut MA, Zonderman AB, Davatzikos C (2003) Longitudinal magnetic resonance imaging studies of older adults: a shrinking brain. J Neurosci 23: 3295–3301.

33. Akdogan I, Kiroglu Y, Onur S, Karabuluti N (2010) The volume fraction of brain ventricles to total brain volume: a computed tomography stereological study. Folia Morphol (Warsz) 69: 193–200.

34. Fjell AM, McEvoy L, Holland D, Dale AM, Walhovd KB (2013) Brain changes in older adults at very low risk for Alzheimer's disease. J Neurosci 33: 8237–8242.

35. Matsumae M, Kikinis R, Morocz IA, Lorenzo AV, Sandor T, et al. (1996) Age-related changes in intracranial compartment volumes in normal adults assessed by magnetic resonance imaging. J Neurosurg 84: 982–991.

36. Ronty H, Ahonen A, Tolonen U, Heikkila J, Niemela O (1993) Cerebral trauma and alcohol abuse. Eur J Clin Invest 23: 182–187.

37. Jennett B, Teasdale G (1981) Intracranial hematoma. In: Jennet B, Teasdale G, editors. Management in head injuries. Philadelphia: F A Davis Company. p. 184.

38. Poyry T, Luoto TM, Kataja A, Brander A, Tenovuo O, et al. (2013) Acute assessment of brain injuries in ground-level falls. J Head Trauma Rehabil 28: 89–97.

39. Ivascu FA, Howells GA, Junn FS, Bair HA, Bendick PJ, et al. (2008) Predictors of mortality in trauma patients with intracranial hemorrhage on preinjury aspirin or clopidogrel. J Trauma 65: 785–788.

40. Downey DM, Monson B, Butler KL, Fortuna GR, Jr., Saxe JM, et al. (2009) Does platelet administration affect mortality in elderly head-injured patients taking antiplatelet medications? Am Surg 75: 1100–1103.

41. Ortel TL (2012) Perioperative management of patients on chronic antithrombotic therapy. Blood 120: 4699–4705.

42. Manchikanti L, Falco FJ, Benyamin RM, Caraway DL, Kaye AD, et al. (2013) Assessment of bleeding risk of interventional techniques: a best evidence synthesis of practice patterns and perioperative management of anticoagulant and antithrombotic therapy. Pain Physician 16: SE261–318.

43. Alghamdi AA, Moussa F, Fremes SE (2007) Does the use of preoperative aspirin increase the risk of bleeding in patients undergoing coronary artery bypass grafting surgery? Systematic review and meta-analysis. J Card Surg 22: 247–256.

44. Sun JC, Whitlock R, Cheng J, Eikelboom JW, Thabane L, et al. (2008) The effect of pre-operative aspirin on bleeding, transfusion, myocardial infarction, and mortality in coronary artery bypass surgery: a systematic review of randomized and observational studies. Eur Heart J 29: 1057–1071.

45. Burger W, Chemnitius JM, Kneissl GD, Rucker G (2005) Low-dose aspirin for secondary cardiovascular prevention - cardiovascular risks after its perioperative withdrawal versus bleeding risks with its continuation - review and meta-analysis. J Intern Med 257: 399–414.

46. Onal IK, Parlak E, Akdogan M, Yesil Y, Kuran SO, et al. (2013) Do aspirin and non-steroidal anti-inflammatory drugs increase the risk of post-sphincterotomy hemorrhage—a case-control study. Clin Res Hepatol Gastroenterol 37: 171–176.

47. Nelson RS, Ewing BM, Ternent C, Shashidharan M, Blatchford GJ, et al. (2008) Risk of late bleeding following hemorrhoidal banding in patients on antithrombotic prophylaxis. Am J Surg 196: 994–999; discussion 999.

48. Otley CC (2003) Continuation of medically necessary aspirin and warfarin during cutaneous surgery. Mayo Clin Proc 78: 1392–1396.

49. Lippe CM, Reineck EA, Kunselman AR, Gilchrist IC (2014) Warfarin: Impact on hemostasis after radial catheterization. Catheter Cardiovasc Interv.

50. Jamula E, Anderson J, Douketis JD (2009) Safety of continuing warfarin therapy during cataract surgery: a systematic review and meta-analysis. Thromb Res 124: 292–299.

51. Nematullah A, Alabousi A, Blanas N, Douketis JD, Sutherland SE (2009) Dental surgery for patients on anticoagulant therapy with warfarin: a systematic review and meta-analysis. J Can Dent Assoc 75: 41.

52. Wallace DL, Latimer MD, Belcher HJ (2004) Stopping warfarin therapy is unnecessary for hand surgery. J Hand Surg Br 29: 203–205.

53. Dietrich W, Dilthey G, Spannagl M, Richter JA (1995) Warfarin pretreatment does not lead to increased bleeding tendency during cardiac surgery. J Cardiothorac Vasc Anesth 9: 250–254.

54. Birnie DH, Healey JS, Wells GA, Verma A, Tang AS, et al. (2013) Pacemaker or defibrillator surgery without interruption of anticoagulation. N Engl J Med 368: 2084–2093.

55. Annala AP, Karjalainen PP, Porela P, Nyman K, Ylitalo A, et al. (2008) Safety of diagnostic coronary angiography during uninterrupted therapeutic warfarin treatment. Am J Cardiol 102: 386–390.

56. El-Jack SS, Ruygrok PN, Webster MW, Stewart JT, Bass NM, et al. (2006) Effectiveness of manual pressure hemostasis following transfemoral coronary angiography in patients on therapeutic warfarin anticoagulation. Am J Cardiol 97: 485–488.

# 22

# Retrospective Cohort Analysis of Chest Injury Characteristics and Concurrent Injuries in Patients Admitted to Hospital in the Wenchuan and Lushan Earthquakes in Sichuan, China

**Xi Zheng[❂], Yang Hu[❂], Yong Yuan, Yong-Fan Zhao***

Department of Thoracic Surgery, West China Hospital, Sichuan University, Chengdu, Sichuan Province, China

## Abstract

*Background:* The aim of this study was to compare retrospectively the characteristics of chest injuries and frequencies of other, concurrent injuries in patients after earthquakes of different seismic intensity.

*Methods:* We compared the cause, type, and body location of chest injuries as well as the frequencies of other, concurrent injuries in patients admitted to our hospital after the Wenchuan and Lushan earthquakes in Sichuan, China. We explored possible relationships between seismic intensity and the causes and types of injuries, and we assessed the ability of the Injury Severity Score, New Injury Severity Score, and Chest Injury Index to predict respiratory failure in chest injury patients.

*Results:* The incidence of chest injuries was 9.9% in the stronger Wenchuan earthquake and 22.2% in the less intensive Lushan earthquake. The most frequent cause of chest injuries in both earthquakes was being accidentally struck. Injuries due to falls were less prevalent in the stronger Wenchuan earthquake, while injuries due to burial were more prevalent. The distribution of types of chest injury did not vary significantly between the two earthquakes, with rib fractures and pulmonary contusions the most frequent types. Spinal and head injuries concurrent with chest injuries were more prevalent in the less violent Lushan earthquake. All three trauma scoring systems showed poor ability to predict respiratory failure in patients with earthquake-related chest injuries.

*Conclusions:* Previous studies may have underestimated the incidence of chest injury in violent earthquakes. The distributions of types of chest injury did not differ between these two earthquakes of different seismic intensity. Earthquake severity and interval between rescue and treatment may influence the prevalence and types of injuries that co-occur with the chest injury. Trauma evaluation scores on their own are inadequate predictors of respiratory failure in patients with earthquake-related chest injuries.

**Editor:** Qinghua Sun, The Ohio State University, United States of America

**Funding:** The authors have no support or funding to report.

**Competing Interests:** The authors have declared that no competing interests exist.

* E-mail: doctorzhaoyongfan@hotmail.com

❂ These authors contributed equally to this work.

## Introduction

In 2008, the devastating Wenchuan earthquake hit China's Sichuan province and led to 69,181 deaths, 18,522 missing and 374,171 injured. Five years later, another violent earthquake hit Sichuan, this time in the Lushan area, leading to at least 196 deaths, 21 missing, and 11,470 injured. The Wenchuan earthquake was rated as 8.0 on the Richter scale, with a maximum intensity of XI on a seismic intensity scale of I–XII defined by the Chinese State Bureau of Quality and Technical Supervision. The Lushan earthquake was rated as 7.0 on the Richter scale with a maximum intensity of IX. Both earthquakes occurred in geologically and demographically similar areas, providing an unusual opportunity to compare the prevalence and types of

casualties in two earthquakes differing primarily in seismic intensity.

Previous studies have reported that chest injuries account for only a small proportion of all earthquake-related injuries, and that most patients with chest injuries present with other, concurrent types of injuries that can significantly affect clinical outcomes [1–3]. These studies have not, however, addressed the question of whether the characteristics of chest injuries or co-occurring injuries vary with earthquake intensity. Addressing this question ideally requires examining two earthquakes that differ in intensity but that affect similar geologic areas with similar types of populations and distributions, and in which the casualties were treated at similar medical facilities. West China Hospital of Sichuan University is roughly equidistant from the epicenters of both earthquakes and was unaffected; it provided medical treatment to more trauma patients in both disasters than other hospitals, altogether 4,092 patients in the Wenchuan earthquake and 400 in the Lushan earthquake. Thus the data collected at West China Hospital on patients treated in both earthquakes provide a unique opportunity to examine the effects of seismic intensity on injury characteristics. Such comparisons may help predict the types of injuries likely to occur in earthquakes of given severity and help administrators allocate limited medical resources appropriately.

We also hoped to take advantage of our data set from two earthquakes in order to verify the efficacy of three types of trauma scoring systems for predicting respiratory failure in patients with chest injuries, all based on the the Abbreviated Injury Scale 2005 (AIS2005): the Injury Severity Score (ISS), the New Injury Severity Score (NISS) and the Chest Injury Index (CII). Our analysis of patients in the Wenchuan earthquake suggested that NISS was superior to the other indices [1,4], so we wished to verify that finding using data from the Lushan earthquake.

## Materials and Methods

The Institutional Review Board of West China Hospital approved the protocol for this retrospective study before it was undertaken; informed consent from participants was ruled unnecessary because we retrospectively analyzed data routinely collected from all inpatients and we analyzed the data anonymously.

Patients from earthquake-affected areas were transported either directly by helicopter from the scene to West China Hospital, or by car or helicopter from field hospitals. All patients admitted to our hospital with possible chest disorders were examined by two thoracic surgeons. Diagnosis of chest injury was made based on physical examination, chest X-ray, computed tomography (CT), fibrobronchoscopy or diagnostic pleuracentesis. All patients with chest injuries were included in our study. Since injuries of the thoracic vertebrae, scapula, and clavicle were treated by orthopedic surgeons, patients with only these injuries but no concurrent chest injury were excluded from our study. Simple contusion of the chest wall and injuries unrelated to the earthquakes, such as spontaneous pneumothorax, were also excluded.

Several items of information were collected from all patients after admission, including age, sex, location where the injury occurred, whether the injury occurred during the primary shock or during aftershocks, the cause and type of injury, diagnosis, duration of mechanical ventilation, and treatment outcome (recovery, deterioration or death). The procedures used to collect these data and update them after the Wenchuan earthquake have been described [4]; the data from patients in the Lushan earthquake were up-dated through 20 July 2013.

Causes of injuries were categorized based on previous studies of earthquakes and reports from the U.S. Centers for Disease Control and Prevention [5]: injuries due to falls, being buried, or being accidentally struck, or other injuries, such as burns, cuts, motor vehicle crashes, and delayed effects of injuries. The cause of injury of patients with multiple injuries were classified based on the cause of the clinically most important injury; for example, patients with multiple injuries due primarily to prolonged burial were classified as having injury due to burial.

In order to estimate the seismic intensity experienced by patients at the time of injury, we used Richter scale data and intensity distribution maps of both earthquakes generated based on Xu et al. [6] and data from the China Earthquake Networks Center. Seismic intensity assesses the intensity of ground shaking and consequences of an earthquake. Seismic intensity usually weakens with increasing distance from the epicenter, except for certain locations where this relationship does not hold. The locations where patients sustained injuries were located on this map and used to explore possible relationships between seismic intensity and the causes and types of injuries. We included in this analysis only patients for whom we obtained reliable information about where they had sustained their injuries.

Chest injuries were assessed using the ISS, NISS, and CII scales as described [4]. Patients who were mechanically ventilated for more than 24 h, either invasively or noninvasively, were diagnosed with respiratory failure.

Data on causes and types of injury in patients from both earthquakes were analyzed using SPSS 17.0 (IBM, Chicago, IL). Differences in continuous variables between patients from the two earthquakes were assessed for statistical significance using Student's t test or the Mann-Whitney U test. Differences in dichotomous variables were analyzed using the chi-squared test or Fisher's exact test. In order to compare the accuracy with which ISS, NISS and CII predict respiratory failure, we calculated receiver operating characteristics (ROC) curves and cut-off values using Medcalc 11.4.2.0 software. A two-sided $p < 0.05$ was considered significant.

## Results

In the Wenchuan earthquake, 1,856 patients were admitted to West China Hospital, and 184 (9.9%) were diagnosed with chest injuries [4,7]. All these patients were admitted after the primary shock; unfortunately patient data were not collected in the wake of the aftershocks. After excluding one woman diagnosed with spontaneous diaphragmatic hernia, we retained 183 in the final analysis. Of these, 165 (90.16%) showed improved and were discharged from our hospital within two months after the quake. A total of 28 patients (15.3%) were diagnosed with chest injuries without concurrent injuries. Thoracic surgical procedures, including closed thoracic drainage, were performed in 69 patients (37.7%). Six of the 183 (3.28%) died, accounting for 18.18% of all the 33 deaths in our hospital in the Wenchuan earthquake [7]. In the Lushan earthquake, 81 of 325 inpatients (24.9%) were diagnosed with chest injuries. Of these, we excluded 7 patients whose injuries were not earthquake-related and 2 patients with simple contusion of the chest wall, leaving 72 patients (22.2%) in the final analysis. None of the patients in our cohort presented with chest injuries exclusively; all had at least one additional injury on admission. Of the total 72 chest injury patients, 67 were injured during the primary shock, and 5 during aftershocks. By 20 July 2013, 60 (83.3%) had shown improvement and had been discharged from our hospital. By this date, no deaths among the patients admitted to our hospital were declared after the earthquake. A total of 15 patients (20.83%) received thoracic surgical procedures.

The trauma patients from both earthquakes had a similar age (p = 0.316) and gender composition (p = 0.397). We categorized each patient by his or her principal type of injury, and found that the frequencies of most types of injury differed significantly between the two earthquakes (Table 1). The frequency of "other" injuries could not be compared because of inadequate sample size. Injuries due to being accidentally struck were among the most frequent injuries in both earthquakes; other frequent causes of injury were being buried (Wenchuan) or falling (Lushan).

Among patients with chest injuries in both earthquakes, the most frequent diagnoses were rib fractures and pulmonary contusions (Table 2). Rib fracture was more frequent in the Wenchuan earthquake, while pulmonary contusion predominated

**Table 1.** Comparison of the causes of chest injury in patients admitted to our hospital in the Wenchuan and Lushan earthquakes.

| Cause of injury[a] | Wenchuan, n (%) | Lushan, n (%) | p* |
|---|---|---|---|
| Being buried | 21 (11.5) | 1 (1.4) | 0.010 |
| Being accidentally struck | 143 (78.1) | 39 (54.2) | <0.001 |
| Falling | 18 (9.8) | 30 (41.7) | <0.001 |
| Other | 1 (0.5) | 2 (2.8) | 0.193 |

[a]Patients with injuries reflecting multiple causes were classified according to the cause of their principal injury.
*Based on the Pearson chi-squared test or Fisher's exact test.

in the Lushan disaster. The frequencies of hemothorax, pneumothorax and sternum fracture differed significantly between the two earthquakes.

Injuries co-occurring with chest injuries were classified into 1 of 6 regions and compared between the two earthquakes (Table 3). Patients with chest injuries presented with concurrent head and spine injuries more often in the Lushan earthquake than in the Wenchuan earthquake.

Next we explored whether chest injury frequency and characteristics were associated with earthquake severity based on data from both earthquakes. We could perform this analysis on only 177 patients because we did not have reliable information about where other patients sustained their injuries. Given this limited sample size, and given the fact that structures in the areas affected by both earthquakes were built to withstand earthquakes up to an intensity of VII (Ministry of Housing and Urban-Rural Development of the People's Republic of China, code of aseismic design of buildings), we divided seismic intensities into two categories, IV–VII and VIII–XI. Types of injury varied with seismic intensity (Table 4): the frequency of being unintentionally struck increased with greater intensity, whereas the frequency of falling decreased. In contrast, the frequencies of different types of chest injury were similar for the two intensity categories (Table 5).

In the Wenchuan earthquake, 38 inpatients with chest injuries (20.7%) suffered from respiratory failure [4]. In the Lushan disaster, 18 of the 72 inpatients with chest injuries (25.0%) developed respiratory failure. Building on our previous work assessing the ability of the ISS, NISS and CII scales to predict

respiratory failure in chest injury patients in the Wenchuan earthquake, we performed the same analysis on Lushan patients. We calculated the area under ROC curves and estimated 95% confidence intervals (95%CI) for all scales (Figure 1 and Table 6). Although NISS was significantly more accurate than the two other scales in our analysis of Wenchuan chest injury patients [4], all three scales performed similarly poorly for Lushan chest injury patients.

## Discussion

Earthquakes are major geological disasters that cause tremendous human and economic losses around the world [8,9]. However, relatively little is known about how earthquake factors such as seismic intensity affect the prevalence and types of casualties. Here we examine the prevalence and causes of different types of chest injury between the more violent Wenchuan earthquake and less violent Lushan earthquake, which affected similar regions of Sichuan province. Our analysis suggests that chest injuries occur more frequently in earthquake victims than previously thought, and that seismic intensity affects causes of chest injury. On the other hand, seismic intensity may not affect types of chest injury. These results may help emergency response centers predict the kinds of patients that they will need to treat and thereby lead to more rational allocation of limited medical resources.

The fact that our hospital was the major provider of medical services to patients in both the Wenchuan and Lushan

**Table 2.** Comparison of the prevalence of types of chest injury among patients admitted to our hospital in the Wenchuan and Lushan earthquakes.

| Chest injury type | Wenchuan, n (%) | Lushan, n (%) | p* |
|---|---|---|---|
| Rib fracture | 161 (88.0) | 39 (54.2) | <0.001 |
| Pulmonary contusion | 117 (63.9) | 57 (79.2) | 0.019 |
| Hemopneumothorax | 39 (21.3) | 9 (12.5) | 0.105 |
| Hemothorax | 33 (18.0) | 1 (1.4) | <0.001 |
| Pneumothorax | 19 (10.4) | 2 (2.8) | 0.047 |
| Fracture of sternum | 4 (2.2) | 7 (9.7) | 0.020 |
| Diaphragmatic hernia | 2 (1.1) | 0 (0.0) | 1.000 |
| Thoracic duct injury | 1 (0.5) | 0 (0.0) | 1.000 |
| Traumatic asphyxia | 1 (0.5) | 0 (0.0) | 1.000 |
| Mediastinal emphysema | 0 (0.0) | 2 (2.8) | 0.079 |
| Mediastinal effusion | 0 (0.0) | 1 (1.4) | 0.282 |

*Based on the Pearson chi-squared test, continuity-corrected chi-squared test or Fisher's exact test.

**Table 3.** Comparison of the prevalence and types of injuries co-occurring with chest injury in patients admitted to our hospital after the Wenchuan and Lushan earthquakes.

| Concurrent injury type[a] | Wenchuan, n (%) | Lushan, n (%) | p* |
|---|---|---|---|
| Brain and skull | 33 (18.0) | 23 (31.9) | 0.016 |
| Face and neck | 8 (4.4) | 5 (6.9) | 0.600 |
| Abdomen | 19 (10.4) | 13 (18.1) | 0.096 |
| Spine and spinal cord | 51 (27.9) | 39 (54.2) | <0.001 |
| Extremities[b] | 113 (61.7) | 35 (48.6) | 0.056 |
| External injuries | 64 (35.0) | 34 (47.2) | 0.070 |

[a]Some patients contained concurrent injuries of multiple types; those patients therefore appear multiple times in the table.
[b]Extremities include the upper and lower limbs, clavicle, scapula, bony pelvis and hip.
*Based on the Pearson chi-squared test or continuity-corrected chi-squared test.

earthquakes gives us a unique opportunity to examine how seismic intensity may affect the prevalence and characteristics of different types of injuries. Normally such comparisons are difficult because the earthquakes being compared differ in numerous respects. In this case, however, both Lushan and Wenchuan counties have similar geologic features and are located at the Longmenshan Fault Zone [10]. Other factors known to affect earthquake losses, such as demographic structure, population density, outbreak time, architectural features and local medical infrastructure, are also similar between the two affected areas [11]. Our hospital is approximately equidistant (100 km) from both epicenters. Thus, the major difference between the two earthquakes in our analysis is seismic intensity, allowing us to draw conclusions about how this parameter may affect casualties admitted to hospital.

Chest injuries were diagnosed in 9.9% of the patients admitted to our hospital in the Wenchuan earthquake [4] and 22.2% in the Lushan earthquake. These incidences are consistent with reports suggesting a 10–15% incidence of chest injuries among trauma patients [12,13]. At the same time, most chest injuries in our patients were minor or moderate and resolved after conservative treatment, as reported in other major earthquakes [2,3,14]. The exception to this, both in our study and previous work, is severe chest injury, especially crushing injuries of the chest, which are associated with high mortality [15–18].

Contrary to our expectations, the incidence of chest injury was higher among patients in the less violent Lushan earthquake than in the more violent Wenchuan disaster, as was the incidence of crushing and other severe chest injuries. In fact, the incidence of chest injury in Lushan is higher than that reported in previous studies of chest injuries in several major earthquakes [1,3,19–21]. We speculate that all these findings reflect the fact that major

transportation networks were more severely disrupted in the Wenchuan disaster, significantly delaying the arrival of patients at our hospital and leading to a larger number of pre-admission deaths due to severe chest trauma. In the Lushan earthquake, in contrast, most transportation networks remained open, facilitating prompt rescue and delivery to our hospital. Therefore we suspect that the data on severe chest injury in our Lushan cohort more accurately reflect what happens in a major earthquake. Previous studies of severe chest injury and other types of severe injury in earthquakes should be interpreted with caution given the risk of underestimating prevalence as a result of missing individuals and pre-admission deaths. Our findings further suggest that prompt rescue and medical attention after destructive earthquakes may save the lives of many patients with severe chest injuries.

Our comparison of the two earthquakes identified several other informative differences. While injuries due to being accidentally struck were the most common type of injury in both earthquakes, injuries due to falls were more frequent in the less intense Lushan earthquake, while injuries due to being buried were more frequent in the more intense Wenchuan disaster. These results can be attributed to seismic intensity since more intense earthquakes like the Wenchuan disaster involve more extensive structural damage, leading to building collapse and increasing the risk of burial. In less intense earthquakes such as Lushan, fewer buildings collapse, so a greater proportion of injuries are due to falls. Only 4 aftershocks at >5.0 on the Richter scale were recorded in the Lushan earthquake, and all were nondestructive. This may explain why only 5 patients in our Lushan cohort (6.9% of the total admitted) were injured during aftershocks; most of these injuries were due to falling or being accidentally struck. These individuals may have been engaging in unsafe behaviors during the disaster, perhaps as

**Table 4.** Relationships between seismic intensity and cause of injury in patients admitted to our hospital after the Wenchuan and Lushan earthquakes.

| Cause of injury, n (%) | Seismic intensity | | p* |
|---|---|---|---|
| | IV–VII | VIII–XI | |
| Being buried | 3 (4.1) | 6 (5.8) | <0.001 |
| Being accidentally struck | 38 (51.4) | 86 (83.5) | |
| Falling | 31 (41.9) | 10 (9.7) | |
| Other | 2 (2.7) | 1 (1.0) | |

*Based on the likelihood ratio of the chi-squared test.

**Table 5.** Relationships between seismic intensity and the prevalence of types of chest injury in patients admitted to our hospital after the Wenchuan and Lushan earthquakes.

| Chest injury type, n (%)[a] | Seismic intensity | | P* |
|---|---|---|---|
| | IV–VII | VIII–XI | |
| Rib fracture | 52 (39.1) | 86 (46.2) | 0.267 |
| Pulmonary contusion | 55 (41.4) | 61 (32.8) | |
| Hemopneumothorax | 11 (8.3) | 21 (11.3) | |
| Hemothorax | 4 (3.0) | 4 (2.2) | |
| Pneumothorax | 5 (3.8) | 11 (5.9) | |
| Fracture of sternum | 6 (4.5) | 3 (1.6) | |

[a]Some patients suffered from more than one type of chest injury and therefore appear multiple times in this table. One patient with diaphragmatic hernia, one with thoracic duct injury, two with mediastinal emphysema and one with mediatinal effusion were not included in the analysis.
*Based on the likelihood ratio chi-squared test.

a result of psychological or physical trauma after the primary shocks [22].

Our findings lead us to recommend the deployment of emergency responders trained in dealing with such critical conditions as crush syndrome, severe infection and brain injuries in the wake of violent earthquakes, where the risk of burial-related injuries is high. In less intense earthquakes, rapid response of psychologists may be particularly important for preventing avoidable injuries due to shock and disorientation.

The most frequent types of chest injury in both earthquakes were rib fractures and pulmonary contusions, similar to the causes of chest injuries in other medical emergencies [23]. Comparing the two earthquakes showed that greater seismic intensity was associated with greater prevalence of rib fractures but lower prevalence of pulmonary contusion. Greater intensity was also associated with higher frequencies of severe injuries like hemothorax and pneumothorax. These findings should be interpreted with caution given the limited sample size, due to lack of reliable data on where most patients sustained their injuries within the earthquake-affected areas. In fact, combining the results of Tables 2 and 5 suggests that seismic intensity may not affect the overall distribution of chest injury types. However, this analysis is based on a crude stratification of intensities into only two categories. Future work should involve many more patients and more detailed stratification of intensity. Despite these limitations, the data suggest that greater proportions of patients in more violent earthquakes may require closed drainage of the pleural cavity. Our lack of statistical power prevents us from drawing any conclusions about a possible relationship between seismic intensity

and rare injuries such as diaphragmatic hernia and thoracic duct injury.

In earthquakes, patients presenting only with chest injury are rare; most chest injuries occur simultaneously with other types of injury [1,3]. Similarly we found that 84.7% of Wenchuan chest injury patients and all Lushan chest injury patients presented concurrently with other types of injury. Since injuries that occur together with chest injuries can affect patient outcomes, we compared the prevalence and types of such concurrent injuries between the two earthquakes. In both disasters, injuries of the face, neck and abdomen were uncommon, and external injuries were frequent but usually mild (Table 3). More than 50% of Wenchuan patients admitted to our hospital [7] and more than 70% of Lushan patients were treated in the orthopedic department, similar to what has been reported in other earthquakes [24]. Injuries of the spine and extremities were the most frequent injuries concurrent with chest injuries. We were surprised to find that the prevalence of concurrent injuries affecting the brain, skull, spine or spinal cord was higher in the less violent Lushan earthquake. Again, the explanation may reflect the fact that many patients with severe injuries of the brain and spinal cord die rapidly, so a greater proportion of such patients in the Wenchuan earthquake may have died before they could be rescued and transported to our hospital. Therefore we recommend the deployment of adequate numbers of orthopedic and neurological specialists to attend to patients with chest injuries in violent earthquakes.

Accurately predicting which earthquake casualties are likely to suffer respiratory failure would significantly aid in emergency triage and allocation of limited medical resources. The three injury

**Table 6.** Comparison of the ability of conventional injury severity scores to predict respiratory failure in patients admitted to our hospital from the Lushan earthquake.

| Scoring system | Cut-off value | Sensitivity (%) | Specificity (%) | AUC | 95%CI |
|---|---|---|---|---|---|
| ISS | 14 | 100.0 | 40.7 | 0.713[a] | 0.594–0.813 |
| NISS | 28 | 55.6 | 81.5 | 0.720 | 0.601–0.819 |
| CII | 18 | 44.4 | 75.9 | 0.590[b] | 0.468–0.705 |

Abbreviations: AUC, area under the ROC curve; CII, chest injury index; ISS, injury severity score; NISS, new injury severity score; 95%CI, 95% confidence interval.
[a]NISS vs. ISS, p = 0.880.
[b]NISS vs. CII, p = 0.136.

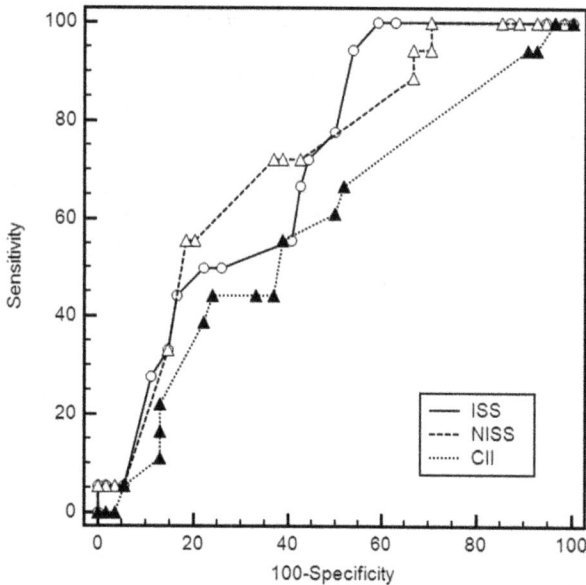

**Figure 1. Receiver operating characteristic (ROC) curves of different trauma scoring systems for predicting respiratory failure in patients admitted to our hospital in the Lushan earthquake.** The solid line indicates the ROC curve for the Injury Severity Score (ISS); the dashed line, the curve for the New Injury Severity Score (NISS); and the dotted line, the curve for the Chest Injury Index (CII) [4].

scales ISS, NISS, and CII, all based on the AIS2005 scale, are widely used to predict survival in disasters, and we recently applied them to the prediction of respiratory failure among Wenchuan chest injury patients [4]. Our results in that study suggested that the NISS was superior to the other scales. When we examined the Lushan cohort, however, all three scales showed unsatisfactory AUC values ranging from 0.590–0.720, compared to values of 0.837–0.893 in the Wenchuan earthquake [4]. While the high sensitivity of ISS may make it useful as a screening method, NISS and CII show poor sensitivity and moderate specificity, limiting their diagnostic usefulness. The AIS2005 scale assesses only injury severity, regardless of how long the patient has had the injury and

what treatments have been administered [25]. Nevertheless, clinicians often use it to predict trauma progression [1,26–28], even though many factors other than injury severity affect such progression. In earthquake-related trauma in particular, factors such as pre-admission treatments, the delay between injury and treatment, and the presence of comorbidities may also affect trauma progression. All these factors may therefore influence the risk of respiratory failure, so we recommend combining conventional injury severity scales with more comprehensive trauma assessment in order to predict respiratory failure in chest injury patients.

Our analysis of patients admitted to our hospital in the Wenchuan and Lushan earthquakes leads us to several conclusions. Previous studies may have underestimated the true incidence of chest injuries in violent earthquakes, and these injuries most frequently involve rib fractures or pulmonary contusions due to being accidentally struck. Greater seismic intensity is associated with lower prevalence of injuries due to falling and higher prevalence of injuries due to being buried. However, seismic intensity does not appear to affect the prevalence and types of chest injury. Earthquake-related chest injuries usually occur together with other injuries, most frequently with orthopedic injuries. The prevalence and types of concurrent injuries may be affected by the delay between rescue and treatment as well as the severity of the earthquake. Injury severity scales by themselves are inadequate for predicting respiratory failure in chest injury patients in earthquakes; more factors should be taken into account when evaluating such trauma.

## Acknowledgments

We thank the public relations department of West China Hospital for help in acquiring data. We would also like to express our gratitude to all doctors and nurses who were involved in rescue work in the two earthquakes.

## Author Contributions

Conceived and designed the experiments: YFZ YH XZ YY. Performed the experiments: XZ YH YY. Analyzed the data: YH XZ YY YFZ. Contributed reagents/materials/analysis tools: XZ YY. Wrote the paper: YH XZ. Revised the manuscript according to the comments of reviewers: XZ YH YY.

## References

1. Toker A, Isitmangil T, Erdik O, Sancakli I, Sebit S (2002) Analysis of chest injuries sustained during the 1999 Marmara earthquake. Surg Today 32: 769–771.
2. Hu J, Guo YQ, Zhang EY, Tan J, Shi YK (2010) Chest injuries associated with earthquakes: an analysis of injuries sustained during the 2008 Wen-Chuan earthquake in China. Surg Today 40: 729–733. doi:10.1007/s00595-009-4130-6.
3. Sato K, Kobayashi M, Ishibashi S, Ueda S, Suzuki S (2013) Chest injuries and the 2011 Great East Japan Earthquake. Respir Investig 51: 24–27. doi:10.1016/j.resinv.2012.11.002.
4. Hu Y, Tang Y, Yuan Y, Xie TP, Zhao YF (2010) Trauma evaluation of patients with chest injury in the 2008 earthquake of Wenchuan, Sechuan, China. World J Surg 34: 728–732. doi:10.1007/s00268-010-0427-2.
5. LeMier M, Cummings P, West TA (2001) Accuracy of external cause of injury codes reported in Washington State hospital discharge records. Inj Prev 7: 334–338.
6. Xu C, Xu X, Zhou B, Yu G (2013) Revisions of the M 8.0 Wenchuan earthquake seismic intensity map based on co-seismic landslide abundance. Nat Hazards: 1–18. doi:10.1007/s11069-013-0757-0.
7. Xie J, Du L, Xia T, Wang M, Diao X, et al. (2008) Analysis of 1856 inpatients and 33 deaths in the West China Hospital of Sichuan University from the

Wenchuan earthquake. J Evid Based Med 1: 20–26. doi:10.1111/j.1756-5391.2008.00010.x.
8. Doocy S, Daniels A, Packer C, Dick A, Kirsch TD (2013) The human impact of earthquakes: a historical review of events 1980–2009 and systematic literature review. PLoS Curr 5. Available: http://www.ncbi.nlm.nih.gov/pmc/articles/PMC3644288/. Accessed 8 January 2014. doi:10.1371/currents.dis.67bd14-fe457f1db0b5433a8ee20fb833.
9. Ratnapradipa D, Conder J, Ruffing A, White V (2012) The 2011 Japanese earthquake: an overview of environmental health impacts. J Environ Health 74: 42–50.
10. Zheng Y, Ge C, Xie Z, Yang Y, Xiong X, et al. (2013) Crustal and upper mantle structure and the deep seismogenic environment in the source regions of the Lushan earthquake and the Wenchuan earthquake. Sci China Earth Sci 56: 1158–1168. doi:10.1007/s11430-013-4641-2.
11. Whitman RV, Anagnos T, Kircher CA, Lagorio HJ, Lawson RS, et al. (1997) Development of a National Earthquake Loss Estimation Methodology. Earthquake Spectra 13: 643–661. doi:http://dx.doi.org/10.1193/1.1585973.
12. Al-Koudmani I, Darwish B, Al-Kateb K, Taifour Y (2012) Chest trauma experience over eleven-year period at al-mouassat university teaching hospital-Damascus: a retrospective review of 888 cases. J Cardiothorac Surg 7: 35. doi:10.1186/1749-8090-7-35.

13. LoCicero J 3rd, Mattox KL (1989) Epidemiology of chest trauma. Surg Clin North Am 69: 15–19.
14. Yoshimura N, Nakayama S, Nakagiri K, Azami T, Ataka K, et al. (1996) Profile of chest injuries arising from the 1995 southern Hyogo Prefecture earthquake. Chest 110: 759–761. doi:10.1378/chest.110.3.759.
15. Gaillard M, Herve C, Mandin L, Raynaud P (1990) Mortality prognostic factors in chest injury. J Trauma 30: 93–96.
16. Demirhan R, Onan B, Oz K, Halezeroglu S (2009) Comprehensive analysis of 4205 patients with chest trauma: a 10-year experience. Interact Cardiovasc Thorac Surg 9: 450–453. doi:10.1510/icvts.2009.206599.
17. Conn JH, Hardy JD, Fain WR, Netterville RE (1963) Thoracic trauma: analysis of 1022 cases. J Trauma 3: 22–40.
18. Shorr RM, Crittenden M, Indeck M, Hartunian SL, Rodriguez A (1987) Blunt thoracic trauma. Analysis of 515 patients. Ann Surg 206: 200–205.
19. Yi-Szu W, Chung-Ping H, Tzu-Chieh L, Dar-Yu Y, Tain-Cheng W (2000) Chest injuries transferred to trauma centers after the 1999 Taiwan earthquake. Am J Emerg Med 18: 825–827. doi:10.1053/ajem.2000.18132.
20. Ghodsi SM, Zargar M, Khaji A, Karbakhsh M (2006) Chest injury in victims of Bam earthquake. Chin J Traumatol 9: 345–348.
21. Ozdogan S, Hocaoglu A, Caglayan B, Imamoglu OU, Aydin D (2001) Thorax and lung injuries arising from the two earthquakes in Turkey in 1999. Chest 120: 1163–1166. doi:10.1590/S1807-59322011000500018.
22. Honma M, Endo N, Osada Y, Kim Y, Kuriyama K (2012) Disturbances in equilibrium function after major earthquake. Sci Rep 2: 749. doi:10.1038/srep00749.
23. Veysi VT, Nikolaou VS, Paliobeis C, Efstathopoulos N, Giannoudis PV (2009) Prevalence of chest trauma, associated injuries and mortality: a level I trauma centre experience. Int Orthop 33: 1425–1433. doi:10.1007/s00264-009-0746-9.
24. Mulvey JM, Awan SU, Qadri AA, Maqsood MA (2008) Profile of injuries arising from the 2005 Kashmir earthquake: the first 72 h. Injury 39: 554–560. doi:10.1016/j.injury.2007.07.025.
25. Baker SP, O'Neill B, Haddon W Jr, Long WB (1974) The injury severity score: a method for describing patients with multiple injuries and evaluating emergency care. J Trauma 14: 187–196.
26. Osler T, Baker SP, Long W (1997) A modification of the injury severity score that both improves accuracy and simplifies scoring. J Trauma 43: 922–925; discussion 925–926.
27. Kimura A, Chadbunchachai W, Nakahara S (2012) Modification of the Trauma and Injury Severity Score (TRISS) method provides better survival prediction in Asian blunt trauma victims. World J Surg 36: 813–818. doi:10.1007/s00268-012-1498-z.
28. Liman ST, Kuzucu A, Tastepe AI, Ulasan GN, Topcu S (2003) Chest injury due to blunt trauma. Eur J Cardiothorac Surg 23: 374–378. doi:10.1016/s1010-7940(02)00813-8.

# 23

# Identification of Serum MicroRNA Signatures for Diagnosis of Mild Traumatic Brain Injury in a Closed Head Injury Model

Anuj Sharma[1ᵒ], Raghavendar Chandran[1,2ᵒ], Erin S. Barry[3], Manish Bhomia[1], Mary Anne Hutchison[3], Nagaraja S. Balakathiresan[1], Neil E. Grunberg[3], Radha K. Maheshwari[1]*

1 Department of Pathology, Uniformed Services University of the Health Sciences, Bethesda, Maryland, United States of America, 2 Biological Sciences Group, Birla Institute of Technology and Science, Pilani, Rajasthan, India, 3 Department of Medical and Clinical Psychology, Uniformed Services University of the Health Sciences, Bethesda, Maryland, United States of America

## Abstract

Wars in Iraq and Afghanistan have highlighted the problems of diagnosis and treatment of mild traumatic brain injury (mTBI). MTBI is a heterogeneous injury that may lead to the development of neurological and behavioral disorders. In the absence of specific diagnostic markers, mTBI is often unnoticed or misdiagnosed. In this study, mice were induced with increasing levels of mTBI and microRNA (miRNA) changes in the serum were determined. MTBI was induced by varying weight and fall height of the impactor rod resulting in four different severity grades of the mTBI. Injuries were characterized as mild by assessing with the neurobehavioral severity scale-revised (NSS-R) at day 1 post injury. Open field locomotion and acoustic startle response showed behavioral and sensory motor deficits in 3 of the 4 injury groups at day 1 post injury. All of the animals recovered after day 1 with no significant neurobehavioral alteration by day 30 post injury. Serum microRNA (miRNA) profiles clearly differentiated injured from uninjured animals. Overall, the number of miRNAs that were significantly modulated in injured animals over the sham controls increased with the severity of the injury. Thirteen miRNAs were found to identify mTBI regardless of its severity within the mild spectrum of injury. Bioinformatics analyses revealed that the more severe brain injuries were associated with a greater number of miRNAs involved in brain related functions. The evaluation of serum miRNA may help to identify the severity of brain injury and the risk of developing adverse effects after TBI.

**Editor:** Baohong Zhang, East Carolina University, United States of America

**Funding:** This study was supported by funding from Congressionally Directed Medical Research Programs (CDMRP), Project# D10_I_AR_J6_855 (PI: Radha K Maheshwari). The funders had no role in study design, data collection and analysis, decision to publish, or preparation of the manuscript.

**Competing Interests:** The authors have declared that no competing interests exist.

* Email: radha.maheshwari@usuhs.edu

ᵒ These authors contributed equally to this work.

## Introduction

Traumatic brain injury (TBI) is one of the signature injuries in the conflicts with Iraq and Afghanistan [1]. Thirty percent of combat troops of Operation Iraqi Freedom (OIF) and Operation Enduring Freedom (OEF) have been diagnosed with mild, moderate, or severe TBI. More TBI cases occur out of the combat zone due to vehicle crashes, falls, sports, and recreational activities, which account for 84% of the total military TBI cases (www.dvbic.org). The Glasgow Coma Scale (GCS) is a standard measure to ascertain the initial severity and prognosis of TBI [2]. Mild TBI (mTBI), which is the most common form of military and civilian TBI, is characterized by loss of consciousness for <30 min and post traumatic amnesia for <24 hr with a GCS of 13–15, and accounts for 77% of the total TBI cases [3]. Diagnosis of mTBI is difficult as the injury may go unnoticed due to the lack of any immediate symptoms and confirmed pathology. Computed tomography (CT) and magnetic resonance imaging (MRI) have limited ability to detect mild brain tissue damage [4–6]. Serum

levels of brain specific/enriched proteins such as S-100β, glial fibrillary acidic protein (GFAP) and its breakdown products, and ubiquitin carboxyl-terminal esterase L1 (UCH-L1) have been proposed as diagnostic markers of severe TBI, but their utility in the diagnosis of mild to moderate TBI is still unknown [7–12]. The majority of mild brain injuries recover spontaneously. However, 10–20% of mTBI patients continue to suffer from post concussive syndrome [3,13–15]. Therefore, it is important to establish diagnostic marker(s) that can distinguish patients with a head injury regardless of the severity of the injury as well as distinguish individuals based on severity of mTBI.

MicroRNAs (miRNA), which are small (19–28 nt) non-coding endogenous RNA, have shown great promise as diagnostic markers of several diseases and disorders [16–18]. Unique changes in the expression of miRNAs in the brain samples after TBI have been reported [19–23]. Redell and group have also investigated the diagnostic potential of the miRNA in severe TBI [20]. To date, a comprehensive evaluation of miRNA as a diagnostic biomarker of mTBI, which also addresses the heterogeneous nature of mTBI, has not been described. The present study was designed to identify serum miRNAs as biomarkers of mild brain injury, which could identify the occurrence of mTBI independent of the severity of the injury within the mild spectrum of TBI.

In this study, a previously described free-fall weight-drop model of mTBI [25] with modifications was used to study the neurobehavioral deficits over a period of 30 days and miRNA modulation during the acute phase of injury. This model resembles the blunt head trauma resulting from a vehicle crash, combat, falls, and other recreational activities. Mice were subjected to an increasing grade of injury within the mild spectrum by varying the weight and height of the falling metal rod, with the most severe being a 3 cm fall height combined with a 333 g weight [25]. The neurobehavioral severity scale-revised (NSS-R) was measured at day 1 post injury, along with open field locomotion (OFL) activity and acoustic startle responses (ASR). NSS-R scores correlated and increased significantly with the grade of injury. OFL activity and startle responses were reduced in the injury groups, except the 2461g/2 cm injury. OFL and ASR activity returned to normal levels by day 14 post injury and remained constant through day 30 post injury measurements. To determine the miRNA changes in the serum during the acute phase of injury, miRNA arrays were performed on serum RNA isolated at 3 hr post injury. Thirteen miRNAs showed similar expression changes among injured mice compared to sham controls. Bioinformatics analyses using the Ingenuity Pathway Analysis (IPA) and DNA Intelligent Analysis (DIANA)-miRPath software showed that the number of significantly modulated serum miRNAs predicted to be involved in brain related functions increased with the severity of the injury.

## Material and Methods

### Animals and Injury

10–11 weeks old C57Bl/6J (Stock# 000664) male mice were obtained from Jackson Laboratories (Bar Harbor, ME). The animals were acclimatized to their new environment for a week and had continuous access to food and water. During the acclimatization period and throughout the experiment, the animals were housed on a reversed light cycle and were handled daily by the laboratory staff. The reverse light cycle was used because mice are nocturnal animals, so the behavioral measures were made during their active periods. Daily handling was done to habituate animals to laboratory staff and handling procedures, thereby reducing any stress associated with handling the animals during the experimental procedures.

**Ethics Statement.** All of the animal experiments were reviewed and approved by the Uniformed Services University of the Health Sciences (USUHS) Institutional Animal Care and Use Committee and were performed in accordance with the Guide for the Care and Use of Laboratory Animals (Committee on Care And Use of Laboratory Animals of The Institute of Laboratory Animal Resources, National Research Council, NIH Publication No. 86-23, revised 1996).

A weight drop injury apparatus (Figure S1A) was custom made by FJB Engineering (330-i North Stone Street Ave., Rockville, MD 20850) based on the description given in Flierl et al. (2009) [25]. The mice were anesthetized using a continuous flow of isoflurane/oxygen mix. The hair on the head was shaved and the animals were placed on the platform where continuous anesthesia was provided through a nose cone. The skin was sterilized using 10% povidone-iodine (Betadine) solution (Purdue Products L.P.,

Stamford, CT). A single cut was made along the mid line of the head to expose the skull. Injury coordinates were: left parietal lobe, 2.5 mm from sagittal suture, and 2.5 mm from lamboid suture (Figure S1B). Injury was induced by a free falling metal rod with a rubber tip of 1 mm diameter (Figure S1A). Rebound injury was minimized by immediately catching the rod after the primary impact. Animals were resuscitated by gently massaging the thorax and providing oxygen through the nose cone. Once continuous breathing resumed, the animals were again put on mild anesthesia using the nose cone. Animals without skull fractures were included in the experiment and the scalp skin was sutured back using Vetbond Tissue Adhesive 1469SB (3 M, St.Paul, MN, USA). The animals were then placed in a cage on a warming mat and were allowed to recuperate from the anesthesia. Injury day was considered as day 0. Sham controls were similarly handled and received only the scalp cut under anesthesia.

### Study Design

The experiment was designed to evaluate the neurobehavioral alteration in the mice following mTBI over a 30 day period and to evaluate the serum miRNA changes of mice at 3 hr post injury.

**Behavior Study.** Multiple smaller cohorts were combined to complete the final analyses. Four different injury groups: 246 g/2 cm (n = 32), 246 g/3 cm (n = 29), 333 g/2 cm (n = 20) and 333 g/3 cm (n = 6) were based on the weight of the impact rod and the height of the fall, respectively. These groups are referred to as injury severity 1 (IS1 = 246 g/2 cm), injury severity 2 (IS2 = 246 g/3 cm), injury severity 3 (IS3 = 333 g/2 cm), and injury severity 4 (IS4 = 333 g/3 cm) through rest of the manuscript. Sham controls (n = 42) were included in the experiment to determine the effect of handling and surgery (scalp cut and suture) on the animals' neurobehavioral responses. In the sham group, animals were handled similar to that of the injured groups except that no injury was made after the scalp cut. The skin was sutured back without making the impact trauma and the animals were allowed to recuperate in the cage similar to the injured animals. An additional control of naïve (n = 25) animals was included to determine the basal level of normal neurobehavioral responses. The naïve group of animals was kept in their housing room and not taken to the surgery room to avoid any stress related to being in the surgery room. Baseline measurements for NSS-R, OFL, and ASR were taken at day 3 (day −3) before the injury (day 0). NSS-R was also measured at day 1 post injury and ASR and OFL were measured at days 1, 14, and 30 post injury.

**MicroRNA Study.** A separate group of animals for all four injuries as described above in the behavior study, were used in the miRNA study (n = 6 each group). In addition, a sham group (n = 6) was included to account for miRNA changes that may occur due to the surgical process such as anesthesia, scalp cut, stress of handling the animal, and sutures. MiRNA expression of injured animals was compared with that of the sham to determine the modulation in miRNA expression due to brain injury.

### Neurobehavioral severity scale-revised (NSS-R)

A revised form of the neurological severity scale (NSS), initially developed for rats, was modified for mice and measured 3 days before the injury (day −3) and at day 1 post injury [26–27]. The NSS-R is a specific, continuous sequence of 10 behavioral tests and observations. This measure was originally designed to model a clinical neurological exam conducted in human neurology patients. This particular sensory-motor assessment scale was based on several previous reports and has been modified to increase standardization and sensitivity [27–32]. Ten tasks assess reflex suppression, general movement, and postural adjustments in response to a challenge. The NSS-R uses a three-point Likert scale, in which a normal, healthy response is assigned a "0," a partial or compromised response is assigned a "1," and the absence of a response is assigned a "2." This three-point scale is clear and reliable and allows for greater discrimination based on sensory-motor responses than do previous scales that used two-point ratings of each response. The NSS-R has a scoring range of 0–20, with higher scores reflecting greater extent of injury. All personnel were blinded to the treatment groups for the NSS-R measurements, but not to the naïve group. Naïve animals did not exhibit a scalp cut and sutures, which were otherwise were present on all the sham and injured animals, and therefore, were easily identifiable. Animals were evaluated on all 10 tasks as listed in Table S1.

## Open Field Locomotion (OFL) test

Open field locomotor activity was measured to evaluate the unconditional behavior of the mouse in its environment. OFL test was performed at 3 days prior to injury (baseline; day −3) and days 1, 14, and 30 post injury. Data collected included horizontal activity for general health and gross motor skills; center time as an index of anxiety-related behavior (where less time spent in the center of the cage is interpreted as more anxiety-related behavior); and vertical activity as an index of depression-related behavior (where less vertical activity may indicate less escape behavior which is interpreted as more depression-related behavior) [33–37]. Locomotor activity was measured using an Omnitech Electronics Digiscan infrared photocell system [Test box model RXYZCM (16 TAO); Omnitech Electronics, Columbus, OH] as described before [38]. One hour activity measurements were obtained during animals' active cycle. Animals were placed singly in a $20 \times 20 \times 30$ cm clear Plexiglas arena covered with a Plexiglas lid with multiple holes to ensure adequate ventilation. A photocell array measured horizontal locomotor activity using 8 pairs of infrared photocells located every 2.5 cm from side-to-side and 16 pairs of infrared photocells located front-to-back in a plane 2 cm above the floor of the arena. A second side-to-side array of 8 pairs of additional photocells located 5.5 cm above the arena floor measured vertical activity. Data were automatically gathered and transmitted to a computer via an Omnitech Model DCM-I-BBU analyzer.

## Acoustic startle reflex (ASR) test

Acoustic startle reflex is a characteristic sequence of involuntary, defensive, muscular responses elicited by a sudden, intense acoustic stimulus. Measurement of acoustic startle response with and without prepulse provides information about information processing and attention [39–43]. ASR was measured 3 days prior to injury (baseline; day −3) and on days 1, 14, and 30 post injury using a Med Associates Acoustic Response Test System (Med Associates, Georgia, VT) consisting of weight-sensitive platforms inside individual sound-attenuated chambers. Each mouse was placed individually in a ventilated holding cage that restricted extensive locomotion, but allowed them to turn around and make small movements. Animal movements in response to stimuli were measured as a voltage change by a strain gauge inside each platform. Responses were recorded by an interfaced Nexlink computer as the maximum response occurring during the no-stimulus periods, during the pre-pulse period, and during the

startle period. Startle stimuli ranged from 100 to 110 dB and were white noise bursts of 20 msec duration sometimes preceded 100 msec by 68, 79, or 90 dB 1 kHz pure tones (pre-pulses). Each stimulus combination was presented six times. The total testing period was about 20 min.

## Behavior Data Analysis

Analysis of covariance (ANCOVA) and repeated measures analysis of covariance (rmANCOVA) were conducted for each of the behavioral variables, covarying for baseline scores to account for any baseline differences. NSS-R data were analyzed by a change score (1 day post injury – Baseline) [44]. OFL data were separated into three subscales: horizontal activity, center time, and vertical activity. The 100 dB ASR data were analyzed. All tests were two tailed using alpha = .05. Data for all the behavior analysis is presented as mean ± standard error mean (SEM).

## MiRNA expression profiles in serum

To determine the effect of acute injury on the circulating miRNA expression profile, serum was collected via cardiac puncture at 3 hr post injury. 600–800 µl of blood was collected in the MiniCollect tube (Cat# 450472, Greiner Bio-One GmbH, Austria) and was allowed to clot at room temperature for 30–45 min. Serum was collected by centrifuging the blood samples at 3000 g/10 min at 4°C and immediately stored at −80°C. Total RNA enriched with miRNA was isolated from serum using miRNeasy Serum/Plasma Kit (Cat# 217184; Qiagen Inc. CA). MiRNA concentration was determined by Bioanalyzer (Agilent Technologies, Inc., Santa Clara, CA). Five ng of miRNA was taken for synthesizing complementary miRNA using the TaqMan MicroRNA Reverse Transcription (RT) Kit (Cat# 4366596; Life Technologies, Carlsbad, CA). For each sample, the following RT reaction mixture was set: 0.27 µl dNTP (100 M), 1 µl RT buffer (10X), 1.2 µl MgCl$_2$ (25 mM), 0.14 µl RNase inhibitor (20 U/µl), 2 µl RT enzyme (50 U/µl), and 1 µl Megaplex RT Primers (either Rodent Primer Pool A [Cat# 4399826] or Rodent Primer Pool B V 3.0 [Cat# 4444299]). Five ng of miRNA in 3 µl volume was then mixed with the above 7 µl RT master mix to make a final reaction volume of 10 µl for each of the Pool A and B reaction. RT reaction was carried out on Veriti 96-Well Thermal Cycler (Life technologies, Carlsbad CA) as: [16°C/2 min; 42°C/1 min; 50°C/1 sec] X 40 cycles; 85°C/5 min; and hold at 4°C. Pre-amplification of the RT reaction was done as follows: Pre-amp master mix was made by mixing 12.5 µl TaqMan Pre-Amp Master Mix (2X) (Cat# 4384266); 2.5 µl of Megaplex Pre-Amp Rodent Primer (either Pool A [Cat# 4399922] or Pool B V 3.0 [Cat# 4444309]); and 5 µl nuclease free water. Five µl of RT reaction of either Pool A or Pool B was mixed with the 20 µl of the above respective Pre-amp master mix. Pre-amp reaction was carried out on Veriti 96-Well Thermal Cycler (Life technologies,

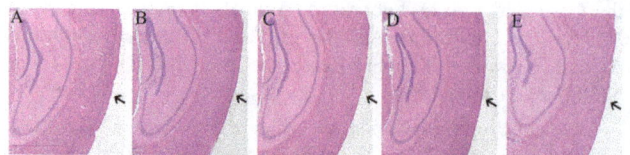

**Figure 1. H&E stained sections of the brain.** Histological evaluation of the brain tissue at the site of injury (arrow) was done to check for the lesion in the brain tissue following mTBI. No significant difference was observed in brain tissue sections between the sham (A), IS1 (B), IS2 (C), IS3 (D) and IS4 (E). Scale is 1 mm.

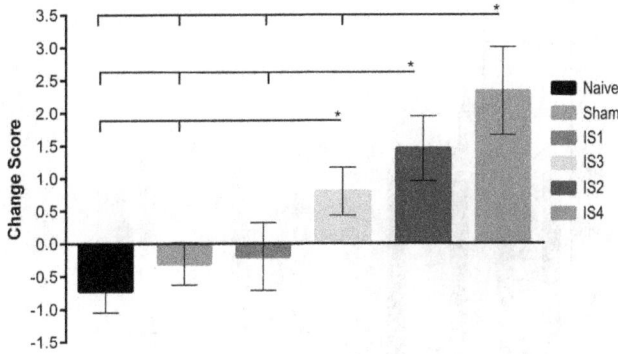

**Figure 2. NSS-R for animals at day 1 post injury.** Change scores between day 1 post injury and baseline were calculated. A gradual, but significant increase in the NSS-R scores were observed day 1 post injury with the increased severity of the injury within the mild spectrum. As expected, naïve and sham groups did not show any increase in their NSS-R scores. No change was observed in the IS1 group. NSS-R score of IS2, IS3, and IS4 groups increased and was the highest among the IS4 group. * P value <0.05.

Carlsbad CA) as: 95°C/10 min; 55°C/2 min; 72°C/2 min; [95°C/15 sec; 60°C/4 min] X 14 cycles; 99.9°C/10 min; and held at 4°C.

MiRNA profile was carried out using the TaqMan Rodent MicroRNA Array Set v3.0 (Life Technologies, Carlsbad, CA) as per manufacturer's protocol. Briefly, for each of the Pool A and B reactions, 9 µl of the pre-amp reaction product was mixed with 450 µl of TaqMan Universal Master Mix, no UNG (Cat# 4440040), and 441 µl of nuclease free water. Each of the reaction mixes was then loaded onto the respective pool's miRNA array plate. PCR reaction was carried out as 94.5°C/10 min; [97.0°C/ 30 sec; 59.7°C/1 min] X 40 cycles on 7900 HT Fast Real Time PCR machine (Life Technologies, Carlsbad, CA).

## Data analysis of miRNA array

MiRNA array threshold cycle (Ct) values were imported into the Real-Time StatMiner Software V.4.5.0.7 (Integromics, Madison, WI) for further analysis. StatMiner software allows merger of both plates A and B of the sample. Samples were grouped according to the weight and the fall height of the injury: IS1, IS2, IS3, IS4, and sham control. Imputation for missing values was skipped, and data were filtered for Ct <36 and "1 or more failure in 6 replicates". Therefore, miRNAs that had Ct value <36 in all the six biological replicates were considered "expressed" and were taken for further analysis. Data were normalized using the "global normalization" as described elsewhere [45]. Relative quantitation (RQ) of the expression data was done over the sham controls and miRNAs that had more than 1.5 fold modulation with a *P value* <0.05 were considered as significantly modulated miRNAs. For the miRNAs where expression was absent (*i.e.*, Ct>36), the fold differences were calculated using the actual Ct value, with the maximum being 40. The "Ct status" is given as "calibrator not detected" or "target not detected" for expression being absent in "sham" or "injured" groups respectively. Ct status was given "valid" when the miRNA expression was detected (Ct<36) in both the "sham" and "injured" groups.

For the identification of miRNAs that may be used as "stably expressed miRNA" for validation of serum miRNA array data, the following approach was taken [46]: Ct values of all miRNAs across the samples, including both the injury and the sham groups, were

taken. Mean and median Ct were calculated for each of the miRNA along with the standard deviation (SD). All miRNAs that had SD values >1 were eliminated. Remaining miRNAs were checked for similar average and median values and those differences greater than 0.5 were eliminated. Remaining miRNAs were checked for the mean Ct range of 14–20 to ensure abundant expression of the miRNA.

## Validation of individual miRNA expression

Expression of miRNAs, miR-214, miR-376a and miR-199a-3p was validated using the singleplex miRNA assay (Life technologies, Carlsbad, CA; Assay# 002306, 001069 and 002304, respectively). MiRNA miR-16 and miR-1937b were used as stable endogenous controls (Life Technologies, Carlsbad, CA; Assay# 000391 and 241023 respectively). A multiplex PCR was performed on 5 ng of miRNA as per manufacturer's protocol. A multiplex RT primer pool was prepared by mixing 10 µl of individual 5 X RT primers for each miRNA. 1X TE was added to make a final volume of 1000 µl. Multiplex RT reaction was set using the TaqMan MicroRNA Reverse Transcription (RT) Kit Cat# 4366596; Life Technologies, Carlsbad, CA) as follows: 6 µl of above multiplex RT primer pool; 0.3 µl of dNTP with dTTP (100 M); 3 µl of RT enzyme (50 U/µl); 1.5 µl of 10X RT buffer; 0.19 µl of RNAse inhibitor (20 U/µl); and 3 µl of RNA (5 ng). RT was carried out on Veriti 96-Well Thermal Cycler (Life technologies, Carlsbad CA) as follows: 16°C/30 min; 42°C/30 min; 85°C/5 min; and held at 4°C. For pre-amplification of RT product, multiplex pre-amplification primer pool was prepared by mixing 10 µl of individual 20X TaqMan assay primer for each miRNA. 1X TE was added to make a final volume of 1000 µl. Pre-amplification reaction was set as follows: 12.5 µl TaqMan Pre-Amp Master Mix (2X) (Cat# 4384266); 3.75 µl of above multiplex pre-amplification primer pool; 3.75 µl nuclease free water; and 5 µl of multiplex RT reaction product. Pre-amp reaction was carried out on Veriti 96-Well Thermal Cycler (Life technologies, Carlsbad CA) as: 95°C/ 10 min; 55°C/2 min; 72°C/2 min; [95°C/15 sec; 60°C/4 min] X 14 cycles; 99.9°C/10 min; and held at 4°C. Individual miRNA real time PCR was set in triplicates as follows: 10 µl of 2X TaqMan Universal Master Mix, no UNG (Cat# 4440040); 1 µl of 20X TaqMan Assay of miRNA; 7.67 µl nuclease free water; and 1.33 µl of multiplex pre-amp product (1:5 diluted). Real Time PCR reaction was carried out as: 50°C/2 min; 95°C/10 min; [95°C/30 sec; 60°C/1 min] X 40 cycles on 7900 HT Fast Real Time PCR machine (Life Technologies, Carlsbad, CA). Three biological repeats were performed for each of the miRNAs and data are presented as fold change values using the comparative Ct method $(2^{-(\text{mean } \Delta\Delta Ct)})$ values.

## Histology of brain sections

Following blood collection for the miRNA study, whole brains were harvested from mice and fixed in 10% normal buffered formalin. Fixed brain tissues were then processed, paraffin embedded, and 5 micron sections were cut at the hippocampus level and stained with H&E (Histoserv Inc., Germantown, MD). Sections were then evaluated under bright field microscopy.

## Results

### Mortality associated with the initial impact increased with the height of fall and rod weight

Animal mortality immediately after the impact with the falling weight increased with increase in the height of the fall and the weight of the rod. The percent mortality was 6.7±2.29, 41.3±5.4, 33.±14.11, and 65.9±11.5 in IS1, IS2, IS3, and IS4, respectively.

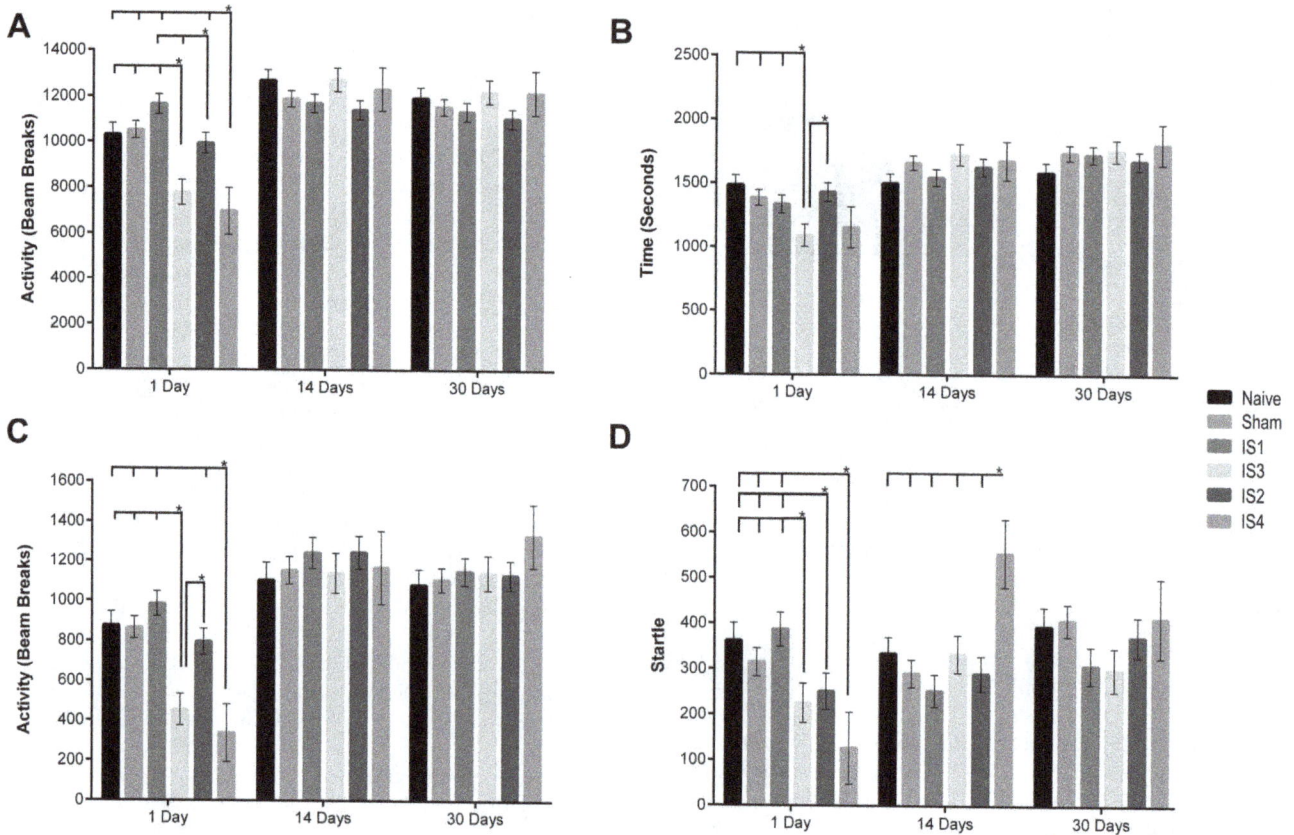

**Figure 3. Neurobehavioral Activity.** OFL test was conducted to evaluate animals' various activities in an open field as a measurement of behavioral deficits. Overall, day 1 showed significant reductions in the activities of injured animals as compared to the naïve and sham controls except for the IS1 group, which was not significantly different from that of naïve and sham groups. (**A**) Horizontal activity was evaluated as an indicator of the overall health. Activity was significantly reduced in the IS3 and IS4 groups. Activity in the IS2 group was significantly reduced as compared to the activity of IS1. Activity of IS1 and IS2 groups were not significantly different from the sham group. (**B**) Time spent in the center of the open field was evaluated as an indicator of anxiety-like behavior. Center time of the animals in IS3 and IS4 groups was reduced as compared to the 246 g injury groups (*i.e.*, IS1 and IS2), sham and naïve animals. The reduction in activity reached significance in the IS3. (**C**) Vertical activity was measured as an indicator of depression-related behavior. Vertical activity of the injured animals was significantly less than that of the sham and naïve animals except the IS1 group. * *P value* <0.05. (**D**) Startle response was measured as an indicator of emotional distress and potential sensory gating impairments. Startle responses of all injured groups, except the IS1 group, were reduced when compared to naïve and sham groups at day 1 post injury. There were no differences between groups at days 14 and 30 post injury, except in the IS4 group where the startle response was significantly higher than all other groups at day 14 post injury. Values are expressed as Mean ± SEM. * *P value* <0.05.

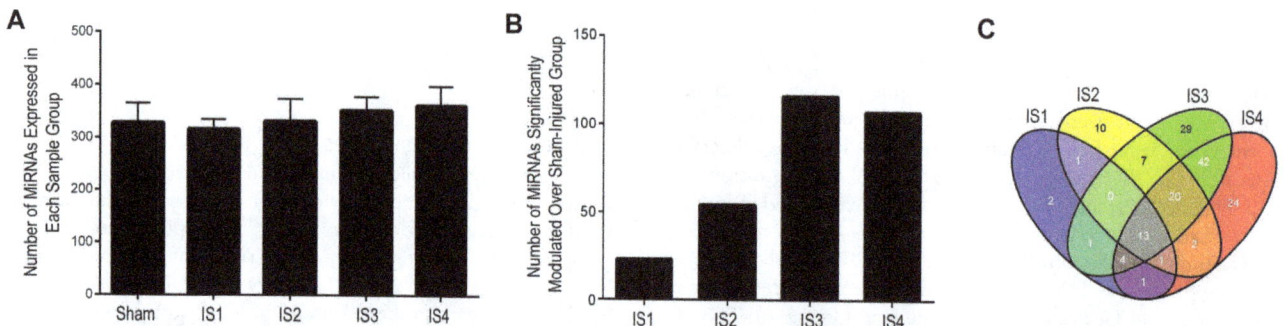

**Figure 4. MiRNA expression pattern.** (A) MiRNAs that show Ct<36 were considered as expressed. The number of miRNAs expressed ranged from 315.83−362.17 with a maximum and minimum numbers detected in IS4 and IS1 respectively. The SD ranged from 19.28−43.37, the maximum being in IS2 and the minimum in IS1. The values are presented as Mean ± SD of the number of miRNAs detected in each group. (B) The number of miRNAs that were significantly modulated (≥1.5 fold; P<0.05) following the injury over the time point matched sham controls increased with the height and weight of the free falling metal rod except in the IS3 group where the number of significantly modulated miRNAs was marginally greater than the IS4 group. (C) Overlapping miRNA data analysis for significantly modulated miRNAs in the injury groups was done using the online Venn diagram generation tool [Oliveros (2007). VENNY. An interactive tool for comparing lists with Venn Diagrams. http://bioinfogp.cnb.csic.es/tools/venny/index.html].

**Table 1.** Significantly modulated miRNA in IS1.

| S. No. | MiRNA | P Value | Fold Difference(log10 [RQ]) |
|---|---|---|---|
| **Calibrator not detected** | | | |
| 1 | mmu-miR-376a | 9.43E-04 | 1.99 |
| 2 | mmu-miR-494 | 1.85E-04 | 1.94 |
| 3 | mmu-miR-297a# | 3.11E-02 | 1.56 |
| 4 | rno-miR-345-3p | 4.78E-03 | 1.08 |
| **Valid** | | | |
| 5 | hsa-miR-214 | 1.82E-03 | 0.58 |
| 6 | mmu-miR-214 | 6.37E-03 | 0.54 |
| 7 | mmu-miR-337-5p | 2.10E-02 | 0.52 |
| 8 | mmu-miR-574-3p | 2.16E-02 | 0.51 |
| 9 | mmu-miR-434-3p | 2.16E-02 | 0.41 |
| 10 | mmu-miR-671-3p | 1.76E-02 | 0.39 |
| 11 | mmu-miR-218 | 4.46E-02 | 0.36 |
| 12 | mmu-miR-676 | 1.58E-02 | 0.33 |
| 13 | mmu-miR-199a-3p | 3.34E-02 | 0.32 |
| 14 | hsa-miR-455 | 4.71E-02 | 0.28 |
| 15 | mmu-miR-322 | 9.85E-03 | −0.34 |
| 16 | mmu-miR-331-3p | 1.99E-02 | −0.35 |
| 17 | hsa-miR-106b# | 2.80E-02 | −0.40 |
| 18 | mmu-miR-106b | 1.41E-02 | −0.47 |
| 19 | mmu-miR-2138 | 5.83E-03 | −0.61 |
| 20 | mmu-miR-31 | 2.16E-02 | −0.85 |
| **Target not detected** | | | |
| 21 | mmu-miR-363 | 4.59E-02 | −1.40 |
| 22 | mmu-miR-181c | 2.86E-02 | −1.66 |
| 23 | rno-miR-196c | 4.66E-02 | −1.81 |

Twenty three miRNA were significantly modulated. Of these 14 were up regulated and 9 were down regulated. Values are given as Log10 of the fold change ($2^{-(mean \Delta\Delta Ct)}$).

No mortality was observed in the injured groups at the later time points in the experiment. Apnea immediately after the impact occurs in rodent model of weight drop injury and resuscitation with oxygen mask and gentle rubbing of the chest cavity improves recovery from the impact [25,47–48]. The immediate mortality in the injury groups may have occurred due to the respiratory arrest upon impact [25]. The High mortality rate in our study as compared to the previously described similar model may be due to the slight modification to the impactor tip. Specifically, a silicon/resin covering was used in the previously described model [25], whereas no such covering was used in our system. H&E staining of the brain section at the hippocampus level (site of injury) did not reveal lesion volume in any of the injured groups, indicating mild brain injury in the animals that survived the initial impact of the injury (Figure 1).

### NSS-R scores increased with the increase in the fall height and weight

NSS-R scores were determined by measuring behaviors of the naïve, sham, and injured animals in a series of 10 tasks to evaluate neurobehavioral effects of acute injury. NSS-R was measured at day −3 (baseline) and day 1 post injury. Significant increases in NSS-R change scores were observed with increasing severity of the injury (Figure 2). There were significant differences among injury groups, $F(5,92) = 6.04$, $P<.001$, $\eta^2 = .247$. NSS-R change scores and group comparisons are presented in Table S2.

### Open field activity of the animals is reduced following the injury

Horizontal activity of the animals was taken as a measure of the overall health of the animals prior to injury and after the injury. Activity was measured as the number of beam breaks during a 1 hr session. Overall, there was a significant Time x Injury interaction, $F(8.33,245.14) = 7.69$, $P<.001$, $\eta^2 = .207$ (sphericity violated, used Greenhouse-Geisser correction). At 1 day post injury, there were significant differences among injury groups, $F(5,149) = 8.46$, $P<.001$, $\eta^2 = .221$ (Figure 3A), such that the activity in IS2, IS3 and IS4 was reduced as compared to the naïve, sham, and IS1 groups. No significant differences were observed among the naïve, sham, and injury groups at 14 and 30 days post injury. Horizontal activity and comparisons among the groups appear in Table S3.

The time spent in the center of the open field was taken as a measurement of anxiety-related behavior. There was a significant effect of Time, $F(2,294) = 16.26$, $P<.001$, $\eta^2 = .100$ (Table S4). There also was a significant Time × Injury interaction, $F(10,294) = 3.45$, $P<.001$, $\eta^2 = .105$. At day 1 post injury, there were significant differences among injury groups, $F(5,148) = 2.97$,

**Table 2.** Significantly modulated miRNA in IS2.

| S.No. | MiRNA | P Value | Fold Difference (log10 [RQ]) |
|---|---|---|---|
| **Calibrator not detected** | | | |
| 1 | mmu-miR-700 | 2.31E-02 | 2.21 |
| 2 | mmu-miR-487b | 2.17E-03 | 1.91 |
| 3 | mmu-miR-376a | 1.11E-03 | 1.70 |
| 4 | mmu-miR-125b | 4.32E-02 | 1.23 |
| 5 | mmu-miR-1932 | 2.25E-02 | 1.17 |
| 6 | mmu-miR-218-1 | 3.42E-02 | 1.05 |
| 7 | mmu-miR-191* | 1.79E-02 | 1.00 |
| **Valid** | | | |
| 8 | mmu-miR-384-5p | 6.70E-03 | 0.73 |
| 9 | hsa-miR-214 | 2.58E-05 | 0.72 |
| 10 | mmu-miR-667 | 5.12E-03 | 0.69 |
| 11 | mmu-miR-218 | 1.82E-04 | 0.64 |
| 12 | mmu-miR-214 | 8.97E-05 | 0.64 |
| 13 | mmu-miR-434-3p | 3.91E-03 | 0.61 |
| 14 | mmu-miR-122 | 1.59E-03 | 0.61 |
| 15 | mmu-miR-34b-3p | 3.05E-03 | 0.60 |
| 16 | mmu-miR-872* | 9.36E-03 | 0.56 |
| 17 | mmu-miR-361 | 8.35E-03 | 0.55 |
| 18 | mmu-miR-485-3p | 2.64E-02 | 0.53 |
| 19 | mmu-miR-574-3p | 2.61E-03 | 0.53 |
| 20 | hsa-miR-9* | 4.56E-02 | 0.52 |
| 21 | mmu-miR-337-5p | 9.90E-03 | 0.49 |
| 22 | mmu-miR-685 | 3.22E-03 | 0.48 |
| 23 | mmu-miR-204 | 1.44E-02 | 0.44 |
| 24 | mmu-miR-376c | 2.57E-02 | 0.43 |
| 25 | mmu-miR-199a-3p | 2.91E-03 | 0.42 |
| 26 | mmu-miR-337-3p | 2.11E-02 | 0.40 |
| 27 | mmu-miR-132 | 4.27E-02 | 0.40 |
| 28 | mmu-miR-671-3p | 1.04E-02 | 0.37 |
| 29 | mmu-miR-152 | 1.58E-02 | 0.36 |
| 30 | mmu-miR-376b* | 1.29E-02 | 0.34 |
| 31 | mmu-miR-212 | 3.85E-02 | 0.32 |
| 32 | mmu-miR-511 | 1.48E-02 | 0.31 |
| 33 | mmu-miR-192 | 2.19E-03 | 0.30 |
| 34 | mmu-miR-145 | 2.81E-02 | 0.25 |
| 35 | mmu-miR-146a | 3.56E-02 | 0.24 |
| 36 | mmu-miR-19b | 3.57E-02 | −0.25 |
| 37 | mmu-miR-322 | 3.22E-02 | −0.26 |
| 38 | hsa-miR-200c | 1.20E-02 | −0.26 |
| 39 | mmu-miR-486 | 2.56E-02 | −0.27 |
| 40 | mmu-miR-1274a | 3.52E-02 | −0.28 |
| 41 | hsa-miR-200b | 4.62E-02 | −0.30 |
| 42 | mmu-miR-2146 | 2.90E-02 | −0.30 |
| 43 | mmu-miR-652 | 1.91E-02 | −0.30 |
| 44 | mmu-miR-18a | 2.17E-02 | −0.34 |
| 45 | hsa-miR-106b* | 9.68E-03 | −0.38 |
| 46 | mmu-miR-451 | 1.48E-02 | −0.42 |
| 47 | mmu-miR-106b | 7.93E-03 | −0.45 |
| 48 | mmu-miR-26b | 3.19E-02 | −0.53 |

**Table 2.** Cont.

| S.No. | MiRNA | P Value | Fold Difference (log10 [RQ]) |
|---|---|---|---|
| 49 | mmu-miR-31 | 1.86E-02 | −1.03 |
| 50 | hsa-miR-875-5p | 4.14E-02 | −3.02 |
| **Target not detected** | | | |
| 51 | rno-miR-196c | 4.67E-02 | −1.53 |
| 52 | mmu-miR-1982.2 | 3.95E-02 | −1.56 |
| 53 | mmu-miR-7a | 8.20E-03 | −1.98 |

Fifty three miRNA were significantly modulated. Of these, 35 were up regulated and 18 were down regulated. Values are given as Log10 of the fold change ($2^{-(\text{mean} \Delta\Delta Ct)}$).

$P = .014$, $\eta^2 = .091$ (Figure 3B), such that the center time was significantly reduced in the IS3 group as compared to the naïve, sham, IS1, and IS2 groups. At 14 and 30 days post injury, no significant differences between the control and injured groups were observed. Center time of each group and comparisons among groups appear in Table S5.

Vertical activity was taken as a measure of depression-related behavior such that less vertical activity is associated with more depression (*i.e.*, learned helplessness). Overall, there was a significant effect of Time, $F_{(2,294)} = 16.20$, $P < .001$, $\eta^2 = .099$ (Table S6). There was also a significant Time x Injury interaction, $F_{(10,294)} = 4.45$, $P < .001$, $\eta^2 = .131$ (Figure 3C). At 1 day post injury, there were significant differences among injury groups, $F_{(5,148)} = 7.32$, $p < .001$, $\eta 2 = .198$, such that the vertical activity in IS3 and IS4 groups was significantly reduced as compared to naïve, sham, IS1, and IS2 groups. No significant differences were observed between naïve, sham, and various injury groups at 14 and 30 days post injury. The vertical activity of each group and comparisons among groups appear in Table S7.

The overall negative effect on general health and vertical activity of the mouse was also evaluated as the percent of animals in injury groups that showed reduced activity compared to the naïve group at day 1 post injury. Each group was evaluated for the number of animals that showed activity less than the lower limit of the baseline activity of naïve animals. Overall, the more severe the injury, the greater percentage of the animals that showed reduced activity in the open field (Figure S2). To eliminate motor activity loss as a cause of reduced activity, animals were subjected to the rotarod test, which showed no significant differences between the various control and injury groups (Figure S3). No apparent signs of pain such as ruffled fur, hunched posture, altered behavior, vocalization, lethargy, tremors, ataxia *etc.* that may affect the activity of the injured mice were observed in the animals.

### Acoustic startle response was reduced in the animals following injury

Startle response of animals to a 100 dB tone was measured and is presented. Overall, when looking at the responses to a 100 dB tone alone, there was a significant Time x Injury interaction, $F_{(10,264)} = 3.72$, $P < .001$, $\eta^2 = .123$, such that a lower startle response was observed in the injured animals at day 1 post injury except in the IS4 group, and the response increased by day 14 and 30 post injury (Figure 3D). At day 1 post injury, there were significant differences among injury groups, $F_{(5,132)} = 3.54$, $P = .005$, $\eta^2 = .118$ (Table S8). On day 14 post injury, there were significant differences among injury groups, $F_{(5,132)} = 2.95$, $P = .015$, $\eta^2 = .100$ (Table S9). No significant differences were

observed between naïve, sham, and various injury groups at 30 days post injury.

### Serum miRNAs are modulated in injured animals

To determine whether miRNAs were modulated after the injury, serum miRNA expression of the injured mice was compared to the serum miRNA expression of the sham mice at 3 hr post injury. The numbers of the miRNA that passed the detection criteria were similar among the injured and sham groups (Figure 4A). However, the number of significantly modulated miRNAs increased with the increasing grade of injury except in the IS4 injury group where the numbers of significantly modulated miRNA were marginally less than the IS3 injury group (Figure 4B). 23 miRNAs (14 up- and 9 down- regulated) were significantly modulated in IS1 injury group (Table 1). 53 miRNAs (35 up- and 18 down-regulated) were significantly modulated in IS2 injury group (Table 2). 116 miRNAs (70 up- and 46 down-regulated) were significantly modulated in IS3 injury group (Table 3). 106 miRNAs (66 up- and 40 down-regulated) were significantly modulated in IS4 injury group (Table 4). Hierarchical clustering of the DDCt values of the expressed miRNAs showed IS3 and IS4 (*i.e.*, 333 g groups) were similar to each other followed by the association with the IS2. The IS1 group clustered away from the rest of the three injury groups (Figure S4). This observation was consistent with the behavior data where the IS1 group did not show any significant differences from the sham group.

### Common miRNA changes regardless of the mTBI severity

To identify miRNAs that may consistently be present regardless of extent or severity of the injury, significantly modulated miRNAs were compared among the injury groups (Figure 4C). 13 miRNAs were found to be modulated in all four injury groups and had similar expression patterns. Nine of the 13 miRNAs were up regulated and 4 were down regulated following injury (Table 5). The Ct values of the modulated miRNAs are given in Table S10.

### Brain function specific miRNAs are modulated following mTBI

The miRNAs common among all mTBI groups were analyzed for their combined effect on functional pathways using the DIANA-miRPath v2.0 [49]. Kyoto Encyclopedia of Genes and Genomes (KEGG) pathways that were most significantly predicted to be affected by the combined effect of the modulated miRNAs were identified. Several brain function related pathways, such as axon guidance, gap junction, dopaminergic synapse, cholinergic synapse, long-term potentiation, tight junction, adherens junction,

**Table 3.** Significantly modulated miRNA in IS3.

| S.No | MiRNA | P Value | Fold Difference (log10 [RQ]) |
|---|---|---|---|
| **Calibrator not detected** | | | |
| 1 | mmu-miR-15a* | 1.8E-13 | 4.57 |
| 2 | mmu-miR-495 | 1.5E-03 | 2.87 |
| 3 | mmu-miR-673 | 3.0E-02 | 2.66 |
| 4 | mmu-miR-433 | 9.8E-04 | 2.63 |
| 5 | mmu-miR-146b | 2.7E-02 | 2.48 |
| 6 | mmu-miR-702 | 2.4E-02 | 2.24 |
| 7 | mmu-miR-10a | 2.6E-02 | 2.22 |
| 8 | mmu-miR-700 | 2.4E-02 | 2.2 |
| 9 | mmu-miR-134 | 1.9E-02 | 2.09 |
| 10 | mmu-miR-487b | 1.3E-03 | 2.01 |
| 11 | mmu-miR-494 | 7.3E-05 | 1.96 |
| 12 | hsa-miR-99b* | 7.7E-03 | 1.87 |
| 13 | mmu-miR-551b | 2.1E-03 | 1.75 |
| 14 | mmu-miR-376a | 7.1E-04 | 1.72 |
| 15 | rno-miR-551B | 5.7E-03 | 1.62 |
| 16 | mmu-miR-434-5p | 2.9E-02 | 1.61 |
| 17 | rno-miR-204* | 1.7E-02 | 1.6 |
| 18 | mmu-miR-467b | 1.6E-02 | 1.6 |
| 19 | mmu-miR-137 | 2.7E-02 | 1.54 |
| 20 | rno-miR-345-3p | 2.0E-03 | 1.41 |
| 21 | mmu-miR-547 | 4.1E-02 | 1.3 |
| 22 | mmu-miR-680 | 4.8E-02 | 1.14 |
| 23 | mmu-miR-218-1* | 3.0E-02 | 1.1 |
| 24 | mmu-miR-345-3p | 3.4E-02 | 1.09 |
| 25 | mmu-miR-295 | 2.6E-02 | 1.09 |
| 26 | rno-miR-351 | 6.3E-03 | 0.89 |
| **Valid** | | | |
| 27 | mmu-miR-122 | 2.2E-04 | 1.24 |
| 28 | mmu-miR-872 | 2.6E-02 | 0.98 |
| 29 | mmu-miR-667 | 7.9E-04 | 0.91 |
| 30 | mmu-miR-214 | 2.4E-07 | 0.88 |
| 31 | mmu-miR-485-3p | 5.1E-04 | 0.83 |
| 32 | mmu-miR-365 | 9.5E-03 | 0.83 |
| 33 | mmu-miR-384-5p | 9.8E-04 | 0.78 |
| 34 | mmu-miR-337-5p | 1.0E-05 | 0.77 |
| 35 | mmu-miR-193* | 7.4E-03 | 0.74 |
| 36 | mmu-miR-671-3p | 2.1E-05 | 0.72 |
| 37 | hsa-miR-214 | 2.5E-05 | 0.71 |
| 38 | mmu-miR-574-3p | 4.2E-05 | 0.71 |
| 39 | mmu-miR-192 | 3.5E-03 | 0.64 |
| 40 | mmu-miR-434-3p | 7.2E-05 | 0.64 |
| 41 | mmu-miR-685 | 3.1E-04 | 0.63 |
| 42 | mmu-miR-193 | 3.5E-02 | 0.62 |
| 43 | mmu-miR-872* | 2.8E-03 | 0.6 |
| 44 | mmu-let-7a* | 4.4E-03 | 0.6 |
| 45 | mmu-miR-410 | 4.8E-03 | 0.58 |
| 46 | mmu-miR-125b-5p | 1.6E-02 | 0.57 |
| 47 | mmu-miR-218 | 1.3E-03 | 0.54 |
| 48 | mmu-miR-34b-3p | 2.5E-04 | 0.54 |

**Table 3.** Cont.

| S.No | MiRNA | P Value | Fold Difference (log10 [RQ]) |
|---|---|---|---|
| 49 | mmu-miR-145 | 1.2E-03 | 0.53 |
| 50 | mmu-miR-500 | 8.2E-05 | 0.51 |
| 51 | mmu-miR-132 | 6.0E-03 | 0.48 |
| 52 | mmu-miR-127 | 3.3E-02 | 0.46 |
| 53 | mmu-miR-125a-5p | 3.1E-03 | 0.46 |
| 54 | mmu-miR-199a-3p | 1.4E-03 | 0.46 |
| 55 | mmu-miR-706 | 2.0E-02 | 0.44 |
| 56 | hsa-miR-671-5p | 1.8E-02 | 0.44 |
| 57 | mmu-miR-152 | 2.4E-03 | 0.44 |
| 58 | mmu-miR-1944 | 4.0E-02 | 0.42 |
| 59 | mmu-miR-361 | 2.7E-02 | 0.38 |
| 60 | mmu-miR-376c | 8.4E-03 | 0.37 |
| 61 | mmu-miR-362-3p | 4.0E-02 | 0.37 |
| 62 | hsa-miR-744* | 7.7E-03 | 0.36 |
| 63 | hsa-miR-455 | 3.0E-02 | 0.35 |
| 64 | mmu-miR-31* | 2.4E-02 | 0.35 |
| 65 | mmu-miR-674* | 4.3E-02 | 0.34 |
| 66 | mmu-miR-204 | 4.2E-03 | 0.32 |
| 67 | mmu-miR-212 | 2.4E-02 | 0.29 |
| 68 | mmu-miR-532-3p | 2.9E-02 | 0.28 |
| 69 | mmu-miR-511 | 2.8E-02 | 0.26 |
| 70 | mmu-miR-1839-3p | 4.9E-02 | 0.19 |
| 71 | mmu-miR-200c | 4.7E-02 | −0.22 |
| 72 | mmu-miR-484 | 2.7E-02 | −0.23 |
| 73 | mmu-miR-18a* | 1.6E-03 | −0.25 |
| 74 | hsa-miR-425 | 4.7E-02 | −0.26 |
| 75 | mmu-miR-1930 | 3.6E-02 | −0.26 |
| 76 | mmu-miR-301a | 4.2E-02 | −0.26 |
| 77 | mmu-miR-2134 | 3.9E-03 | −0.28 |
| 78 | mmu-miR-19b | 1.3E-02 | −0.29 |
| 79 | mmu-miR-222 | 4.6E-02 | −0.31 |
| 80 | mmu-miR-141 | 3.9E-02 | −0.33 |
| 81 | hsa-miR-200c | 2.1E-03 | −0.33 |
| 82 | mmu-miR-106a | 2.0E-02 | −0.34 |
| 83 | mmu-miR-130b | 5.5E-03 | −0.34 |
| 84 | mmu-miR-486 | 1.7E-02 | −0.35 |
| 85 | mmu-miR-17 | 9.6E-03 | −0.39 |
| 86 | mmu-miR-331-3p | 1.3E-02 | −0.41 |
| 87 | mmu-miR-652 | 7.1E-03 | −0.41 |
| 88 | mmu-let-7d | 7.6E-03 | −0.41 |
| 89 | mmu-miR-17* | 9.6E-03 | −0.43 |
| 90 | mmu-miR-16 | 2.7E-02 | −0.43 |
| 91 | hsa-miR-421 | 6.9E-04 | −0.43 |
| 92 | mmu-miR-345-5p | 2.4E-03 | −0.43 |
| 93 | mmu-miR-18a | 1.6E-03 | −0.43 |
| 94 | mmu-miR-103 | 2.1E-02 | −0.44 |
| 95 | mmu-miR-25 | 4.3E-03 | −0.47 |
| 96 | mmu-miR-93 | 4.8E-03 | −0.47 |
| 97 | mmu-miR-140 | 1.7E-02 | −0.48 |

**Table 3.** Cont.

| S.No | MiRNA | P Value | Fold Difference (log10 [RQ]) |
|---|---|---|---|
| 98 | mmu-let-7i | 1.5E-03 | −0.48 |
| 99 | mmu-miR-20a | 8.0E-04 | −0.48 |
| 100 | mmu-miR-20b | 2.5E-02 | −0.49 |
| 101 | mmu-miR-340-5p | 2.0E-02 | −0.5 |
| 102 | mmu-miR-186* | 1.6E-02 | −0.51 |
| 103 | mmu-miR-301b | 7.0E-03 | −0.54 |
| 104 | mmu-miR-15b | 5.0E-04 | −0.54 |
| 105 | mmu-miR-26a | 4.1E-03 | −0.57 |
| 106 | mmu-miR-142-3p | 4.2E-03 | −0.6 |
| 107 | mmu-miR-26b | 7.4E-03 | −0.63 |
| 108 | hsa-miR-106b* | 5.9E-05 | −0.64 |
| 109 | mmu-miR-451 | 5.0E-05 | −0.78 |
| 110 | mmu-miR-106b | 4.2E-05 | −0.83 |
| 111 | mmu-miR-31 | 2.4E-02 | −0.87 |
| 112 | hsa-miR-875-5p | 2.5E-02 | −3.16 |
| **Target not detected** | | | |
| 113 | rno-miR-196c | 2.2E-02 | −1.39 |
| 114 | mmu-miR-463 | 2.2E-03 | −1.75 |
| 115 | mmu-let-7e | 3.7E-02 | −1.98 |
| 116 | mmu-miR-363 | 4.4E-03 | −2.95 |

One hundred and sixteen miRNA were significantly modulated. Of these, 70 were up regulated and 46 were down regulated. Values are given as Log10 of the fold change $(2^{-(\text{mean } \Delta\Delta Ct)})$.

and long-term depression, were found to be targeted by the modulated miRNAs (Figure S5). Specific analysis of the axon guidance pathway, previously reported as affected upon TBI, showed that the number of the miRNAs predicted to be involved in this pathway increased with the severity of the injury (Figure 5). The combined effect of modulated miRNAs on functional pathways using the DIANA-miRPath v2.0 [49] was also performed for the significantly modulated miRNAs common among the three injury groups that showed significant change in NSS-R, OFL, and ASR tests (*i.e.*, IS2, IS3, and IS4) (Table S11). The axon guidance pathway, along with several other brain related function pathways, was one of the most affected KEGG Pathway (Figure S6). Unique miRNAs that were modulated only in the IS1 group (Table S12), which did not show any significantly difference in NSS-R and OFL tests, showed long-term potentiation pathways as the most affected pathway by DIANA-miRPath v2.0 analysis (data not shown).

Correlation analysis of the modulated miRNAs and their validated targets by the IPA software revealed a direct relation with validated targets of six of the modulated miRNAs to the axon guidance pathway (Figure 6). Because behavioral analysis showed symptoms of depression in the injured animals, a correlation analysis of the modulated miRNAs with depression-related pathways was performed, this showed their direct effect on the depression-related validated targets (Figure 6). The molecular pathway for sensorimotor impairments was also predicted to be targeted by the significantly modulated miRNAs (Figure 6). This correlates with the NSS-R and ASR measurements that also showed sensorimotor impairments. The expression profile of 3 out of 13 commonly modulated miRNAs, miR-199-3p, miR-214, and miR-376a that have been shown to be important in brain related

processes and functions was also validated using the singleplex miRNA assay (Life Technologies, Carlsbad, CA) (Figure 7).

## Stable miRNA expression in serum

To identify miRNAs that can be used for validating the expression data of the miRNA array, miRNAs that exhibited stable expression in the serum, irrespective of the sham or injury group, were identified. 18 miRNAs were identified that showed stable Ct values across the sham and injury groups with SD <1 (Table S13). One of the miRNAs (miR-16) has been described as stable serum miRNA in other studies [50]. Therefore, miR-16 (Mean Ct = $15.54\pm0.91$) along with another miRNAs, miR-1937b (Mean Ct = $14.91\pm0.90$) were taken for use as endogenous controls in the miRNA expression validation experiments. Similar results were obtained with either of the selected stable miRNAs (data not shown) and data presented here used miR-16 as the stable endogenous miRNA. MiR-1937b is no longer considered a miRNA as it is a tRNA-derived small RNA fragment (tRF) (http://www.mirbase.org/cgi-bin/mirna_entry.pl?acc=MI0009938). Therefore, miR-1937b (like non-coding small nuclear RNA U6), presents a target that is of non-miRNA origin and may be useful as stable endogenous small RNA to validate miRNA expression in serum.

## Discussion

MTBI is a heterogeneous injury that can range from no clinical symptoms to development of post concussive syndrome (PCS) after injury. Rapp and Curly [51] describe mTBI as an event that may lead to the development of neurological disorders. The heterogeneous nature of mTBI makes it difficult to diagnose, based exclusively on current behavioral and neurocognitive analyses

**Table 4.** Significantly modulated miRNA in IS4.

| S. No. | MiRNA | P Value | Fold Difference (log10 [RQ]) |
|--------|-------|---------|------------------------------|
| **Calibrator not detected** | | | |
| 1 | mmu-miR-15a* | 2.14E-13 | 4.47 |
| 2 | mmu-miR-129-3p | 6.98E-05 | 3.37 |
| 3 | hsa-miR-149 | 7.43E-03 | 3.33 |
| 4 | mmu-miR-187 | 1.92E-03 | 3.22 |
| 5 | mmu-miR-433 | 7.82E-04 | 2.87 |
| 6 | mmu-miR-34c | 1.08E-04 | 2.81 |
| 7 | mmu-miR-146b | 2.44E-02 | 2.52 |
| 8 | hsa-let-7e* | 3.67E-07 | 2.27 |
| 9 | mmu-miR-10a | 2.49E-02 | 2.23 |
| 10 | mmu-miR-134 | 2.06E-02 | 2.07 |
| 11 | mmu-miR-494 | 1.42E-04 | 2.02 |
| 12 | rno-miR-204* | 5.97E-03 | 1.97 |
| 13 | mmu-miR-383 | 3.11E-03 | 1.89 |
| 14 | mmu-miR-487b | 2.96E-03 | 1.87 |
| 15 | mmu-miR-376a | 4.14E-03 | 1.68 |
| 16 | mmu-miR-137 | 2.01E-02 | 1.65 |
| 17 | rno-miR-345-3p | 5.67E-04 | 1.61 |
| 18 | mmu-miR-381 | 3.45E-03 | 1.60 |
| 19 | mmu-miR-455 | 3.32E-02 | 1.59 |
| 20 | hsa-miR-99b* | 1.94E-02 | 1.58 |
| 21 | mmu-miR-125b* | 3.70E-02 | 1.28 |
| 22 | mmu-miR-345-3p | 2.48E-02 | 1.17 |
| 23 | mmu-miR-218-1* | 4.93E-02 | 0.98 |
| 24 | rno-miR-351 | 8.86E-03 | 0.86 |
| **Valid** | | | |
| 25 | mmu-miR-122 | 5.56E-05 | 1.41 |
| 26 | mmu-miR-667 | 9.46E-04 | 1.19 |
| 27 | mmu-miR-365 | 2.39E-03 | 0.93 |
| 28 | mmu-miR-34b-3p | 6.71E-04 | 0.91 |
| 29 | mmu-miR-485-3p | 3.61E-04 | 0.84 |
| 30 | mmu-miR-214 | 4.42E-07 | 0.80 |
| 31 | mmu-miR-204 | 1.71E-04 | 0.77 |
| 32 | hsa-miR-214 | 1.03E-05 | 0.75 |
| 33 | mmu-miR-193* | 1.37E-03 | 0.74 |
| 34 | mmu-miR-384-5p | 2.60E-02 | 0.74 |
| 35 | mmu-miR-125b-5p | 2.47E-03 | 0.70 |
| 36 | mmu-miR-194 | 1.78E-03 | 0.69 |
| 37 | mmu-miR-127 | 1.59E-02 | 0.69 |
| 38 | mmu-miR-671-3p | 1.94E-04 | 0.69 |
| 39 | mmu-miR-434-3p | 1.61E-03 | 0.67 |
| 40 | mmu-miR-199a-3p | 1.01E-04 | 0.62 |
| 41 | mmu-miR-132 | 6.76E-03 | 0.61 |
| 42 | mmu-miR-410 | 2.09E-02 | 0.60 |
| 43 | mmu-miR-872* | 8.59E-03 | 0.58 |
| 44 | mmu-miR-192 | 3.06E-04 | 0.57 |
| 45 | mmu-miR-145 | 1.40E-03 | 0.56 |
| 46 | hsa-miR-671-5p | 4.68E-03 | 0.53 |
| 47 | mmu-miR-574-3p | 1.26E-03 | 0.53 |

**Table 4.** Cont.

| S. No. | MiRNA | P Value | Fold Difference (log10 [RQ]) |
|---|---|---|---|
| 48 | mmu-miR-532-5p | 1.23E-02 | 0.52 |
| 49 | mmu-miR-337-5p | 5.90E-03 | 0.52 |
| 50 | mmu-miR-375 | 4.70E-02 | 0.50 |
| 51 | mmu-miR-218 | 7.99E-04 | 0.50 |
| 52 | mmu-let-7a* | 5.98E-03 | 0.49 |
| 53 | hsa-miR-455 | 2.99E-03 | 0.49 |
| 54 | mmu-miR-500 | 2.66E-03 | 0.46 |
| 55 | mmu-miR-1944 | 1.63E-02 | 0.45 |
| 56 | mmu-miR-685 | 1.30E-03 | 0.43 |
| 57 | mmu-miR-148a | 1.47E-03 | 0.42 |
| 58 | mmu-miR-212 | 3.16E-02 | 0.41 |
| 59 | mmu-miR-224 | 6.52E-03 | 0.40 |
| 60 | mmu-miR-676 | 2.96E-03 | 0.40 |
| 61 | mmu-miR-152 | 9.64E-03 | 0.40 |
| 62 | mmu-miR-200a | 4.06E-02 | 0.39 |
| 63 | hsa-miR-744* | 1.19E-02 | 0.36 |
| 64 | mmu-miR-497 | 9.60E-03 | 0.35 |
| 65 | mmu-miR-532-3p | 2.04E-02 | 0.30 |
| 66 | mmu-miR-133a | 4.79E-02 | 0.27 |
| 67 | mmu-miR-19b | 2.20E-02 | −0.27 |
| 68 | mmu-miR-28 | 1.19E-02 | −0.27 |
| 69 | mmu-miR-18a* | 1.54E-02 | −0.30 |
| 70 | mmu-miR-301a | 2.62E-02 | −0.32 |
| 71 | mmu-miR-18a | 2.96E-02 | −0.32 |
| 72 | mmu-miR-15b | 7.79E-03 | −0.34 |
| 73 | mmu-miR-879* | 4.04E-02 | −0.35 |
| 74 | mmu-miR-191 | 2.35E-03 | −0.35 |
| 75 | mmu-let-7i | 2.49E-02 | −0.35 |
| 76 | mmu-miR-222 | 1.42E-02 | −0.35 |
| 77 | mmu-let-7d | 1.78E-02 | −0.36 |
| 78 | hsa-miR-106b* | 1.21E-02 | −0.36 |
| 79 | mmu-miR-93 | 2.02E-02 | −0.36 |
| 80 | mmu-miR-106a | 2.31E-02 | −0.37 |
| 81 | mmu-miR-16* | 1.54E-02 | −0.39 |
| 82 | mmu-miR-25 | 3.56E-02 | −0.39 |
| 83 | mmu-miR-130b | 2.38E-02 | −0.40 |
| 84 | mmu-miR-2134 | 2.10E-02 | −0.41 |
| 85 | mmu-miR-17 | 4.15E-03 | −0.43 |
| 86 | mmu-miR-16 | 3.14E-02 | −0.43 |
| 87 | mmu-miR-15a | 2.51E-02 | −0.44 |
| 88 | rno-miR-148b-5p | 1.10E-02 | −0.45 |
| 89 | mmu-miR-451 | 1.04E-02 | −0.51 |
| 90 | mmu-miR-340-5p | 1.11E-02 | −0.53 |
| 91 | mmu-miR-20a | 3.68E-03 | −0.53 |
| 92 | hsa-miR-421 | 5.54E-04 | −0.53 |
| 93 | mmu-miR-26b | 1.48E-02 | −0.57 |
| 94 | mmu-miR-1274a | 2.25E-02 | −0.60 |
| 95 | mmu-miR-186 | 3.50E-02 | −0.60 |
| 96 | mmu-miR-142-3p | 4.12E-03 | −0.61 |
| 97 | mmu-miR-17* | 4.59E-03 | −0.62 |

**Table 4.** Cont.

| S. No. | MiRNA | P Value | Fold Difference (log10 [RQ]) |
|---|---|---|---|
| 98 | mmu-miR-301b | 2.02E-03 | −0.66 |
| 99 | mmu-miR-26a | 1.46E-03 | −0.66 |
| 100 | mmu-miR-186* | 2.64E-03 | −0.67 |
| 101 | mmu-miR-106b | 1.92E-03 | −0.68 |
| 102 | mmu-miR-31 | 1.59E-02 | −0.86 |
| 103 | hsa-miR-875-5p | 1.02E-02 | −3.75 |
| **Target not detected** | | | |
| 104 | rno-miR-196c | 4.12E-02 | −1.80 |
| 105 | mmu-miR-363 | 1.33E-02 | −2.38 |
| 106 | mmu-miR-2138 | 4.71E-02 | −2.52 |

One hundred and six miRNA were significantly modulated. Of these, 66 were up regulated and 40 were down regulated. Values are given as Log10 of the fold change $(2^{-(mean\ \Delta\Delta Ct)})$.

[51]. Biochemical assays for brain related proteins in serum, such as GFAP, UCH-L1 and S100β, are either not sensitive or selective for mTBI [7–12]. Therefore, a more reliable and sensitive molecular assay is needed to accurately diagnose mTBI. In this experiment, acute phase miRNA changes in the serum were measured to determine the feasibility of using miRNA as diagnostic markers of mTBI.

Increasing grades of mTBI were induced by a weight drop device by increasing the height and weight of the falling rod. Injuries were characterized by the sensory motor responses designed to model clinical neurological examination and indicated the injuries to be within the mild spectrum of TBI [26–27]. Consistent with mTBI, histological analysis of the brain showed no gross pathological changes following the injury. Behavior impairments such as depression and loss of interest have been described in patients with mTBI [52]. Reduced escape behavior, measured in terms of vertical activity of the animal in an open field apparatus, can be a measure of depression-related behavior [53–

55]. Transient, but significant depression-related behavior in terms of reduced vertical activity was observed in the injured animals at day 1 post injury, which recovered over time. A general negative impact on the overall health of the animals was also observed at day 1 post injury, indicated by the reduction in horizontal activity of the injured animals. Sensory gating impairments have also been reported in mTBI [56]. Increase in the OFL activity of the animals at the later time points of day 14 and day 30 as compared to day 1 activity was interesting. We hypothesize that the naïve and sham control animals remember being in the chambers and that the other animals, due to injury, may not remember the chamber as well and spend more time exploring. ASR is a complex behavior that engages higher brain functions and is related to information processing [39,41,57–58]. A significantly reduced startle response was observed in animals with injury, such that the greater the injury severity, the less startle response was observed. The parietal lobe, where the injury was centered, is involved in the sensorimotor information processing [59]. It is suggested that the

**Table 5.** Common MiRNA among all injury groups.

| S. No. | MiRNA | IS1 | IS2 | IS3 | IS4 |
|---|---|---|---|---|---|
| 1 | mmu-miR-376a | 1.99 | 1.70 | 1.72 | 1.68 |
| 2 | hsa-miR-214 | 0.58 | 0.72 | 0.71 | 0.75 |
| 3 | mmu-miR-214 | 0.54 | 0.64 | 0.88 | 0.80 |
| 4 | mmu-miR-337-5p | 0.52 | 0.49 | 0.77 | 0.52 |
| 5 | mmu-miR-574-3p | 0.51 | 0.53 | 0.71 | 0.53 |
| 6 | mmu-miR-434-3p | 0.41 | 0.61 | 0.64 | 0.67 |
| 7 | mmu-miR-671-3p | 0.39 | 0.37 | 0.72 | 0.69 |
| 8 | mmu-miR-218 | 0.36 | 0.64 | 0.54 | 0.50 |
| 9 | mmu-miR-199a-3p | 0.32 | 0.42 | 0.46 | 0.62 |
| 10 | hsa-miR-106b* | −0.40 | −0.38 | −0.64 | −0.36 |
| 11 | mmu-miR-106b | −0.47 | −0.45 | −0.83 | −0.68 |
| 12 | mmu-miR-31 | −0.85 | −1.03 | −0.87 | −0.86 |
| 13 | rno-miR-196c | −1.81 | −1.53 | −1.39 | −1.80 |

Thirteen miRNAs were commonly modulated among all the injury groups. Of these, 9 were up regulated and 4 were down regulated. Values are given as Log10 of the fold change $(2^{-(mean\ \Delta\Delta Ct)})$.

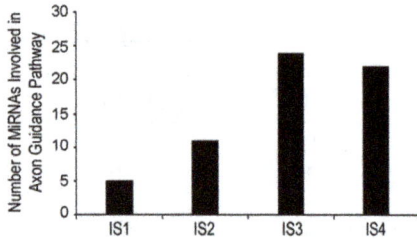

**Figure 5. Involvement of significantly modulated miRNA in axon guidance pathway.** Quantitative bioinformatics analysis on the number of miRNA involved in the axon guidance pathway was done using IPA. The number of the significantly modulated miRNAs that were predicted to modulate axon guidance pathway increased with the severity of the injury.

right inferior parietal lobe plays a role in auditory signal processing and integration of sensory and motor functions [39,59–60]. This observation indicates the diffuse nature of the injury that may also affect central brain functions. Many individuals, who suffer with mTBI do not exhibit neurobehavioral alterations and acute symptoms of mTBI, such as headaches, sleep disturbance and depression or recover spontaneously from the injury [13–15]. A similar observation was made in the current experiment, where the percent of animals' OFL activity in the mildest of mild injury group (*i.e.*, IS1) was similar to sham and naïve control groups. Other groups, with a more severe form of the mild injury, however, showed greater reduction in the percent activity than the sham and naïve groups.

MiRNA changes in the serum have been suggested as a potential marker of disease and injury [16–18]. MiRNA modulations in the serum of TBI patients have been reported. Down regulated expression of has-mir-16, and has-mir-92 and increased levels of has-mir-765 correlated with the severe TBI, however, their utility in diagnosing mTBI was limited [24]. Earlier we have also reported the modulation of let-7i in the serum and cerebrospinal fluid of rats following blast injury [22]. Modulation of miRNA expression in the brain following TBI has been shown before [19-23]. Some of the miRNAs (mir-21, mir-34a, mir-27b, mir-9, mir-874, mir-223, mir-144 and mir-153) that were reported to increase in the brain after moderate to severe TBI [20–21,23,61–62] did not show significant modulation in the serum in our experiment. Mir-497 and mir-149, which were up regulated in IS4 group, were earlier reported to also increase in the brain after TBI [23,63]. Mir-451 and mir-340-5p, which were shown to be up regulated in the brain post TBI, were down regulated in our experiment [19,61]. Despite the difference in the tissue being analyzed after the TBI, some common targets of modulated miRNAs were observed. Earlier studies found apoptosis as one of the cellular process targeted by the miRNAs modulated in the brain following TBI [19–21]. Apoptosis was predicted to be affected by the modulated miRNAs in this experiment as well. BDNF, which was identified as a predicted target of one of the down regulated miRNA mir-106 in this experiment, was also identified as target of the modulated miRNAs following TBI in an earlier study [19].

Two main observations were made in the current experiment. First, the number of miRNAs that were significantly modulated post injury increased with the severity of the injury. Second, thirteen common miRNAs were significantly modulated in all the

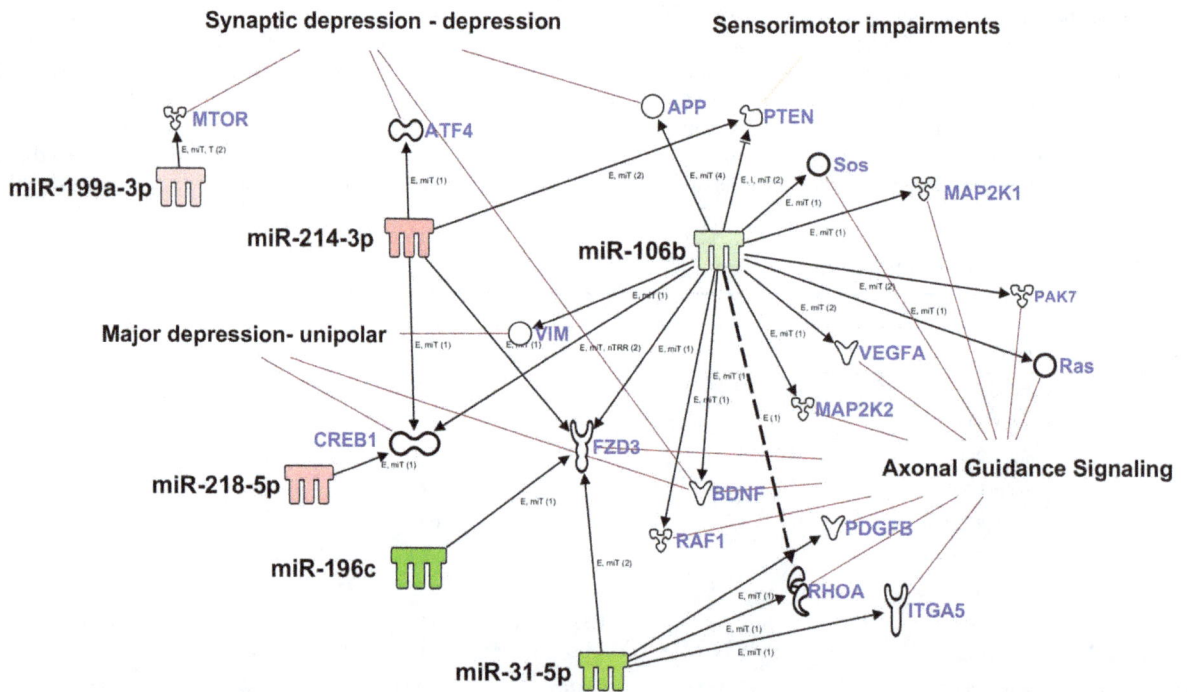

**Figure 6. IPA Analysis for effect of significantly modulated miRNAs common among all four injury groups on brain functions related pathways.** MiRNAs common to all four injury groups were taken and their targets and pathway analysis in relation to brain related functions were performed. My Pathway tool of IPA software was used to build the custom pathway using miRNAs that show experimentally validated targets by overlaying with 1) depression, 2) sensorimotor function and the 3) axon guidance pathway molecules. Of the 13 common modulated miRNAs, only 6 miRNAs were found to have experimentally validated targets that are predicted to modulate axon guidance, synaptic depression and sensorimotor impairments.

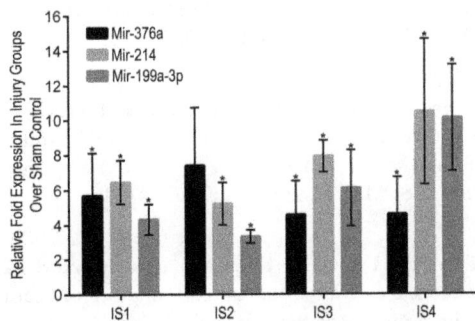

**Figure 7. Expression of miRNAs in individual real time PCR assay.** The fold upregulation of three miRNAs, miR-376a, miR-214 and miR-199a-3p, in the injury groups over the sham mice was validated using the individual real time PCR assays. Similar to the miRNA arrays, expression of the three miRNAs was found to be up regulated in the injured groups over the sham animals. Data presented is the fold up regulation ($\pm$ SEM; *$P<0.05$) calculated from the mean DDCt value obtained from three biological samples for each injury group. Statistical significance was calculated using the individual Ct values obtained from the three biological replicates for each injury group.

four injury groups compared to the sham controls. Functional analysis to identify the combined effect of modulated miRNAs showed that eight of the thirteen miRNAs may play a role in CNS related pathways, such as synaptic depression, sensorimotor impairments and the axon guidance pathway (Figure 5, Figure S5). Vimentin (VIM) and phosphatase and tensin homolog (PTEN), targets of the significantly down regulated miRNA mir-106b, expression has been shown to increase in the brain post TBI and has been related to inflammatory cell proliferation and differentiation and neuronal survival and neurite integrity, respectively [64–67]. Brain-derived neurotrophic factor (BDNF) and Amyloid precursor protein (APP), also targets of mir-106b, have been shown to increase post TBI [68–69]. BDNF has been reported to have a neuroprotective effect post TBI [68,70]. The role of APP is, however, debated as some studies have shown APP association with neuronal loss and others have shown APP as neuroprotective [71–74]. Axon guidance includes axon outgrowth, repulsion, and attraction, which plays an important role in neuronal functions and axonal regeneration. Axonal injury is prevalent in TBI [75–78]. Axon guidance and synaptic plasticity is affected post TBI and positive regulation of axon guidance has been suggested to result in better functional outcomes [79–81]. Elevated levels of axon related proteins, such as neurofilament heavy chain, Tau, S100B and myelin basic protein in the serum, have also been suggested as potential biomarkers of mTBI [82]. Two of the significantly up regulated miRNAs that were validated using the singleplex miRNA assay, have been shown to play a role in neuronal differentiation and CNS development. Normal miR-376a expression has been shown to be involved in the early fetal brain development, whereas accumulation of unedited miR-376a has been linked to neurodevelopmental disorders and increased metastasis potential of gliomas [83–86]. MiR-214 has also been shown to enhance neurite outgrowth and its expression is up regulated during the mouse cortical neuron, embryonic stem cells development, and at the early developmental stages in embryonic retina [87–88]. However, miR-214 levels have been shown to decrease in the neurons of the dorsal root ganglion after an injury to the sciatic nerve [89]. MiR-376a was also up regulated in the serum of rats exposed to blast induced moderate TBI [22]. Down regulated mir-106b and up regulated miR-376a and miR-214 along with other modulated miRNAs at the acute stage of injury,

may reflect the metabolic active state of neural tissue engaged in the immediate response to injury that involve neuroprotection, synaptic plasticity, axonal damage/regeneration, and neurogenesis.

Endogenous neurogenesis and neuronal maturation have been proposed as keys to recovery and as therapeutic targets after TBI. TBI is often followed by the increase in endogenous neuronal progenitor cells proliferation and migration, neuronal differentiation, and neurogenesis [90–96]. Proliferating neuroprogenitor cells differentiate into immature neurons post TBI but fail to develop further into the mature neurons [91,97]. A small subset of newborn granular neurons, however, has been observed in the brain after TBI, though the formation of these neurons is not significantly enhanced [97–98]. Dash and group also reported development of mature neurons in the dentate gyrus of the hippocampus one month after the TBI [96]. To determine if bioinformatics analysis targeting the axon guidance pathway may be exploited for predicting the severity of the injury, significantly modulated miRNA in each injury groups were analyzed by IPA for their predicted involvement in modulating axon guidance pathway. The number of miRNAs that are predicted to modulate axon guidance pathway related brain functions increased with the severity of the injury, suggesting an enhanced effect of injury on molecular functions associated with the axon guidance and neurogenesis (Figure 5). Long-term studies are needed to evaluate development of chronic pathologies such as axon damage, synapse and blood brain barrier functions in the brain following injury in this model of mTBI. However, the quantitative bioinformatics analysis of the modulated miRNAs relating to their potential CNS involvement can be helpful to identify the severity of the injury at early time points after the injury. In conclusion, a cohort of 13 serum miRNAs identified in this study, may be used as acute biomarkers of mTBI regardless of any neurobehavioral or cognitive alterations following the injury. Future studies will be needed to validate this cohort of 13 miRNAs as acute biomarkers of mTBI in the other animal models of injury and in the human mTBI. In addition, further behavioral studies will be needed to identify the long-term cognitive deficits and/or sleep disorders in the mTBI model described in this study. Such long-term studies will also be able to determine the prognostic value of the miRNAs identified in this study as acute biomarkers of mTBI.

## Supporting Information

**Figure S1  Closed head injury (CHI) device.** (A) CHI device was custom made based on the design of CHI device described by Flierl *et. al.* (2009) [30]. Injury was induced by a metal rod of specific weight falling under gravity. The rod can be set for a specific height using the holding grooves made 0.5 cm apart. The rod was released using a pneumatic control operated by a foot pedal. The tip of the rod was fitted with a rubber tip (1 mm in diameter/1 mm in length). (B) Site of the injury was over the parietal lobe, 2.5 mm from the sagittal and lamboid suture.

**Figure S2  Animal activity in an open field test.** Percentage of the animals that show reduced activity within each of the controls and the injury groups was evaluated. The lowest baseline horizontal and vertical activity values (beam breaks) in the naïve group were used as reference numbers. Animals exhibiting activity lower than the reference number were identified and were used to calculate the percentage of the animals within a group that exhibited reduced activity on day 1 post injury ([Number of animals that exhibited reduced activity in a group/total number of the animals in the group]*100). Data showed that as the grade of the injury increased, a higher percentage of the animals showed reduced activity.

## Figure S3 Motor activity post injury.
Animals were subjected to the rotarod test to evaluate the motor activity deficits post injury using a Med Associates rat rotarod (Med Associates, Inc., St. Albans, VT). Animals were placed on an accelerating (4–40 rpm) rotating rod (7.0 cm diameter) for a maximum period of 5 min and the time spent on the rod by each animal was measured. Three attempts of 5 min each were given to each animal and the mean time spent was calculated. Data presented here is the change scores between 1 day, 14 day and 30 day post injury and baseline (Mean time spent at each time point- mean time spent at BL measurement). No significant differences were found in the motor activity of the injured mice compared to the naïve or the sham groups at any time point measured.

## Figure S4 Hierarchical clustering (HC) of DDCt values.
HC of DDCt of miRNAs calculated over the sham controls showed 333 g injury groups (i.e., IS3 and IS4) clustering together followed by IS2 and IS1 respectively. HC indicates that more severe of the injuries with in the mild spectrum showed close association.

## Figure S5 Brain functions related pathways targeted by the significantly modulated miRNAs common among all the four injury groups.
Thirteen common miRNAs that were significantly modulated among all the four injury groups were analyzed for their combined effect on KEGG pathways using DIANA-miRPath v2.0 software [50]. Eight of the significantly modulated miRNAs, miR-106b, miR-199a-3p, miR-214, miR-218, miR-31, miR-434-3p, miR-671-3p, and miR-574-3p were predicted to significantly modulate several nervous system function and disease related pathways.

## Figure S6 Brain functions related pathway targeted by the significantly modulated miRNAs unique to the injury groups with the neurobehavioral alterations.
Nineteen miRNAs that were significantly modulated among all the three injury groups, which demonstrated alteration in the neurobehavioral functions (i.e., IS2, IS3 and IS4) were analyzed for their combined effect on the significant modulation of KEGG pathways using DIANA-miRPath v2.0 software [44].

## Table S1 List of the tasks performed for determining NSS-R scores.

## Table S2 NSS-R change scores.
NSS-R change scores of the individual groups are given and its significance with the other groups in the study is indicated. Values are expressed as mean ± SEM. * P value significant <0.05.

## Table S3 The horizontal activity in OF.
The horizontal activity (number of beam breaks) of the individual groups is given and its significance with the other groups in the study is indicated. Values are expressed as mean ± SEM. * P value significant <0.05.

## Table S4 The center time spent over the time period of the study.
The center time of the animals (in seconds) from all

groups over the period of the study is given. Values are presented as mean ± SEM. * * P value significant <0.05.

## Table S5 The center time of the animals in OFL.
The time spent in the center (in seconds) is given for each of the groups and its comparison with the other groups is given. Values are presented as mean ± SEM. * P value significant <0.05.

## Table S6 The vertical activity over the time period of the study.
The vertical activity of the animals (number of beam breaks) from all the groups over the period of the study is given. Values are presented as mean ± SEM. * * P value significant < 0.05.

## Table S7 The vertical activity in OFL.
The vertical activity of the animals (number of beam breaks) in each group and its comparison with the other groups for day 1 is given. Values are presented as mean ± SEM. * P value significant <0.05.

## Table S8 Day 1 ASR.
ASR response of the animals in each groups and its comparison with the other groups is given. Values are presented as mean ± SEM. * P value significant <0.05.

## Table S9 Day 14 ASR.
ASR response of the animals in each groups and its comparison with the other groups is given. Values are presented as mean ± SEM. * P value significant <0.05.

## Table S10 Average Ct values for the common miRNAs.
Average Ct value for each of the miRNA in the injury and the sham control group indicate their abundance in the sample. High expression = Ct ranging from 11–15; Good expression = Ct ranging from 16–20; Moderate expression = Ct ranging from 21–25; Low Expression = Ct ranging from 26–30; and Rare expression = Ct ranging from 31–35.

## Table S11 MiRNAs present only in the injury groups that demonstrate behavior changes.
Nineteen miRNAs were significantly modulated in the injury group that showed significant behavior alterations. Of these 14 were up regulated and 5 were down regulated. Two miRNAs, mmu-miR-487b and mmu-miR-218-1* were expressed only in the injured animals and not in the sham-injured animals i.e., "calibrator not detected". For all other miRNAs Ct value was <36 in both, the injured and the sham-injured groups. Values are given as log10 of the fold change $(2^{-(\text{mean }\Delta\Delta Ct)})$.

## Table S12 MiRNA present only in the injury groups that do not demonstrate behavior changes.
Two miRNAs, miR-297a* and miR-181c were found to be significantly modulated in the IS1 injury group, which did not demonstrate any significant neurobehavioral and cognitive changes as compared to the sham injury group. "Calibrator not detected" is the miRNA which is expressed only in the injured animals and not in the un-injured sham animals. "Target not detected" is the miRNA that was expressed only in the un-injured sham animals and not in the injured animals. In such case the Ct value for non-detected miRNA was taken as 40 followed by the fold change and statistical analysis.

**Table S13 Selection of the endogenous control miRNA.** The most stable miRNA were selected based on their Ct values across the samples (n = 30). Ct for each miRNA from all the samples, irrespective of the injury or control group, were taken and Ct values with a SD <1 were selected. Mean Ct were calculated to determine the abundance of miRNAs in the serum samples. To ensure that there are no outliers, median Ct was also calculated. MiRNA that showed similar mean and median Ct values were then selected. MiRNA that show more abundance *i.e.*, Ct <25 were considered for determining a candidate stable endogenous miRNA in validation experiments.

## Acknowledgments

Authors would like to acknowledge Dr. Amanda Fu for her help with animal surgeries; Mr. Kevin Cravedi, Dr. Angela Yarnell, Dr. Paridhi Gupta, and Ms. Manoshi Gayen for their help with the animal behavior experiments. Authors would also like to acknowledge Dr. Joseph McCabe, Program Director for Neuroprotection & Modeling, The Center for Neuroscience & Regenerative Medicine, USUHS, Bethesda, MD, for his help in establishing the CHI machine in the CNRM and for providing the operational support.

**Author Disclosure Statement**

The opinions expressed herein are that of the author(s), and are not necessarily representative of those of the Uniformed Services University of the Health Sciences (USUHS), CDMRP, BITS Pilani, the Department of Defense (DOD), the United States Army, Navy; or Air Force.

## Author Contributions

Conceived and designed the experiments: AS RC NEG RKM. Performed the experiments: AS RC ESB MKB MAH. Analyzed the data: AS RC ESB NSB. Contributed reagents/materials/analysis tools: RKM NEG. Wrote the paper: AS NEG RKM.

## References

1. Risdall JE, Menon DK (2011) Traumatic brain injury. Philosophical transactions of the Royal Society of London Series B, Biological sciences 366: 241–250.
2. Teasdale G, Jennett B (1976) Assessment and prognosis of coma after head injury. Acta neurochirurgica 34: 45–55.
3. Fischer H (2013) U.S. Military Casualty Statistics: Operation New Dawn, Operation Iraqi Freedom, and Operation Enduring Freedom. CRS Report for Congress. Prepared for Members and Committees of Congress: Congressional Research Service. pp. 1–12.
4. Belanger HG, Vanderploeg RD, Curtiss G, Warden DL (2007) Recent neuroimaging techniques in mild traumatic brain injury. The Journal of neuropsychiatry and clinical neurosciences 19: 5–20.
5. Niogi SN, Mukherjee P, Ghajar J, Johnson C, Kolster RA, et al. (2008) Extent of microstructural white matter injury in postconcussive syndrome correlates with impaired cognitive reaction time: a 3T diffusion tensor imaging study of mild traumatic brain injury. AJNR American journal of neuroradiology 29: 967–973.
6. Yuh EL, Cooper SR, Ferguson AR, Manley GT (2012) Quantitative CT improves outcome prediction in acute traumatic brain injury. Journal of neurotrauma 29: 735–746.
7. Vos PE, Jacobs B, Andriessen TM, Lamers KJ, Borm GF, et al. (2010) GFAP and S100B are biomarkers of traumatic brain injury: an observational cohort study. Neurology 75: 1786–1793.
8. Thelin EP, Johannesson L, Nelson D, Bellander BM (2013) S100B Is an Important Outcome Predictor in Traumatic Brain Injury. Journal of neurotrauma 30: 519–528.
9. Papa L, Lewis LM, Falk JL, Zhang Z, Silvestri S, et al. (2012) Elevated levels of serum glial fibrillary acidic protein breakdown products in mild and moderate traumatic brain injury are associated with intracranial lesions and neurosurgical intervention. Annals of emergency medicine 59: 471–483.
10. Papa L, Lewis LM, Silvestri S, Falk JL, Giordano P, et al. (2012) Serum levels of ubiquitin C-terminal hydrolase distinguish mild traumatic brain injury from trauma controls and are elevated in mild and moderate traumatic brain injury patients with intracranial lesions and neurosurgical intervention. The journal of trauma and acute care surgery 72: 1335–1344.
11. Papa L, Akinyi L, Liu MC, Pineda JA, Tepas JJ 3rd, et al. (2010) Ubiquitin C-terminal hydrolase is a novel biomarker in humans for severe traumatic brain injury. Critical care medicine 38: 138–144.
12. Brophy GM, Mondello S, Papa L, Robicsek SA, Gabrielli A, et al. (2011) Biokinetic analysis of ubiquitin C-terminal hydrolase-L1 (UCH-L1) in severe traumatic brain injury patient biofluids. Journal of neurotrauma 28: 861–870.
13. Pogoda TK, Hendricks AM, Iverson KM, Stolzmann KL, Krengel MH, et al. (2012) Multisensory impairment reported by veterans with and without mild traumatic brain injury history. Journal of rehabilitation research and development 49: 971–984.
14. Theeler BJ, Flynn FG, Erickson JC (2012) Chronic daily headache in U.S. soldiers after concussion. Headache 52: 732–738.
15. Kiraly M, Kiraly SJ (2007) Traumatic brain injury and delayed sequelae: a review–traumatic brain injury and mild traumatic brain injury (concussion) are precursors to later-onset brain disorders, including early-onset dementia. TheScientificWorldJournal 7: 1768–1776.
16. Mayr M, Zampetaki A, Willeit P, Willeit J, Kiechl S (2013) MicroRNAs within the continuum of postgenomics biomarker discovery. Arteriosclerosis, thrombosis, and vascular biology 33: 206–214.
17. Allegra A, Alonci A, Campo S, Penna G, Petrungaro A, et al. (2012) Circulating microRNAs: new biomarkers in diagnosis, prognosis and treatment of cancer (review). International journal of oncology 41: 1897–1912.
18. Wahid F, Shehzad A, Khan T, Kim YY (2010) MicroRNAs: synthesis, mechanism, function, and recent clinical trials. Biochimica et biophysica acta 1803: 1231–1243.
19. Redell JB, Liu Y, Dash PK (2009) Traumatic brain injury alters expression of hippocampal microRNAs: potential regulators of multiple pathophysiological processes. Journal of neuroscience research 87: 1435–1448.
20. Redell JB, Zhao J, Dash PK (2011) Altered expression of miRNA-21 and its targets in the hippocampus after traumatic brain injury. Journal of neuroscience research 89: 212–221.
21. Lei P, Li Y, Chen X, Yang S, Zhang J (2009) Microarray based analysis of microRNA expression in rat cerebral cortex after traumatic brain injury. Brain research 1284: 191–201.
22. Balakathiresan N, Bhomia M, Chandran R, Chavko M, McCarron RM, et al. (2012) MicroRNA let-7i is a promising serum biomarker for blast-induced traumatic brain injury. Journal of neurotrauma 29: 1379–1387.
23. Truettner JS, Alonso OF, Bramlett HM, Dietrich WD (2011) Therapeutic hypothermia alters microRNA responses to traumatic brain injury in rats. Journal of cerebral blood flow and metabolism: official journal of the International Society of Cerebral Blood Flow and Metabolism 31: 1897–1907.
24. Redell JB, Moore AN, Ward NH 3rd, Hergenroeder GW, Dash PK (2010) Human traumatic brain injury alters plasma microRNA levels. Journal of neurotrauma 27: 2147–2156.
25. Flierl MA, Stahel PF, Beauchamp KM, Morgan SJ, Smith WR, et al. (2009) Mouse closed head injury model induced by a weight-drop device. Nature protocols 4: 1328–1337.
26. Grunberg NE, Yarnell AM, Hamilton KR, Starosciak AK, Chwa A, et al. (2011) A revised neurological severity scale for rodents.. Annual Meeting of Society for Neuroscience. Washington, D.C.
27. Sharma P, Su YA, Barry ES, Grunberg NE, Lei Z (2012) Mitochondrial targeted neuron focused genes in hippocampus of rats with traumatic brain injury. International journal of critical illness and injury science 2: 172–179.
28. Shohami E, Novikov M, Bass R (1995) Long-term effect of HU-211, a novel non-competitive NMDA antagonist, on motor and memory functions after closed head injury in the rat. Brain research 674: 55–62.
29. Hamm RJ (2001) Neurobehavioral assessment of outcome following traumatic brain injury in rats: an evaluation of selected measures. Journal of neurotrauma 18: 1207–1216.
30. Marti M, Mela F, Fantin M, Zucchini S, Brown JM, et al. (2005) Blockade of nociceptin/orphanin FQ transmission attenuates symptoms and neurodegeneration associated with Parkinson's disease. The Journal of neuroscience: the official journal of the Society for Neuroscience 25: 9591–9601.
31. Yarnell AM, Shaughness MC, Barry ES, Ahlers ST, McCarron RM, et al. (2013) Blast traumatic brain injury in the rat using a blast overpressure model. Current protocols in neuroscience/editorial board, Jacqueline N Crawley [et al] Chapter 9: Unit 9 41.
32. Xing G, Barry ES, Benford B, Grunberg NE, Li H, et al. (2013) Impact of repeated stress on traumatic brain injury-induced mitochondrial electron transport chain expression and behavioral responses in rats. Frontiers in neurology 4: 196.
33. Bowen DJ, Eury SE, Grunberg NE (1986) Nicotine's effects on female rats' body weight: caloric intake and physical activity. Pharmacology, biochemistry, and behavior 25: 1131–1136.
34. Elliott BM, Faraday MM, Phillips JM, Grunberg NE (2004) Effects of nicotine on elevated plus maze and locomotor activity in male and female adolescent and adult rats. Pharmacology, biochemistry, and behavior 77: 21–28.
35. Faraday MM, O'Donoghue VA, Grunberg NE (2003) Effects of nicotine and stress on locomotion in Sprague-Dawley and Long-Evans male and female rats. Pharmacology, biochemistry, and behavior 74: 325–333.
36. Grunberg NE, Bowen DJ (1985) The role of physical activity in nicotine's effects on body weight. Pharmacology, biochemistry, and behavior 23: 851–854.

37. Morse DE, Davis HD, Popke EJ, Brown KJ, O'Donoghue VA, et al. (1997) Effects of ddC and AZT on locomotion and acoustic startle. I: Acute effects in female rats. Pharmacology, biochemistry, and behavior 56: 221–228.

38. Hamilton KR, Starosciak AK, Chwa A, Grunberg NE (2012) Nicotine behavioral sensitization in Lewis and Fischer male rats. Experimental and clinical psychopharmacology 20: 345–351.

39. Acri JB, Grunberg NE, Morse DE (1991) Effects of nicotine on the acoustic startle reflex amplitude in rats. Psychopharmacology 104: 244–248.

40. Alain C, He Y, Grady C (2008) The contribution of the inferior parietal lobe to auditory spatial working memory. Journal of cognitive neuroscience 20: 285–295.

41. Swerdlow NR, Caine SB, Braff DL,Geyer MA (1992) The neural substrates of sensorimotor gating of the startle reflex: a review of recent findings and their implications. Journal of psychopharmacology (Oxford, England) 6: 176–190.

42. Acri JB, Morse DE, Popke EJ, Grunberg NE (1994) Nicotine increases sensory gating measured as inhibition of the acoustic startle reflex in rats. Psychopharmacology 114: 369–374.

43. Faraday MM, Rahman MA, Scheufele PM, Grunberg NE (1998) Nicotine administration impairs sensory gating in Long-Evans rats. Pharmacology, biochemistry, and behavior 61: 281–289.

44. Allison PD (1990) Change Scores as Dependent Variables in Regression Analysis. Sociological Methodology 20: 93–114.

45. D'Haene B, Mestdagh P, Hellemans J, Vandesompele J (2012) miRNA expression profiling: from reference genes to global mean normalization. Methods in molecular biology (Clifton, NJ) 822: 261–272.

46. Deo A, Carlsson J, Lindlof A (2011) How to choose a normalization strategy for miRNA quantitative real-time (qPCR) arrays. Journal of bioinformatics and computational biology 9: 795–812.

47. Marmarou A, Foda MA, van den Brink W, Campbell J, Kita H, et al. (1994) A new model of diffuse brain injury in rats. Part I: Pathophysiology and biomechanics. Journal of neurosurgery 80: 291–300.

48. Foda MA, Marmarou A (1994) A new model of diffuse brain injury in rats. Part II: Morphological characterization. Journal of neurosurgery 80: 301–313.

49. Vlachos IS, Kostoulas N, Vergoulis T, Georgakilas G, Reczko M, et al. (2012) DIANA miRPath v.2.0: investigating the combinatorial effect of microRNAs in pathways. Nucleic acids research 40: W498–504.

50. Song J, Bai Z, Han W, Zhang J, Meng H, et al. (2012) Identification of suitable reference genes for qPCR analysis of serum microRNA in gastric cancer patients. Digestive diseases and sciences 57: 897–904.

51. Rapp PE, Curley KC (2012) Is a diagnosis of "mild traumatic brain injury" a category mistake? The journal of trauma and acute care surgery 73: S13–23.

52. Bryan CJ, Clemans TA, Hernandez AM, Rudd MD (2013) Loss of consciousness, depression, posttraumatic stress disorder, and suicide risk among deployed military personnel with mild traumatic brain injury. The Journal of head trauma rehabilitation 28: 13–20.

53. Katz RJ, Roth KA, Carroll BJ (1981) Acute and chronic stress effects on open field activity in the rat: implications for a model of depression. Neuroscience and biobehavioral reviews 5: 247–251.

54. Seligman ME, Maier SF (1967) Failure to escape traumatic shock. Journal of experimental psychology 74: 1–9.

55. Overmier JB, Seligman ME (1967) Effects of inescapable shock upon subsequent escape and avoidance responding. Journal of comparative and physiological psychology 63: 28–33.

56. Kumar S, Rao SL, Nair RG, Pillai S, Chandramouli BA, et al. (2005) Sensory gating impairment in development of post-concussive symptoms in mild head injury. Psychiatry and clinical neurosciences 59: 466–472.

57. Lee Y, Lopez DE, Meloni EG, Davis M (1996) A primary acoustic startle pathway: obligatory role of cochlear root neurons and the nucleus reticularis pontis caudalis. The Journal of neuroscience: the official journal of the Society for Neuroscience 16: 3775–3789.

58. Koch M, Schnitzler HU (1997) The acoustic startle response in rats–circuits mediating evocation, inhibition and potentiation. Behavioural brain research 89: 35–49.

59. Freund HJ (2003) Somatosensory and motor disturbances in patients with parietal lobe lesions. Advances in neurology 93: 179–193.

60. Leung AW, Alain C (2011) Working memory load modulates the auditory "What" and "Where" neural networks. NeuroImage 55: 1260–1269.

61. Liu L, Sun T, Liu Z, Chen X, Zhao L, et al. (2014) Traumatic Brain Injury Dysregulates MicroRNAs to Modulate Cell Signaling in Rat Hippocampus. PloS one 9: e103948.

62. Sabirzhanov B, Zhao Z, Stoica BA, Loane DJ, Wu J, et al. (2014) Down-regulation of miR-23a and miR-27a following Experimental Traumatic Brain Injury Induces Neuronal Cell Death through Activation of Proapoptotic Bcl-2 Proteins. The Journal of neuroscience: the official journal of the Society for Neuroscience 34: 10055–10071.

63. Bao TH, Miao W, Han JH, Yin M, Yan Y, et al. (2014) Spontaneous Running Wheel Improves Cognitive Functions of Mouse Associated with miRNA Expressional Alteration in Hippocampus Following Traumatic Brain Injury. Journal of molecular neuroscience: MN.

64. Moon C, Ahn M, Kim S, Jin JK, Sim KB, et al. (2004) Temporal patterns of the embryonic intermediate filaments nestin and vimentin expression in the cerebral cortex of adult rats after cryoinjury. Brain research 1028: 238–242.

65. Hausmann R, Betz P (2001) Course of glial immunoreactivity for vimentin, tenascin and alpha1-antichymotrypsin after traumatic injury to human brain. International journal of legal medicine 114: 338–342.

66. Wang G, Jiang X, Pu H, Zhang W, An C, et al. (2013) Scriptaid, a novel histone deacetylase inhibitor, protects against traumatic brain injury via modulation of PTEN and AKT pathway: scriptaid protects against TBI via AKT. Neurotherapeutics: the journal of the American Society for Experimental NeuroTherapeutics 10: 124–142.

67. Goh CP, Putz U, Howitt J, Low LH, Gunnersen J, et al. (2014) Nuclear trafficking of Pten after brain injury leads to neuron survival not death. Experimental neurology 252: 37–46.

68. Yang K, Perez-Polo JR, Mu XS, Yan HQ, Xue JJ, et al. (1996) Increased expression of brain-derived neurotrophic factor but not neurotrophin-3 mRNA in rat brain after cortical impact injury. Journal of neuroscience research 44: 157–164.

69. Van Den Heuvel C, Lewis S, Wong M, Manavis J, Finnie J, et al. (1998) Diffuse neuronal perikaryon amyloid precursor protein immunoreactivity in a focal head impact model. Acta neurochirurgica Supplement 71: 209–211.

70. Griesbach GS, Hovda DA, Molteni R, Gomez-Pinilla F (2002) Alterations in BDNF and synapsin I within the occipital cortex and hippocampus after mild traumatic brain injury in the developing rat: reflections of injury-induced neuroplasticity. Journal of neurotrauma 19: 803–814.

71. Itoh T, Satou T, Nishida S, Tsubaki M, Hashimoto S, et al. (2009) Improvement of cerebral function by anti-amyloid precursor protein antibody infusion after traumatic brain injury in rats. Molecular and cellular biochemistry 324: 191–199.

72. Murakami N, Yamaki T, Iwamoto Y, Sakakibara T, Kobori N, et al. (1998) Experimental brain injury induces expression of amyloid precursor protein, which may be related to neuronal loss in the hippocampus. Journal of neurotrauma 15: 993–1003.

73. Corrigan F, Thornton E, Roisman LC, Leonard AV, Vink R, et al. (2014) The neuroprotective activity of the amyloid precursor protein against traumatic brain injury is mediated via the heparin binding site in residues 96-110. Journal of neurochemistry 128: 196–204.

74. Corrigan F, Vink R, Blumbergs PC, Masters CL, Cappai R, et al. (2012) Characterisation of the effect of knockout of the amyloid precursor protein on outcome following mild traumatic brain injury. Brain research 1451: 87–99.

75. Hanell A, Clausen F, Djupsjo A, Vallstedt A, Patra K, et al. (2012) Functional and histological outcome after focal traumatic brain injury is not improved in conditional EphA4 knockout mice. Journal of neurotrauma 29: 2660–2671.

76. Takeuchi S, Nawashiro H, Sato S, Kawauchi S, Nagatani K, et al. (2013) A better mild traumatic brain injury model in the rat. Acta neurochirurgica Supplement 118: 99–101.

77. Selwyn R, Hockenbury N, Jaiswal S, Mathur S, Armstrong RC, et al. (2013) Mild traumatic brain injury results in depressed cerebral glucose uptake: An (18)FDG PET study. Journal of neurotrauma 30: 1943–1953.

78. Johnson VE, Stewart W, Smith DH (2013) Axonal pathology in traumatic brain injury. Experimental neurology 246: 35–43.

79. Schirmer L, Merkler D, Konig FB, Bruck W, Stadelmann C (2013) Neuroaxonal regeneration is more pronounced in early multiple sclerosis than in traumatic brain injury lesions. Brain pathology (Zurich, Switzerland) 23: 2–12.

80. Urrea C, Castellanos DA, Sagen J, Tsoulfas P, Bramlett HM, et al. (2007) Widespread cellular proliferation and focal neurogenesis after traumatic brain injury in the rat. Restorative neurology and neuroscience 25: 65–76.

81. Frugier T, Conquest A, McLean C, Currie P, Moses D, et al. (2012) Expression and activation of EphA4 in the human brain after traumatic injury. Journal of neuropathology and experimental neurology 71: 242–250.

82. Rostami E, Davidsson J, Ng KC, Lu J, Gyorgy A, et al. (2012) A Model for Mild Traumatic Brain Injury that Induces Limited Transient Memory Impairment and Increased Levels of Axon Related Serum Biomarkers. Frontiers in neurology 3: 115.

83. Goossens K, Mestdagh P, Lefever S, Van Poucke M, Van Zeveren A, et al. (2013) Regulatory microRNA network identification in bovine blastocyst development. Stem cells and development.

84. Kawahara Y, Zinshteyn B, Sethupathy P, Iizasa H, Hatzigeorgiou AG, et al. (2007) Redirection of silencing targets by adenosine-to-inosine editing of miRNAs. Science (New York, NY) 315: 1137–1140.

85. Ekdahl Y, Farahani HS, Behm M, Lagergren J, Ohman M (2012) A-to-I editing of microRNAs in the mammalian brain increases during development. Genome research 22: 1477–1487.

86. Choudhury Y, Tay FC, Lam DH, Sandanaraj E, Tang C, et al. (2012) Attenuated adenosine-to-inosine editing of microRNA-376a* promotes invasiveness of glioblastoma cells. The Journal of clinical investigation 122: 4059–4076.

87. Chen H, Shalom-Feuerstein R, Riley J, Zhang SD, Tucci P, et al. (2010) miR-7 and miR-214 are specifically expressed during neuroblastoma differentiation, cortical development and embryonic stem cells differentiation, and control neurite outgrowth in vitro. Biochemical and biophysical research communications 394: 921–927.

88. Decembrini S, Bressan D, Vignali R, Pitto L, Mariotti S, et al. (2009) MicroRNAs couple cell fate and developmental timing in retina. Proceedings of the National Academy of Sciences of the United States of America 106: 21179–21184.

89. Zhang HY, Zheng SJ, Zhao JH, Zhao W, Zheng LF, et al. (2011) MicroRNAs 144, 145, and 214 are down-regulated in primary neurons responding to sciatic nerve transection. Brain research 1383: 62–70.

90. Rice AC, Khaldi A, Harvey HB, Salman NJ, White F, et al. (2003) Proliferation and neuronal differentiation of mitotically active cells following traumatic brain injury. Experimental neurology 183: 406–417.

91. Yi X, Jin G, Zhang X, Mao W, Li H, et al. (2013) Cortical endogenic neural regeneration of adult rat after traumatic brain injury. PloS one 8: e70306.

92. Zhang L, Yan R, Zhang Q, Wang H, Kang X, et al. (2013) Survivin, a key component of the Wnt/beta-catenin signaling pathway, contributes to traumatic brain injury-induced adult neurogenesis in the mouse dentate gyrus. International journal of molecular medicine 32: 867–875.

93. Itoh T, Satou T, Hashimoto S, Ito H (2005) Isolation of neural stem cells from damaged rat cerebral cortex after traumatic brain injury. Neuroreport 16: 1687–1691.

94. Zheng W, ZhuGe Q, Zhong M, Chen G, Shao B, et al. (2013) Neurogenesis in adult human brain after traumatic brain injury. Journal of neurotrauma 30: 1872–1880.

95. Rola R, Mizumatsu S, Otsuka S, Morhardt DR, Noble-Haeusslein LJ, et al. (2006) Alterations in hippocampal neurogenesis following traumatic brain injury in mice. Experimental neurology 202: 189–199.

96. Dash PK, Mach SA, Moore AN (2001) Enhanced neurogenesis in the rodent hippocampus following traumatic brain injury. Journal of neuroscience research 63: 313–319.

97. Gao X, Chen J (2013) Moderate traumatic brain injury promotes neural precursor proliferation without increasing neurogenesis in the adult hippocampus. Experimental neurology 239: 38–48.

98. Bye N, Carron S, Han X, Agyapomaa D, Ng SY, et al. (2011) Neurogenesis and glial proliferation are stimulated following diffuse traumatic brain injury in adult rats. Journal of neuroscience research 89: 986–1000.

# Permissions

The contributors of this book come from diverse backgrounds, making this book a truly international effort. This book will bring forth new frontiers with its revolutionizing research information and detailed analysis of the nascent developments around the world.

We would like to thank all the contributing authors for lending their expertise to make the book truly unique. They have played a crucial role in the development of this book. Without their invaluable contributions this book wouldn't have been possible. They have made vital efforts to compile up to date information on the varied aspects of this subject to make this book a valuable addition to the collection of many professionals and students.

This book was conceptualized with the vision of imparting up-to-date information and advanced data in this field. To ensure the same, a matchless editorial board was set up. Every individual on the board went through rigorous rounds of assessment to prove their worth. After which they invested a large part of their time researching and compiling the most relevant data for our readers.

The editorial board has been involved in producing this book since its inception. They have spent rigorous hours researching and exploring the diverse topics which have resulted in the successful publishing of this book. They have passed on their knowledge of decades through this book. To expedite this challenging task, the publisher supported the team at every step. A small team of assistant editors was also appointed to further simplify the editing procedure and attain best results for the readers.

Apart from the editorial board, the designing team has also invested a significant amount of their time in understanding the subject and creating the most relevant covers. They scrutinized every image to scout for the most suitable representation of the subject and create an appropriate cover for the book.

The publishing team has been an ardent support to the editorial, designing and production team. Their endless efforts to recruit the best for this project, has resulted in the accomplishment of this book. They are a veteran in the field of academics and their pool of knowledge is as vast as their experience in printing. Their expertise and guidance has proved useful at every step. Their uncompromising quality standards have made this book an exceptional effort. Their encouragement from time to time has been an inspiration for everyone.

The publisher and the editorial board hope that this book will prove to be a valuable piece of knowledge for researchers, students, practitioners and scholars across the globe.

# List of Contributors

**Hong-wei Chen**
Department of Orthopedics, Wenzhou Medical College-Affiliated Yiwu Central Hospital, Yiwu, Zhejiang, China

**Guo-dong Liu**
Department 8, Research Institute of Surgery, Daping Hospital, Third Military Medical University, Chongqing, P.R.China

**Li-jun Wu**
Department of Orthopedics, Wenzhou Medical College-Affiliated Second Hospital, Wenzhou, Zhejiang, China; Institute of Digital Medicine, Wenzhou Medical College, Wenzhou, Zhejiang, China

**Karin Kiechle and Karl Kanz**
Department of Trauma Surgery, Klinikum der Universität München, Ludwig-Maximilians Universität, München, Germany

**Jeffrey J. Bazarian, Kian Merchant-Borna and Brian Blyth**
Department of Emergency Medicine, University of Rochester Medical Center, Rochester, New York, United States of America

**Veit Stoecklein**
Department of Neurosurgery, Klinikum der Universität München, Ludwig- Maximilians Universität, München, Germany

**Eric Rozen**
Department of Athletics and Recreation, University of Rochester, Rochester, New York, United States of America

**Jason H. Huang and Samantha Dayawansa**
Department of Neurosurgery, University of Rochester Medical Center, Rochester, New York, United States of America

**Peter Biberthaler**
Department of Trauma Surgery, Technical University of Munich, München, Germany

**Peter M. Kreuzer, Martin Schecklmann, Susanne Staudinger and Berthold Langguth**
Department of Psychiatry and Psychotherapy, University of Regensburg, Regensburg, Germany,

**Michael Landgrebe**
Department of Psychiatry and Psychotherapy, University of Regensburg, Regensburg, Germany Department of Psychiatry, Psychosomatic Medicine and Psychotherapy, Sozialstiftung Bamberg, Bamberg, Germany

**Michael E. Hoffer**
Spatial Orientation Center, Department of Otolaryngology, Naval Medical Center San Diego, San Diego, California, United States of America

**Carey Balaban**
Departments of Otolaryngology, Neurobiology, Communication Sciences and Disorders, and Bioengineering, University of Pittsburgh, Pittsburgh, Pennsylvania, United States of America

**Martin D. Slade**
Department of Internal Medicine, Yale University, New Haven, Connecticut, United States of America

**Jack W. Tsao**
Wounded, Ill and Injured Directorate (M9), US Navy Bureau of Medicine and Surgery, Washington, D.C., United States of America

**Barry Hoffer**
Department of Neurosurgery, Case Western University, Cleveland, Ohio, United States of America

**Newton Cho, Khizer Amin, Mariam Shirazi, Matthew C. Wong and Kelly Russell**
Injury Prevention Research Office, S t. Michael's Hospital, University of Toronto, Toronto, Canada

**Michael D. Cusimano**
Injury Prevention Research Office, St. Michael's Hospital, University of Toronto, Toronto, Canada Division of Neurosurgery, St. Michael's Hospital, University of Toronto, Toronto, Canada

**Steven R. McFaull and Minh T. Do**
Health Surveillance and Epidemiology Division, Public Health Agency of Canada, Ottawa, Canada

**Soo Chin Kim and Sun-Won Park**
Department of Radiology, Seoul Metropolitan Government - Seoul National University Boramae medical center, Seoul, Korea Department of Radiology, Seoul National University College of Medicine, Seoul, Korea

**Inseon Ryoo**
Department of Radiology, Seoul National University College of Medicine, Seoul, Korea
Department of Radiology, Korea University Guro Hospital, Seoul, Korea

**Seung Chai Jung**
Department of Radiology, Seoul National University College of Medicine, Seoul, Korea
Department of Radiology, Asan Medical Center, Seoul, Korea

**Tae Jin Yun, Seung Hong Choi, Ji-hoon Kim and Chul-Ho Sohn**
Department of Radiology, Seoul National University College of Medicine, Seoul, Korea
Department of Radiology, Seoul National University Hospital, Seoul, Korea

**Andrew B. Newberg, Andrew Gepty and Nancy Wintering**
Myrna Brind Center of Integrative Medicine, Thomas Jefferson University, Philadelphia, Pennsylvania, United States of America

**Mijail Serruya**
Department of Neurology, Thomas Jefferson University, Philadelphia, Pennsylvania, United States of America

**Charles Intenzo**
Department of Radiology, Thomas Jefferson University, Philadelphia, Pennsylvania, United States of America

**Todd Lewis**
Magee Rehabilitation Hospital, Philadelphia, Pennsylvania, United States of America

**Daniel Amen**
Amen Clinics, Inc., Newport Beach, California, United States of America

**David S. Russell**
Institute for Neurodegenerative Disorders, New Haven, Connecticut, United States of America
Yale University School of Medicine, New Haven, Connecticut, United States of America

**Junpei Yamamoto and Takaki Miwa**
Department of Otorhinolaryngology, Kanazawa Medical University, Ishikawa, Japan

**Hideaki Shiga**
Department of Otorhinolaryngology, Kanazawa Medical University, Ishikawa, Japan
Department of Quantum Medical Technology, Graduate School of Medical Science, Kanazawa University, Ishikawa, Japan

**Kohshin Washiyama, Kichiro Koshida and Ryohei Amano**
Department of Quantum Medical Technology, Graduate School of Medical Science, Kanazawa University, Ishikawa, Japan

**Junichi Taki, Koichi Okuda and Seigo Kinuya**
Department of Biotracer Medicine, Graduate School of Medical Science, Kanazawa University, Ishikawa, Japan

**Sakae Kinase**
Risk Analysis and Applications Research Group, Nuclear Safety Research Center, Japan Atomic Energy Agency, Ibaraki, Japan

**Naoto Watanabe and Hisao Tonami**
Department of Diagnostic and Therapeutic Radiology, Kanazawa Medical University, Ishikawa, Japan

**Mitsuru Furukawa**
Headquarter, Kanazawa University, Ishikawa, Japan

**Shao-Hua Su, Fei Wang, Jian Hai, Ning-Tao Liu, Fei Yu, Yi-Fang Wu and You-Hou Zhu**
The Department of Neurosurgery, Tongji Hospital, Tongji University School of Medicine, Shanghai, China

**Yi-Chou Chen and Thomas A. Stoffregen**
School of Kinesiology, University of Minnesota, Minneapolis, Minnesota, United States of America

**Ting-Hsuan Hung**
Office of Institutional Research, Edgewood College, Madison, Wisconsin, United States of America

**Tzu-Chiang Tseng**
Graduate Institute of Sport Coaching Science, Chinese Cultural University, Taipei, Taiwan

**City C. Hsieh**
College of Well Being, YuanPei University, HsinChu, Taiwan

**Fu-Chen Chen**
Department of Recreation Sport and Health Promotion, National Pingtung University of Science and Technology, Pingtung, Taiwan

**Veerajalandhar Allareddy, Rahimullah Asad, David G. Speicher and Alexandre T. Rotta**
Department of Pediatric Critical Care, Rainbow Babies and Children's Hospital, Case Western Reserve University School of Medicine, Cleveland, Ohio, United States of America

**Min Kyeong Lee and Romesh P. Nalliah**
Department of Dental Medicine, Harvard University, Boston, Massachusetts, United States of America

**Sankeerth Rampa**
Department of Public Health, Texas A & M University, College Station, Texas, United States of America

**Veerasathpurush Allareddy**
Department of Dentistry, University of Iowa, Iowa City, Iowa, United States of America

**Martin Gerdin and Johan von Schreeb**
Health Systems and Policy, Department of Public Health Sciences, Karolinska Institutet, Stockholm, Sweden

**Nobhojit Roy**
Health Systems and Policy, Department of Public Health Sciences, Karolinska Institutet, Stockholm, Sweden
Department of Surgery, Bhabha Atomic Research Centre Hospital, Mumbai, India
School of Habitat, Tata Institute of Social Sciences, Mumbai, India

**Göran Tomson**
Health Systems and Policy, Department of Public Health Sciences, Karolinska Institutet, Stockholm, Sweden
Medical Management Centre, Department of Learning, Informatics, Management and Ethics, Karolinska Institutet, Stockholm, Sweden

**Satish Dharap and Vineet Kumar**
Department of Surgery, Lokmanya Tilak Municipal Medical College and General Hospital, Mumbai, India

**Monty Khajanchi**
Department of Surgery, Seth G. S. Medical College & King Edward Memorial Hospital, Mumbai, India

**Li Felländer Tsai**
Division of Orthopedics and Biotechnology, Department of Clinical Science Intervention and Technology, Karolinska Institutet, Stockholm, Sweden

**Max Petzold**
Centre for Applied Biostatistics, Occupational and Environmental Medicine, Sahlgrenska Academy at University of Gothenburg, Gothenburg, Sweden

**Joseph Jonathan Lee, Arturo Gonzalez-Izquierdo and Ruth Gilbert**
Institute of Child Health, University College London, London, United Kingdom

**Qian Wen, Chao-Ying Zhou, Ming-Qian Zhou, Wei Luo and Li Ma**
Institute of Molecular Immunology, Southern Medical University, Guangzhou, People's Republic of China

**Dan Jin**
Department of Orthopaedics and Traumatology, Nanfang Hospital, Southern Medical University, Guangzhou, People's Republic of China

**Chungui Xu, Yanhua Wang, Na Han, Yuhui Kou, Xiaofeng Yin, Peixun Zhang, Tianbing Wang, Dianying Zhang and Baoguo Jiang**
Department of Trauma and Orthopaedics, Peking University People's Hospital, Beijing, China

**Sarah Derrett, Ari Samaranayaka, Suzanne Wilson, John Langley, Rebbecca Lilley and Gabrielle Davie**
Injury Prevention Research Unit, Department of Preventive and Social Medicine, Dunedin School of Medicine, University of Otago, Dunedin, New Zealand,

**Shanthi Ameratunga**
School of Population Health, Faculty of Medical and Health Sciences, University of Auckland, Auckland, New Zealand

**Ian D. Cameron**
Rehabilitation Studies Unit, Sydney Medical School, University of Sydney, Sydney, Australia,

**Emma Wyeth**
Te Roopū Rangahau Hauora Māori a Ngāi Tahu (Ngāi Tahu Māori Health Research Unit), Department of Preventive and Social Medicine, Dunedin School of Medicine, University of Otago, Dunedin, New Zealand

**Jeffrey J. Bazarian, Kian Merchant-Borna and Beau Abar**
Emergency Medicine, University of Rochester School of Medicine and Dentistry, Rochester, New York, United States of America

**Tong Zhu**
Imaging Sciences, University of Rochester School of Medicine and Dentistry, Rochester, New York, United States of America

**Jianhui Zhong**
Imaging Sciences, Biomedical Engineering, and Physics, University of Rochester, Rochester, New York, United States of America

**Damir Janigro**
Cleveland Clinic Lerner Research Institute, Cleveland, Ohio, United States of America

**Eric Rozen**
Athletics and Recreation, University of Rochester, Rochester, New York, United States of America

**Andrew Roberts**
University of Rochester, Rochester, New York, United States of America

**Hannah Javien**
Hamilton College, Clinton, New York, United States of America

**Eric G Blackman**
Physics and Astronomy, University of Rochester, Rochester, New York, United States of America

**Annemieke C. Scholten, Juanita A. Haagsma, Ed F. van Beeck and Suzanne Polinder**
Department of Public Health, Erasmus University Medical Center, Rotterdam, The Netherlands

**Martien J. M. Panneman**
Research Department, Consumer and Safety Institute, Amsterdam, The Netherlands

**Oluwaseye Ayoola Ogun, Kristen L. Janky, Edward S. Cohn and Yunxia Wang Lundberg**
Boys Town National Research Hospital, Omaha, Nebraska, United States of America

**Bela Büki**
Department of Otolaryngology, Karl Landsteiner University Hospital Krems, Krems an der Donau, Austria

**Ajai K. Malhotra, Stephanie R. Goldberg, Nancy R. Martin, Luke G. Wolfe, Mark M. Levy, Vishal Khiatani, Todd C. Borchers, Therese M. Duane, Michel B. Aboutanos and Rao R. Ivatury**
Department of Surgery, Virginia Commonwealth University, Richmond, Virginia, United States of America

**Laura McLay**
Department of Biostatistics, Virginia Commonwealth University, Richmond, Virginia, United States of America

**C. Michael Dunham, Gregory S. Huang and Renee Merrell**
Trauma/Critical Care Services, St. Elizabeth Health Center, Youngstown, Ohio, United States of America

**David A. Hoffman**
Division of Cardiology, St. Elizabeth Health Center, Youngstown, Ohio, United States of America

**Laurel A. Omert**
CSL Behring, King of Prussia, Pennsylvania, United States of America

**David J. Gemmel**
Medical Education and Statistics, St. Elizabeth Health Center, Youngstown, Ohio, United States of America

**Xi Zheng, Yang Hu, Yong Yuan and Yong-Fan Zhao**
Department of Thoracic Surgery, West China Hospital, Sichuan University, Chengdu, Sichuan Province, China

**Anuj Sharma, Manish Bhomia, Nagaraja S. Balakathiresan and Radha K. Maheshwari**
Department of Pathology, Uniformed Services University of the Health Sciences, Bethesda, Maryland, United States of America

**Raghavendar Chandran**
Department of Pathology, Uniformed Services University of the Health Sciences, Bethesda, Maryland, United States of America
Biological Sciences Group, Birla Institute of Technology and Science, Pilani, Rajasthan, India

**Erin S Barry, Mary Anne Hutchison and Neil E. Grunberg**
Department of Medical and Clinical Psychology, Uniformed Services University of the Health Sciences, Bethesda, Maryland, United States of America

# Index